The Sheep

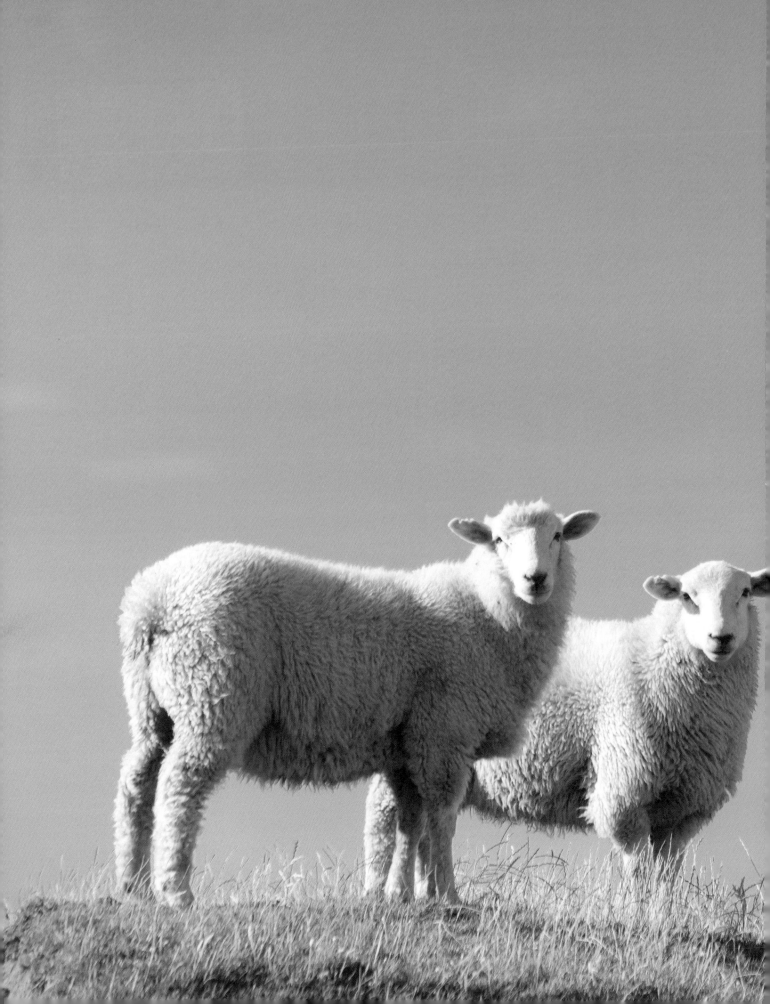

The Sheep
Health, Disease and Production

DM WEST, AN BRUÈRE & AL RIDLER

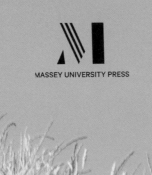

MASSEY UNIVERSITY PRESS

First published in 1993 by the New Zealand Veterinary Association
This fourth revised edition published in 2018 by Massey University Press
Reprinted 2022
Private Bag 102904, North Shore Mail Centre
Auckland 0745, New Zealand
www.masseypress.ac.nz

Text copyright © DM West, AN Bruère and AL Ridler 2017
Images copyright © DM West, AN Bruère and AL Ridler, except for pp. 2–3, 8, 16, 39, 40, 62, 76, 92, 111, 112, 156, 187, 188, 205, 206, 234, 252, 257, 258, 264, 269, 270, 282, 291, 292, 308, 330, 342, 356: copyright © iStock

Design by Sarah Elworthy

The moral right of the authors has been asserted

All rights reserved. Except as provided by the Copyright Act 1994, no part of this book may be reproduced, stored in or introduced into a retrieval system or transmitted in any form or by any means (electronic, mechanical, photocopying, recording or otherwise) without the prior written permission of both the copyright owner(s) and the publisher.

A catalogue record for this book is available from the National Library of New Zealand

Printed and bound in China by 1010 Printing Asia Ltd

ISBN: 978-0-9951001-1-4

Contents

Acknowledgements 6

Preface 7

Chapter 1 Introduction 8

Chapter 2 Genital soundness in the ram and diseases of the genitalia 16

Chapter 3 Factors affecting lamb production and the investigation of poor lambing 40

Chapter 4 Abortion in ewes 62

Chapter 5 Lamb survival and lamb mortality 76

Chapter 6 Hogget growth, pneumonia and diseases of hoggets 92

Chapter 7 Clinical aspects of trace-element requirements of grazing ruminants with particular reference to sheep and cattle 112

Chapter 8 Internal parasites 156

Chapter 9 Metabolic disorders 188

Chapter 10 Poor thrift in adult ewes 206

Chapter 11 Foot diseases and lameness 234

Chapter 12 Eye diseases 252

Chapter 13 Caseous lymphadenitis 258

Chapter 14 Diseases of the mammary gland 264

Chapter 15 Clostridial diseases 270

Chapter 16 Other causes of sudden death including salmonellosis, *Histophilus somni*, septicaemia, redgut, enteric listeriosis and anthrax 282

Chapter 17 Neurological disorders 292

Chapter 18 Disorders of the skin and wool 308

Chapter 19 External parasites 330

Chapter 20 Miscellaneous diseases of sheep 342

Chapter 21 Exotic diseases 356

Index 395

About the authors 407

Acknowledgements

From its first publication in 1993, *The Sheep: Health, Disease and Production* has proven a valuable and popular reference for New Zealand veterinarians, veterinary students and farmers. Its publication has been made possible because of the expert and readily given advice of a number of colleagues and the invaluable skill and experience of Dr Peter Jolly and the staff at the New Zealand Veterinary Association.

We gratefully acknowledge the advice given by Professors Keith Thompson, Bill Pomroy, Kevin Stafford and Steve Morris of Massey University and Professor Gareth Bath of the Republic of South Africa on both the initial publication and subsequent editions.

We also thank all those colleagues who have provided photographs and personal descriptions of diseases, which add realism to the text. In this respect, special mention is made of the professional artwork of Peter Parkinson, which has so effectively embellished the text, which would have otherwise been less easy to understand. Also, the assistance given by Stefan Smith with photograph selection is acknowledged.

A special thanks is given to all the many loyal farmers who, over many years, have given us unstinting friendship, time and access to their flocks and properties for both student teaching and research. Without their generosity much of the knowledge and experience reported in this book would not have been gained.

Preface

This book is about sheep health and the diagnosis of sheep diseases, with a specific emphasis on commercially farmed sheep in New Zealand. It describes the common to less-common diseases seen in New Zealand; where necessary, reference is made to diseases of other countries. The final section of the book deals with exotic sheep diseases in detail, so that New Zealand-trained veterinarians and farmers can appreciate their potential threat to the livestock industries of this country.

Where considered appropriate, reference is made to historical events in the discovery of new diseases in this country. We can all profit by researching the experiences of these earlier authors who, by today's standards, worked with very limited and basic diagnostic facilities. They were keen clinical observers, and we are indebted to them for their detailed and accurate reports of the many diseases recorded for the first time in New Zealand.

Present-day veterinarians now have an extensive knowledge of most sheep diseases and how these can be diagnosed and controlled. In addition, a highly effective range of animal health products is available for both treatment and prevention of disease, with particular emphasis on the latter. Thus, sheep farmers are better able than ever to farm for maximum production through the maintenance of good animal health. New diseases and problems will arise, but with advancing technology their solution is ever more likely.

In the second edition of this book, published in 2002, new sections on *Salmonella* Brandenburg and foot and mouth disease were added and there was considerable extension of the section on transmissible spongiform encephalopathies (scrapie, bovine spongiform encephalopathy and human infection).

In the third and fourth editions of this book, many new references were added and the new data they describe has been written into the text. In addition, a wider range of illustrations and colour photographs has been used to enhance the text descriptions and there is increased use of tables.

This book is written and intended to be used as a reference for veterinary students, veterinarians and livestock farmers. The authors recommend its use by farmers, both to help them to understand the health problems that may affect sheep production and also to encourage a more informed relationship with their veterinarian.

Some commercial products available in New Zealand are mentioned in the text to assist local readers. Mention or exclusion of any particular product carries with it no endorsement or otherwise by the authors or the publisher.

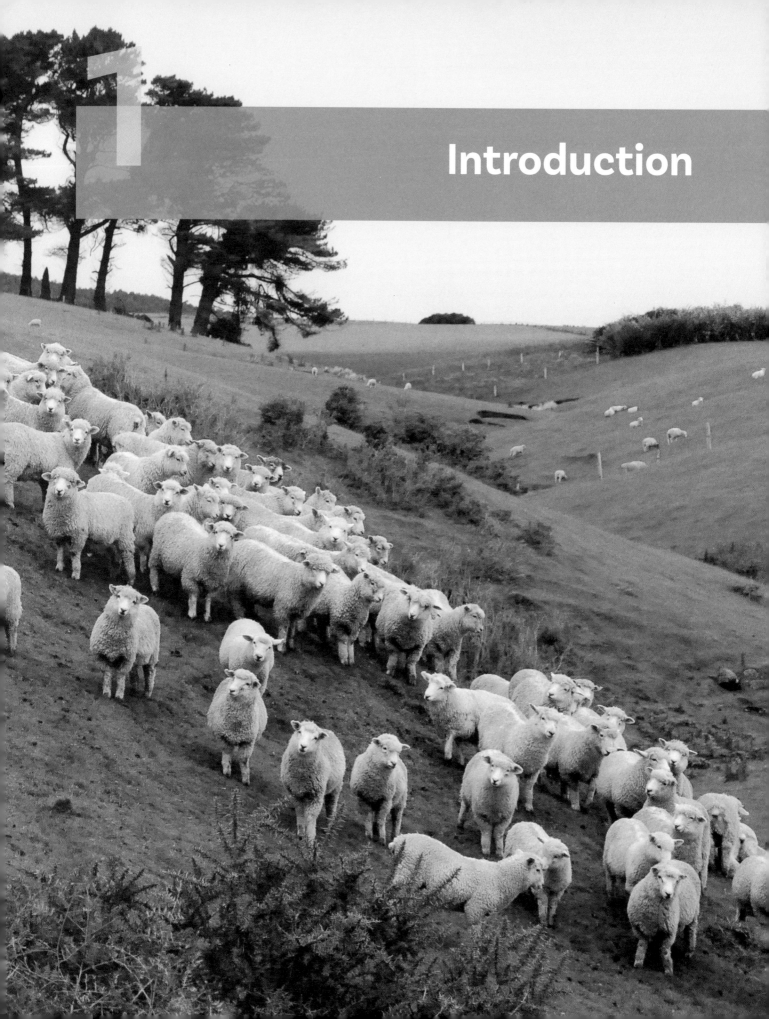

1 Introduction

Despite a large reduction in sheep numbers in the past 30 years, New Zealand is still more heavily stocked with sheep than most other important sheep-producing countries, and from European colonisation in the early 19th century onwards sheep have played a significant role in our country's economy. The flock of 200 Merinos established on Mana Island in 1832 by John Wright is believed to be our first commercial sheep farm. For the rest of the 19th century, with the influx of European colonists came also large numbers of sheep; mainly from Britain, but, from 1850 onwards, many shipments of Merino sheep also came from Australia. The first million was reached by 1857, and by 1880 the sheep population had reached 13 million, which were mainly of Spanish Merino derivation.

A number of British breeds, such as the Southdown, English Leicester, Cheviot, Border Leicester, Lincoln and Romney Marsh, were also imported but in smaller numbers. The Romney Marsh, first imported in 1853, was gradually modified by New Zealand breeders; it was eventually renamed the New Zealand Romney and became the foundation breed of the country's mainly dual-purpose sheep population. By the end of the century, over 2.5 million hectares of New Zealand native pasture had been replaced by English grasses and clover and around 20 million sheep were being farmed, of which only 6 million were Merinos. Cross-breeds such as the halfbred and Corriedale (Lincoln or English Leicester rams over Merino ewes) were developed, and later other popular breeds such as the Perendale and Coopworth were derived from cross-breeding Cheviot and Border Leicester rams with the Romney. Today, approximately 8% of New Zealand's sheep population consists of Merinos and other fine-wool breeds and crosses; these are mainly grazed on the drier hill country of the South Island. They still flourish as producers of fine wools suitable for clothing manufacture, and a number of Merino breeders have developed niche overseas markets for their wool, where it is used to make high-quality clothing.

More recently, as well as the predominance of the Romney and its derivatives, there has been an increased use of two-, three- and four-breed composite sheep. These have incorporated the use of 'exotics' — the Finn, East Friesian and Texel — cross-breeding with the Romney, Coopworth or Perendale. Other breeds, including the Suffolk and Poll Dorset, have become popular as terminal sires. Wool, pelts and tallow were the first main export products of the sheep industry, but, following the successful shipping of frozen carcasses to London in 1882, sheep meat exports soon became a significant part of the country's export earnings. As an example, in 2015 over 40% of the 21 million lambs slaughtered for the meat trade were exported to the European Union.

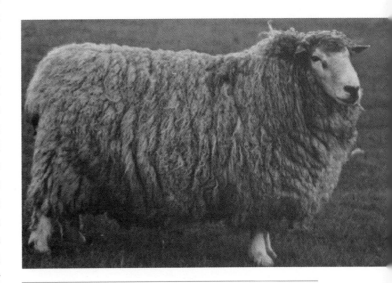

Figure 1.1 Typical Romney Marsh or Kent sheep (1920s).

In spite of depressed meat and wool prices at times, and fluctuations in sheep numbers, the sheep industry has shown some remarkable improvements in productivity. Outstanding advances include, firstly, the improvement in the national lambing percentage (lambs docked to ewes mated), which was almost static at between 95% and 103% until the early 1990s; in 2015 it reached 127%. A second advance is the faster growth rates of young sheep — and hence the higher slaughter weight of export lamb — which has gone from 14.0 kg in 1993 to 18.3 kg in 2015. Finally, the increased number of ewe hoggets being mated (estimated at about 30%) has increased the gross reproductive performance of many flocks. These improvements are largely the result of a better understanding of the role of nutrition in reproduction and in growth and development, breed improvements, cross-breeding and significant developments in the understanding and control of animal health and disease; all of which can be attributed to a combined effort by animal scientists, veterinarians and farmers.

For a thorough overview of sheep production in New Zealand, readers are directed to the 'Sheep Production' chapter of the book *Livestock Production in New Zealand*, edited by Kevin Stafford and published by Massey University Press (2017).

The role of the veterinary profession

New Zealand veterinarians have always been actively involved in taking new animal health information to the farmer, ensuring its correct application and monitoring the results.

Historically a small cadre of earlier veterinarians, mainly associated with the Department of Agriculture, diagnosed and solved many of our animal disease problems. The first government veterinarian was John Gilruth, a Scot, who arrived in New Zealand in 1893 and was put in charge of the veterinary division of the Department of Agriculture. He soon recruited staff who, like him, travelled the country assessing the disease situation of its farm animals. Gilruth published leaflets for farmers and initiated the annual reports of the Veterinary Division of the Department of Agriculture, with the first report being published in 1893. By 1899 Gilruth's veterinary staff numbered four, and by 1902 he had a staff of 24 qualified field veterinarians. He established diagnostic laboratory services which first operated from a small room in Government House. These limited facilities were abandoned in 1905 when the diagnostic station and farm at Wallaceville were opened.

With the development of the veterinary club system under Alan Leslie — another determined Scot — in the late 1940s and through the 1950s, there was a rapid infusion of young and enthusiastic veterinarians into nearly every rural district of New Zealand. Veterinary services to sheep farms as well as dairy farms began in earnest, and areas of the country with significant sheep populations soon had well-established services.

The rapid expansion of field veterinary services to sheep farmers has been assisted greatly by the pharmaceutical industry, which has produced an increasing range of sheep vaccines, anthelmintics, antibiotics and endocrine products. Notable among the vaccines were the clostridial vaccines (which were vastly improved and dispensed in combination), Salmonella vaccine and the abortion-preventing vaccines for toxoplasmosis and campylobacteriosis. The improved anthelmintics have included fine-particle phenothiazine, methyridine and later the benzimidazoles, macrocyclic lactones and amino acetonitrile derivatives. With parasite control being an established part of grassland farming, the development and correct use of these latter products has been vital to the maintenance of stock health (see Chapter 8). There have also been outstanding developments in external parasite control (see Chapter 19).

The discovery of trace-element diseases caused by dietary deficiencies of copper, cobalt, iodine and selenium were of great significance to animal health. More recently, the extent of the 'subclinical' effects of selenium and cobalt has been appreciated, and widespread preventive procedures are now undertaken regularly on many New Zealand farms. This extension in use of trace elements has largely resulted from the development of very effective and readily available diagnostic tests with which they can be monitored. Their concentrations can be measured in a variety of animal tissues, animal fodder and soil, if necessary, so that an investigation can be completed within one or two days. Previously it took weeks for some test results to be obtained.

The 1950s and onwards were notable for many

improvements to veterinary services to farmers. New government diagnostic services were established at Whangarei, Ruakura, Palmerston North, Lincoln and Invermay in addition to the Central Animal Health Laboratory at Wallaceville. These are now all privately operated enterprises, except for the Investigation and Diagnostic Centre at Wallaceville. The highly sophisticated services offered by these laboratories are essential to most veterinary investigations, and the costs are now accepted by farmers as a normal part of farm expenditure. Previously such services were given to farming at no cost.

In 1963, New Zealand began training its own veterinarians. The veterinary science degree at Massey University has always had a large sheep-health component, commensurate with the size of the sheep industry and its significance to the New Zealand economy. As training for young veterinarians, the course has emphasised the application of knowledge in a preventative manner. As well as the undergraduate course, many doctoral and masterate studies on sheep health and disease have been completed. Some of the important subjects relating to sheep researched by postgraduates include: brucellosis control, anthelmintic resistance, trace-element studies, foot diseases, chorioptic mange, abortion, tooth abnormalities, pneumonia, Johne's disease, chromosome studies, leptospirosis, hogget lambing, neosporosis and ewe longevity.

In 1998, animal production scientists from the previous Faculty of Agriculture at Massey University were amalgamated with members of the previously named Faculty of Veterinary Science to form the Institute of Veterinary, Animal and Biomedical Sciences (IVABS). This proved a progressive move, particularly in the production animal area, where it brought two closely related disciplines together and advanced research and teaching of the many subjects where animal production and animal health are inextricably related.

The Sheep Society of the New Zealand Veterinary Association (now the Society of Sheep and Beef Cattle Veterinarians, NZVA) was the first specialised branch of the Veterinary Association and was formed in 1970. Since then it has brought interested veterinarians together at its annual conference and published regular proceedings. It has also contributed to and hosted International Sheep Veterinary Congresses.

In addition, the Australian and New Zealand College of Veterinary Scientists (ANZCVSc) gives formal opportunity to veterinarians who wish to establish their expertise in sheep health, to study for and pass examinations for either membership or fellowship of the College. The New Zealand Veterinary Association through VetLearn provides online courses and VetScholar programmes, which enable veterinarians to update their knowledge in their own time. The SciQuest resource includes tens of thousands of references from New Zealand journals on animal health and disease and is vital for research in these areas.

This summary of developments in sheep health and disease in New Zealand demonstrates that the profession is able to provide a high-quality, expert animal health service to New Zealand sheep farmers. In spite of economic fluctuations that have affected the incomes of sheep farmers from time to time, the application of sound veterinary advice is always vital if animals are to be healthy and produce their best.

This text, which is largely based on the undergraduate course that has evolved at Massey since 1967, has been produced to emphasise the clinical aspects of sheep health that the veterinarian can apply in the field. Knowledge and experience are essential for the specialist veterinarian before regular animal health programmes can be effectively developed. The operator must have both of these attributes. He/she must be thoroughly conversant with the sheep industry and target performance data. With this in mind, the authors have gone to considerable trouble to emphasise the different disease areas and give examples, where possible, of typical disease problems and how these may be dealt with.

The general principles of flock and herd investigation

Definition of 'disease'

For production animals, the term 'disease' refers not only to animals that are clinically ill but also to those animals or groups of animals that do not reach target performance. Thus, as well as being able to recognise animals affected with a particular disease, it is also necessary to investigate conditions such as hogget ill thrift, in which young sheep fail to achieve a satisfactory growth rate. In some instances the farmer may not recognise any abnormality unless the productivity of the animals is monitored closely and a comparison made with both local and national data, for example average weaning weights, lambing performance, numbers of dry ewes and wool weights.

The importance of the clinical procedure

Most animal health programmes stem from an initial clinical investigation during which the observant veterinarian identifies a need for further investigation or monitoring of the flock, and with this the farmer will gain confidence in the veterinarian's ability as an animal health professional adviser. Thus it is imperative that the first job is done well!

The diagnosis, treatment and control of production animal diseases are very dependent on the results of the clinical investigation of the animals on the farm, their management and the environment. The principles of this basic but vital procedure may be applied, with modification, to nearly every veterinary investigation. Therefore it is essential that newly qualified veterinarians develop these skills and continually hone them as new knowledge and technology become available.

The procedure

Flock and herd investigations can be described under the following headings:
1. History
2. Examination of the environment
3. Examination of the animals
4. Use of ancillary aids
5. Data analysis and decision making
6. Reporting back and further monitoring.

1. History

In flock and herd problems a two-phase approach is commonly used. Firstly, dealing with the problem at hand; and secondly, as appropriate, expanding this into a whole-farm approach. In either case it is essential to keep a permanent record for future use. The initial data include the following items:

A clear definition of the problem
- Concentrate on the problem at hand, as this is what the farmer expects.
- Be tactful. You may be appalled by the poor condition of the animals or the state of their environment, but be careful not to offend your client. Be understanding — your client may have personal problems of which you are unaware (e.g. financial problems, family illness, etc.).
- Separate the owner's observations from his/her interpretations.
- Obtain a clear time sequence of events leading to the problem. Obtain dates if possible from the farm diary.
- Avoid using slang terms like 'crook' animals. Show concern.
- Determine the losses to date:
    * Morbidity rate — % affected animals
    * Case mortality rate — % affected animals that have died as a result of the condition
    * Population mortality rate — % exposed animals that die due to the condition.
- Determine prior treatment and control procedures, if any.
- Obtain a history of the management of the animals, in relation to nutrition, feeding and reproduction (if mature animals).
- Without prejudice, assess the ability and experience of the farmer. Remember, farmers are very intelligent people. Many have tertiary qualifications and are very experienced in business matters.
- In most investigations the history taking occurs throughout the visit and is often ongoing. With time, a good client–veterinarian relationship will develop. An experienced veterinarian with long-term knowledge of his/her client's property and its animals is an invaluable asset to the farmer. A 'local' veterinarian with experience and accumulated knowledge is a unique expert among farm advisers.

Property profile
When investigating flock and herd problems it is important for the veterinarian to have a sound understanding of the overall farm enterprise, the level of production and the financial performance. It is not always possible to collect a full range of data on the initial visit, and usually several visits are necessary for completion of the profile. The following and rather full format lists the data that need to be gathered for a full farm profile, and will greatly assist animal health investigations on that property. It can also

be readily computerised for a permanent record.
- Situation, e.g. Rongotea district, Manawatu.
- Land elevation above sea level. For comparative analysis the farm may be classed into one of the following categories:
  * Flat
  * Flat 50% hill 50%
  * Rolling hill country
  * All hill
- Effective farm area in hectares.
- Farm class or type (1–8).
- Main soil types or type (soil tests may be needed).
- Subdivision, number of paddocks; a farm plan is helpful, if available.
- Stock classes, stocking rate, sheep to cattle ratio. The stock unit (SU) conversion relates the energy requirements of various classes of stock to the requirements of one breeding ewe (55 kg) producing one lamb per annum. However, for individual properties stock units will vary depending on the mature liveweight of animals and stock performance (e.g. lambing percentage, growth rates). They are calculated for the winter tally (1 July). Stock unit measurements used in New Zealand may differ slightly between agricultural organisations, but based on the 55 kg ewe rearing one lamb equivalent, the approximate conversion factors incorporated for recording purposes are given in Table 1.1.

Stock class	Number of stock units (SU)
Ewes	1
Hoggets	0.7–1
Wethers	0.7
Rams	1
Breeding cows	6
Rising 2-year-old cattle	4–5
Rising 1-year-old cattle	3.5–4

Table 1.1
Stocking rate conversion factors based on a 55 kg ewe rearing one lamb equivalent.

Reproductive performance and mating management

In addition to the mating information, such as numbers of rams used and timing of ram introduction, the tallies of ewes and lambs at specific times of the year are recorded. From these figures, the lambing performance (lambs docked/ewes mated), ewe mortality, lamb mortality and various classes of dry ewe can be calculated. Ram examination data will be part of reproductive information and is dealt with in detail in Chapter 2. Similar data may also be collected about beef cattle on the property.

Other available animal health information

The farmer may already have considerable animal health information that may eventually prove useful in your investigations, and this may be worth collating. This will include such items as:

- Sheep or cattle disease recognised previously.
- Vaccination information — diseases vaccinated against, frequency, timing and vaccines used.
- Internal parasite control — the importance of internal parasite control in relation to the efficiency of New Zealand sheep farming is paramount (see Chapter 8). Times of drenching, anthelmintics used, classes of animals treated and the presence of special parasites such as liver fluke should be noted.
- Bodyweights and body condition scores (BCS) — one of the most useful aids in studying poor flock performance is the regular weighing and BCS of the various classes of sheep. Many farmers have this information. Bodyweight is correlated with both reproduction and wool growth (see Chapters 3 and 6).
- Trace elements — it is useful to find out what, if any, micro-element deficiencies occur on the property. Record how trace elements have been administered, products used for prevention and how frequently they have been used.
- Fertiliser usage — it may be possible to obtain information on fertiliser usage. Regular topdressing is an integral part of New Zealand grassland farming and a variety of fertilisers are used. These contain various mixes of phosphate, sulphur, calcium, nitrogen, potassium and trace elements (see Chapter 7).

2. Examination of the environment

The importance of examining the environment is often overlooked. The examination begins as you enter the property and should extend well beyond the immediate vicinity of the woolshed or dairy shed. Eventually a farm walk or motorbike ride should be undertaken to assess the topography, soil type, feed availability and water supply. This also gives you a better appreciation of how well feed supplies are being used and what are available for the future.

3. Examination of the animals

In most instances the examination of the animals (flock and individuals) begins during the history taking. Observation of the animals at a distance as well as close up is important and is often overlooked by inexperienced veterinarians. Don't be in a rush to get your hands on the animal(s) or wield the postmortem knife before you view the whole scene. Observation skills are an essential part of your investigative approach. They develop over time and eventually become second-nature to the investigation. Where appropriate, the clinical examination of individual animals must not be overlooked even though you may be investigating a flock problem.

The distance examination

The flock should be examined as a whole while in the paddock or holding pen. Specific things to observe include:

- size, approximate weight and variation in size within the flock
- fleece — look for abnormalities such as flystrike, dermatophilosis or wool derangement
- evidence of lameness
- evidence of diarrhoea (dags, faecal staining of hocks)
- photosensitivity
- listening for coughing
- whether any individuals appear abnormal (e.g. depressed, separated from flock, showing nervous signs, recumbent).

Weighing and body condition scoring a number of sheep is another useful aid during a flock investigation (see Chapter 6).

Individual animal clinical examination

Even if a disease condition is affecting an entire flock, it is usual for variations to occur in the severity of the disease between individual animals. If individual animals appear abnormal, they should be examined in more detail as this may provide important clues about the disease process. A basic clinical examination does not take long to perform and should include the measurement of cardinal signs, examination of teeth and mucous membranes, assessment of hydration and auscultation of the lung fields and rumen. In some cases a more thorough clinical examination may be required, or a briefer version of the clinical examination tailored to the presenting problem may be performed (e.g. in a lameness investigation, the clinical examination may consist primarily of examination of the feet).

'Normal' values for sheep are as follows:
- temperature: 39.5°C +/− 0.5°C
- heart rate: 70–90/min
- respiration rate: 15–70/min
- rumination rate: 3–4/min
- mucous membranes (third eyelid or gums): pale pink
- hydration status: can be assessed by tenting the upper eyelid.

Note that during clinical examination sheep are usually stressed or anxious and so heart rate and respiration rate are frequently elevated as a result.

Postmortem examination

Postmortem examination of affected animals can be an extremely valuable part of an investigation. Not only does it allow identification of lesions that may be specific to a certain disease, but it also gives an opportunity to collect samples such as liver (e.g. for trace-element analysis), gastrointestinal tract (e.g. for worm counts) or specific samples for microbiology (e.g. gut contents for *Salmonella*) or histopathology (e.g. ileum or lymph node for Johne's disease). It is ideal to necropsy as many animals as possible/practical. Generally the animals selected are those that have already died, preferably selecting the most recently dead. If animals are severely affected and likely to die they may be euthanased for postmortem examination.

4. Use of ancillary aids

Further diagnostic tests are an important part of most flock/herd investigations. For diagnostic tests to be interpreted meaningfully it is necessary to collect the correct samples

and the appropriate number of samples for the test to be undertaken. The following are examples of diagnostic tests commonly used in herd or flock investigations:
- Assessing the trace-element status from blood, serum and liver samples (see Chapter 7).
- Assessing the parasite burden using faecal egg counts, worm burdens, faecal egg count reduction tests and larval culture (see Chapter 8).
- Serology, e.g. rams for brucellosis (see Chapter 2).
- Microbiology, e.g. intestinal contents for *Salmonella* spp, etc.
- Haematology/biochemistry, e.g. anaemia associated with haemonchosis, or elevated liver enzymes from facial eczema.
- Samples for histopathology, e.g. Johne's disease.
- Pasture and soil samples to assess the fertility level. These are often interpreted in conjunction with other consultants such as soil scientists.

5. Data analysis and decision making

As with all veterinary examinations, the veterinarian is required to make a decision. This falls into the area of tentative diagnosis, prognosis and therapy.

One of the first steps is to decide whether an abnormality is present and to define it in regard to the pattern of occurrence, the group affected and the costs of the problem. Many production-animal problems are multifactorial and a single specific aetiology cannot be defined. Nevertheless it is necessary to outline a course of action, usually involving some intervention or change in management, and to monitor the result. In some situations it may be appropriate to conduct a response trial.

6. Reporting back and further monitoring

Before leaving the farm it is essential to discuss with the owner the action recommended. Results of diagnostic tests can be reported by phone, fax or email. If these are not available, decisions should be confirmed in writing. The report is most valuable and is an essential record for future use by the farmer and veterinarian.

In addition, before leaving the farm the appropriate time for the next visit should be discussed with the farmer. Many herd or flock problems will not be solved by a single visit and will require further visits to monitor the progress of any action. For instance, the use of copper therapy in cattle — should this be repeated? As the results of your investigation become available, the advice may need to be modified. Thus, monitoring should be part of many flock or herd investigations and forms the basis for ongoing animal advisory services.

REFERENCES

Bell KJ, Swan RA, Chapman HM. A cost-effective study of sheep flock health and production programmes. *Proceedings of the International Conference on Veterinary Preventive Medicine and Animal Production, Australian Veterinary Journal,* 142, 1985

Bruère AN, West DM. Preparing today's undergraduates for the challenges of sheep production medicine in the 1980s. *Proceedings of the International Conference on Veterinary Preventive Medicine and Animal Production, Australian Veterinary Journal,* 131, 1985

Cranston L, Ridler A, Greer A, Kenyon P. Sheep production. In: *Livestock Production in New Zealand.* Edited by Stafford KJ. Massey University Press, Auckland, New Zealand, pp 86-124, 2017

Farquharson BC. Use of computers in animal health. *Proceedings of the 16th Seminar of the Society of Sheep and Beef Cattle Veterinarians, New Zealand Veterinary Association,* 133-36, 1986

Grant IM, Watts TJ, Allworth MB, Morley FHW, Caple IW. Sheep flock health and production: the Mackinnon project of the University of Melbourne Veterinary School. *Proceedings of the International Conference on Veterinary Preventive Medicine and Animal Production, Australian Veterinary Journal,* 142, 1985

McNeill PH, Rhodes AP, Willis BH. A flock health and production service for New Zealand. Veterinary Services Council, New Zealand, 1984

Morris ST. Economics of sheep production. Edited by Stuen S and Ulvund MJ. *Proceedings of the 7th International Sheep Congress, Norway,* 12-16 June, pp 29-32, 2009

Quinlivan TD. Achievements of the Sheep and Beef Cattle Society NZVA in its first 25 years. *Proceedings of the 25th Seminar of the Society of Sheep and Beef Cattle Veterinarians, New Zealand Veterinary Association,* 1-20, 1995

Tenquist JD. *Wallaceville Laboratory. An anecdotal history.* MAF Technology, Wallaceville Animal Research Centre, PO Box 40063, Upper Hutt, New Zealand, 1990

West DM. Sheep health and production in New Zealand. *Proceedings of the 19th Seminar of the Society of Sheep and Beef Cattle Veterinarians, New Zealand Veterinary Association,* 3-6, 1989

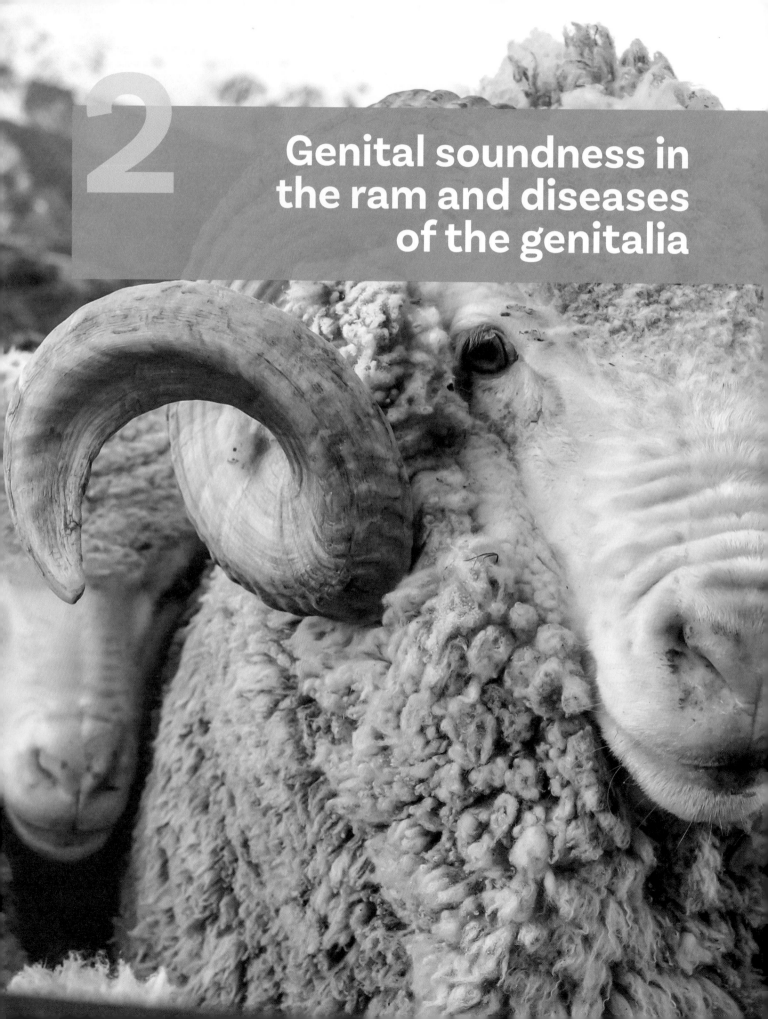

2 Genital soundness in the ram and diseases of the genitalia

The veterinary inspection of rams for breeding soundness prior to either sale or mating is now practised in many sheep-raising countries. In New Zealand it has been a routine procedure on many sheep farms since the 1950s and has not only proven to be of significant value in animal health improvement, but has also become a traditional annual contact for sheep farmer and veterinarian.

Prior to the introduction of ram soundness examinations, little was known of diseases such as ovine brucellosis and epididymitis caused by other organisms. In Australia and New Zealand, effective control programmes for ovine brucellosis are operating and the disease has now been eliminated on many farms. In addition, examination of rams prior to mating leads to some confidence in using relatively low ram : ewe ratios (e.g. 1 : 100), reducing the cost of purchasing and feeding extra rams.

The aim of any ram breeder or commercial sheep farmer should be to use rams which are free from known disease and defects that are likely to impair successful mating. Such rams should be able to produce good-quality semen continuously over the mating period. It should be emphasised that ram soundness examinations are not a finite guarantee of fertility. A small number of rams can pass a soundness examination and still have poor fertility. Fortunately these rams seem to be rare.

The examination

Reasons for undertaking breeding soundness examinations

Some of the more common reasons for undertaking genital or breeding soundness examinations of rams include:
- Pre-mating — generally 1–2 months prior to the start of mating
- Pre-sale or post-purchase
- In response to a reproductive problem

The specific method of ram examination will vary depending on the individual circumstances, but the following descriptions are intended to cover the more common situations.

History

In instances where an individual ram has not performed well, a detailed history of the case and flock is essential. This will often help in the interpretation of the findings of the clinical examination. As sperm production takes approximately 60 days, determining whether any rams have shown illness, been transported or shown lameness in the past two months is important. In all ram examinations a clear identification (usually by metal ear tag) is necessary. If a certificate is to be provided, a more detailed description of the rams will be necessary. Temporary spray or raddle marks on a ram's wool are not an acceptable means of identification and should not be used.

General clinical examination

Rams should be evaluated from a distance for signs of illness or lameness. Body systems other than the genitalia should be examined for abnormalities, especially where individual stud rams are involved. In particular, any sign of lameness, ill health or abnormality should be noted along with the body condition score (BCS) of the ram. During pre-mating breeding soundness examinations, the recommended ram BCS is 3.5–4 out of 5.

When a large group of rams is examined, for example young rams before sale, then only those rams showing ill health are subjected to closer examination. In commercial flocks, culling of rams is usually based on age, condition,

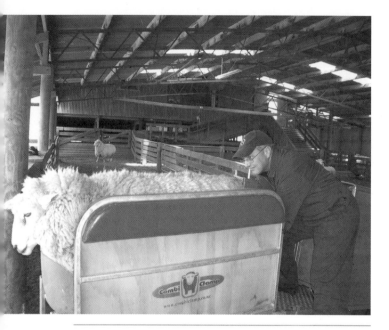

Figure 2.1 Soundness examination of a ram in a 'Combi Clamp'.

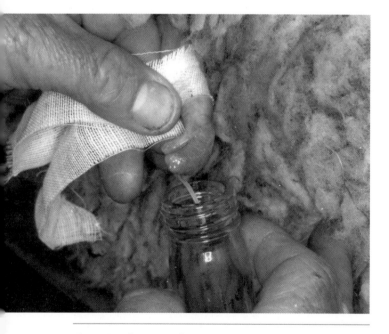

Figure 2.2 The penis of a ram held by a clean gauze bandage with the urethral process inserted into a universal container ready for semen collection.

teeth wear and feet abnormalities. These should be considered along with the examination of the genitalia.

Genitalia examination

A carefully conducted examination of the genitalia is an essential part of the ram breeding soundness examination, and in most cases it is sufficient to predict the likely fertility of a ram without the need for semen evaluation. It is generally easiest to examine rams when they are in the standing position. The operator should stand directly behind the animal and firstly assess the external scrotal skin to evaluate wool length and presence or absence of lesions. Palpation of the scrotal contents should be undertaken using both hands, beginning by palpation of the neck of the scrotum and the scrotal cord followed by palpation of the testes and epididymides. The scrotal contents should be evaluated for symmetry, testicular size and tone, and lesions within the structures. Further details on normal genital parameters and genital abnormalities can be found later in this chapter.

Some veterinarians have found that the examination of rams can be very effectively done using a handling system that clamps or holds individual sheep. With large numbers of rams it makes the process less physical and 300 rams an hour can be examined by an experienced operator (see Figure 2.1).

In routine examinations of large numbers of rams the penis is not usually examined unless there are obvious visible abnormalities of the prepuce. However, in cases of individual rams or particularly valuable animals, the penis should be examined. This is done with the animal in the sitting position.

Other supplementary tests

Semen collection and evaluation

In most situations a careful history, general clinical examination as appropriate and careful genital examination are sufficient for evaluating the soundness of rams for breeding. Semen evaluation can be of value where doubt exists or poor reproductive performance is being investigated, when one ram is to be mated individually to a group of ewes, or when a ram is of particular value. The collection procedure is relatively easy and quick. Semen can be collected from a ram either by electro-ejaculation, using an artificial vagina, or from a ewe's vagina after service. The reason for collection varies but the common reasons are to assess the ram's fertility, to culture for bacteriology and for artificial insemination.

In Australia and New Zealand, most ram semen samples are obtained by use of an electro-ejaculator. This procedure should only be undertaken by a trained veterinarian. For effective collection, the ram should be restrained on its side with the legs held so that the semen container (Figure 2.2) is not kicked away during collection. When the cleaned and gel-covered probe has been inserted carefully into the ram's rectum, the 'on' button is pressed for the count of 4 seconds and then turned off for the same interval. In most cases a good semen sample will be obtained after 2–3 such stimulations. If not, the ram should be released and a further attempt made later.

Ram semen is very susceptible to cold shock and all collecting tubes and pipettes used to handle the semen should be warm if the semen is to be assessed or used for artificial insemination. The common assessment of ram's semen is on volume (only if collected by artificial vagina) density, motility, morphology and live : dead ratio. Some of these can be assessed without the aid of a microscope.

An approximate estimate of concentration can be made by visual appraisal:

Thick creamy	3×10^9 ml
Creamy	2×10^9 ml
Thick milky	1×10^9 ml
Milky	0.5×10^9 ml
Cloudy water	$<0.1 \times 10^9$ ml

In most cases an estimation of motility is required shortly after collection of the sample — in the field, this means having a microscope set up close to where the sample is collected. Measurement of other parameters such as morphology and sperm density can be done back at the veterinary practice or at a diagnostic laboratory.

It should be recognised that evaluation of semen characteristics is a relatively specialised task and additional reading or training is recommended prior to undertaking it. Unless expertly executed, semen evaluation can lead to quite erroneous conclusions about the suitability of a particular ram for mating. The quality of the sample obtained should be carefully considered in relationship to the history and clinical findings. While one good sample is usually diagnostic, one unsatisfactory sample could be due to the technique of collection and may have to be repeated, especially if the physical examination and history does not support the finding.

Serving behaviour

In general, mating behaviour of rams has seldom been incriminated as a cause of infertility, although some rams perform better than others when mated to large groups of ewes. Serving capacity tests, similar to those used for beef bulls, have been designed and used for rams, but the relationship between pen mating tests and flock fertility is poor, especially for British breeds of sheep.

However, occasionally the mating behaviour of rams, especially two-tooth rams, may be associated with poor reproductive performance. The practice of managing young rams in isolation from ewes may contribute to such instances.

Categories of soundness

For clinical differentiation, the following categories of ram soundness or unsoundness are suggested for general use. A **genitally sound ram** is one that has no congenital, physical or genital abnormalities, or any condition that in its progression will cause a ram to become incapable of service. It must be remembered that, technically, a ram can only be classed as sound at the time of examination.

For practical purposes of ram inspection, three separate degrees of breeding soundness are recognised.

1. The **sound ram**, which is free from all defects of the genitalia and, as far as can be gauged by clinical examination, is sound for mating and to be sold.
2. The **temporarily unsound ram**, which has some defect that can be treated to restore the ram to full soundness.
3. The **permanently unsound ram**, in which the defect or disease will permanently impair the performance of the ram.

Timing of the examination

The timing of the ram examination is very important. Rams should be inspected at least one month before the mating season. The owners of stud ram flocks and commercial ram-producing flocks must supply, to their clients, rams not only of sound genetic background but also of good fertility and free from the major defects described below. Further, in order that information can be gathered on the overall incidence of genital disease (e.g. cryptorchidism) in a given stud flock, the first veterinary inspection should take place soon after the ram lambs have been weaned. If the rams are not inspected until near to the time of sale, then a biased picture of the problems of that flock may be presented.

For a variety of reasons, as many as 20% of ram lambs bred for sale may be culled before the two-tooth stage. Into this culled group frequently go, for example, cases of cryptorchidism and monorchidism, so that the farmer becomes less conscious of the persistent prevalence of these and other conditions within the flock. In addition, the reduction in the size of the ram hogget flock to be wintered has obvious advantages to the breeder in terms of feed conservation. There is also nothing more annoying to a ram breeder than to have a 'beautiful' two-tooth ram culled just prior to the annual sales with a defect that could have been detected months earlier.

At least one or two inspections of rams between weaning and the two-tooth stage not only acquaints the flock owner with any problems but also enables control measures to be taken if a disease is detected. Regular examination and record keeping also provide important local and national data from which priorities for research can be established. In the case of flock rams used on commercial sheep farms, at least one annual examination at least 1–2 months prior to mating will ensure that animals are in rising health and free from known disease. Likewise, treatment and replacement of defective rams can take place in plenty of time to ensure sound rams for mating.

Specific conditions that may contribute to genital unsoundness in the ram

The conditions described in the following sections may be considered as causing either temporary or permanent unsoundness in the ram.

The prepuce and penis

Conditions of the prepuce and penis are relatively uncommon in rams. As a consequence, examination of these areas do not form part of routine ram soundness examinations and they are only examined if a problem is noted or suspected. Shearing damage to the prepuce may occur occasionally. Apart from general conditions such as phimosis, congenitally deformed or small penis and hypospadias, two conditions are of particular importance in the ram: obstruction of the urethral process and balano-posthitis. Of the congenital conditions, hypospadias is the most common.

Examination of the penis

The examination of the penis of the ram requires the animal to be held in a sitting position with its forelegs held securely by an assistant. The examiner must then secure the penis near to the sigmoid flexure with one hand and move it out of the prepuce, where it is held firmly by the other hand. If the penis is to be held out for a period (e.g. for semen collection), a piece of soft gauze bandage should be carefully held around the neck of the penis by the fingers and thumb.

Hypospadias

Hypospadias is a congenital anomaly in rams and other mammals, in which the urethra opens onto the perineum so that urine is constantly dribbled down the perineum and crutch region. It is seen in young rams at an early age and because of the constant crutch staining it can attract striking flies. Such animals are best culled.

Damage and obstruction of the urethral process

Damage to the urethral process in rams can occur during shearing. Its subsequent effect on fertility is largely unknown, but it does represent a defect and should certainly be noted in stud or valuable rams. Blockage of the urethral process with calculi is common in housed, concentrate-fed rams. As a result, the urethral process frequently becomes necrotic and sloughs off. The necrosis can extend to involve the glans penis as well.

Balano-posthitis

The most common condition affecting the penis and prepuce of rams is balano-posthitis or pizzle rot. It is caused directly by a bacterium, probably *Corynebacterium renale*, which grows profusely in alkaline urine. Such urine is produced readily by sheep fed a protein-rich diet. Improved New Zealand pastures are therefore highly conducive to this disease at many times of the year. From the urea excreted in the urine as a result of such a diet, the causal bacterium produces ammonia. Ammonia is cytotoxic and has a direct scalding effect on the penis and prepuce, producing the characteristic signs of pizzle rot. It is particularly common in wethers because the penis does not develop fully and wethers urinate into the prepuce.

The disease can be transmitted freely between ewes, rams, wethers and lambs. Cattle can also become affected and act as carriers.

Clinical findings

Balano-posthitis is easy to detect. It usually starts as a small ulcer that develops near the external orifice of the prepuce. As the disease progresses, scabs develop over these ulcers and the prepucial opening, and the internal prepucial membranes may become involved. The latter may become necrotic and slough, producing foul-smelling pus and necrotic material within the prepuce.

If the prepucial opening remains blocked by scabs on the external prepuce, the necrotic material and accumulated urine cause the prepuce to swell. With such severe internal lesions the ram or wether may have difficulty urinating, and in very severe cases the penis cannot be extruded or may even slough. The animal may die of uraemia.

Rams do not usually develop severe internal lesions as seen in wethers and in most cases the lesions are confined to the external prepuce.

Treatment and prevention

It should be emphasised that this disease can be prevented. This can be done by ensuring that infected animals are isolated from other mating animals (e.g. wethers kept separated from rams). Infected rams should be treated and cured well before the mating season. It is also highly desirable to eliminate the conditions under which the causative bacterium flourishes. This can be done by keeping male animals carefully shorn around the prepuce. Any stained wool from this area should be destroyed and not left to contaminate the environment. At certain times of the year it may be necessary to carefully restrict the diet of male animals in order to produce acid urine, which will automatically clear minor lesions of pizzle rot. In the case of these mild external lesions (posthitis), a few days of restricted diet, confinement to the woolshed, hay feed and ad libitum water will usually effect a cure without the need for topical medication.

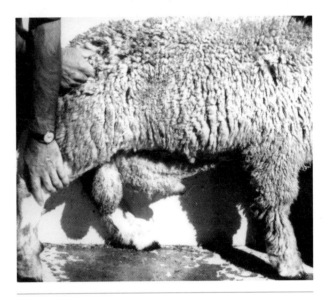

Figure 2.3 (a) Advanced balano-posthitis in a ram, showing blocking of the external prepucial orifice and urine accumulation.

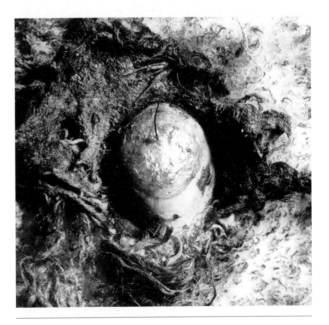

Figure 2.3 (b) External lesions of balano-posthitis. Note stained wool around the prepuce.

With severe internal lesions as well (balano-posthitis), it may be necessary to dose the ram with ammonium chloride (1–3 g) in water, two to three times daily, and in addition to irrigate the prepuce with suitable antiseptic solutions. In severe cases it may be necessary to incise the prepuce to allow drainage of urine and pus. In such cases the urethral process and penis are frequently damaged, and the ram becomes permanently unsound.

In Australia, testosterone treatment was once used to prevent balano-posthitis in wethers but has now largely fallen out of favour as a treatment. In New Zealand its use has never been extensive, probably because of smaller numbers of wethers farmed. It is now no longer available. Testosterone injections do not prevent scabs forming on the external prepuce, but do prevent the development of internal prepucial lesions.

The scrotum

Three important features should be noted in the examination of the scrotum: wool length, the presence or absence of scrotal abscesses, and chorioptic mange.

Wool length

It is important to ensure that rams with woolly scrota (e.g. Romneys, Merinos, Corriedales) do not carry excess wool during the mating season. Wool length can affect testes size by interfering with spermatogenesis. The optimum wool length is about 0.5–1.0 cm at mating.

Scrotal abscesses

Abscesses occur in rams frequently as a result of shearing cuts, and are a common cause of both temporary and permanent unsoundness. They should be treated carefully, as they tend to extend to deeper structures and may permanently damage the genitalia. They can be easily confused with acute cases of epididymitis in which the infected epididymis has burst to the exterior.

Chorioptic mange

Chorioptic or scrotal mange is one of the primary diseases affecting the external genitalia of rams. The causative mites (*Chorioptes bovis*) live and feed on the skin of sheep, goats, cattle and horses. Their life cycle is about three weeks from the egg to the larval stage to the egg-laying female. The disease is not confined solely to the ram but is probably widespread in both sexes in most sheep flocks.

The mites are usually found on the lower half of the body, particularly on the scrota of rams, around the dew claws and the brisket and often on the poll. Many sheep have mites but don't have mange, but when mange does occur it is generally on those areas of the body on which the mites concentrate. Paradoxically, however, in individual sheep the extent of the mange is not necessarily related to mite numbers. Mildly infested sheep may have the most severe mange. Rams without lesions of chorioptic mange are just as likely to be infected with mites as those with lesions. Furthermore, rams with old, inactive lesions may be free of mites.

Severe mange on the scrotum will reduce fertility and may even cause temporary or permanent infertility. Outbreaks of scrotal mange can be quite explosive and unpredictable, and under suitable conditions will persist over long periods of time. Control is therefore of considerable importance to the ram breeder.

Lesions of chorioptic mange should be diagnosed as either active or inactive. Active lesions when rubbed usually produce a marked nibbling or biting response by the ram. Active lesions when scraped or manipulated leave a bleeding area or at least a noticeable hyperaemia. Such areas may be pinhead size or larger. If such lesions are found, the ram is temporarily unsound and should be treated. Severe lesions covering approximately more than half of the scrotum usually render animals totally unsuitable for mating during that season and may even make them permanently unsound. It is important to remember that animals without lesions may carry mites and this must be considered when giving advice on treatment and control.

Control and treatment

Treatment can be applied either locally to the affected scrotum, or generally by dipping with a suitable parasiticide of which the organophosphorus compounds are most widely used. Topical treatment is satisfactory for individual cases, but for flock treatment the use of dipping at the higher recommended strengths of insecticide are most appropriate. Although no official claims have been made by the manufacturers, some veterinarians and farmers believe that ivermectin and possibly moxidectin either given orally or by injection aid in the treatment and control of mange. In ram hoggets there is frequently a build-up in the mite population during winter so that the preventive spraying of these animals is a wise recommendation to ram breeders.

The testes

Testis size

The size of a ram's testicles may vary considerably and is affected by age, health and season. It is clinically difficult to differentiate testicular atrophy from testicular hypoplasia, unless the former is associated with an obvious defect such as concurrent epididymitis. Furthermore, the inexperienced veterinarian must be acquainted with the seasonal variation of testes size, which is particularly noticeable in the Romney.

A sound ram at the height of the breeding season should have large oval testes that are firm to the touch and of equal size. However, in the non-breeding season the testes may reduce by up to 30%, and spermatogenesis is markedly reduced. There is some debate about what constitutes a 'satisfactory' scrotal circumference, but it is generally recommended that for mature rams a figure of ≥ 32 cm is used, while for rising two-tooth rams examined prior to sale (14–16 months of age) a satisfactory scrotal circumference is ≥ 28 cm. However, veterinarians should use their common sense in interpreting scrotal circumference and consider other relevant factors such as age, breed, season, testicular tone, health status, BCS and other abnormalities.

Large testicles produce more sperm per day than small testicles, and in normal rams each gram of testicular tissue produces approximately 20×10^6 sperm per day. As many examinations will be carried out on ram hoggets, some of which are actually still completing puberty, it is pertinent to remember the following points.

During the first few weeks of post-natal life, the weight of a ram's testes increases slowly relative to the more rapid changes in bodyweight. When bodyweight increases beyond 20 kg (weaning), testicular weight increases at a greater rate, maximum growth taking place between 24 and 27 kg. Puberty is reached at approximately 140 days of age (approximately January) and 35 kg bodyweight. However, there are wide between-breed differences (e.g. Suffolk 112 days; Merino 225 days). Increased testicular size implies increased spermatogenesis.

It must also be remembered that occasionally one testis in the ram descends before the other. Also, there is sometimes a size difference between the testes during puberty, which becomes inapparent at maturity. It is possible that these cases are related to the occurrence of cryptorchidism, and had the descent of the testes been delayed further, they may not have passed through the inguinal ring and into the scrotum. Hence, in young rams caution must be exercised when determining if a ram is sound based on uneven testes size or uneven testicular descent.

In the examination of the testes of the mature ram it is necessary to ensure that both size and tone are adequate. The ram with large symmetrical testes free from defects is likely to produce semen of good quality, while the ram with small, non-resilient testes is likely to produce poor-quality semen. In fact, the manual examination of ram genitalia is considered much more important and is generally more relevant to fertility prediction than a single semen examination. Semen examination, unless expertly executed, can lead to erroneous conclusions on the suitability of a particular ram for mating.

In addition to testes size and tone, the epididymis must be examined, especially the head and tail of the epididymis. The spermatic cords are also examined, particularly for firm swellings that may denote an abscess of the superficial inguinal lymph nodes or even a varicocele (the latter are relatively rare in British breeds of sheep but not uncommon in the Merino).

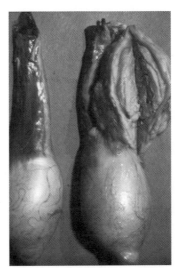

Figure 2.4 Abscess of the inguinal lymph node.

Testicular atrophy and testicular degeneration

Testicular atrophy can be seen in association with systemic disease and other chemical and physical factors. Many cases of testicular atrophy are unilateral (affecting one testis only) and result from an epididymitis of the organ. Such atrophy is permanent.

However, testicular degeneration may occur in a mild transitory form where there is only slight seminal degeneration for a short period. It may also be severe and prolonged with grossly abnormal semen being produced. In extreme cases, the seminal degeneration may be so severe that it becomes irreversible and the testis will atrophy.

The majority of cases of testicular degeneration result from an increase in testicular temperature. The normal heat-loss mechanisms fail to cope with the heat gained, and seminal degeneration occurs.

Spermatogenesis in the ram is most efficient when the internal temperature of the testis is about 4°C below the body temperature. This lowered temperature is maintained by several complex scrotal mechanisms involving blood flow in the pampiniform plexus and the raising and lowering of the testis by the cremaster muscles. There are genetic differences between rams in their ability to control testis temperature. The following circumstances can result in increased testicular temperature which may lead to seminal degeneration:

- hot weather
- physical exertion
- any scrotal thickening, e.g. chorioptic mange
- fever
- flystrike
- over-fatness
- heavy wool cover of the scrotum
- rugging
- housing in conditions that allow little air movement around the scrotum and where the humidity is high
- unfavourable transport conditions, e.g. overcrowding, hot weather.

Seminal degeneration is frequently reported in rams prepared for sales, shows and export. In many cases the rams have left few, if any, progeny after their first year of mating but in subsequent seasons have performed adequately.

Clinical features of testicular degeneration

Testicular degeneration does not affect the health of the ram; usually if they are stud rams they are in excellent condition and usually carrying an exceptional fleece of wool.

With mild testicular degeneration the testes will be bilaterally symmetrical but reduced in size and will tend to be soft and even flabby. The semen may only show slight changes in consistency and several examinations may be required for its evaluation.

As the degeneration becomes more severe, testis size is reduced further, the testes tend to feel long and non-resilient and the quality of the semen is changed markedly. The severity of testicular degeneration and the time taken for recovery depends on the severity of the cause and the time the testis is exposed to heat insult.

An example of testicular degeneration in its simplest form is shown in Figure 2.5.

Following a sudden insult to the testes, evidence of seminal degeneration will usually not show up for several days as the semen in the epididymis usually remains unaffected. The signs of sperm deterioration are usually seen after about a week. Following a serious seminal degeneration it may take three months or more for sperm production to become normal. The spermatogenic cycle (spermatogonia to mature sperm) takes approximately two months in the ram.

However, in making a prognosis for an individual case, great care must be taken as complete recovery may be over many months. Some almost hopeless cases have made a recovery eventually, probably because the basal sperm cells (spermatogonia) appear to be quite resistant to complete destruction by overheating. The later semen elements, spermatocytes, spermatids and sperm, are, on the other hand, very susceptible to degeneration following heat change.

In the practical situation the picture of testicular degeneration is complex. Causal factors that tend to increase testicular temperature may act continuously or intermittently. They may act for a short time only, for instance when a woolled ram is left standing on a truck on a hot day, or when full-woolled rams are being prepared for sale or showing. Further, individual rams will respond in different ways to the same set of factors.

Diagnosis of testicular degeneration

The diagnosis of testicular degeneration can be made by physical examination and semen examination. Mild cases of testicular degeneration cannot be detected by physical examination alone and may escape notice, but they are likely to recover, given time.

Treatment of testicular degeneration

Treatment for testicular degeneration is to shear the ram, put him onto grass feeding only, and maintain him in cool conditions. To assess whether a ram is recovering from testicular degeneration it may be necessary to collect a number of semen samples over a period of time. Fortunately, most rams recover before mating in autumn.

Prevention of testicular degeneration in rams

There is something of a dilemma in preparing rams for showing and sale. To obtain good sale prices, rams are usually fed well from an early age to increase their size and are presented for sale in full wool. Ram sales are usually held in summer. These factors can have a stressful effect on the ram's reproductive system but can be modified to reduce the likelihood of seminal damage occurring.

The following are practical recommendations that can be made to the ram breeder:
- Shearing of the scrotum does decrease the problem and assists the ram to maintain optimum testicular temperature.
- Ensure that rams always have access to shade.
- Avoid housing rams in enclosed buildings that do not allow a good air flow around the ram.
- Avoid confining rams in full wool in summer in small pens with no shade.
- Take particular care when transporting rams to and from sales or shows to avoid overheating. It is when the truck is stationary that a lot of damage can occur.
- Apart from shows and sales, when transporting rams during hot summer weather it is preferable to shear them beforehand, or at least shear the belly and scrotum.
- Ensure that sales and shows are conducted in buildings that prevent overheating of rams.
- When buying rams the purchaser should carefully feel the scrotal contents or seek veterinary advice.

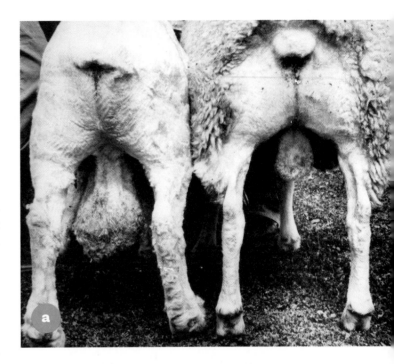

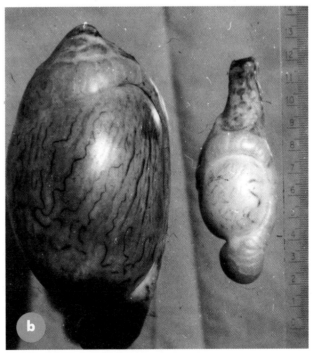

Figure 2.5 Examples of extreme testicular degeneration compared with normal **(a)** in live sheep and **(b)** at autopsy.

The scrotal circumference for mature Romney rams should be in the following range:

	Mean (cm)	Range (cm)
November	32	29–35
March	35	33–40

Testicular hypoplasia

As well as decreased testis size associated with seminal degeneration, there are a variety of conditions in which the testes of rams are hypoplastic as a result of genetic or developmental defects. Such defects are usually permanent, and in many cases affected animals will not breed. Distinct forms of testicular hypoplasia are listed below:

- Unilateral testicular hypoplasia.
- Testicular hypoplasia due to cryptorchidism and monorchidism.
- Primary micro-orchidism (XXY chromosomal complement, the equivalent of Klinefelter's syndrome in humans).
- Micro-orchidism of unknown aetiology.
- Hypo-orchidism in association with segmental aplasia of the epididymis.
- Bilateral epididymal spermiostasis.
- Hypo-orchidism and inguinal hernia.
- Hypo-orchidism in association with varicocele.

The many types of hypo-orchidism may need particular investigation to determine their aetiology. For example, in valuable rams chromosome analysis may reveal individual cases of primary micro-orchidism in which a ram has two X chromosomes as well as a Y chromosome.

Cryptorchidism and monorchidism

The diagnosis of cryptorchidism and monorchidism (one or both testes not in the scrotum) presents no difficulties. Occasionally one or both testes can be palpated in the inguinal canal, having made a partial descent. Both conditions are inherited and in Merino rams they are associated with polledness. The culling of such rams is advisable, as although many rams with one testis descended will breed, their use, even in commercial flocks, is not recommended as they are likely to breed a proportion of ram lambs that are also cryptorchids. Australian work suggests that unilateral testicular hypoplasia and cryptorchidism have the same hereditary basis. There is some suggestion that the same may also be true of the Romney breed.

Other testicular defects, such as segmental aplasia, bilateral spermiostases and varicocele, are rare in New Zealand rams and in many cases do not present a difficult clinical problem to diagnose.

Epididymitis

Epididymitis is usually caused by either *Brucella ovis* or the Gram-negative pleomorphic bacteria (*Actinobacillus seminis, Histophilus somni*) and is a common cause of ram wastage and rejection in New Zealand and Australia. The detection of palpable lesions of epididymitis presents few problems to the experienced veterinarian but it is important that the cause is diagnosed. This involves a consideration of the history of the problem, the age of the rams affected, the number affected, and the use of further diagnostic tests. These most commonly include serology and occasionally microbiology from semen ejaculates and the histopathology of affected gonads. In rams, vasectomy often also results in lesions of epididymitis and it is important to exclude this; exclusion is usually by history and presence of a scar at the surgery site.

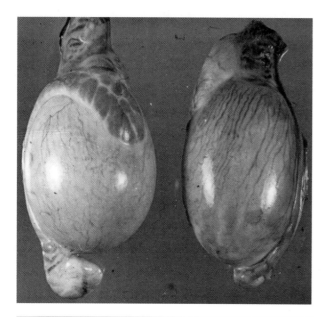

Figure 2.6 Segmental aplasia: normal testis and epididymis (left); the tail of the epididymis (right) is incomplete.

Brucella ovis infection of sheep

Infection with *Brucella ovis* may result in chronic lesions of the male genital tract, which often lead to reduced fertility. The disease is transmitted mainly through rams having sexual contact and by transmission from infected to non-infected rams serving the same ewe. Eradication can be successfully achieved by a test and cull procedure. Simple control measures enable continued freedom from disease.

Brucellosis as a cause of epididymitis in rams was discovered first in New Zealand and Australia. It has involved the rural veterinarian in a tremendous amount of clinical work and has been brought under control by a voluntary accreditation scheme for stud and commercial sheep flocks. This has been made possible by the pioneering work of Crawford, Buddle and others and the development of accurate serological tests for its diagnosis. For this reason it is pertinent to record a brief history of brucellosis in sheep in New Zealand and Australia.

History

In 1942, Gunn, Sanders and Granger reported an incidence of approximately 5.5% of rams examined that had a clinical abnormality which they called epididymitis with spermatocoele. This came from an extensive fertility study of over 9000 rams in Queensland and New South Wales. No bacterial cause was attributed to these lesions at that time, but retrospectively it is highly likely that a significant proportion was caused by *B. ovis*.

Later, in New Zealand, Crawford (1949) expressed concern about the prevalence of epididymitis in rams in the Gisborne district. His clinical studies concluded that the disease was affecting the lambing percentage in a number of flocks that he examined.

During 1953, the physical and metabolic characteristics of the organism associated with epididymitis in rams were described both in New Zealand and Australia. Further work by Buddle and Boyes in New Zealand led Buddle to confirm in 1956 that the organism was a member of the genus *Brucella* but it was shown to have different characteristics to the three 'classical Brucella' (*B. abortus*, *B. melitensis* and *B. suis*). He suggested that the new variant be given the name *Brucella ovis*.

In the 1980s a nationwide voluntary accreditation scheme was developed and now the majority of pedigree flocks and a small number of commercial flocks are accredited free.

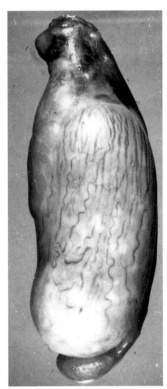

Figure 2.7 Misshapen undescended testis (partial cryptorchid).

Host animals

Brucella ovis is a disease primarily of sheep, although naturally occurring infection has been recognised in farmed deer in New Zealand. Experimentally, laboratory animals, white-tailed deer and goats have been infected, but natural infection of these species has not been documented.

Prevalence

The prevalence of brucellosis differs widely between individual flocks of rams. In Tasmania, for example, when a programme using serological testing was begun in 1959, 18% of all ram flocks were affected with a prevalence of infection ranging from 10% to 74%. Similar ranges of prevalence were observed in New Zealand, but exact information is difficult to obtain because surveys were generally limited in time and locality.

It has been suggested that the prevalence of *B. ovis* infection may have declined under the impact of control measures used in New Zealand. In the decade 1954–1964, 39% of specific pathogens isolated from ram testicles submitted to New Zealand diagnostic stations were *B. ovis*, but in 1965–1966 only 7% were *B. ovis*. From a postal survey conducted in 1982 the prevalence of infection at first testing was found to range from 0% to 75% in 49 flocks undertaking accreditation schemes. The overall prevalence of infection in rams in New Zealand was estimated to be approximately 3%, with the average prevalence within infected flocks being 5% for stud farms and 11% for commercial flocks.

By 1987, physical examination of rams' genitalia from the farms that had entered voluntary *B. ovis* control schemes suggested a marked reduction in the prevalence of the disease. Of 111,000 rams which were palpated, only 1.1% had epididymitis and this was caused principally by Gram-negative pleomorphic bacteria. In stud flocks only 631 samples out of 51,000 submitted were seropositive for *B. ovis* (1.1%).

While data are no longer kept on *B. ovis* prevalence, the disease is likely to be uncommon. However, outbreaks still occur and vigilance is required from veterinarians and farmers to maintain disease-free status in individual flocks.

The organism

Brucella ovis is a small Gram-negative coccobacillus. It is an obligatory pathogen which is most commonly associated with sheep, particularly rams. However, it is also recognised as causing disease in deer. It is a rough organism. This characteristic distinguishes it from the other naturally occurring members of the *Brucella* genus except *B. canis*, which also occurs as a rough organism naturally. The rough *Brucellas* are antigenically different in their (surface) lipopolysaccharides from the smooth *Brucellas* and this difference allows quick serological differentiation of these two types of organism and their infections in a range of tests.

Brucella ovis appears to be a relatively genetically stable organism and only two types have been identified.

Pathogenesis
Pathogenesis in the ram

The organism can enter the body through any mucous membrane. Experimentally, infection has been produced by infecting conjunctival, penile, preputial, vaginal, rectal and nasal mucosae. It has also been produced by intravenous, intratesticular and subcutaneous inoculation, through shearing wounds inflicted with contaminated hand-pieces and orally.

After infection, the organism remains localised for some time in the mucous membrane and the local lymph node. During this phase, the body's defence mechanism may overwhelm the organism, resulting in a transient infection only, or the infection may progress to a bacteraemic phase. At the end of the bacteraemic phase, the organism will have localised in the epididymis and accessory sex glands and sometimes in testicles, kidneys, liver, spleen and lungs.

Pathological changes are generally confined to the epididymis and accessory sex glands. The earliest lesions usually develop in the tail of the epididymis and this is also where the majority of gross lesions develop. Lesions of the head and body of the epididymis are less common. Large lesions may develop very rapidly and it is not unusual to find lesions measuring 2–3 cm in a ram which was clinically normal a few days earlier. The lesions may persist as granulomas or develop into abscesses. These abscesses may contain large amounts of creamy yellow pus. Older lesions become progressively more caseated and fibrotic and eventually become entirely fibrotic or may contain small granules of inspissated or calcified material. A few lesions may resolve, leaving only small lesions that are difficult to detect by palpation.

These lesions begin as an inflammation of the interstitium of the tubules with oedema and lymphocyte infiltration. Later, the tubular epithelium itself becomes infiltrated with lymphocytes and with other cells like neutrophils. Finally, the epithelium becomes hyperplastic. This leads to narrowing or even blocking of the lumen of the tubule, resulting in sperm stasis and leakage of sperm into the surrounding tissue which acts as a foreign body; hence, at necropsy, granulomas, haemorrhages, adhesions and abscesses can be found.

Inflammatory changes have also been found elsewhere in the genital tract, especially in the accessory glands. These lesions are less severe and more difficult to detect.

Depending on the location and severity of the changes, the inflammation of the genital tract can result in semen of inferior quality. The reduced semen quality is characterised by lower sperm counts, sometimes aspermia, lower sperm motility and a higher number of abnormal spermatocytes. Pus is sometimes noticeable, and neutrophils and other cells are often seen in semen smears. Once infected, rams are likely to remain infected for life. Similar effects on semen quality and pathological lesions are found in infected stags, although the epididymal lesions tend to be more difficult to palpate and many stags appear to resolve the infection within a year.

Pathogenesis in the ewe

The pathogenesis in the ewe is less well defined. The most likely way of infection is by mating. After experimental intravaginal infection, it has been possible to isolate *B. ovis* from the vagina and the blood for several months, although in most cases the infection has resolved by the time of the next oestrous period. Conjunctival instillation and intravenous inoculation have also been able to produce (transient) infections.

Following experimental infection of pregnant ewes, localisation of the bacteria takes place in the placenta, leading to placentitis and endometritis. Depending on the stage of gestation and the severity of the lesions, either the ewe aborts or gives birth to small, weak lambs. However, under field conditions abortions are very rarely a feature of *B. ovis* infections, possibly because under field conditions infection is more likely at mating than mid-pregnancy.

Transmission

Natural infection by *B. ovis* has been recorded in sheep and now deer. Infected rams can excrete the organism in their semen for at least two years and in some cases probably indefinitely. Hence, the disease is considered to be venereal in nature and can be spread among young rams, probably by sodomy or by sniffing or licking infected semen.

The role of the ewe in the spread of the disease is not clear and is probably not important except as a temporary mechanical carrier after mating with an infected ram. Ewes mated to infected rams can become infected, develop serological titres and in a few instances produce dead lambs with grossly diseased placentae. However, even in flocks with a high proportion of actively infected rams, infection in the ewe is transient and rarely persists from one breeding season to the next. This point is now supported from clinical data where *Brucella*-free rams have not become infected when introduced to ewe flocks which in previous years had been exposed to rams infected with *B. ovis*.

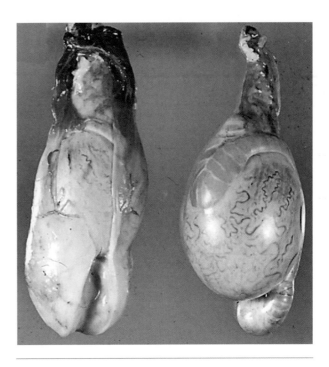

Figure 2.8 (a) Advanced epididymitis due to *B. ovis* infection (left), normal testis (right).

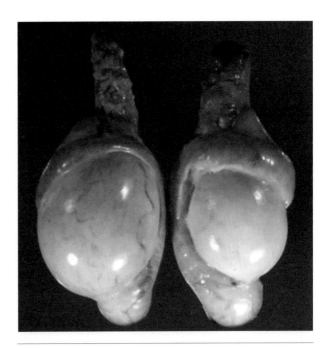

Figure 2.8 (b) Epididymitis due to *B. ovis* infection (right), normal testis (left). Note the reduced size of the affected testis.

Rams can become infected by mating with a ewe previously served by an infected ram during the same oestrous period and also by direct contact with other infected rams. Transmission among rams probably increases as sexual activity increases towards the mating season and will be further influenced by the gathering into flocks of rams from different sources. Once a ram is infected with *B. ovis*, a detectable antibody response usually develops in 3–6 weeks and the organism can usually be isolated from semen after about 4–5 weeks.

While transmission of *B. ovis* occurs between rams and stags by direct contact, there is no evidence of transmission between rams or stags by grazing paddocks that have been recently stocked by infected animals, or by grazing in paddocks adjacent to infected animals.

The effect of Brucella ovis infection

Rams infected with *B. ovis* can produce semen of variable quality. Since the effect of the infection on semen quality depends on the stage of infection and the extent and severity of the lesions (e.g. unilateral and small or bilateral and blocking), much variation in semen quality is found between infected rams and even between ejaculates from the same animal. Semen quality from infected rams ranges from aspermia to apparently normal.

Because of the many factors that contribute to the fertility (lambing percentage) of a flock it is difficult to predict precisely what effect rams infected with *B. ovis* will have on the final number of ewes that conceive. Further, the practice of over-mating (i.e. using more rams than may be required) may mask the effect in some flocks. However, field data have shown that using infected rams for mating generally reduces the lambing performance of the ewes and may produce a protracted lambing season.

The impact becomes much clearer when greater importance is attached to the fertility of individual rams or where farmers wish to use a low ram : ewe ratio. In these situations it is vital that the fertility of individual rams is not adversely affected.

The only way to eliminate this risk is by eradicating *B. ovis* from the whole flock. If this approach is followed, the economic impact can be measured in the (perpetual) yearly ram wastage, and its associated costs, that would occur under the alternative approach of palpation and culling. In the long term, in nearly all cases the cost of culling rams with lesions will exceed the cost of eradication, especially since the disease can spread rapidly and often reaches infection rates of 60% and higher.

Along with reduced ram wastage, the policy of complete eradication adds the advantages of a shorter lambing period, better lambing percentage and the use of fewer rams. Since freedom from *B. ovis* is a mandatory requirement for most export rams, an accredited-free flock has a competitive edge over flocks of unknown status.

Diagnosis

In flocks with established infections, palpation will often lead to a presumptive diagnosis when it reveals a considerable number of rams with epididymis. Palpation is usually the first and most important clinical procedure in the diagnosis of epididymitis (and eventually brucellosis) in a flock. Indeed, on a flock basis, particularly when a number of mature rams have palpable lesions, a confirmed diagnosis of brucellosis is almost inevitable.

The presumptive diagnosis can be confirmed by serological testing. In flocks with established infections, serological testing of the whole flock will normally reveal many more infected animals. It should be realised that not all of these positive rams will be shedders, the percentage of (potential) shedders being reported as 40% for low-titered reactors to 100% for high-titered ones, with an average figure of 80%.

A variety of serological tests have been reported. Among them are the gel diffusion test (GDT), several modifications of the complement fixation test (CFT) and the enzyme-linked immunosorbent assay (ELISA). At present, the CFT is regarded as the method giving the optimal combination of sensitivity and specificity. This test is used in several countries in accreditation and eradication schemes. The ELISA test provides similar accuracy and can also be used in accreditation schemes. The GDT has a very high specificity of around 100% but a low sensitivity of only around 92%, and is only really used when it is necessary to confirm cases of *B. ovis* infection.

Seroconversion occurs from about 3 weeks after inoculation or infection. Most animals will have developed good titres by 4–5 weeks. Over time a gradual decrease of titres takes place to a level at which they are sustained. The sensitivities of the CFT and the ELISA have been assessed at 97–98% and the specificities at around 99%.

In chronically infected ram flocks, using both serological tests together increases the likelihood of identifying infected rams. The ELISA test is also used when samples are anticomplementary in the CFT (0.8% of submitted samples). False-positive reactions occur and it has been found that their occurrence is negatively correlated with titre. If a flock has a history of being non-infected, then a few low-titre reactions to the CFT are probably non-specific. However, if the flock is clearly infected, the reactions must be interpreted more strictly.

Other ancillary diagnostic methods available are:

- **Culture of semen** — in infected rams, *B. ovis* can usually be isolated from semen samples; but it should be noted that one negative culture has limited significance. Nevertheless, in problem flock investigations semen culture is a useful diagnostic aid and if positive provides unequivocal evidence of infection. *Brucella ovis* can survive in semen for at least 4 days at room temperature. However, as samples become older, isolation becomes more difficult since they become increasingly contaminated by other organisms. A selective medium should be used for initial isolation and the laboratory should be forewarned about sample submission.
- **Microscopic examination of semen** — the presence of abnormal cells in semen smears after staining with the modified Ziehl-Neelsen method may be an aid in diagnosis. Many infected animals have high numbers of white blood cells in their semen and in some this is even visible to the naked eye as pus. Especially in these samples, the chance of finding the organism with a staining method is high.
- **Histopathology of the genital tract** — since *B. ovis* can frequently be isolated from accessory glands, specimens for bacteriological examination should include testicles, epididymides, seminal vesicles, bulbourethral glands and ampullae.

A multiplex PCR for the detection of *B. ovis, Actinobacillus seminis* and *Histophilus somni* in ram semen has been developed in Australia. Its use could be complementary or an alternative to semen and other biological samples for the detection of these organisms.

Finally, it should be emphasised that a combination of tests should be used in the diagnosis of brucellosis to ensure that uncertain cases are clearly defined. One ram that may be a *B. ovis* shedder but is missed, or carelessly left in a flock of 'clean rams' simply because one test was uncertain, can lead, in a short time, to costly contamination of other rams.

Control and eradication

Since the ewe plays no role of significance in the transmission of *B. ovis* outside the mating season, the eradication of *B. ovis* focuses on its detection in rams.

Eradication by test and slaughter

Brucella ovis can be eradicated from flocks and areas by a test and cull procedure. Infected rams are detected by scrotal palpation and serum testing (CFT and possibly ELISA). Once a flock is confirmed as being infected, rams that react to the serological tests, or have epididymitis, should be culled. The remaining rams are retested at about monthly intervals until a clear test is obtained. A further free test at an interval of at least 60 days should ensure that no animal in the incubation stage has gone undetected.

The number of tests required before a flock is freed from *B. ovis* infection depends on the number of rams initially infected, the length of time the flock has been infected, and the accuracy of sampling and testing. Usually one to three tests are necessary to detect all infected animals in a flock. In some cases, the so-called problem flocks, a higher number of tests is necessary. A reason for this can be the presence of one or more shedders with low antibody levels that are sometimes below detection level. Use of both the CFT and ELISA tests in series or parallel is recommended for chronically infected flocks, where infection has been present for greater than a year, to increase the likelihood of detecting all infected rams. This may expedite a quick clearance of the disease from the flock.

A second reason for slow progress in eradication is the rapid spread of the disease through the ram flock. This will occur because of high sexual activity in the mating season. It will be of further importance whenever there is homosexual activity prior to the mating season or when rams are brought together from different sources. Hence, the best progress in eradication can be made during the time of the year when rams are least sexually active, i.e. winter and spring.

Finally, the practising veterinarian must ensure that the farmer has completely mustered all rams for testing, that these are correctly identified (ear tags), that all reports are clearly and accurately completed before samples are submitted for laboratory testing and that infected rams are culled promptly.

Eradication by total replacement

In flocks where the prevalence of *B. ovis* is very high and a suitable source of *B. ovis*-free rams is available, the most appropriate action may be to replace all the rams.

Eradication by managing a 'two-flock' system

Because *B. ovis* is essentially a disease of rams, it is possible to eradicate the infection from the farm by running two separate flocks of rams, one of which is known to be free and the other known or suspected of being infected. Strict separation between the two ram flocks must continue for the whole year, including mating, and this requires a very high level of management. Each year the number of rams in the 'infected' flock is reduced as they age and the number in the 'free' flock is increased with the addition of brucellosis-free two-tooths. On some farms, it may be appropriate to keep the 'infected' group of rams for a shorter period (perhaps one mating season) before they are culled. In general, 'two flock' systems are very hard to manage and breakdowns can occur unless they are very carefully supervised.

Eradication using a combination of methods

Occasionally, it is appropriate to use a combination of the eradication methods explained previously. For instance, if *B. ovis* can be clearly identified as infecting a specific subgroup of rams on a farm, the most appropriate action may be to dispose of that subgroup.

It is also common when conducting eradication procedures by testing and culling to maintain known *B. ovis*-free rams, such as recent purchases, separate from the group of rams under investigation (i.e. a 'two-flock' system). If the test and slaughter programme becomes protracted, there is then the option either to continue with the 'two flock' system or, alternatively, to dispose of the infected sub-flock.

Sheep Brucella ovis flock accreditation scheme

In the 1980s a nationwide voluntary flock accreditation scheme was developed (see the flowchart). The vast majority of pedigree flocks, and a small number of commercial flocks, are part of this scheme.

Dealing with possible Brucella ovis breakdowns

Although the CFT has a high specificity (approximately 99%), false-positive reactions do occur. The difficulty is to distinguish these false reactions from true infections due to the introduction of *B. ovis* into accredited-free flocks.

If positive serological results are obtained from an accredited-free flock, the testing veterinarian should obtain further blood samples from reacting rams and investigate the possible routes of introduction of infection. The original and follow-up blood samples are subjected to a range of serological tests, including CFT, ELISA and GD tests. The results from this serological panel are compared with published results of false-positive and false-negative samples (Hilbink et al., 1993, Figure 2.9). Of the 97 false-positive CF tests, 32 also gave false reactions in the ELISA. In these situations the GD test proved to be the most useful discriminating test, as all 97 false-positive CF test reactors were negative in the GD test and of the 45 true CF test reactors only three were negative in the GD test.

In doubtful cases, additional tests such as semen culture or in extreme cases necropsy may be indicated. The need for careful follow-up to minimise the effects of such cases for ram breeders has been emphasised (West, 2000a).

Brucella ovis infection in deer

In 1996, *B. ovis* infection was recognised as causing disease in deer in New Zealand and since then further naturally occurring cases have been identified. Stags can become infected either by contact with infected rams or by contact with other infected stags, and it is likely that transmission occurs by sniffing or licking infected semen. While it has not been demonstrated experimentally, it is possible that infected stags could transmit the disease back to rams. The disease in stags has similar effects to that in rams with lesions in the epididymes, seminal vesicles and ampullae, and an overall decrease in semen quality. However, in contrast to the disease in rams, it appears that the majority of stags resolve the infection within a year and semen quality returns to normal. Deer farmers wishing to remain free of this disease should not mix rams of unknown *B. ovis* status with stags and test introduced stags before mixing.

1. Owner elects to join the scheme

This is an industry-based scheme and participation of ram flock owners is voluntary. The veterinary practitioner is responsible for carrying out all testing of rams for B. ovis and certifying the flock when it is free. All costs of examination and testing should be borne by the owner.

2. Accreditation test

To fulfil the requirements for accreditation the veterinarian is to:

(a) Check that no new rams, other than from accredited-free flocks, have been introduced within the previous two months.

(b) Palpate the scrotal contents and blood sample and serologically test all rams and teasers over the age of 15 months and rams under 15 months which have been used for mating.

(c) Palpate the scrotal contents of all sale rams within three months of sale for breeding purposes. Blood sample and serologically test any with lesions of epididymitis.

Inf? — Yes → 5. Eradication testing; No → 3. Flock accredited

5. Eradication testing

Should B. ovis infection be diagnosed and should the owner wish to proceed towards accreditation, then a B. ovis eradication programme should be implemented on the farm under the supervision of the veterinarian. The eradication programme should be adapted to the particular flock circumstances on the property concerned.

The flock may be accredited when:

(a) All rams and teasers 15 months of age and over, and any younger than 15 months which have been used for mating, have had two consecutive negative blood tests no less than 60 days and not more than 180 days apart.

(b) All sale rams have undergone scrotal palpation within three months of sale for breeding purposes, and any with lesions of epididymitis have been negative to serology.

Further details on the *Brucella ovis* accreditation scheme can be obtained from the Society of Sheep and Beef Cattle Veterinarians, New Zealand Veterinary Association.

For non-accredited-free flocks, determining the extent and frequency of B. ovis testing in individual flocks should be determined by the veterinarian based on risk assessment.

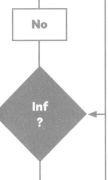

Inf? — No → back to 2. Accreditation test; Yes → continue eradication

4. Annual re-accreditation test

(a) All stud rams and teasers over the age of 15 months and stud rams less than 15 months of age which have been used for mating: scrotal palpation and bloods for serology.

(b) Commercial rams over the age of 15 months: scrotal palpation of all rams, bloods from the whole flock or 20 rams, whichever is the least, and any ram with epididymitis.

(c) Scrotal palpation of all sale rams within three months of sale for breeding purposes. Blood sample any with lesions of epididymitis.

3. Flock accredited

The veterinarian issues a Certificate of Accreditation (available from approved laboratories) to flock owner. Accreditation will be valid for a period of one year from the date of testing.

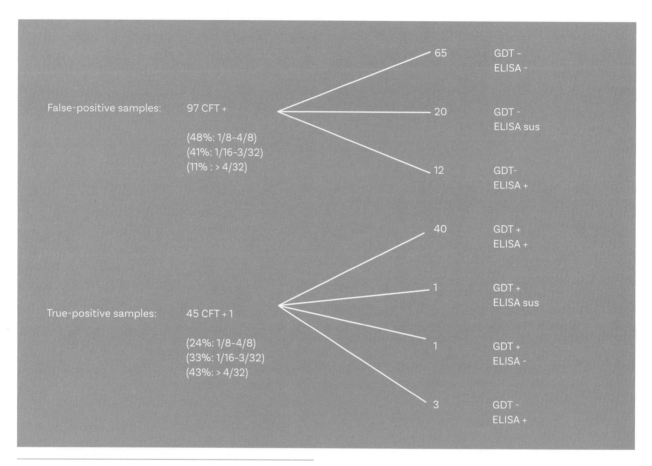

Figure 2.9 Analysis of comparative testing for *Brucella ovis* on questionable reactors in re-accreditation submissions from accredited *B. ovis*-free flocks (from Hilbink et al., 1993).

Gram-negative pleomorphic infection: *Actinobacillus seminis/Histophilus somni*

The organisms

An acute epididymitis affecting mainly young rams and associated with a Gram-negative pleomorphic organism was first reported in New Zealand in 1955. It has also been reported in Australia, South Africa and several other sheep-raising countries.

Subsequently a variety of organisms with very similar characteristics have been isolated from the lesions of young rams with epididymitis. These include: *Actinobacillus seminis, Aggregatibacter actinomycetemcomitans, Actinobacillus*-like organisms, *Histophilus ovis, Haemophilus somnus* and *Haemophilus agni*. In general it appears that these organisms fall into two groups. *Histophilus ovis, Haemophilus somnus* and *Haemophilus agni* share similar morphological, biochemical and serological properties and are now considered by many bacteriologists to belong to a single species. In this book they are referred to as *Histophilus somni*. The other group will be referred to as *Actinobacillus seminis*. Thus the term Gram-negative pleomorphic bacteria refers to *A. seminis/H. somni*.

Histophilus somni has also been associated with septicaemia and acute death of lambs (see Chapter 16) but the relationship between genital infection and septicaemia is unclear.

Occurrence and prevalence

On individual farms the incidence can be quite high and

can lead to the regular annual loss of a significant number of ram lambs or ram hoggets. There are reports of flocks in New Zealand with an annual wastage of young rams from 3% to 10%. The national prevalence of the disease has not been determined in Australia and New Zealand, but in mixed-aged rams in South Africa a very high incidence and wide distribution of infection has been found. In one study 74.8% of 409 flocks examined had rams infected with *A. seminis/H. somni* and 61.1% of these flocks had rams with epididymal lesions.

Studies in New Zealand have shown that it is possible to culture *A. seminis/H. somni* for several months from the semen of as many as 95% of ram hoggets in some flocks. However, the significant point is that only a low proportion (1–10%) of these 'temporary carriers' develop clinical lesions of epididymitis. Among older rams the disease appears to be rare.

Infection and transmission

Little is known about how rams become infected and how the infection is transmitted from year to year. In affected flocks nearly all young rams at six months of age have been found to be shedding *A. seminis/H. somni* in their semen, although the site of the infection has not been established. In some it could be relatively superficial, in the lower urethra or prepucial area.

Fortunately, as mentioned previously, only a small proportion of rams develop lesions of epididymitis and the majority of rams become free of genital infection by 15 months of age, which is about the time of sale.

Two suggestions on transmission and pathogenesis of the disease have been made. The first suggests that the ram lamb acquires the organism from the ewe *in utero* due to systemic spread of the organism. It has been proposed that the invasion of the placenta and foetus occurs late in pregnancy and that the organism is harboured in the lamb in its genital tract in the subclinical or latent phase. The second, and perhaps more likely, means of infection is that the preputial cavity of the young ram becomes invaded by organisms from the environment, particularly around yards and buildings. It is then considered that the infection travels in a retrograde fashion to the accessory sex glands and occasionally the epididymis. It has been shown that leuteotrophic hormone enhances retrograde movement and this hormone increases at the time of puberty.

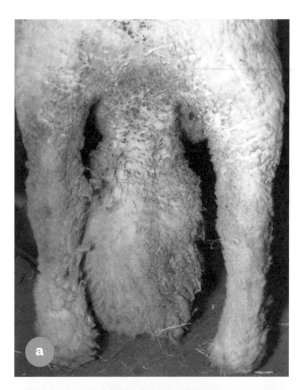

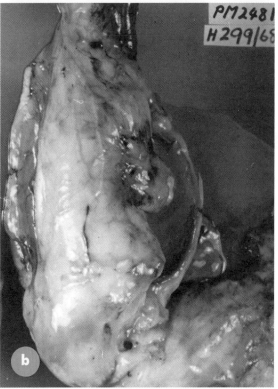

Figure 2.10 Acute epididymitis caused by *A. seminis*: **(a)** in live sheep; **(b)** postmortem, note ruptured testicle and discharged pus.

Clinical features

It must be re-emphasised that epididymitis caused by *A. seminis/H. somni* occurs commonly in young rams during and immediately following puberty (6–15 months of age). Many rams excrete the organism for a period in their semen, but in only a few do lesions of epididymitis develop (Figure 2.10).

A variety of clinical signs may occur. In some rams there is a severe systemic reaction associated with the development of an acute and severe epididymitis. Frequently, affected rams will isolate themselves from the flock, tend to stop grazing, walk with difficulty and become recumbent. In some cases the swelling is quite severe and the abscess formed in the epididymis and testes will burst to the exterior and discharge thick, glairy pus. In others the swelling may subside and leave a permanently swollen epididymis and atrophied testicle rendering the ram permanently unsound.

Many rams have infection in the accessory sex glands and duct system but show no obvious clinical lesions. However, the semen quality of such rams is often affected and pus and other inflammatory exudate are present in the ejaculate. Surprisingly, most rams in the latter category do recover, semen quality returns to normal and the organism may no longer be detected. Occasionally, persistently infected rams have been identified for up to two years.

Diagnosis

Lesions of epididymitis can be readily detected by palpation. Subclinical cases and carrier rams are more difficult to detect and can only be found by the bacteriological examination of carefully collected semen samples. Serology has not proven to be useful, as many rams do not seroconvert until lesions of epididymitis are obvious. Diagnosis is essentially a diagnosis of exclusion by ruling out other causes of epididymitis (*B. ovis* and vasectomy).

Control

There is no simple procedure yet available to control *A. seminis/H. somni* infections. This is a problem primarily of ram breeding flocks, as the condition is seldom of concern to commercial sheep farmers.

If the organism does gain entry to the ram at puberty, lack of good environmental hygiene is probably very important in aiding the spread of the disease. The tendency of ram lambs to congregate in groups in paddocks may be an important contributing factor to the spread of the disease. Therefore care should be taken to avoid holding rams in dirty yards and sheds, and the latter need to be cleaned regularly. Frequent paddock changes may also be important where large flocks of ram lambs are being reared.

Alternatively, several flocks may be grazed in an effort to disperse the animals while they are vulnerable to infection. Administering antibiotics to all ram lambs before puberty has not proven to be successful and when subsequently sampled the number of rams that carry the infection was not altered. However, long-term feeding of low dosages of antibiotics has reduced the incidence of clinically affected rams in some flocks in the United States.

In problem flocks, it can be anticipated that most ram lambs around the time of puberty will be excreting the organisms in their semen and it is possible that the widespread use of ram lambs for mating increases the level of infection, but not enough is known at present to be positive about this. It is generally recommended that rams known to be excreting the organisms in their semen should not be used as ram breeding sires; this *may* reduce the problem but will not eliminate it.

An American report has shown that an autogenous, multivalent, adjuvant bacterin was effective in reducing the clinical incidence of epididymitis. Such a vaccine is not available in New Zealand.

REFERENCES

Al-Katib WA, Dennis SM. Pathological changes in accessory sex organs of rams following experimental infection with *Actinobacillus seminis*. *New Zealand Veterinary Journal* 56, 319-25, 2008

Bailey KM. Naturally acquired *Brucella ovis* infection in deer. *Surveillance* 24, 10-11, 1977

Bruère AN, Marshall RB, Ward DPJ. Testicular hypoplasia and XXY sex chromosome complement in two rams: The ovine counterpart of Klinefelters syndrome in man. *Journal of Reproduction and Fertility* 19, 103-8, 1969

Bruère AN. Some clinical aspects of hypo-orchidism (small testes) in the ram. *New Zealand Veterinary Journal* 18, 189-98, 1970

Bruère AN. The segregation patterns and fertility of sheep heterozygous and homozygous for three different Robertsonian translocations. *Journal of Reproduction and Fertility* 41, 453-64, 1974

Bruère AN. Examination of the ram for breeding soundness. In: *Current Therapy in Theriogenology*, edited by Morrow DA. WB Saunders & Co, Philadelphia, USA, 1986

Bruère AN, West DM. Effectiveness of the New Zealand brucellosis control scheme for sheep. *Proceedings of the New Zealand Society of Animal Production* 47, 49-52, 1987

Bruère AN, West DM, McLachlan NJ, Edwards JD, Chapman HM. Genital infection of ram hoggets associated with a Gram-negative pleomorphic organism. *New Zealand Veterinary Journal* 25, 191-3, 1977

Buddle MB. Observations on the transmission of *Brucella* infection in sheep. *New Zealand Veterinary Journal* 3, 10-19, 1955

Buddle MB. Production of immunity in rams against *Brucella ovis* infection. *New Zealand Veterinary Journal* 10, 111-13, 1962

Buddle MB, Calverley FK, Boyes BW. *Brucella ovis* vaccination of rams. *New Zealand Veterinary Journal* 11, 90-3, 1963

Bulgin MS. Epididymitis in rams and lambs. *Veterinary Clinics of North America: Food Animal Practice* 6, 3, 683-8, 1990

Crawford R, Jebson JL, Murray MD. Chorioptic mange in the scrotum of rams. *New Zealand Veterinary Journal* 18, 209-10, 1970

Dodd DC, Hartley WJ. Specific suppurative epididymitis in rams. *New Zealand Veterinary Journal* 3, 105-10, 1955

Gunn RMC, Sanders RN, Granger W. Studies in infertility in sheep. *Bulletin of Council for Scientific and Industrial Research*, Melbourne, No. 148, 1942

Hartley WJ. Pathology of *Brucella ovis* infection in the pregnant ewe. *New Zealand Veterinary Journal* 9, 115-20, 1961

Hartley WJ, Jebson JL, McFarlane D. Some observations on the natural transmission of ovine brucellosis. *New Zealand Veterinary Journal* 3, 5-10, 1955

Hilbink F, Wright M, Ross G. Use of the double immunologel diffusion test and enzyme-linked immunosorbent assay to distinguish false from true reactors in the complement fixation test for *Brucella ovis*. *New Zealand Veterinary Journal* 41, 111-15, 1993

Jebson JL, Hartley WJ, McClure TJ, McFarlane D. Pathology of brucellosis in rams in New Zealand. *New Zealand Veterinary Journal* 3, 100-4, 1955

Lees WV, Meek AH, Rosendal S. Epidemiology of *Haemophilus somnus* in young rams. *Canadian Journal of Veterinary Research* 54, 331-6, 1990

McMillan KR, Southcott WH. Aetiological factors in ovine posthitis. *Australian Veterinary Journal* 49, 405-8, 1973

McRae K. Chorioptic mange in sheep flocks — epidemiology and control. *Proceedings of the Sheep and Beef Cattle Veterinarians, New Zealand Veterinary Association* 4, 29-36, 1974

Noseworthy CM. Studies on the Gram-negative pleomorphic organism associated with epididymitis in rams. *MVSc thesis*, Massey University, Palmerston North, New Zealand, 1984

Quinlivan TD. Breeding soundness in the ram: A review of the proceedings and resolutions from two seminars held in 1964 and 1969. *New Zealand Veterinary Journal* 18, 233-40, 1970

Reichel MP, Ross G, Drake J, Jowett JH. Performance of an enzyme-linked immunosorbent assay for the diagnosis of *Brucella ovis* infection in rams. *New Zealand Veterinary Journal* 47, 71-4, 1999

Rhodes AP. The effect of chorioptic mange on ram fertility. *PhD Thesis*, Massey University, Palmerston North, New Zealand, 1971

Rhodes AP. Seminal degeneration associated with chorioptic mange of the scrotum of rams. *Australian Veterinary Journal* 51, 428-32, 1975

Ridler AL. *Brucella ovis* infection in New Zealand. *New Zealand Veterinary Journal* 50 (Supplement), 96-8, 2002

Ridler AL, West DM. Effects of *Brucella ovis* infection on semen characteristics of 16-month-old red deer stags. *New Zealand Veterinary Journal* 50, 19-22, 2002

Ridler AL, West DM, Stafford KJ, Wilson PR, Fenwick SG. Transmission of *Brucella ovis* from rams to red deer stags. *New Zealand Veterinary Journal* 48, 57-9, 2000

Ridler AL, West DM, Stafford KJ, Wilson PR. Persistence, serodiagnosis and effects on semen characteristics of artificial *Brucella ovis* infection in red deer stags. *New Zealand Veterinary Journal* 54, 85-90, 2006

Ridler AL, West DM. Control of *Brucella ovis* infection in sheep. *Veterinary Clinics of North America: Food Animal Practice* 27, 61-66, 2011

Ridler AL. *Brucella ovis* — an update on control. *Proceedings of the Society of Sheep and Beef Cattle Veterinarians NZVA*, 4.10.1-4.10.6, 2012

Ridler AL, Smith SL, West DM. Ram and buck management. *Animal Reproduction Science* 130, 180-3, 2012

Ridler AL, Smith SL, West DM. Seroconversion and semen shedding in rams experimentally infected with *Brucella ovis*. New Zealand Veterinary Journal 62, 47-50, 2014

Ris DR. The complement fixation test for the diagnosis of *Brucella ovis* infection in sheep. New Zealand Veterinary Journal 22, 143-6, 1974

Ris DR, Hamel KL, Long DL. Comparison of an enzyme-linked immunospecific assay (ELISA) with the cold complement fixation test for the serodiagnosis of *Brucella ovis* infection. New Zealand Veterinary Journal 32, 18-20, 1984

Saunders VF, Reddacliff LA, Hornitsky M. Multiplex PCR for the detection of *Brucella ovis*, *Actinobacillus seminis* and *Histophilus somni* in ram semen. Australian Veterinary Journal 85, 72-7, 2007

Scales GH, Hondelink GJ. Control of ovine posthitis in Merinos grazing improved pastures in South Island High Country. New Zealand Veterinary Journal 23, 78-80, 1975

Southcott WH. Etiology of ovine posthitis: Description of a causal organism. Australian Veterinary Journal 41, 193-200, 1965a

Southcott WH. Epidemiology and control of ovine posthitis and vulvitis. Australian Veterinary Journal 41, 225-34, 1965b

Surveillance

(1975): 1:18	*Brucella ovis* serology and vaccination
(1975): 1:19-20	'Actinobacillus-like' epididymitis
(1975): 5:17-18	Epididymitis in rams
(1975): 5:20	Corynebacterial epididymitis in the ram
(1977): 1:3-4	Observations on *Brucella ovis* infection in sheep
(1977): 1:19	*Actinobacillus*-type epididymitis
(1977): 4:24-6	Controlling *Brucella ovis* infection
(1982): 2:30	Ovine brucellosis — negative serology in clinical cases
(1982): 3:6-9	Ovine brucellosis control: An overview of 49 flocks
(1982): 4:13-14	The incidence and activity of epididymitis in young stud rams in Ashburton County
(1983): 4:3-4	Survival of *Brucella ovis* in semen
(1987): 2:12	*Brucella ovis* accreditation
(1988): 1:12	Brucellosis not a disease of goats in New Zealand
(1989): 16:(3)7	Brucellosis eradication scheme
(1991): 18(4):10	*Brucella ovis* voluntary accreditation scheme

Tekes L, Hajtos I. Trials with Enzyme-Linked Immunosorbent Assay (ELISA) for the diagnosis of subclinical genital infection in rams caused by *Histophilus ovis* and *Actinobacillus seminis*. Journal of Veterinary Medicine 37, 549-55, 1990

Webster MC. *Actinobacillus seminis*-like bacteria in rams. Proceedings of the Sheep and Beef Cattle Society, New Zealand Veterinary Association 10, 51-5, 1980

West DM, Bruce RA. Observations on the eradication of *Brucella ovis* infection from a ram flock. New Zealand Veterinary Journal 39, 29-31, 1991

West DM, Bruère AN. Accreditation for freedom from ovine brucellosis. New Zealand Veterinary Journal 27, 263-5, 1979

West DM, Bruère AN. The *Brucella ovis* complement fixation test. New Zealand Veterinary Journal 31, 124-6, 1983

West DM, Stafford KJ, Alley MR, Badcoe LM, Hilbink F, Compton CWR. Serological and necropsy findings for rams infected with *Brucella ovis* which were not identified by the complement fixation test. New Zealand Veterinary Journal 41, 82-6, 1993

West DM. Sheep *Brucella ovis* flock accreditation scheme: An update for participating veterinarians. Proceedings of the Society of Sheep and Beef Cattle Veterinarians, New Zealand Veterinary Association 30, 61-8, 2000

West DM. *Brucella ovis* control: Dealing with problem flocks. Proceedings of the Society of Sheep and Beef Cattle Veterinarians, New Zealand Veterinary Association 30, 51-60, 2000

Worthington RW. Serology as an aid to diagnosis uses and abuses. New Zealand Veterinary Journal 30, 93-7, 1982a

Worthington RW. The complement fixation test for *Brucella ovis*. New Zealand Veterinary Journal 30, 159-60, 1982b

Worthington RW, Cordes DO. The complement fixation test for *Brucella ovis*. New Zealand Veterinary Journal 29, 63, 1981

Worthington RW, Hilbink F. *Brucella ovis* Testing Programme — recorded information. Proceedings of the Sheep and Beef Cattle Society, New Zealand Veterinary Association 18, 189-200, 1988

Worthington RW, Weddell W, Penrose ME. A comparison of three serological tests for the diagnosis of *B. ovis* infection in rams. New Zealand Veterinary Journal 32, 58-60, 1984

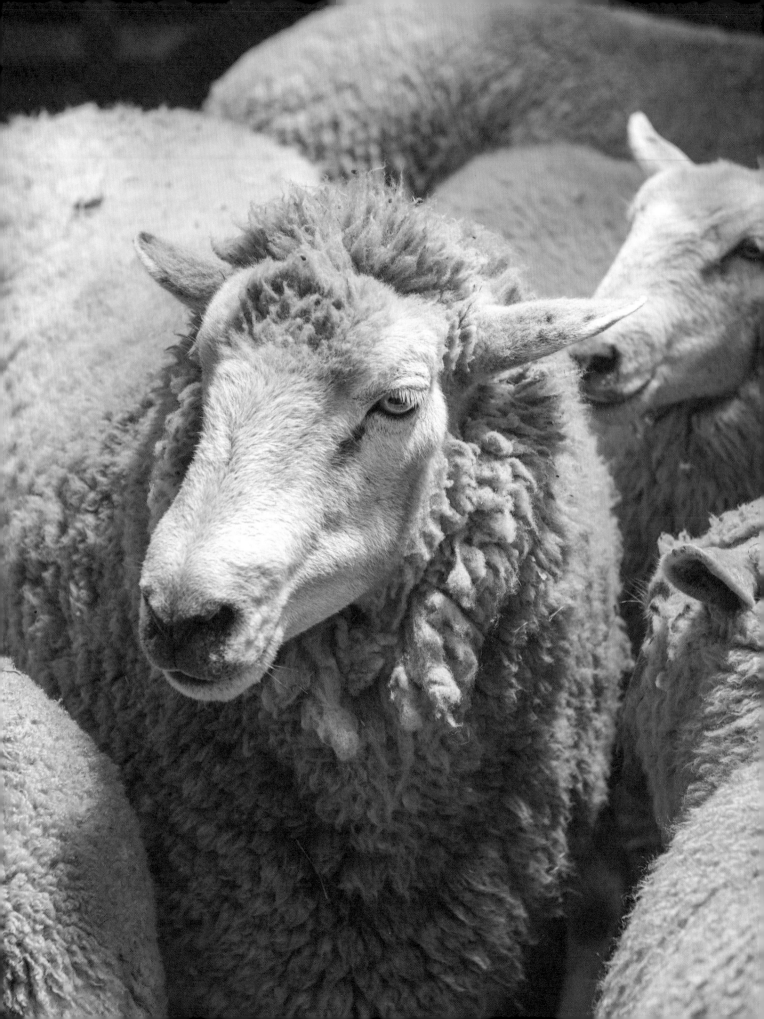

3 Factors affecting lamb production and the investigation of poor lambing

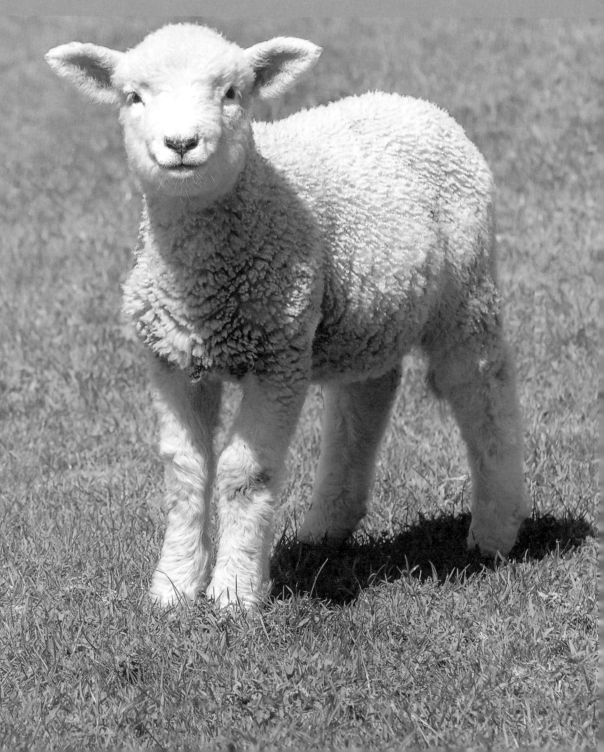

Improved lambing percentage is an important factor in achieving high sheep farm productivity. Reproductive rates of some New Zealand sheep are not high in comparison with some overseas countries. Reference to the New Zealand Meat and Wool Board's Economic Survey shows that the reproductive performance of the national sheep flock increased significantly during the late 1990s. Before that time the national mean lambing percentage fluctuated between 95% and 103% for several decades. It has since risen to above 120% in most recent years. However, the average lambing percentage for different regions may range from 90% to 130%. Further, there are some very high-performing flocks returning lambing percentages of over 180% lambs born and surviving.

The reasons for this varied national performance are complex, and some of the factors such as topography and weather cannot be controlled other than to attempt to modify their effects. An important concept to recognise is that the number of lambs docked or weaned is an end point in a chain of events beginning before mating. Even early events such as the pattern of hogget growth can have a subsequent effect on reproductive performance, but the two most important periods are undoubtedly around the time of joining and lambing. The discrepancy between conception rates and lambs born has been highlighted in recent years by the now common use of ultrasound scanning to diagnose pregnancy and parity of mated ewes.

Various studies have defined the reproductive performance of New Zealand flocks and a modified version of a study in the North Island is presented in Figure 3.1.

Figure 3.1 shows that of the 180 potential lambs at joining only 120 were present at docking, meaning that a third of the potential lambs had been lost. When investigating problems of low lamb production it is important to know the levels of 'acceptable' loss and how management and

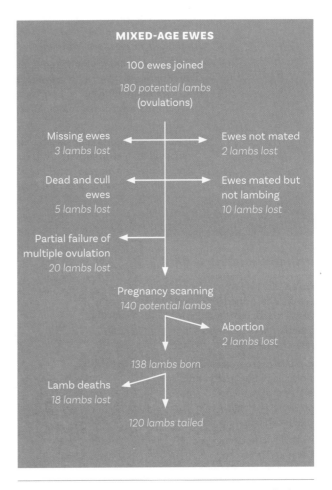

Figure 3.1 The reproductive performance of 25 sheep flocks in the North Island (modified from Knight TW, Moore RW, McMillan W, 1982).

environmental factors can affect the number of potential lambs lost and hence the eventual lambing percentage.

The various stages in the reproductive process include oestrus, ovulation, fertilisation, embryo and foetal development, birth and growth. Each is a distinct process and management of the ewe may influence any one of these processes, thereby influencing the performance of the ewe.

The veterinarian with a sound knowledge of all these areas and with a special training in diseases such as abortion and ram soundness is ideally placed to investigate poor reproductive performance. With this in mind it is important to summarise each stage of this process with special reference to the data a veterinarian should collect in any clinical investigation of poor reproductive performance.

Oestrous activity

The ovarian follicular activity of breeding ewes continues at a high level throughout the year. Throughout anoestrus and on each day of the oestrous cycle, some ovarian follicles mature to within 48–96 hours of ovulation. However, during the non-breeding season these mature follicles do not ovulate but instead undergo atresia. In the transition from anoestrus to the breeding season the sensitivity of the hypothalamus–pituitary to oestradiol reduces and the tonic luteinizing hormone pulses increase, eventually resulting in ovulation.

During the breeding season, ewes exhibit oestrus approximately every 17 days unless they are pregnant (common range 16–20 days). Mature ewes stay on heat for about 24 hours (common range 12–36 hours) while two-tooth ewes stay on heat for a shorter time (common range 1/2–24 hours). Generally a proportion of Romney ewes display oestrus in February but maximum reproductive activity does not occur until April and May (Table 3.1).

In many flocks, especially in the North Island, rams are joined with the ewes in March and in some flocks as early as February. The incidence of oestrus recorded in North Island flocks over the mating period is, however, much lower than in the South Island and much of this observed difference is undoubtedly due to the earlier joining. In their survey of North and South Island flocks Kelly and Knight (1979) showed that almost twice as many ewes mated during the first cycle in the South Island flocks. The date rams were joined with ewes on average was 8 March in the North and 18 April in the South (see Table 3.2).

Clearly, delaying the date of mating in the North would

Time of mating period	Percentage ewes in oestrus	Conception rate
18 January–4 February	-	-
4 February–21 February	0.5	0.0
21 February–9 March	8.5	29.4
9 March–26 March	41.0	62.8
26 March–12 April	88.0	77.6
12 April–29 April	95.2	81.6
29 April–16 May	93.7	81.9
16 May–2 June	89.2	82.9
2 June–19 June	90.7	82.1

Table 3.1 The pattern of reproductive performance of five Romney flocks in the Manawatu (from Quinlivan and Martin, 1971).

Ewes first mated in	South Island %	North Island %
Cycle 1	92.4	47.5
Cycle 2	6.9	33.4
Cycle 3	0.3	17.4
Not mated	0.4	1.4
Return to service – cycle 1	9.7	13.3
Failing to lamb	4.0	8.1

Table 3.2 Mating performance of North Island and South Island sheep flocks (from Allison, 1983).

allow more ewes to be mated during the first and second cycles, and would result in a less protracted lambing and also a lower return-to-service rate. Hence the recording of the mating dates and the length of the mating period are essential data to the veterinarian's investigation.

Factors affecting the breeding season of the ewe

The following factors may affect the breeding season of the ewe:
- breed of sheep
- farm latitude
- farm altitude
- age of ewe
- presence of the ram
- photoperiod control and melatonin
- stress
- hormonal induction of oestrus

Breed of sheep

There is considerable variation both between and within breeds in the duration of the breeding season. In general, breeds of high-country origin have short seasons, while lowland breeds have longer seasons. The season is roughly symmetrical around the shortest day. The Merino and Dorset Horn breeds are two with very long breeding seasons. The Dorset Horn, for example, may have from 10 to 17 oestrous periods in a year while a mountain breed such as the Welsh Mountain (not found in New Zealand) may have between 4 and 9 oestrous periods. In some countries, breeds such as the Merino and Persian sheep are reported to breed all year round. The New Zealand Romney and its derivatives, the Perendale and the Coopworth, and the newer composite sheep, have shorter breeding seasons with fewer oestrous periods.

Latitude

The latitude of the farm may affect the oestrous period, which is clearly shown by the significant difference in the time of joining rams with ewes throughout New Zealand. This fact was highlighted from New Zealand Romney Survey data in which the country was divided into distinct geographical regions for recording. In area 1, which is mainly north of Auckland, rams and ewes were often mated in February and the majority by mid-March. In areas 4 and 5, which represents much of the South Island, joining was, by contrast, generally after the middle of March and mainly at the beginning of April. It is interesting that the percentage of ewes mated to first service was found to be significantly higher in the southern districts than in the north.

Altitude

As with latitude, the pattern of oestrus varies with altitude. On farms situated above 1500–2000 feet (450–600 m), the onset of oestrus in ewes is later with a shorter period of peak activity and an earlier decline in the proportion of ewes in oestrus. In the study reported by Quinlivan and Martin (1971), maximum oestrous responses (or submission rates) of 95% and higher were first observed on low-altitude farms between 26 March and 4 April and on high-altitude farms between 12 and 20 April (see Figure 3.2). From 16 May the submission rate on high farms fell. This, coupled with the lower reproductive performance both early and late in the season, emphasises the importance of time of joining of the rams, particularly on high-altitude farms where the time for effective mating and maximum reproductive efficiency is restricted.

Age effect and mating ewe hoggets

Compared with older ewes, young ewes (hoggets and maiden two-tooths) cycle later, stay on heat for a shorter time, are less active in seeking out the ram, have lower ovulation rates and have higher rates of

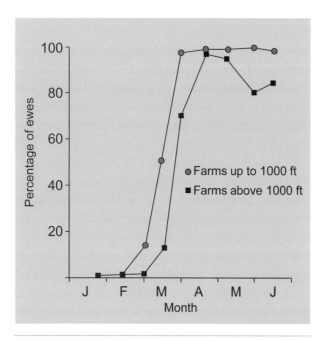

Figure 3.2 Proportions of ewes that exhibited oestrus on farms at low and high altitudes (from Quinlivan and Martin, 1971).

embryo loss. For these reasons younger age groups are often mated separately from the mixed-age ewes and a greater percentage of rams are joined with them. When investigating low reproductive performance in a flock, it is important to obtain the age structure of the flock and to analyse the performance of the hoggets, two-tooth ewes and mixed-age ewes separately.

Ewe hoggets have the potential to be successfully mated at 6–9 months of age. The additional lambs and higher net profit make this activity attractive to sheep farmers. With the introduction of Finn and East Friesian genetics into Romney-based flocks, lambing performance can be significantly improved in this age group of sheep. In general, hogget lambing can be highly effective if the hoggets are well grown to reach puberty, and also well fed throughout pregnancy and lactation so that they will reach acceptable two-tooth mating weights.

Extensive data are now available that provide a valuable guide to achieving maximum results from hogget mating and are comprehensively reviewed in the book *Hogget Performance — Unlocking the Potential*, available from Beef and Lamb New Zealand. They are summarised as follows:

- Individual ewe hoggets should be well grown and a *minimum* of 40 kg at the start of the breeding period. Trial work has shown that for every kg increase in bodyweight above 36 kg, the lambing percentage increases by approximately 2% (Table 3.3).
- Ewe hoggets should be under a sound parasite control programme.
- It is generally recommended that ewe hoggets be mated later, perhaps early May and definitely separately from other ewes.
- Vasectomised rams are often used to advantage to stimulate oestrus 17 days prior to mating. Even used at relatively high ratios of teasers to ewe hoggets (1 : 200), it has been shown that the teaser rams had a beneficial effect on lambing performance, up to 16% in some trials. It is suggested that a ratio of 1 : 100 is probably most suitable.
- Ewe hoggets do not actively seek out the ram, so it is recommended that they be mated at a higher ratio of mature rams (mating ram lambs to ewe hoggets is not recommended) than adult sheep. Use a ratio of 1 : 50 to 1 : 100 of mature rams during mating.
- Use a condensed mating period of 17–34 days. For well-grown hoggets 70–90% should be mated in 1.5 to 2 cycles and 50–90% of them should be in lamb. Again, Finn and East Friesian genetics should improve the mating performance (Table 3.3).
- Vaccination against common causes of abortion, campylobacteriosis and toxoplasmosis is recommended. See Chapter 4.
- Ultrasound pregnancy diagnosis is advisable to ensure that pregnant hoggets can be adequately fed, especially those carrying twins. Hoggets should be managed separately from other flocks during lambing and lactation.
- Shearing hoggets before mating (at least 4–5 weeks earlier) is recommended.
- Mate ewe hoggets in small mobs, no more than 500, and in small paddocks — 8 ha or less. Use flat or rolling country by preference.
- Aim for daily liveweight gains of 100–150 g/day throughout pregnancy.

Presence of the ram (ram effect)

It has long been recognised that vasectomised 'teaser' rams will stimulate a synchronised oestrus in ewes early in the breeding season and the mechanisms involved have now been outlined. If used, teaser rams should be introduced to the ewes 17 days before the intended start of mating.

The proportion of ewes responding after ram introduction varies greatly; breed of ram and ewe, and time of year, are important factors influencing the response. A prerequisite for a response is that ewes are isolated from rams for a period (approximately 21 days) before ram introduction. Knight (1983) has described the sequence of events that occur following the introduction of rams. Within 10–30 minutes of ram introduction there is an increase in the tonic luteinizing hormone pulses which leads to a preovulatory luteinizing hormone surge by 27–36 hours. The ewes have a silent ovulation (i.e. ovulation without behavioural oestrus) within 3–4 days. In 40–60% of these ewes the corpus luteum formed after the silent ovulation is maintained for the normal duration and first oestrus and ovulation occurs 18–20 days after ram introduction. In the remaining ewes the corpus luteum does not develop properly and regresses by day 6–8 to be replaced by a silent ovulation. The corpus luteum formed from this second silent ovulation is maintained for the normal duration to give a second peak of oestrus about day 22–24. Thus we have two peaks of oestrous activity spaced out over 6–8 days and occurring 18––26 days after the time of ram introduction. Once the ewes have commenced their own breeding cycles the presence of the ram cannot affect them in this way.

The stimulus from the ram is due to pheromones present in the ram's wool and wool wax. Bucks are equally effective as rams at stimulating ewes. Although the teaser rams are often introduced to the ewes for longer periods, only 48 hours of exposure is sufficient to initiate the ovulating response.

If it is important to advance the date of lambing in a flock, ram synchronisation perhaps offers the most effective way of achieving this. However, the effects of teaser rams are variable and are likely to result in only a four- to five-day advance of the mean lambing date. Dorset rams have been shown to be more effective teasers than Romney rams. In addition there is evidence to suggest that entire rams are more effective than vasectomised rams and that some strains of Dorset rams are better than others.

Variable	Increase in lambing %
Vaccination for toxoplasmosis and campylobacteriosis (abortion)	5.2
Weight of hogget at mating (kg)	
<36	Reference
37–40	8.6
41–44	13.8
45–48	20.1
>49	25.5
Breed of hoggets	
Romney	Reference
¼ Finn or East Friesian	13.5
½ Finn or East Friesian	23.1
Coopworth	10.8

Table 3.3 Major factors affecting the lambing percentage of live hoggets and the expected increase in performance associated with each of them (from Kenyon et al., 2004).

CASE EXAMPLE

To avoid flystrike problems with later lambs, the owner of a North Island hill-country property at Hunterville was joining the rams with the ewes on 1 March and mating for three 17-day periods. The majority of the farm was above 500 m and the early joining had resulted in 15% of the two-tooths being dry/dry (not lambing). In fact, the farmer was withdrawing the rams on 20 April at a time of maximum oestrous response.

In the first year of the investigation, mating had already taken place (starting on 1 March) and 18% of the two-tooths were dry/dry that year. However, in subsequent years mating was delayed by three weeks and the number of dry/dry two-tooths was reduced to 5–6%.

CASE EXAMPLE

The following is an example of the use of teasers in a flock. Normally the rams on this coastal farm were joined with the ewes on 1 February. As ram harnesses were used it was possible to assess from the farmer's recorded data that approximately 60% of his flock was pregnant by 18 March. In the following year teasers were introduced in early February and entire rams were joined on 21 February (a delay of 21 days). The submission rates were high (over 75% in the first 20 days) and by 11 March 60% of the flock were pregnant. Although joining had been delayed by three weeks, the mean lambing date was not altered. This condensing of tupping and lambing has a number of significant advantages. Feed for flushing and lambing can be used to maximum advantage, a more even line of lambs can be produced and there is three weeks less time spent on the lambing beat.

This case study helps to emphasise the practical fact that a number of farmers join the rams with the ewes too early in the season, resulting in a spread lambing and in too many dry ewes. This is particularly so in the North Island and although the reasons advanced for early joining — viz. to lamb early so that lambs can be weaned before the pasture deteriorates and to get a proportion of them to killing weights to catch the premium for early lambs — appear valid at first sight, advancing the joining date does not necessarily result in a corresponding advancement of the mean lambing date.

Photoperiod control and melatonin

Photoperiod has a major influence on the breeding season of ewes, but the confining of ewes to a darkened shed each day is generally impractical. However, the discovery that melatonin is the hormone responsible for the photoperiod-induced changes in the hypothalamus–pituitary has provided an alternative means of controlling the ewes' breeding season.

Melatonin is released from the pineal gland 10 minutes after darkness and returns to basal levels 10 minutes after the onset of light. Australian work has indicated that when melatonin incorporated into sheep nuts was fed 8 hours before darkness for 10 weeks to ewes, oestrous activity occurred at least 21 days earlier than in control ewes and the lambing percentage was increased. The treatment has been simplified to a single subcutaneous implant (Regulin) and has returned good results in Merino and Merino cross-bred sheep. However, the results of trials with Romney and Coopworth ewes in New Zealand have only had limited success. Nearly all trials involving the treatment of these breeds for a December joining have shown little effect. Latter treatments involving late January joining have shown a small advancement of the breeding season and increased conception rates. The effectiveness of Regulin treatment depends on the genotype of the sheep and its sensitivity to induction or its depth of anoestrus.

Stress

Oestrus in sheep can be affected significantly by stress. One of the main stress effects is produced by shearing sheep either before or during the mating period. Work at Ruakura Animal Research Centre has demonstrated the dramatic cessation of oestrous activity when sheep were shorn during the tupping period (see Figure 3.3).

Further work with two-tooth ewes has shown that this age group is even more adversely affected. Shearing the latter sheep even as early as four weeks before the joining date caused a major spread of lambing and a delay equivalent to between one and two oestrous periods.

Shearing is not the only stress experienced by ewes, and severe adverse weather conditions can also suppress behavioural oestrus significantly (see Table 3.4).

Hormonal induction of oestrus

Ewes can be induced to breed out of their normal season

to assist in the year-round supply of prime lambs. The standard procedure is to treat ewes with a progestagen incorporated into an intravaginal device for 11–14 days. At withdrawal of the progestagen the ewes may be injected with pregnant mare serum gonadotrophin (PMSG), depending on the season, and oestrus occurs 25–72 hours later. As the ewes begin oestrus at a similar time, a high ram : ewe ratio of 1 : 10 is recommended. Unfortunately hormonal treatment in this way reduces the fertility of ewes and conception rates are lower (40–50%) than for the normal breeding season (80–90%), depending on how far out of season it is. In addition, many of the ewes that are stimulated into oestrus revert to anoestrus if they fail to conceive at the induced oestrus. Inducing some ewes to display oestrus by the use of hormones can stimulate other ewes to begin cycling, especially if this is done closer to the time of the natural mating season.

Ovulation

The ovulation rate at joining determines the maximum number of lambs that can be produced or the potential lambing performance. High ovulation rates are the key to high lambing percentages, as between 60% and 70% of the variation between flocks in lamb docking percentage can be accounted for by differences in ovulation rate. Thus the most critical time in the reproductive cycle of the ewe is the 3–6 weeks before the joining period and over the joining period, when the ovulation rate will be determined.

It is possible to accurately assess the ovulation rate by endoscopically examining approximately 100 ewes in a flock. In practice such a procedure may not be possible or even desirable. An alternative is to assess the fecundity by

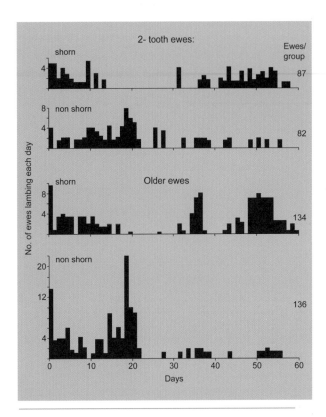

Figure 3.3 Number of ewes lambing each day during the 60-day lambing period (after Welch et al., 1979).

Table 3.4 Effect of fasting and shearing on bodyweight, oestrus and ovarian activity in four groups of 10 ewes mated during cold weather (MacKenzie et al., 1975).

	Group and treatment			
	1 (HW)	2 (HS)	3 (LW)	4 (LS)
Initial bodyweight (kg) at beginning	55.5	55.3	55.3	55.6
Bodyweight (kg) at commencement of ovulation	56.2	54.6	48.6	47.9
Failure of oestrus	-	4	3	7
Silent heats	-	2	1	6

HW = feeding *ad lib*, unshorn; HS = feeding *ad lib*, shorn;
LW = fasted, unshorn; LS = fasted, shorn

ultrasound pregnancy diagnosis. It is a distinct advantage to have this data when investigating low lambing performance.

The ovulation rate may be influenced by a number of factors, which include the following:
- bodyweight and nutrition of the ewe at mating
- time of the breeding season
- age of the ewe
- genetic factors
- mating on lucerne and phyto-oestrogens in subterranean clovers
- mycotoxins
- level of nutrition during rearing
- premating shearing
- immunisation against ovarian steroids
- premating parasite burdens of ewes.

Effect of bodyweight and nutrition of the ewe at mating

Ewe liveweight and nutrition at mating are important factors affecting ovulation rate, and much of the variation in reproductive performance between flocks can be explained by nutrition prior to mating. In the 1960s, Coop produced figures of a 6% increase in twinning for every 10 lb increase in liveweight at mating (i.e. a 1.3% rise per 1 kg). More-recent work has indicated that the response may vary with the breed of sheep (Finn and Booroola sheep being relatively unresponsive) and may be greater than that recorded by Coop, in some instances. Figures of a 1.8%, 2.6% and 3.7% increase in twinning per 1 kg liveweight have been recorded (Figure 3.4). Below 40 kg mean liveweight, barrenness increases significantly. Coop also recorded a dynamic effect estimated to be about a 1% increase in twinning for each week of flushing.

The complex relationships between nutrition, liveweight, changes in liveweight and ovulation rate have been studied in detail at Ruakura by Rattray et al. (1983). This work has emphasised that to achieve good ovulation rates, not only is it important to reach good mating weights but it is also important to have the ewes on a rising plane of nutrition. The researchers emphasised the benefit of weight gain and the detrimental effect of weight loss.

- Heavy ewes have a higher percentage of multiple ovulations than light ewes (other things being equal) and in general a rise of 1.5–2% per 1 kg liveweight is expected.
- Liveweight gain is beneficial and liveweight loss is detrimental to ovulation rate.
- Light ewes are more responsive than heavy ewes to weight gain, but by the same token it is more detrimental for light ewes to lose weight.

To obtain a flushing response, a minimum period of three weeks of high-level feeding immediately prior to ram introduction is required. This will give a three-week carry-over period during which time most of the ewes should be mated.

While the work at Ruakura has highlighted the importance of flushing ewes, the amount of feed required to achieve this is often underestimated. Furthermore there are seasons and districts when summer–autumn rainfall is completely inadequate to provide optimum pasture for ewes at this time of year. Supplementary feeds such as silage or crops may be used in some districts but such a practice could jeopardise winter feed supplies. Note that for flocks with very high reproductive performance, flushing ewes may not necessarily be desirable.

When investigating a problem of low lamb production,

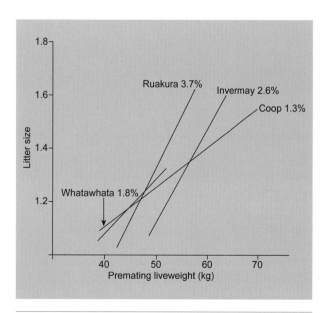

Figure 3.4 The relationship between premating liveweight of ewes and litter size — between flock basis (from Allison and Kelly, 1978). The % values indicate the percentage increase in twinning per extra kilogram of liveweight.

an important parameter to measure is the bodyweight and condition of ewes close to mating. The importance of feeding ewes at this period to achieve a good bodyweight, and some liveweight gain or at least a reduction of weight loss, cannot be overemphasised. In addition, it is useful to weigh two-tooth ewes separately from the older sheep; if their weights are low, it would indicate that hogget growth rates have been poor and the latter animals should also be examined to ensure a better performance in the following season.

Figure 3.5 clearly demonstrates the importance of maintaining a good bodyweight and condition score on ewes over the summer post-weaning period and throughout the reproductive period (mating to lambing). To achieve this, farmers may have to manage ewes of relatively poorer condition separately from those of good bodyweight over the summer post-weaning period. Thus the ewes of minimum bodyweight would in fact be brought up to the bodyweight of the rest of the flock, and all ewes would be mated at the optimum bodyweight or condition score needed to achieve high reproductive performance.

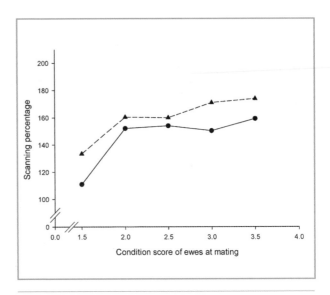

Figure 3.5 The relationship between condition score of composite two-tooth (Comp TT; •) and mixed-aged Romney ewes (Rom MA; ▲) at mating and subsequent scanning percentage (from Kenyon et al. 2004a).

Time of the breeding season
The time of the breeding season also influences the ovulation rate. Generally the ovulation rate is low early in the breeding season, rises to a peak and then decreases towards the end of the breeding season. The majority of farmers attempt to join the rams at the time when most of the ewes are entering their second oestrous cycle.

Age of the ewe
Two-tooth ewes have lower ovulation rates than older ewes.

Genetic factors
The ovulation rate varies between breeds, for instance the Finnish Landrace sheep (Finn) has very high ovulation rates. Litter size exceeds 200% with litters of four lambs being quite common. While few farmers in New Zealand run pure Finns, the number of Finn cross-bred sheep has increased as farmers seek more fecund ewes.

There are two major fecundity genes that have been discovered in New Zealand: the Booroola gene and the Inverdale gene.
1. The Booroola gene was discovered in prolific Merinos; each copy of the gene has an additive effect. Heterozygous ewes with one copy of the gene shed 2–5 eggs while homozygous ewes with two copies of the gene shed 5–10 eggs. There has been little use of the Booroola gene in New Zealand commercial flocks, possibly because of the management difficulties associated with the major shift in ovulation rate with different copies of the gene.
2. The Inverdale gene is located on the X chromosome, and DNA testing can be used to identify carrier sheep. There is difficulty in managing an X-linked gene as a ram carrying the gene passes it on to all of his daughters and none of his sons. A ewe with one copy of the gene passes it on to half of her offspring of either sex. Females homozygous for the Inverdale gene have ovarian hypoplasia, or what has been termed streak ovaries, and are infertile. Ewes with a single copy of the gene have an increased ovulation rate of about one egg, which results in an increased litter size of about 0.6. Thus, it would be possible to increase litter size by mating a carrier ram to normal ewes; the resulting ewe lambs will all be carrier ewes which could be mated to terminal sires and their progeny sold.

Mating on lucerne and phyto-oestrogens in subterranean clovers

Flushing and mating ewes on lucerne has been shown to depress the lambing percentage by some 10–40% due to a depression in ovulation rate. Barrenness is increased but only slightly (2%). Coumesterol has been identified as the main oestrogenic compound in lucerne, which increases markedly when lucerne plants are affected with fungal disease, aphid attack or are in flower. In general, it is recommended that ewes should be removed from lucerne at least 14 days before mating, but because the major effect is a reduction in ovulation rate they can be returned to lucerne after tupping.

Phyto-oestrogens in subterranean clovers (*Trifolium subterraneum*) and medics (*Medicago* spp) have a marked effect on the reproduction of sheep. However, unlike Western Australia where these effects are well known, the effects of phyto-oestrogens on sheep reproduction in New Zealand are somewhat uncertain. The main subterranean clovers on the drier hill country of the North Island have moderate to low concentrations of phyto-oestrogens. In wetter regions, red clovers (*Trifolium pratense*) are grown and some of these have significant levels of phyto-oestrogens.

Some work has indicated that ewes grazing Pawera red clover before and during mating had fewer ewes mated, a lower ovulation rate, fewer ewes lambing and fewer twins. Further work has shown that histological analysis of cervix samples of aged hill-country ewes from North Island farms have 17% moderate changes to their cervix, which is indicative of phyto-oestrogen damage. Further, udder development in young animals and teat growth in wethers from some areas of New Zealand also suggests phyto-oestrogen involvement.

Mycotoxins

Several mycotoxins are capable of producing a marked depression of reproductive performance in the ewe. These include the following:

1. Pithomyces chartarum

Pithomyces chartarum, the fungus-producing sporidesmin that is the causative agent of facial eczema, has a twofold effect in reproduction. In addition to the obvious effects of facial eczema on reproductive loss through reduced bodyweight or even death of ewes, there are direct effects on ewes suffering from subclinical facial eczema. An increase of 200 IU gamma glutamyl transferase (GGT) per litre serum over joining may decrease ewes ovulating (–4%), ewes ovulating multiples (–3% to –6%), ewes lambing (–3% to –5%) and ewes lambing multiples (–4% to –5%). Lamb birthweights may also be decreased (see the section of facial eczema, Chapter 18).

Subclinical facial eczema in hoggets may reduce lambing of two-year-old ewes by 6% for every 200 IU GGT per litre serum, while in mature ewes subclinical facial eczema delays the onset of the breeding season, reduces the number of oestrous cycles and may hasten the end of the breeding season by 20 days. Hence, particularly in North Island flock investigations, it is important for any veterinary examination to obtain a good history of previous occurrences of facial eczema in the flock.

2. Zearalenone-induced infertility of sheep

The effect of zearalenone on the reproductive performance of New Zealand sheep grazing on pasture was first reported by Jagusch et al. (1980). It was suggested that some substance, 'Factor G', in pasture was responsible for losses in reproductive potential that could not be attributed to facial eczema. Subsequent research confirmed the original work and identified zearalenone intoxification as a major cause of reduced lambing percentages in North Island flocks.

Zearalenone is a fungal toxin produced by the fungus known as *Fusarium*. Zearalenone is oestrogenic in activity. The *Fusarium* found in pasture is generally saprophytic and tends to grow preferentially on dead litter, similar to *Pithomyces chartarum*. The fungi grow most during late summer and autumn (March to May) under warm, dry conditions, but the widespread distribution of toxic pasture suggests that the conditions required for fungal growth are not particularly restrictive. Survey data by Garthwaite et al. (1994) reported toxic levels of zearalenone in autumn on some New Zealand pastures from Northland to Southland. Nine per cent of over 6000 samples tested had zearalenone at high enough levels for ewe fertility to be depressed, and another 35% were from paddocks where flocks would be 'at risk'. This widespread March to May distribution of zearalenone in pasture of course coincides almost precisely with the New Zealand annual mating period for sheep. Other fungi (*Acremonium*), common in New Zealand pastures, may also produce zearalenone.

The structure of zearalenone and its breakdown products are similar to that of the reproductive steroid hormones. This enables them to bind to oestrogen receptors of mammals, interfering with the signal transduction and control of endogenous oestrogens. In adult sheep, the primary effect of zearalenone is to reduce ovulation and fertilisation rates. Before mating it also may alter oestrous behaviour by decreasing the cycle length and increasing the duration of oestrus. The longer the exposure and the higher the daily dose of zearalenone, the greater the effect on fertility.

The extent of the effect and its duration on ewe reproduction will depend on both the quantity of zearalenone ingested and the period over which it was ingested. A feeding period of only 5 days at a level of 6 mg/ewe/day has been shown to significantly reduce ovulation rates, and the effects of as little as 1 mg/ewe/day ingested for 20 days reduced ovulation rates by 20%. This depression of ovulation may carry over for at least one oestrous cycle after the ingestion of zearalenone has ceased. Further, the effects of prolonged feeding of affected pasture for 20–40 days may persist over at least two cycles. In general, the effect is a depression of lambing rate of about 5% for every 1 mg/ewe/day of zearalenone eaten in a short period (5–7 days) and about twice this for longer (20-day) periods. The fertility of rams is apparently unaffected.

Measuring the amount of zearalenone in pasture can be diagnostically helpful, but sheep urine testing is the best indicator that toxic levels of zearalenone have been ingested. Urine samples should be collected from 12–15 ewes using the partial smother technique (this involves holding a hand over the sheep's nostrils to produce a brief suffocation), and an equal quantity from each ewe pooled for a single test. The amount of zearalenone is corrected for urine concentration by measuring the zearalenone to creatinine ratio. An example of a farm survey of mean zearalenone : creatinine ratios in the urine of New Zealand sheep flocks is shown in Table 3.5.

Prevention of the detrimental effects of zearalenone on sheep fertility is difficult. Several avenues have been suggested, none of which have easy or even realistic field use. Androstenedione immunogens (Androvax, Ovastim) have been suggested as a means of increasing ovulation rate to overcome the negative effect of zearalenone, but were experimentally ineffective. The use of alternative crops such as chicory or brassicas may be useful, but the economics of growing these on a large scale would be difficult.

It was noticed by Smith et al. (1990) that some ewes continued to ovulate multiples in spite of ingesting high levels of zearalenone, suggesting that some sheep may be genetically resistant to zearalenone effects and that genetic selection of this could be a means of control in the long term. Research work based on the measurement of the zearalenone : creatinine ratio in urine in experimental flocks has shown promise. A simple challenge-test could be offered to breeders, using the same test structure already used for testing rams for facial eczema tolerance (Ramguard).

Table 3.5 Mean urine zearalenone : creatinine (Z : Cr) ratios in New Zealand sheep flocks and estimated zearalenone intakes and risk categories (from Towers, 1996).

Z : Cr* ratio	Percentage of flocks				Zearalenone intake** (mg per day)	Expected reduction in lambing percentages
	1991	1992	1993	1994		
0–12.5	32	56	68	50	0–1	0–5
12.5–25	36	35	27	27	1–3	5–25
>25	32	9	5	23	>3	15–50
	n = 53	*n* = 226	*n* = 379	*n* = 61		

*   µmole zearalenone per mole creatinine
**   estimated from urinary Z : Cr ratio

Level of nutrition during rearing

Ovulation rate is influenced by the pattern of early growth. Sheep that are reared on a high level of nutrition until 12 months of age have higher ovulation rates than sheep reared on a low level of nutrition, even where subsequent adult nutrition removes liveweight differences. Similar studies at Whatawhata Research Station emphasised that hogget weights were generally too light and that it is important to rear ewe hogget replacements well.

Premating shearing

Shearing two-tooth ewes before mating generally increases their lambing percentage slightly, but shearing should be undertaken carefully and well before the date of joining. Because shearing stimulates appetite it is necessary to have adequate feed available to achieve a beneficial effect. If feed is limited, shearing may prove detrimental.

Immunisation against ovarian steroids

The immunisation of ewes to produce antibodies against the ovarian steroid androstenedione has given increases in the percentage of lambs born of up to 40% with an average response of approximately 22%. Two commercial products are available, Androvax Plus® (MSD Animal Health) and Ovastim® injection for sheep (Virbac New Zealand Ltd) (polyandroalbumin *syn* ovandrotone albumin). These products are safe to use but are designated PAR class 1 because without proper application they could cause significant animal welfare problems related to inadequate feed supply for the extra lambs.

When androstenedione is linked to a heterologous protein, a steroid–protein conjugate is produced which is able to stimulate the immune system of treated ewes. The antibodies produced have the ability to bind to free androstenedione present in the blood, thus reducing the level of biologically available androstenedione. This alters the feedback of ovarian hormones on the pituitary gland, allowing it to secrete additional amounts of ovary-stimulating hormones. The immunisation programme alters ovarian activity for a short period (45–50 days) and antibody levels continue to decline so that they are very low at the time of lambing.

In the first year two injections are required. The timing of these is important and differs slightly between the two products, so the vaccine instructions must be carefully followed. The first injection must be given 6–10 weeks before joining. The second injection must be given 3–6 weeks after the first and 3–4 weeks before joining. During the 4–6 weeks after the booster injection, the antibody levels fall but they are often so high that no follicular oestradiol is produced and this means that in the first few weeks after the booster dose many ewes may not show oestrus (Figure 3.6). Therefore the timing of joining after the booster dose is critical because early injection has been known to drop the lambing performance significantly. Treated ewes should be identified so that they can be treated with only one injection if mated the following year. In the second and subsequent years one injection only is required, 3–6 weeks before joining.

Although these products have a number of advantages, their use also presents significant husbandry challenges. Flock management and nutrition is more difficult and demanding, particularly under pasture grazing systems, because of increased multiple births. Adequate pasture must be available to feed the extra lambs and maintain ewe bodyweight for the next mating. Ultrasound pregnancy diagnosis may be a useful procedure to use in flocks that have been immunised because it enables multiparous ewes to be given preferential feeding. It must be emphasised that immunisation, while being a useful tool to increase

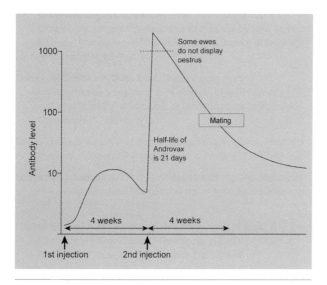

Figure 3.6 Antibody levels after sensitising and booster injections of Androvax (from Hudson and McNatty, 2002).

lamb production, is not a substitute for poor reproductive performance, low bodyweight or inadequate nutrition. Initially it is probably wise to only treat a proportion of the flock to ensure that feed resources are not over-extended by the extra lambs.

Premating parasitic burdens of ewes

In the 1970s, analysis of 81 field trials involving more than 62,000 ewes showed that ewes given a single anthelmintic drench during the 6 weeks before the start of the mating season produced a mean of 3.6% more lambs (range −11% to +20%) due to increased twinning. Flocks with a mean faecal egg count above 100 eggs per gram were positively correlated with an increase in fertility. Other factors including location, fertility level, liveweight of the flock and the timing of treatment or type of drench were not important. However, there have been many changes in sheep production systems in New Zealand since that time, so while many farmers continue to routinely drench their ewes prior to mating ('pre-tup drench'), this blanket approach is difficult to justify.

It is now recommended that adult ewes are not routinely drenched but that premating drenching decisions can be made based on the internal parasite status of the flock (faecal egg counts, grazing management, season, evidence of parasitism, sheep/cattle ratio) and farmers' objectives.

In some situations, only treating a proportion of the flock with anthelmintics, such as two-tooths or ewes in poorer body condition, may be appropriate. It should be noted that unnecessary drenching of ewes is costly and likely to contribute to anthelmintic resistance.

Fertilisation

Fertilisation rates in New Zealand sheep flocks are generally high and failure of fertilisation makes only a small contribution to reproductive wastage when measured by failure to produce a lamb, since many ewes have a second and sometimes a third opportunity to conceive during the mating period. An exception to this is flocks joined early in the breeding season where a large proportion of ewes may not be first mated until the last cycle of mating. Levels of barrenness in New Zealand sheep flocks are generally less than 8%, with factors other than failure of fertilisation contributing to this value (e.g. embryonic mortality).

Levels of barrenness can be influenced by factors such as ram soundness, ram percentage, the choice of mating paddocks and the duration of the joining period.

Ram soundness (see Chapter 2)

One point of note is that the duration of spermatogenesis is around 2 months, and all the spermatozoa the ram will ejaculate in a normal mating period are already in formation in the testes the day he is introduced to the ewes. Thus, rams should be prepared well before the breeding season to increase their sperm production.

Ram percentage

Generally rams are joined at a rate of between 1 and 2 rams per 100 ewes, and this ratio usually gives a satisfactory result. However, the rate actually used may vary depending on flock size, terrain, time of joining, breed of sheep and the age of ewes. Although some rams can be joined with many more ewes, there may be a reduction in the percentage of ewes mated in the first 16 days and in the mean number of rams mating each ewe.

Allison (1977) demonstrated that increasing the number of ewes per ram from 200/4 to 400/4 and from 240/4 to 720/4 resulted in a decrease in reproductive performance (Table 3.6). In these trials the two-tooth ewes were affected before the older ewes.

When investigating problems of low reproductive performance it is important to ensure that there are adequate rams to cover the ewes. Extra consideration should be given to younger age groups such as ewe hoggets and two-tooth ewes. These age groups should preferably be mated separately and with higher ram ratios.

Choice of paddock and paddock size

When considering the optimum paddock in which to mate ewes, consideration should be given to reducing flock dispersion to enable maximum contact between the ewes and the rams. This will not only ensure that ewes in oestrus are detected by the ram, but also that these ewes are served a number of times, preferably by more than one ram. Where unsatisfactory mating paddocks cannot be avoided, a higher ram to ewe ratio is recommended.

Ratio rams/ewes	Age of ewes	No. of records	17-day submission	Mean no. rams mating each ewe	% returning to service
4/200	Two-tooths Mixed age	100 100	90.0 98.0	2.86 2.67	15.6 16.3
4/400	Two-tooths Mixed age	200 199	71.5 96.0	1.94 2.64	18.9 13.6
4/240	Two-tooths Mixed age	60 172	88.3 97.1	3.04 2.88	9.4 18.6
4/720	Two-tooths Mixed age	179 530	79.9 90.2	2.33 2.29	14.7 19.7

Table 3.6 Percentage of ewes mated in the first 17 days, the percentage returning to service and the mean number of rams mating each oestrous ewe (from Allison, 1977).

Duration of the joining period

Under optimal mating conditions it is anticipated that between 95% and 98% of ewes should be pregnant at the end of a 34- to 40-day mating period. Because it is desirable that replacement stock be derived from ewes that conceive early in the breeding season, the mating period is often restricted in stud and some commercial properties to 34 days or even less. Subsequently a harnessed ram or a prime lamb sire (terminal sire) may be used and the progeny culled. Commercial properties usually leave the rams with the ewes for a longer period than stud properties, especially with two-tooth ewes.

The use of ram harnesses

The use of a harness and coloured crayon to detect mating patterns within a flock is a common technique. A representative sample of mixed-age ewes and two-tooth ewes can be mated separately to harnessed rams and this will provide information on submission rates and return rates. At intervals of 14–16 days the colour of the crayon should be changed so that ewes returning to the ram are marked with a different colour. The harness must be carefully fitted to the ram, ensuring that it is comfortable and is positioned correctly to mark the ewe. Problems of the harness chafing or slipping should be checked regularly, but these will be minimised if the rams have a fleece length of 1–2 cm. Care must be taken in interpreting the results of crayon marking, as very light marks may go undetected (especially if the ewes are woolly) and not all ewes that are marked necessarily produce a lamb. It is unwise to cull unmarked ewes as not pregnant, as some crayons do not mark very well during cold weather or a harness may slip or fall off. Ram harnesses are also used as an aid to separate the flock into early and late lambers and thus better utilise feed resources in the critical period prior to lambing. Some farmers choose to only use harnesses for the third cycle, to identify late-lambing ewes.

Embryonic mortality

There are many reports on the extent of wastage that occurs in the period of early embryogenesis; that is from fertilisation to days 20–30 of pregnancy. During this period there is slow growth of the embryo up to day 10–11 of pregnancy, followed by rapid increases in size and commencement of implantation. An estimated 20–30% of fertilised eggs are usually lost. The many ova or embryos that die by day 12 cause no disturbance of the normal cycle length, but those that survive beyond this time prevent regression of the corpus luteum.

The majority of embryonic deaths occur before day 18 and most ewes, even in experiencing a long cycle, will be remated within the normal joining period. A significant part of the basal embryonic loss is inevitable and even desirable in disposing of unfit genetic material. However, the level of embryonic loss varies considerably between farms, and this together with the many factors that are known to influence embryonic mortality indicate possible scope for reduction, but not elimination, of this source of wastage.

Embryonic loss can be influenced by the following:
- age of ewe
- genotype
- nutrition
- selenium deficiency
- high temperature
- stress
- infectious causes — toxoplasmosis, hairy shaker disease

Age of ewe

Embryonic mortality is much higher in young sheep (hoggets and two-tooths) than older ewes, and is one of the main reasons for the lowered reproductive performance of two-tooth compared with mixed-age ewes. This is possibly due to issues with quality of the ova and/or oviduct.

Genotype

Differences in embryonic mortality have been found in ewes mated to specific lines of rams selected within a breed and between breeds.

Area	Mating periods — 16 day intervals			Failed to exhibit oestrus
	1	2	3	
Northern North Island	73.8	23.2	2.0	1.0
Southern North Island	64.9	31.3	3.2	0.6
Mid Canterbury North Otago	83.3	13.8	2.3	0.6
Southland	84.1	13.8	1.7	0.4

Table 3.7 Percentage rate at which ewes were mated for first time (from Quinlivan and Martin, 1971).

Area	% ewes returned		% ewes pregnant	
	Period 1	Period 2	Period 1	Period 2
Northern North Island	31.6	29.4	50.4	32.9
Southern North Island	26.9	24.9	47.4	36.4
Mid Canterbury North Otago	27.7	31.0	60.3	25.4
Southland	19.9	24.1	67.2	23.2

Table 3.8 Percentage ewes returned and conceived of ewes mated (from Quinlivan and Martin, 1971).

Nutrition

Severe short-term under-nutrition within 21 days of gestation can cause a measurable level of embryo mortality, particularly in two-tooth ewes. In mature ewes, prolonged but moderate feed restriction from about day 90–100 of pregnancy is unlikely to reduce lambing percentages. In contrast it has been shown that high-plane feeding can reduce embryo survival by suppressing the level of circulating progesterone in the ewe.

Selenium deficiency

In New Zealand there are areas where a reduced fertility condition characterised by a high incidence of barren ewes can be eliminated by a single dose of selenium (Se) before mating. Similarly, studies in the UK have demonstrated improved pregnancy rates in response to Se supplementation. Although the major selenium responsive areas have been mapped, much of New Zealand is considered marginal for selenium with deficiencies being more evident in some years. Analysis of blood and liver selenium levels provides information on the selenium status of the flock; where levels are low, selenium is usually administered to the ewes before mating (see Chapter 7).

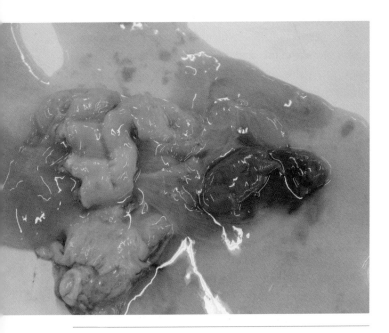

Figure 3.7 Embryonic loss shown by a partially autolysed foetus in the process of resorption.

High temperature

Continuous high temperatures have been shown to cause embryonic death in early pregnancy, the greatest effect being during the first week after mating. Heat-induced embryo mortality is not considered a problem in New Zealand and, due to diurnal variation, is only considered of importance in the subtropical sheep-breeding area of Australia.

Stress

Embryonic mortality has been shown to increase markedly (approximately double) in the following circumstances:
- if ewes are given daily injections of 60 IU ACTH (adrenocorticotropic hormone) for 20 days after mating
- if ewes are exposed to 6 hours of artificial rainfall daily for either days 1–10 or 11–20 after mating
- if ewes are subjected to management stress such as mustering, yarding, weighing or transport for 4–6 hours daily for either days 1–10 or 11–20 after mating.

This work emphasises the importance of careful handling of ewes during the tupping period; every effort should be made to avoid stress and to keep any interference to a minimum.

Infectious causes

Infection with toxoplasmosis and hairy shaker disease virus (see Chapter 4) can cause embryonic loss, although foetal and lamb losses are more usual. In many instances the contribution of these two infections to embryonic loss is difficult to diagnose, especially in the absence of abortions. Serology of the ewe is difficult to interpret because in the case of toxoplasmosis, antibody titres are common and for hairy shaker disease antibodies may relate to pestivirus infection unrelated to the event. A live attenuated *Toxoplasma* vaccine is available and in some flocks its use has reduced the number of dry/dry two-tooth ewes.

The widespread use of ultrasound pregnancy testing has identified higher than expected rates of foetal death and resorption of foetuses older than 30 days in some flocks. It appears that maiden ewes, particularly ewe hoggets, are more commonly affected. The ewes are not seen to abort and without the aid of ultrasound scanning would have been classed as dry/dry ewes, i.e. did not become pregnant. They otherwise appear to remain healthy. In most cases no infectious agents have been identified, although *Neospora caninum* or *Leptospira interrogans* serovar Pomona may be involved in some cases (see Chapter 4). In one study, affected hoggets had a reduction in weight gain in the month preceding the foetal loss compared with hoggets that retained pregnancy, but it is unknown whether this was a cause or a consequence of the foetal loss.

Placental development

Placental development begins about 30 days after conception and is largely completed by 90 days of gestation. Underfeeding of the ewe during early pregnancy can reduce the number of cotyledons and the size of the placentae, thus reducing the supply of nutrients to the lamb and causing lower lamb birthweights. If ewes lose 5 kg or more in the first 90 days of pregnancy, lamb birthweights (especially from multiple-bearing ewes) will be reduced regardless of late-pregnancy nutrition.

Ultrasound pregnancy diagnosis

Ultrasound pregnancy diagnosis has become routine on many New Zealand sheep farms, although a nationwide survey in 2012 suggested that around a quarter of farmers are still not utilising this technology. Garrick (1998) outlined the potential benefits of sheep pregnancy diagnosis (Figure 3.8). Many of these benefits are small, and whether they occur or not depends on the lambing percentage of the flock and the management skill of the farmer. However, collectively the benefits can be significant. As well as helping monitor reproductive performance on farms, pregnancy testing can aid in the diagnosis of reproductive problems or in research of embryonic loss.

A further benefit of ultrasound pregnancy scanning is that it focuses attention on the discrepancy between the number of lambs present at scanning and the number actually docked. Surveys have allowed the docking percentage to be predicted from the scanning percentage for different breeds (Figures 3.9 and 3.10).

Termination of pregnancy

Mismating due to rams gaining access to ewes during the breeding season is an occasional problem for which

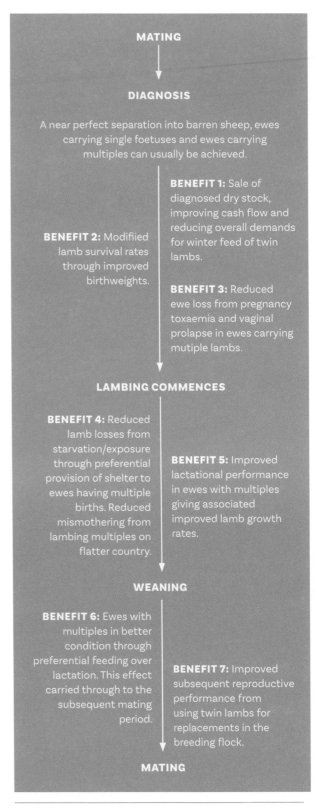

Figure 3.8 An overall view of the productive benefits of ultrasound pregnancy diagnosis (from Garrick, 1998).

termination of pregnancy is requested. It is often desirable that the ewes can be quickly re-mated to the correct ram within the same breeding season. In ewes, progesterone produced by the corpus luteum is essential for maintaining pregnancy only during about the first 50 days of gestation. Beyond about 50 days of gestation the placenta alone produces sufficient progesterone to maintain pregnancy. Even during the first 50 days of pregnancy a luteolytic dose of prostaglandin may not be effective in inducing abortion, possibly because the foetus produces an ovine trophoblast protein that blocks the action of prostaglandin. While a single dose using 250 μg cloprosterol is likely to be effective in most ewes in the first 50 days of pregnancy, two doses spaced 2 weeks apart is likely to be more reliable.

The injection of 15–20 mg of oestradiol benzoate or 8–16 mg of the short-acting glucocorticoid dexamethasone into ewes at days 141–145 of gestation will induce an early lambing. Where intensive lambing indoors is practised,

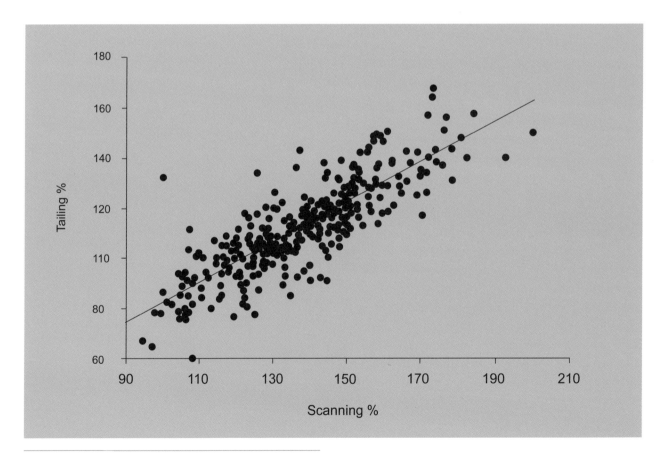

Figure 3.9 Tailing % vs scanning % (all data 1995–98) in Marlborough sheep flocks (Anderson and Sewell, 2000).

ewes can be treated to lamb during daylight hours but accurate mating dates are essential. The use of such techniques is not advised for normal farm conditions.

Conclusion

There is now a considerable body of scientific information that can be used to increase the reproductive performance of individual flocks. Veterinarians should become more actively involved in applying this knowledge. When investigating problems of low lamb production, it must be appreciated that lambing percentage is the end result of many factors exerting varying effects at different stages in the reproductive process. Thus there are a number of 'causes' involved. Correction of these problems will only be achieved by regular farm visits, careful investigation and data collection.

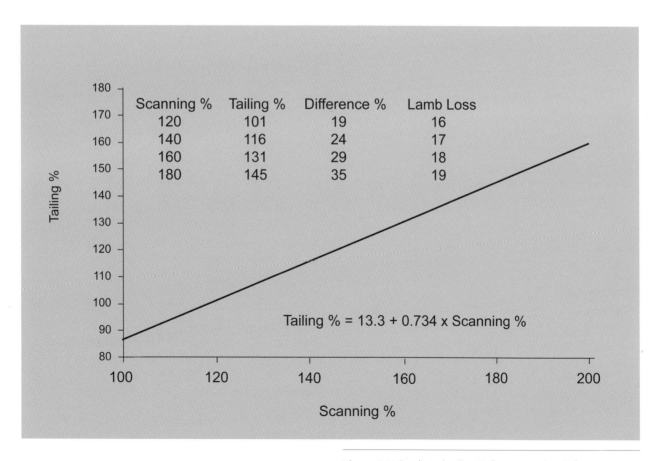

Figure 3.10 Predicted tailing % from scanning % for Marlborough sheep flocks (Anderson and Sewell, 2000).

REFERENCES

Allison AJ. Flock mating in sheep 2. Effect of number of ewes per ram on mating behaviour and fertility of two-tooth and mixed-age Romney ewes run together. *New Zealand Journal of Agricultural Research* 20, 123-8, 1977

Allison AJ. Review: The management of mating for maximum fertilisation and conception. *Proceedings of the Society of Sheep and Beef Cattle Veterinarians, New Zealand Veterinary Association* 13, 76-90, 1983

Allison AJ, Kelly RW. Some effects of liveweight and breed of ewe on fertility and fecundity. *Proceedings of the Society of Sheep and Beef Cattle Veterinarians, New Zealand Veterinary Association* 8, 24-30, 1978

Allison AJ, Stevenson JR, Kelly RW. Reproductive performance and wool production of Merino and high fertility strain (Booroola and Merino ewes). *Proceedings of the New Zealand Society of Animal Production* 37, 230-2, 1977

Anderson PVA, Sewell J. The significance and use of sheep scanning data. *Proceedings of the Society of Sheep and Beef Cattle Veterinarians, New Zealand Veterinary Association* 30, 31-6, 2000

Ch'ang TS, Rae AL. The genetic basis of growth, reproduction and maternal environment in Romney ewes. 1. Genetic variation in hogget characters and fertility of the ewe. *Australian Journal of Agricultural Research* 21, 115-29, 1970

Coop IE. Liveweight-productivity relationships in sheep I: Liveweight and Reproduction. *New Zealand Journal of Agricultural Research* 5, 249-64, 1962

Coop IE. The influence of liveweight on wool production and reproduction of high country flocks. *New Zealand Journal of Agricultural Research* 9, 165-71, 1966

Corner-Thomas RA, Kenyon PR, Morris ST, Ridler AL, Hickson RE, Greer AW, Logan CM, Blair HT. Brief communication: Ewe ultra-sound pregnancy diagnosis and its use by New Zealand farmers. *Proceedings of the New Zealand Society of Animal Production* 74, 65-7, 2014

Doney JM, Smith WF, Gunn RG. Effects of post-mating environmental stress or administration of ACTH on early embryonic loss in sheep. *Journal of Agricultural Science, Cambridge* 87, 133-6, 1976

Edney TN. Early embryonic death and subsequent cycle length in the ewe. *Journal of Reproduction and Fertility* 13, 437-43, 1967

Edwards SJ, Juengel JL. Limits on hogget lambing: The fertility of the young ewe. *New Zealand Journal of Agricultural Research* 60, 1-22, 2017

Fielden ED, Smith JF. Reproductive management of grazing ruminants in New Zealand. *New Zealand Society of Animal Production*, Occasional Publication No. 12, 1998

Garrick DJ. The potential benefits of knowing the pregnancy status of ewes. *Proceedings of the Society of Sheep and Beef Cattle Veterinarians, New Zealand Veterinary Association* 28, 203-18, 1998

Geenty K (Ed). *Making every mating count.* Beef and Lamb New Zealand, 2013

Geldard H, Scaramuzzi RJ, Wilkins JF. Immunisation against polyandroalbumin leads to increases in lambing and tailing percentages. *New Zealand Veterinary Journal* 32, 2-5, 1984

Gunn R, Doney JM, Smith WF. Fertility in Cheviot ewes 3. The effect of level of nutrition before and after mating on ovulation rate and early embryo mortality in South Country Cheviot. *Proceedings of the New Zealand Society of Animal Production* 29, 25-31, 1979

Hudson N, McNatty K. Androvax. *Proceedings of the Society of Sheep and Beef Cattle Veterinarians, New Zealand Veterinary Association* 32, 255-60, 2002

Kelly CM. Current aspects of the use of ovandrotone-albumin as a fecundity improver in sheep. *Proceedings of the Society of Sheep and Beef Cattle Veterinarians, New Zealand Veterinary Association* 15, 23-39, 1985

Kenyon PR, Morel PCH, Morris ST. Effect of liveweight and condition score of ewes at mating, and shearing mid-pregnancy, on birthweights and growth rates of twin lambs to weaning. *New Zealand Veterinary Journal* 52, 145-9, 2004

Kenyon PR, Morel PCH, Morris ST. The effect of individual liveweight and condition score of ewes at mating on reproductive and scanning performance. *New Zealand Veterinary Journal* 52, 230-5, 2004

Kenyon PR, Morel PCH, Morris ST, West DM. The effect of individual liveweight and use of teaser rams prior to mating on the reproductive performance of ewe hoggets. *New Zealand Veterinary Journal* 53, 340-3, 2005

Kenyon PR, Morel PCH, Morris ST, West DM. Effect of the age of rams on reproductive performance of ewe hoggets. *New Zealand Veterinary Journal* 55, 184-7, 2007

Kenyon PR, Morris ST, Revell DK, McCutcheon SN. Shearing during pregnancy — review of a policy to increase birthweight and survival of lambs in New Zealand pastoral farming systems. *New Zealand Veterinary Journal* 51, 200-7, 2003

Kenyon PR, Pinchbeck GL, Perkins NR, Morris St, West DM. Identifying factors which maximise the lambing performance of hoggets: A cross sectional study. *New Zealand Veterinary Journal* 52, 371-7, 2004

Kenyon PR (Ed). *Hogget performance — unlocking the potential.* Beef and Lamb New Zealand, 2012

Knight TW. Influencing the onset of ovarian activity. *Proceedings of the Society of Sheep and Beef Cattle Veterinarians, New Zealand Veterinary Association* 13, 16-20, 1983

Knight TW. Reproductive wastage: A guide to fundamental research: A New Zealand perspective. In: *Reproductive Physiology of Merino Sheep: Concepts and Consequences*, edited by CM Oldman, GB Martin, IW Purvis. University of Western Australia, Perth, 1990

Knight TW, Moore RW, McMillan WH. In: Shimmins M (ed). *The Whatawhata Way: An integrated approach to hill country* *farming in New Zealand*. P41. Agricultural Promotion Associates Ltd, Wellington, New Zealand, 1982

Lewis KHC. Ewe fertility response to premating anthelmintic drenching. *New Zealand Journal of Experimental Agriculture* 3, 43-7, 1975

MacKenzie AJ, Thwaites CJ, Edney TN. Oestrous, ovarian and adrenal response of the ewe to fasting and cold stress. *Australian Journal of Agricultural Research* 26, 545-51, 1975

Morris ST. Production and management consequences of out-of-season lambing. *Proceedings of the Society of Sheep and Beef Cattle Veterinarians, New Zealand Veterinary Association* 27, 65-71, 1997

Quinlivan TD, Martin CA. Oestrous activity and lamb production in the NZ Romney ewe. *Australian Journal of Agricultural Research* 22, 497-511, 1971

Rattray PV, Jagusch KT, Smeaton DC. Interactions between feed quality, feed quantity, body weight and flushing. *Proceedings of the Society of Sheep and Beef Cattle Veterinarians, New Zealand Veterinary Association* 13, 21-34, 1983

Ridler AL, Corner-Thomas RA, Kenyon PR, Griffiths KJ. Investigation of plasma progesterone and liveweight in ewe lambs affected by fetal loss. *New Zealand Veterinary Journal* 65, 34-8, 2017

Shallard K. The use of androstenedione to increase the lamb drop. *Proceedings of the Society of Sheep and Beef Cattle Veterinarians, New Zealand Veterinary Association* 15, 40-4, 1985

Smith JF. A review of recent developments on the effect of nutrition on ovulation rate (the flushing effect) with particular reference to research at Ruakura. *Proceedings of the New Zealand Society of Animal Production* 51, 15-23, 1991

Smith JF, Morris CA. Review of zearalenone studies with sheep in New Zealand. *Proceedings of the New Zealand Society of Animal Production* 66, 306-10, 2006

Towers NR. Zearalenone induced infertility in sheep. *Proceedings of the Society of Sheep and Beef Cattle Veterinarians, New Zealand Veterinary Association* 22, 159-78, 1992

Towers NR. Oestrogenic fungal toxins affecting sheep and cattle production. *Proceedings of the Society of Sheep and Beef Cattle Veterinarians, New Zealand Veterinary Association, Pan Pacific Conference* 26, 43-58, 1996

Towers NR. Mycotoxin poisoning in grazing livestock in New Zealand. *Proceedings of the New Zealand Society of Animal Production* 66, 300-6, 2006

Welch RAS, Kilgour R, Robinson GA, Smith ME, Williams ET. The effect of shearing ewes during the mating period on the subsequent lambing pattern. *Proceedings of the New Zealand Society of Animal Production* 39, 100-2, 1979

4 Abortion in ewes

The national incidence of abortions in New Zealand sheep flocks is quoted at 1–2%, but with a total annual production of millions of lambs this represents a considerable loss. In many cases the incidence of abortion within a flock is low, but when uterine infection is introduced into a fully susceptible flock it may rise as high as 70%. Because most abortions are seen in late pregnancy, even a few losses can have a profoundly worrying effect on the farmer.

The most common causes of ovine abortion in New Zealand are *Campylobacter fetus fetus* and *Toxoplasma gondii*, although in southern areas of the country *Salmonella* Brandenburg is also a major abortive agent. Less common causes of infectious abortion include *Listeria, Yersinia, Bacillus, Leptospira* and hairy shaker disease. There is also a possibility that *Neosporum caninum*, a well-established cause of abortion in cattle, may be associated with some abortions in sheep. Stress, plant and chemical toxins may also cause abortion but tend to be very uncommon and sporadic. As a country we are fortunate to be free from enzootic abortion caused by *Chlamydophila abortus* and abortion caused by *Salmonella abortus ovis*, which are major causes of ovine abortion overseas.

Campylobacteriosis

Abortion caused by *C. f. fetus* is often referred to as campylobacteriosis. It was previously called vibriosis or vibrio. *Campylobacter f. fetus* abortion usually occurs during the last 6 weeks of pregnancy, but infection may also cause early neonatal loss. Following abortion, affected ewes usually remain fertile and immune to infection in subsequent years. In most cases the ewe remains healthy, although a small proportion of aborting ewes may develop metritis resulting in severe illness and/or death.

Campylobacteriosis occurs in most sheep-raising countries of the world and a high prevalence has been reported throughout New Zealand.

Aetiology

In sheep, *Campylobacter* abortion is caused by *C. fetus* subspecies *fetus* (not *C. fetus venerealis*, as in cattle). There are a number of strain types of this organism present in New Zealand. *C. jejuni* and, rarely, *C. coli*, found in the intestinal tract of sheep, cattle, dogs and cats and other animals, are occasional causes of abortion in sheep.

Transmission

The infection is transmitted to susceptible animals by ingestion of contaminated feed or water, or by direct contact with infected foetuses or foetal membranes. The latter may become a source of infection for mechanical transmission of the agent by shepherds. Venereal transmission of *C. f. fetus* does not occur as it does with *C. f. venerealis* of cattle.

Carrion-eating birds such as the North American magpie (*Pica pica*) and ravens (*Corvus corone corone*) in Britain have been shown to spread infection. The New Zealand magpie (*Gymnorhina tibicen*) does not scavenge or eat carrion and is not likely to spread infection. However, the black-backed gull (*Larus dominicanus*) is seen frequently scavenging in lamb paddocks and may be a mechanical vector, as may be the Australasian harrier hawk (*Circus approximans*).

Introduced carrier sheep may bring an infection to a flock and an abortion storm may follow in younger sheep or older sheep that have no immunity.

Pathogenesis

Abortions usually appear in the last third of pregnancy from 7 to 25 days after infection. Campylobacter infection has not been associated with early embryonic loss and 'barren ewes'.

The organism may persist in the intestinal tract of sheep, but the length of persistence has not been well defined. It has been found in the bile, gall bladder and intestines of sheep of 3 months to 8 years of age. After initial infection, a bacteraemia occurs for 10–14 days followed by placental localisation of the infection if the animal is pregnant. Bacterial growth is greatly enhanced by nutrients in the placenta. The bacteria invade the placenta causing an acute inflammatory response with areas of necrosis of both foetal and maternal tissues. The foetus is invaded and necrotic foci may develop in a range of organs including liver and lungs.

Foetal death is followed by abortion, which occurs between 1 and 3 weeks after exposure to the organism. An unknown proportion of infected animals may become intestinal carriers and this may allow the infection to persist in a flock from year to year.

Clinical features

The farmer may find aborted foetuses or may simply see affected ewes with a blood-stained perineal region. Occasionally foetal membranes may protrude from the vulva. The disease is often of a cyclical nature, and high-density winter grazing may produce a high level of infection in the environment and challenge to susceptible ewes. As stated, the abortions occur mainly after the third month of pregnancy and mainly in maiden ewes.

The aborting ewe rarely shows any systemic effect. Secondary metritis may on occasion develop and cause chronic ill health. *Campylobacter f. fetus* may persist in the uterine discharge for up to 6 weeks.

Some ewes carry infected lambs to full term, when they are either born dead or weak. Such ewes usually produce insufficient milk to raise a lamb. It has been suggested that *C. f. fetus* may be responsible for high perinatal lamb losses on some properties.

Diagnosis and pathology

Gross lesions of *C. f. fetus* infection in the lamb are variable and not specific. The placenta may be oedematous and/or hyperaemic and is often opaque. The foetus will usually have serosanguinous subcutaneous oedema and similar fluid in the body cavities, as is usual in most intrauterine deaths. Some foetuses may be mummified. About 26% of infected foetuses show liver lesions that are characteristic of *C. f. fetus*. These are pale white-yellow, 2–15-mm-diameter circular areas of necrosis.

Culture of the organism is possible from foetal stomach contents, the placenta and vaginal discharges. The organism can frequently be identified by direct microscopic examination of foetal stomach contents, using a dark-field microscope. Organism typing and histological examination of the placenta and foetus may also be required to confirm a diagnosis.

Control

Control during an outbreak is based on preventing access of animals to infection and/or eliminating the infection. As the organism is spread mainly by the ingestion of contaminated grass, reducing the exposure to such areas should reduce the spread of disease. This is best achieved by reducing the stocking density and, if possible, removing stock from contaminated pasture. The prompt recognition and removal of aborting ewes and aborted foetuses are necessary. Careful attention to hygiene is necessary to prevent the mechanical spread of the infection on clothing and equipment. Vaccination may also be used in the face of an abortion storm, either alone or in combination with antibiotics. Under such circumstances, for the vaccine to be effective it is important that the first dose be given 6 weeks before the due date of lambing or as early as possible in the outbreak.

In some cases, the organism may be eliminated from carrier animals and animals incubating the infection by treatment with antibiotics. Antibiotic therapy has been used successfully in some cases. The dose rates are usually higher than recommended therapeutic doses. This strategy may be useful for reducing further abortions in high-value ewes.

Prevention of *C. f. fetus* infection can be achieved by the use of an adjuvant prepared vaccine of killed ovine cultures of *C. f. fetus*. Some vaccines contain *C. f. jejuni* antigen as well as *C. f. fetus* antigen.[1] However, the significance of *C. f. jejuni* as a regular cause of abortion in sheep has not been substantiated, even though it has been isolated occasionally from aborted foetuses. The vaccine is injected subcutaneously in the neck region. Previously

---

1 Campylovexin® (Virbac New Zealand Ltd), Campyvax4® (MSD Animal Health)

unsensitised ewes are given a sensitiser dose pre-tupping and a booster dose 4–8 weeks later. In subsequent years the same sheep are given a booster dose either pre-tup or at ram withdrawal. In some flocks, only the maiden ewes are vaccinated rather than the whole flock of ewes. Such a regimen appears to have been successful in preventing further outbreaks of campylobacteriosis, although in flocks where the challenge is likely to be high (e.g. strip-grazing with very high stocking densities, grazing vaccinated and non-vaccinated ewes together), an annual booster may be necessary.

Toxoplasmosis

Toxoplasmosis is of major importance in many countries as a cause of abortion in sheep. In New Zealand its occurrence is widespread. It can occur concurrently with other infections (e.g. *Campylobacter fetus fetus*).

Aetiology and pathogenesis

The causative protozoan parasite *Toxoplasma gondii* is an obligate intracellular parasite with a two-stage asexual life cycle which can take place in warm-blooded animals, and a coccidian-type sexual life cycle which is confined to the intestines of members of the cat family. It is relevant to ovine toxoplasmosis that wild rodents and birds can harbour bradyzoites (asexual part of cycle) in tissue cysts within brain and muscle. In addition, infection in mice can also be passed from generation to generation without causing significant illness, thus helping to maintain a long-lasting reservoir of infection for cats.

It is cats that can amplify and spread the infection in their faeces in the form of many millions of very resistant oocysts. In general, younger rather than older cats pose the greatest threat. The degree of contamination that is theoretically possible by *Toxoplasma gondii* oocysts in cat faeces is shown in Table 4.1.

After ingestion of feed or water contaminated with *Toxoplasma* oocysts, susceptible sheep become, and remain, infected for life. Infection of the ovine placenta and foetus (conceptus) occurs only when the initial infection establishes in susceptible pregnant sheep, following the ingestion of oocysts.

The oocysts excyst in the digestive tract and the released sporozoites penetrate the cells lining the gut so that tachy-

> **CASE EXAMPLE**
>
> At the beginning of July a farmer yarded 330 mixed-age ewes, due to lamb in 3–4 weeks' time, for crutching and clostridial vaccination. The ewes had not been vaccinated against *Campylobacter fetus fetus*. Just prior to returning the ewes to their paddock, the farmer noticed that one had aborted in the yards. Over the following three weeks, 90 of the 330 ewes aborted, with all the ewes remaining healthy. Three foetuses were submitted for examination and *C. f. fetus* was isolated from the stomach contents of all three.
>
>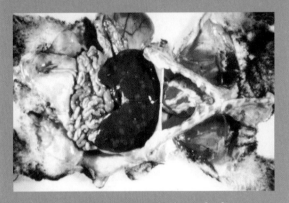
>
> **Figure 4.1** Necrotic lesions in the liver of a foetus infected with *Campylobacter fetus fetus*.

Oocysts in cat faeces ~1 million/gram

50 g of cat faeces in 10 tonnes of feed

5000 oocysts/kg feed

(NB: 200 oocysts will infect one ewe)

Therefore 25 infective doses/kg feed

Table 4.1 The degree of contamination of sheep feed theoretically possible by *Toxoplasma gondii* oocysts in cat faeces (after Buxton, 1989).

zoites eventually reach and infect the placenta and foetus.

Toxoplasma gondii has been isolated from ram semen, and it has been recognised that in New Zealand ewes, seroconversions often occur during the mating period. It has been suggested that infection of rams, with transmission to the ewe during mating, may also be an important route of spread, as well as from cat faeces.

Clinical features

As in campylobacteriosis, few overt signs of disease are seen in sheep. An observant farmer may see a small amount of blood and mucus discharging from the vulva as a sign that an abortion has occurred. In general, infection early in pregnancy is likely to cause foetal resorption, with the ewe subsequently returning to oestrus or becoming a dry/dry ewe for that season. Infection late in pregnancy (day 120 onwards) will usually result in the birth of a normal lamb which may be infected or become immune. Infection in mid-pregnancy (days 60–120) will cause foetal death, mummification and abortion. The time from infection occurring to abortion is up to 40 days. An increased number of dry/dry ewes, particularly two-tooths, found at weaning, may retrospectively help to support a diagnosis of toxoplasmosis. Obviously, important aspects to be considered are the presence of breeding populations of wild cats, especially in hay barns where kittens may contaminate hay that is subsequently spread on pasture.

Diagnosis and pathology

Diagnosis of the disease in sheep is usually possible from the gross pathology of the placental cotyledons. These show numerous grey-white (1–3 mm) foci of necrosis (strawberry cotyledons; Figure 4.4). Foetuses may also be mummified in utero.

A sensitive method of confirming a diagnosis is the histopathological examination of the placental cotyledons and the foetal brain, lung and liver for characteristic microscopic lesions. It should be noted that the above examinations also apply to goats, although it is frequently difficult to obtain a goat placenta as they are more prone to eat them than the ewe.

Serological methods of confirming a diagnosis include the dye test, indirect fluorescent antibody test, indirect haemagglutination test, ELISA and the latex agglutination test. The most common of these used by diagnostic

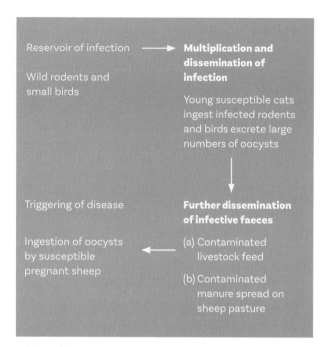

Table 4.2 The spread of toxoplasmosis to sheep.

	DAY
Oocysts ingested	0
Infection in mesenteric lymph nodes	4
Febrile response	5–12
Parasitaemia	5–12
Toxoplasma in uterine caruncular septa	10
Toxoplasma in placental trophoblast cells	10
Toxoplasma-specific foetal antibody	30

Table 4.3 Pathogenesis of toxoplasmosis in pregnant sheep.

laboratories is the indirect fluorescent antibody test (IFAT), performed on foetal heart blood or thoracic fluid. If testing ewes, paired sera several weeks apart should be collected to show that significant rises in antibody titres occurred during pregnancy. This has little practical use clinically.

Control

Once an outbreak of toxoplasmosis has started there is little that can be done other than to observe sensible precautions such as disposing of dead lambs and infected placentae and disinfecting contaminated pens where necessary. Sheep-to-sheep transmission is not thought to occur. The organism appears susceptible to sulphonamides and even single injections of trimethoprim and sulphadiazine (Tribrissen injection 48%) at 60 mg/kg may be useful in valuable sheep.

In New Zealand a live attenuated *Toxoplasma* vaccine is available (Toxovax, MSD Animal Health), which was developed at the Wallaceville Animal Research Centre. A single dose of 2 ml is injected intramuscularly into the neck of each sheep. Non-pregnant, healthy ewes can be vaccinated at any time, but not closer than 4 weeks before the onset of mating. If teaser rams are used prior to mating, the vaccine should be given at least 4 weeks before teaser introduction. The vaccine must not be used in pregnant stock or within 4 weeks of mating. The vaccine is required only once in the sheep's lifetime. Because the vaccine contains a live organism it has a short shelf life of 30 days, must be protected from heat and light and must not be frozen. The vaccine is also suitable for use in goats.

Measures to limit the breeding of cats and to maintain the number of adults at a low level sufficient to control vermin are helpful. Wild cats may need to be culled. The maintenance of adult neutered cats in a healthy state reduces the chance of recrudescence of *Toxoplasma* infection and re-excretion of oocysts.

Overseas it has been shown that chemoprophylaxis using monensin (15 mg/head/day) or decoquinate fed to ewes during pregnancy produced a significant reduction in *Toxoplasma*-induced perinatal mortality. Monensin fed judiciously can provide a relatively inexpensive control of toxoplasma in pregnant sheep and goats; however, it would have little use in New Zealand where sheep are seldom fed concentrated feed.

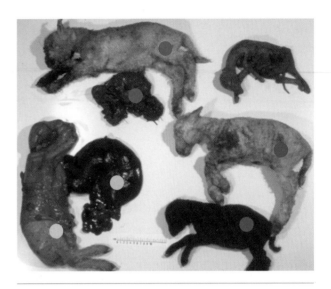

Figure 4.2 A range of aborted foetuses following abortion due to *Toxoplasma gondii*. Foetuses with the same coloured dots are twins — often one twin is relatively normal while the other is mummified.

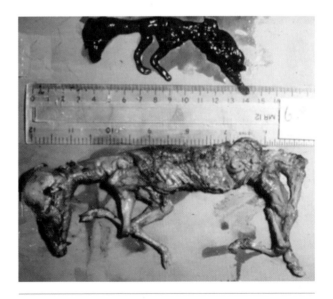

Figure 4.3 Two mummified foetuses following *Toxoplasma gondii* abortion.

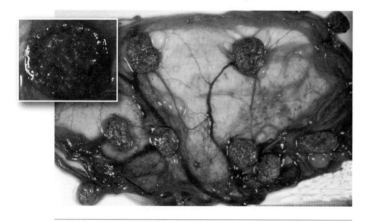

Figure 4.4 'Strawberry cotyledons' – areas of necrosis.

A cyclical pattern of the disease seems to have emerged, as expected with the disease having become endemic. It is now likely that in some cases farmers feel they can recognise the disease and do not seek veterinary or laboratory assistance in diagnosis. To date, cases in sheep have not been reported in the North Island of New Zealand.

Aetiology and pathogenesis

Ewes are infected by direct contact with aborted foetuses/placentae or by ingestion of contaminated feed. The organism probably has an environmental survival of four or more months and sheep that survive become intestinal carriers for up to six months. Thus carrier sheep are likely to be important for introduction of infection into a flock. Black-backed gulls (*Larus dominicanus*) have been shown to carry large numbers of organisms, with up to 25 million organisms per gram of intestinal contents reported. Excretion of the organism in the faeces of black-backed gulls may enable introduction onto a new property. Farmers and vehicles are likely to be important vectors in the transmission of disease. It has also been isolated from sheep yard dust.

In general, farms with high stocking rates that use intensive grazing systems appear to be the worst affected by *S*. Brandenburg abortions. This suggests that high stocking density is an important precipitating factor.

Clinical features

Both two-tooth and mixed-age ewes are affected, but the majority of abortions are in multiple-lamb-bearing ewes. Ewes in late pregnancy become dull and fevered and abort putrid, late-term lambs that have been dead at least a day. Around half of the aborting ewes subsequently develop severe necrotising metritis and die. Occasionally ewes may develop severe diarrhoea before death. Some ewes have only a short-term dullness and their lambs are born dead, or small and weak.

Combined farm data from the late 1990s showed that on average 3–4% of the flock aborted (range 0.2–25%) over a period of around 30 days (range 7–75 days). Without treatment, 30–50% of aborting ewes subsequently died.

Diagnosis and pathology

Aborted foetuses have advanced autolysis with swollen, macerated livers and the placenta is necrotic. Postmortem

Zoonosis

Toxoplasma gondii is zoonotic, although clinical disease in humans is uncommon. The prevalence of human subclinical disease with development of serum antibodies is relatively common in New Zealand. Humans can become infected by ingestion of oocysts following accidental ingestion of infected cat faeces, or by ingestion of bradyzoites in raw meat. Ingestion of tachyzoites in aborted placentae may also be a risk for humans, although the likelihood of transmission by this route is very low. Clinical disease in adults is characterised by fever and lymphadenitis. Infection of pregnant women may result in congenital infection, and this may result in abortion, stillbirth or birth of a child with central nervous system defects and other permanent damage.

Salmonella Brandenburg

In 1996 *Salmonella* Brandenburg, a *Salmonella* serotype that had previously only caused sporadic disease in many species, was isolated from aborting and dying ewes in mid-Canterbury. Subsequently, cases have been reported in Canterbury, Otago and Southland. In areas where the disease has already occurred, the severity of the clinical disease can be less than in areas where it occurs for the first time. Abortion or enteritis due to *S*. Brandenburg infection have also been reported in other species such as cattle, horses and dogs. Enteritis has been reported in humans.

examination of dead ewes reveals an acute suppurative necrotising metritis. *Salmonella* Brandenburg can be cultured from foetal stomach contents or liver, clean placentae or vaginal swabs. Histologically the placenta shows early acute placentitis and capillaries are packed with organisms.

Treatment

Parenteral long-acting oxytetracycline given early in the course of the disease usually prevents ewe death, but will not prevent abortion. It is not recommended to vaccinate during an outbreak.

Control

Vaccination

The original *Salmonella* vaccine was designed to protect against enteric salmonellosis (see Chapter 16) and contained inactivated strains of *S. typhimurium, S.* Hindmarsh and *S. bovis-morbificans*. Since the advent of *S.* Brandenburg abortions in ewes, inactivated *S.* Brandenburg has been added to the vaccine (Salvexin +B, MSD Animal Health). This vaccine can be used to protect against *S.* Brandenburg abortion and enteric salmonellosis, but it is important to recognise that the ideal timing of vaccination differs for the two different syndromes.

To protect against *S.* Brandenburg abortion, it is recommended that all ewes receive a sensitiser dose with a booster 4–6 weeks later. In subsequent years an annual booster should be given. The timing of this vaccine is important and it is recommended that ewes are vaccinated in early pregnancy, with the second vaccination given at least 2–3 weeks before the period of greatest risk (e.g. at ram introduction and then ram removal, or at ram removal and then 4–6 weeks later). The vaccine gives increased, but not complete, protection; in the face of heavy challenge, abortions and ewe deaths may still occur. It does, however, reduce faecal shedding of the organism and so reduces environmental contamination. Therefore it is important to also try to reduce other predisposing factors.

Other control methods

Ewes farmed intensively, particularly where mob stocking/strip-grazing is practised, appear to be more susceptible to the disease. In cases of an outbreak, spreading ewes out and reducing stocking density may decrease the numbers affected, although this is not always the case. It is also advisable to minimise pre-lambing yarding and general stress where possible.

As a likely means of disease introduction is carrier animals, it is advisable to avoid purchasing stock from properties known to be affected by *S.* Brandenburg.

Environmental contamination should be minimised by procedures such as rapid disposal of aborted foetuses and placentae, quarantine of aborted ewes, good hygiene of clothing, equipment and vehicles, and visiting non-affected mobs before affected mobs so as not to transfer infection. Control of scavenging birds such as black-backed gulls is also warranted. *S.* Brandenburg is zoonotic and workers should undertake appropriate hygiene procedures when dealing with sick animals.

CASE EXAMPLE

In mid-August, while shifting ewes onto a new break of grass, a Southland farmer noticed that a few were lethargic and slow to move. These ewes aborted shortly afterwards. Over the following three weeks, of the 4450 ewes on the property 320 aborted and 150 ewes subsequently died. The aborted foetuses autolysed rapidly, had a putrid smell and had swollen livers. *Salmonella* Brandenburg was isolated from foetal stomach contents. Necropsy of dead ewes revealed a severe, acute metritis and associated septicaemia.

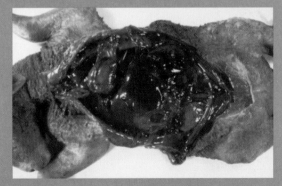

Figure 4.5 An autolysed foetus aborted due to *Salmonella* Brandenburg.

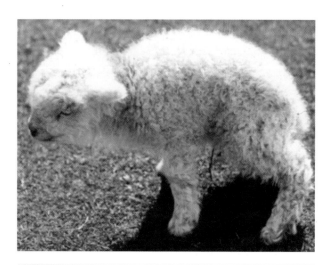

Figure 4.6 Live lamb affected with hairy shaker disease. Note the hairy appearance and dark wool on the neck.

foetuses may be aborted. Postpartum sepsis is rare.

Live lambs that are hairy and stunted are frequently produced. They also show chorea, which becomes worse with stimulation, and sometimes they have abnormal pigmented patches of the fleece. Many such lambs die from malnutrition, but some survive and fatten and the chorea frequently decreases with age. The tremor seen in such lambs is almost absent at rest or sleep. In New Zealand, one case of a fatal mucosal disease-like condition has been reported soon after weaning in surviving lambs with hairy shaker disease. This syndrome has also been reported overseas, and the disease can be reproduced experimentally.

When hairy shaker disease occurs it can be economically very serious for the farmer in that season. Some examples of outbreaks from the South Island emphasise this point. Both involve the mixing of infected and susceptible flocks at, or soon after, mating.

Hairy shaker disease (border disease)

The pestivirus infection known as hairy shaker disease has been diagnosed as a cause of abortion mainly in the Otago–Southland region and less frequently in the rest of New Zealand.

Aetiology

The causative organism is one or more of the pestiviruses closely related to those of bovine viral diarrhoea. The virus affects all ages of pregnant ewe.

Transmission

Infection is via the mucous membranes of susceptible animals, and the disease may be introduced to a flock by clinically normal ewes and rams. Lambs that survive after showing signs of hairy shaker disease and affected ewes are potential sources of infection, although the ewes will breed again satisfactorily the next season.

Clinical features

A wide range of clinical features are seen in hairy shaker disease. Embryonic death shown by late return to oestrus is frequently a feature. Abortion of mummified foetuses may occur, or if late in pregnancy small, usually hairy,

Pathology and diagnosis

In affected lambs, there is a fall in the ratio of secondary to primary wool follicles and, as a consequence, a proportional increase in heavy medullated fibres. There is retardation of the central nervous system, which shows a deficiency of myelin; there is an increase in glial cells; and, rarely, macroscopic cavitation of cerebral white matter is seen.

The diagnosis of hairy shaker disease can be made through the clinical findings, histopathological examination of well-preserved foetal brain or testing foetal spleen with the bovine virus diarrhoea antigen ELISA. The cotyledons of aborted foetuses are considered to be rounded, small and pale. The serology of ewe blood can be used, although interpretation may be difficult because the pestivirus infection may be unrelated to the event.

Control

Control of pestivirus abortion is achieved by avoiding exposure of susceptible ewes to the infection when they are pregnant, especially during tupping and also over the first three months of gestation.

Advice given to a farmer at the time of an outbreak may include:
- Cull any lambs severely affected with hairy shaker disease soon after birth.

- Attempt to fatten mildly affected lambs for slaughter.
- Buy in ewe replacements this year rather than retaining any of the current ewe lambs.
- Any female stock purchased should be mixed with the flock at least 4 weeks before tupping.
- Cull any ewes that produce hairy shakers in two consecutive years. This obviously requires a good means of ewe identification.

This simple strategy should lead ultimately to an extremely low incidence of hairy shaker disease. It has also been suggested mixing a few 'hairy shakers' with the ewe hoggets if these are to be retained in the flock.

Long-term control depends on flock management, either to prevent infection entering or to ensure that breeding animals are exposed to infections early in their life, when they are not pregnant.

Helicobacter spp

For some time *Helicobacter* spp have been suspected as the cause of some undiagnosed abortions, particularly in the southern half of the South Island. In 2016, stored samples from undiagnosed abortions were tested retrospectively and *Helicobacter* spp (*H. bilis* and *H. trogontum*) were identified from 16% of the affected farms. Samples from control flocks were negative for *Helicobacter*. This suggests that *Helicobacter* spp are a likely cause of abortion in New Zealand.

Field reports would suggest that *Helicobacter* spp are most likely associated with abortion in the third trimester of pregnancy and with the birth of weak lambs. Aborted placentae and foetal livers have lesions very similar to those seen in *Campylobacter fetus fetus* abortions. Work is being undertaken to produce a commercially available diagnostic test.

Neospora caninum

The protozoan *Neospora caninum* readily causes abortion in cattle. There are also reports of natural infections in sheep, causing mortality in newborn lambs and congenital infection in naturally exposed sheep. Further, in both New Zealand and overseas experimental work, infection with tachyzoites has been shown to cause abortion at various

Case 1: Canterbury fat-lamb farmer

Following the purchase of a new block of land, the farmer mixed sheep from the new block with his own flock four weeks after tupping. Four to six weeks before the expected lambing date, about 10% of his ewes aborted. The cause was not identified. A further 50% of the ewes produced full-term lambs with clinical signs resembling those of hairy shaker disease. Many of the lambs were typically small, hairy and trembling with patches of brown pigments in their fleece. Other showed some of these signs only.

These findings suggest that the home flock had been infected by mixing it with the new flock four weeks after tupping. The occurrence of only a few clinical cases in the new flock suggests that the virus had been present in the new flock for some time, allowing a natural immunity to develop.

Case 2: Gore sheep farmer

On a farm near Gore with 1100 ewes, 300 aborted or produced small, hairy lambs that season.

These hairy lambs showed the classical conformation and fleece characteristics of hairy shaker disease. On questioning the farmer, it seemed that hairy shaker disease was endemic on the farm, since a few 'hairy fellas' were born every year. However, this year the farmer had bought in more than 700 replacement ewes (he was changing over from Perendales to Romney ewes) in four or five different batches at tupping time.

A traceback indicated that hairy shaker disease had not been experienced by any of the farms of origin of these ewes. After running with bought-in rams for 4-5 weeks, they were mixed with the farmer's own ewes. Abortions occurred and weak hairy lambs were born only in the bought-in Romneys and not in the homegrown Perendales. Thus it seemed that 'clean' bought-in ewes contracted the disease in the first few weeks of their pregnancy.

levels up to 50% and in extreme cases 100%. In an extensive serological and postmortem examination of some aborted lambs in one New Zealand survey (Howe et al., 2012), good circumstantial evidence suggested the possible association of *N. caninum* with both the aborting ewes and its presence in some of the pregnant ewes. In some of the aborted lambs where brain tissue was obtained, the presence of both degeneration and DNA strongly suggested that *Neospora* may have been involved in some of the abortions. These reports of both overseas and New Zealand sheep abortion investigations suggest that *N. caninum* is worthy of further consideration when investigating an abortion outbreak in sheep, particularly in maiden ewes when no other pathogen likely to have caused the losses is identified.

The pathogenesis of *Neospora* infection is complex. Although PCR and DNA tests can be used to detect the parasite in blood, foetal brain and uterine tissue, the timing of sampling from blood may be critical. Blood samples taken at the time of the detection of reabsorbing fetuses and abortions may more accurately reflect the organism's involvement in the abortions. Cattle studies have shown that *Neospora* DNA disappears from the circulation soon after an abortion has occurred and it is possible that a similar disappearance occurs in sheep.

Other infectious agents

Other infectious agents isolated from aborted lambs include *Bacillus licheniformis, Listeria monocytogenes, Listeria ivanovii, Pasteurella, Staphylococcus, Streptococcus* and *Yersinia pseudotuberculosis*. Usually these cause only sporadic losses, although in some cases losses may be high. *Bacillus* or *Listeria* abortions are often associated with feeding poor-quality baleage or silage.

Leptospira interrogans serovar Pomona has been reported to cause ovine abortion overseas, and was associated with mid-gestational foetal losses in hoggets on a New Zealand farm. *Brucella ovis* has been associated with abortion but this is very rare.

Non-infectious causes

Laboratory diagnoses of non-infectious causes of abortion in sheep are rare. Lincoln Animal Health Laboratory has reported ergot abortion after ewes were fed 'cleanings' from a seed-dressing plant. There is also anecdotal evidence of macrocarpa causing abortion. Abortions may also occur as a result of trauma to the ewe's abdomen, e.g. at crutching or when mobs are crowded through narrow gateways, or secondary to disease in the ewe such as pregnancy toxaemia, although such instances are rare.

Nitrate poisoning and foetal abnormalities (and abortion?) in sheep

In 1974, AM Day presented a paper to the Sheep and Beef Cattle Society of the New Zealand Veterinary Association in which were reported five outbreaks of arthrogryposis where up to 4% of lambs born were affected. These losses occurred in ewe flocks affected by nitrate poisoning during early to mid-gestation. Increased numbers of dry ewes were also reported.

In 1990, Gumbrell presented seven reports of farms in Canterbury where, following high autumn nitrate levels in various plants, deformed lambs were born in the following spring and there were increased numbers of dry ewes in the affected flocks.

The various feeds incriminated in these occurrences included rape (*Brassica napus*), new grass (ryegrass), short-rotation ryegrass, green oats, grass and turnips. The main feature of all these outbreaks were lambs that were born with twisted limbs, undershot lower jaws through to severe arthrogryposis. In some flocks up to 33% of the ewes were dry. The period of pregnancy when the ewes were exposed to high nitrate levels in their feed was usually at about the two months stage or earlier.

Laboratory tests showed no evidence of Akabane virus infection. It has been suggested that exposure of pregnant ewes to high levels of nitrate may result in early abortion. If exposure occurs around 60 days of gestation, the foetus may suffer from the effects of hypoxia resulting from the methaemoglobinaemia of nitrate poisoning.

Exotic diseases causing abortion in sheep

A range of diseases that occur overseas can cause significant abortion in sheep; some of these are described in Chapter 21. The list includes:

- enzootic abortion due to *Chlamydophila* (*Chlamydia*) *abortus*
- Rift Valley fever
- Wesselbron disease
- Akabane disease
- tick-borne fever
- brucellosis due to *Brucella melitensis*
- salmonellosis, particularly *Salmonella abortus-ovis*
- Q-fever (*Coxiella burnetii*).

Some of these are unlikely to occur in New Zealand because of the lack of insect vectors and other factors. However, Animal Health Laboratories has constantly checked for such important diseases as enzootic abortion of ewes, salmonellosis and *B. melitensis*.

The clinical investigation of abortion in sheep

Sheep farmers, particularly those in intensive farming areas, are quite sensitive about abortion in their ewe flocks. Experience with abortion investigations and the continual submission of abortion material for laboratory testing confirms this.

It is unlikely that a significant (over 5%) outbreak of abortion would not be investigated by a veterinarian, with samples being submitted for testing. Therefore it is most important that a good clinical procedure is followed to ensure that a diagnosis is reached and the best possible advice is given to the farmer.

The following is a summary of the routine procedure that should be followed in significant abortion investigations.

History

First and foremost a full history of the case must be taken:
- Has an abortion outbreak occurred before on the property?
- Have stock been bought in?
- Which group is the problem confined to?
- Are the two-tooths mixed with the older ewes?
- Are ewe hoggets mated?
- Is stock kept at a high density?
- Are the ewes vaccinated for campylobacteriosis?
- Are the ewes vaccinated for toxoplasmosis?
- Are the ewes vaccinated for *Salmonella* Brandenburg?

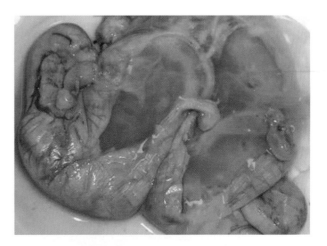

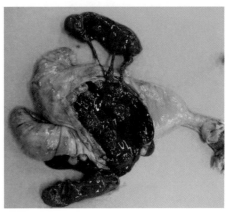

Figure 4.7 Dead resorbing foetuses possibly due to *Neospora caninum*.

- Are the ewes showing any systemic signs such as illness or death?
- What state are the aborted foetuses in when expelled (fresh or autolysed)?

It is vital to visit the farm and discuss the problem with the farmer to get a full appreciation of each particular situation, i.e. farm topography, management methods and general stock health.

Clinical examination

Initially necropsies should be carried out on the farm, if lambs and/or ewes are available; often, tentative diagnoses can be made at this stage based on the history, the clinical picture and the necropsy findings (e.g. campylobacteriosis or *S.* Brandenburg). If animals are not available or if doubt still exists, the farmer can bring further foetuses into the clinic. Ideally a minimum of 10 foetuses and membranes from reasonably fresh cases should be collected for such an examination. These should be examined for gross lesions and the best four or five sampled. The best samples to take are fresh and fixed cotyledons. From the foetus, fresh stomach contents and heart blood or thoracic fluid should be collected along with fresh and fixed brain, lung, liver and spleen. Costs for examination will vary according to the laboratory.

A firm diagnosis should be possible following laboratory examination of these samples. Further sampling at 10-day intervals may be warranted, if the diagnosis remains unclear or if it is suspected that more than one infectious agent is present.

REFERENCES

Anderson P. The implications of *Campylobacter* infections in ewe flocks. *Proceedings of the Society of Sheep and Beef Cattle Veterinarians, New Zealand Veterinary Association* 31, 31-40, 2001

Bailey KM. Sheep abortion outbreak associated with *Salmonella* Brandenburg. *Surveillance* 24, 10-11, 1997

Bailey KM. *Campylobacter* species in sheep. *Surveillance* 24, 14-15, 1997

Bailey K. *Salmonella* Brandenburg — Canterbury 2008. *The Society of Sheep and Beef Cattle Veterinarians NZVA Newsletter*, No. 35, 20, 2009

Barlow RM, Gardiner AC, Nettleton PF. The pathology of a spontaneous and experimental mucosal disease like syndrome in sheep recovered from clinical border disease. *Journal of Comparative Pathology*, 93, 451-61, 1983

Buxton D. Toxoplasmosis and neosporosis. In: *Diseases of Sheep* (3rd ed), edited by Martin WB and Aitken ID. Oxford, Blackwell Scientific Publications, 2000

Buxton D. Diagnosis of chlamydial and *Toxoplasma* abortion. *Proceedings of the Society of Sheep and Beef Cattle Veterinarians, New Zealand Veterinary Association* 2, 324-9, 1989

Clark RG, Fenwick SG, Nicol CM, Marchant RM, Swanney S, Gill JM, Holmes JD, Leyland M, Davies PR. *Salmonella* Brandenburg — emergence of a new strain affecting stock and humans in the South Island of New Zealand. *New Zealand Veterinary Journal* 52, 26-36, 2004

Clark RG, Gill JM. A review of sheep abortions in Otago and Southland. *VetScript* 15, 18-19, 2002

Day AM. Arthrogryposis, infertility and nitrate poisoning. *Proceedings of the Society of Sheep and Beef Cattle Veterinarians, New Zealand Veterinary Association* 4, 43-5, 1974

Dennis SM. *Vibrio fetus* infection in sheep. *Veterinary Record* 7, 69-82, 1961

Dubey JP, Towle A. *Toxoplasmosis in sheep: A review and annotated bibliography.* Commonwealth Institute of Parasitology, St Albans, UK, 1986

Gardner DE. Abortion associated with mycotic infection in sheep. *New Zealand Veterinary Journal* 15, 85-6, 1967

Gill J, Clark G. *Salmonella* Brandenburg update from Otago and Southland. *The Society of Sheep and Beef Cattle Veterinarians NZVA Newsletter*, No.35, 20-1, 2009

Gill J, Haydon TG, Rawdon G, McFadden AMJ, Ha HJ, Shen Z, Pang J, Swennes AG, Paster BJ, Dewhirst FE, Fox JG, Spence RP. *Helicobacter bilis* and *Helicobacter trogontum*: Infectious causes of abortion in sheep. *Journal of Veterinary Diagnostic Investigation* 28, 225-34, 2016

Gumbrell RC. Sheep abortions — what we do not have. *Surveillance* 15, 17-18, 1988

Gumbrell RC. Nitrate poisoning and foetal abnormalities in sheep. *Surveillance* 17, 10-11, 1990

Gumbrell RC, Saville DJ, Graham CF. Tactical control of ovine Campylobacter abortion outbreaks with a bacterin. *New Zealand Veterinary Journal* 44, 61-3, 1996

Hartley WJ. Some investigations into the epidemiology of ovine toxoplasmosis. *New Zealand Veterinary Journal* 14, 106-17, 1961

Hartley WJ. Experimental transmission of toxoplasmosis in sheep. *New Zealand Veterinary Journal* 9, 1-6 (correction 9: 47), 1961

Hartley WJ, Boyes BW. Incidents of ovine perinatal mortality in New Zealand with particular reference to intra-uterine infections. *New Zealand Veterinary Journal* 12, 33-6, 1964

Hartley WJ, Kater JC. Perinatal disease conditions of sheep in New Zealand. *New Zealand Veterinary Journal* 12, 49-57, 1964

Hartley WJ, Marshall SC. Toxoplasmosis as a cause of ovine perinatal mortality. *New Zealand Veterinary Journal* 5, 119-24, 1957

Hill, Fl. AgriQuality disease reports: Ovine abortions, nitrate in feed and Salmonella isolates. *VetScript* 12, 14-5, 1999

Howe L, Collett MG, Pattison RS, Marshall J, West DM, Pomroy WE. Potential involvement of Neospora caninum in naturally occurring ovine abortions in New Zealand. *Veterinary Parasitology* 185, 64-71, 2012

Jensen Rue, Miller VA, Hammarlund MA, Graham WR. Vibrionic abortion in sheep: 1. Transmission and immunity. *American Journal of Veterinary Research* 18, 326-9, 1957

Jensen Rue, Miller VA, Morbello JA. Placental pathology of sheep with vibrionic abortion in sheep: 1. Transmission and immunity. *American Journal of Veterinary Research* 22, 326-9, 1961

Kerslake J, Perkins NR, Davies PR. *Salmonella* Brandenburg in sheep: Case-control survey of sheep in New Zealand. *New Zealand Veterinary Journal* 54, 125-31, 2006

Li H, McFarlane RG, Wagner J. Vaccination of pregnant ewes against infection with *Salmonella* Brandenburg. *New Zealand Veterinary Journal* 53, 416-22, 2005

Mannering S, Fenwick S, Marchant R, Perkins N, West D. *Campylobacter fetus* subsp. *fetus* abortions in sheep: PFGE strain typing of isolates from 1999 and 2000. *Proceedings of the Society of Sheep and Beef Cattle Veterinarians, New Zealand Veterinary Association* 31, 23-30, 2001

Mannering SA, West DM, Marchant R, Fenwick SG, O'Connell K. *Campylobacter fetus* subsp. *fetus* abortion in sheep: A study of strain types and vaccine protection. *Proceedings of the Society of Sheep and Beef Cattle Veterinarians, New Zealand Veterinary Association* 33, 115-20, 2003

Marchant R. The use of vaccine to reduce the impact of *S.* Brandenburg disease in sheep. *Proceedings of the Society of Sheep and Beef Cattle Veterinarians, New Zealand Veterinary Association* 32, 161-70, 2002

McFarlane D, Salisbury RM, Osborne HG, Jebson JL. Investigation into sheep abortion in New Zealand during the 1950 lambing season. *Australian Veterinary Journal* 28, 221-6, 1952

Orr M, Roe AR. A mucosal disease-like condition in lambs with hairy shaker disease. *New Zealand Veterinary Journal* 41, 152, 1993

Orr M. Animal Health Laboratory Network — sheep abortion cases 1996. *Surveillance* 24, 9-10, 1997

Porter WL, Lewis KHC, Manktelow BW. Hairy shaker disease of lambs: Acquired immunity, abortion and transmission via mucous membranes. *New Zealand Veterinary Journal* 20, 4-7, 1972

Porter WL, Lewis KHC, Manktelow BW. Hairy shaker disease of lambs: Further studies on acquired immunity, abortion and effects on foetal growth. *New Zealand Veterinary Journal* 20, 4-7, 1972

Quinlivin TD, Jopp AJ. A survey on the incidence and cause of ovine abortion in Hawkes Bay. *New Zealand Veterinary Journal* 30, 65-8, 1982

Ridler AL, Corner-Thomas RA, Kenyon PR, Griffiths KJ. Investigation of plasma progesterone and liveweight in ewe lambs affected by fetal loss. *New Zealand Veterinary Journal* 65, 34-8, 2017

Roe A. *Salmonella* Brandenburg: A practitioner's perspective. *Proceedings of the Society of Sheep and Beef Cattle Veterinarians, New Zealand Veterinary Association* 29, 23-8, 1999

Shortridge EH. Toxoplasmosis in cats in New Zealand. *New Zealand Veterinary Journal* 16, 129-30, 1968

Smibert RM. *Vibrio fetus var intestinalis* isolated from fecal and intestinal contents of clinically normal sheep: 1. Isolation of microaerophilic vibrios. *American Journal of Veterinary Research* 26, 315-9, 1965

Surveillance

(1975) (3): 13	Toxoplasma abortion
(1977) (1): 19	Ergot abortion in sheep
(1980) (4): 19	*Campylobacter* abortion in sheep
(1981) (4): 21	*Yersinia pseudotuberculosis* as a cause of abortion
(1982) (3): 16	Listeria abortions in goats
(1983) (4): 10	Sheep abortion: Tactical control of *Campylobacter fetus fetus* abortion with campylovexin bacterin
(1986) (2): 8	Sheep abortion: *Campylobacter* control: Hairy shaker disease
(2006) (4): 33	Listeria abortion

Teale AJ, Blewett DA, Miller JK. Experimentally induced toxolasmosis in young rams: the clinical syndrome and semen secretion of *Toxoplasma*. *Veterinary Record*, 111, 53-5, 1982

Te Punga WA. Toxoplasmosis in sheep: 2. Serological response in the early stages of infection. *New Zealand Veterinary Journal* 12, 153-5, 1964

Te Punga WA, Penrose ME. Toxoplasmosis in sheep: 1. Naturally occurring heat-stable and heat-labile antibodies, and accessary factor-like activity in sheep sera. *New Zealand Veterinary Journal* 12, 1502, 1964

Waldhalm DG, Mason DR, Meinershagen WD, Scrivener LH. Magpies as carriers of ovine *Vibrio fetus*. *Journal of the American Veterinary Medical Association* 144, 497-500, 1964

Watson WA, Hunter D, Bellhouse R. Studies on vibrionic infection of sheep and carrion crows. *Veterinary Record* 81, 220-6, 1967

West DM. Ovine abortion in New Zealand. *New Zealand Veterinary Journal* 50 (Suppl.), 93-5, 2002

West DM, Collett MG, Perkins NR, Christodoulopoulos G, Morris ST, Kenyon PR. Investigations of foetal loss in maiden ewes. *Proceedings of the Society of Sheep and Beef Cattle Veterinarians of the New Zealand Veterinary Association* 34, 147-60, 2004

Weston JF. Dose-titration challenge of pregnant hoggets with *Neospora caninum* tachyzoites. *Proceedings of the Society of Sheep and Beef Cattle Veterinarians, New Zealand Veterinary Association* 37, 137-45, 2007

Wilkins MF, O'Connell EO, Te Punga WA. Toxoplasmosis in sheep: Effect of a killed vaccine on lambing losses caused by experimental challenge with *Toxoplasma gondii*. *New Zealand Veterinary Journal* 35, 31-4, 1987

Wilkins MF, O'Connell EO, Te Punga WA. Toxoplasmosis in sheep III: Further evaluation of the ability of a live *toxoplasma gondii* vaccine to prevent lamb losses and reduce congenital infection following experimental oral challenge. *New Zealand Veterinary Journal* 36, 86-9, 1988

Wilkins MF. Toxoplasmosis — role of the ram. *Proceedings of the Society of Sheep and Beef Cattle Veterinarians, New Zealand Veterinary Association*, 32, 189-96, 2002

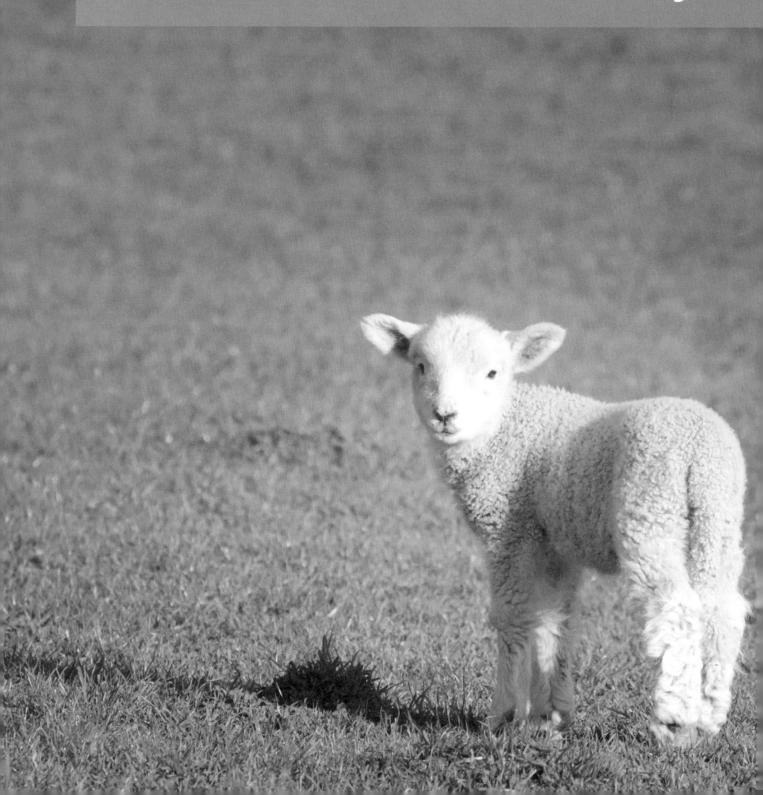

5

Lamb survival and lamb mortality

In New Zealand it is estimated that between 5% and 25% of lambs die before they are weaned, with the majority dying during the perinatal period. This significant loss was first highlighted by McFarlane (1955), who conducted extensive lamb mortality surveys that formed the basis for future investigations. With the widespread use of ultrasound pregnancy scanning, farmers are more aware of these losses. While some of these losses may be due to foetal resorption or abortion, on most properties the majority of the losses are due to lamb mortality at or after birth. Clearly this represents a significant financial loss not only to the individual farmer but also to the sheep industry.

Lamb losses and survival rates in New Zealand are somewhat anecdotal and are usually highlighted by media attention following severely inclement weather which may occur during lambing. With increased pregnancy rates now recorded at scanning and the higher national lambing percentages overall, the lamb mortality rate has also increased. Lamb survival varies widely between flocks, as can be seen from the data shown in Table 5.1.

These data emphasise this high production wastage. It is also of significance that the New Zealand lamb survival data are comparable to the results reported for more-intensive overseas lambing systems in the UK and USA. It is also interesting that the overseas surveys also showed the same variations between farms within each survey, i.e. high and low survival rates.

Investigation of lamb loss

In most cases veterinary assistance to investigate lamb loss problems is requested when a large number of dead lambs are seen during the lambing period and the cause (e.g. inclement weather) is not evident. Frequently the request for help does not come until after docking when the farmer finds a much lower percentage of lambs than in previous years, or there is a large discrepancy between the ultrasound scanning percentage and the docking percentage. Alternatively, at docking or weaning the number of wet/dry ewes may be high, suggesting that more lambs than usual have died. Thus it is often a retrospective investigation and in many cases the information will be incomplete, inaccurate and perhaps even exaggerated.

When investigating a high lamb mortality rate, a careful consideration of flock history and a wide range of necropsies on dead lambs must be undertaken. Often the losses are due to a number of inter-related factors rather than a single straightforward problem.

Estimation of losses

To define the magnitude of the problem, an estimate of the number of lambs lost is required. Where information is available and appropriate, data should be collected on the number of ewes mated, scanning percentage, number of lambs born, number of lambs tailed and number of lambs weaned. It is also useful to determine the number of dry/dry ewes (ewes that do not give birth to a lamb), which can be done either at scanning or prior to lambing, and the number of wet/dry ewes (ewes that do give birth to a lamb or lambs, which do not survive), which can be done at docking or weaning by palpation of the udder.

Another aid to diagnosis is the age marking of ewes, usually done with a coloured ear-tag system or by ear marking with either one or two notches from different parts of the ear. Such identification will enable the investigator to check two-tooth ewes against mixed-age ewes and so on. It will also give information on any ewe wastage that has occurred after mating and up to weaning.

Author and date	Breed of ewe	No. of ewes or lambs	Survival (% of lambs born)			
			mean	single	twin	triplet
Dalton et al., 1980	Coopworth	1532	85	87	78	
	Perendale	1776	87	89	81	
	Romney	1170	76	78	65	
Rohloff et al., 1982		96 farms	86–91	91	93	82
Scales et al., 1986†	Romney	516	81	83	81	58
Knight et al., 1988	Marshall Rom, Rom	1860	83	85	81	
Nicoll et al., 1999	Rom, Texel	16863	85	88	84	65
Tarbotton & Webby, 1999*†	Rom, Coop	2624	82	93	78‡	
Smeaton et al., 1999*	Rom x Finn	1250	90≠98§			
Litherland et al., 1999*†	Rom x Coop, Rom					
	— early	766	88		88	
	— late	510	79		79	
Jopson et al., 2000	Coopworth	817	77–93			
Kenyon et al., 2002	Romney	1030	79	83	80	59
Thomson et al., 2004	Mixed breeds	3376	87	90	88	76
Everett-Hincks, 2004	Coopworth-stud	~4000	89	89	94	78

Data published 1980 to 2004 for different breeds of ewes. Lamb survival measured from birth to weaning. When original data uses different beginning and end points the data have been corrected based on values from the paper by Nicoll et al., 1999.

* Data from scanning and assumed 4% loses from scanning to lambing; based on Nicoll et al., 1999.

† Data only up to docking, and assumed loss from docking to weaning of 3% for singles, 4% for twins, and 9% for triplets; based on Nicoll et al., 1999.

‡ Includes triplets.

§ There were a range of treatments, and data were not broken down into birth ranks.

Table 5.1 Lamb survival data from New Zealand (Muir et al., 2005).

History

A thorough history is essential when investigating lamb losses. Broad areas that should be included in the history are:

- breed of ewes and rams
- recent weather conditions
- paddock-, date- or ewe-age-related patterns to the lamb deaths
- feeding and management over pregnancy and lambing
- vaccination history (*Campylobacter,* toxoplasmosis, *Salmonella* Brandenburg and *Clostridia*)
- trace-element supplementation (iodine, selenium).

Diagnostic procedure

To determine the major causes of loss, postmortem examination of lambs needs to be carried out. It may be possible in some cases to conduct a significant survey of dead lambs during the season in which the problem has occurred. However, if the problem is presented retrospectively a full lamb mortality survey will need to be planned for the following season.

It cannot be emphasised too strongly that the more dead lambs that are submitted for examination from a problem property, the greater the chance of diagnosing the causes of death. If a wide sample of lambs is not included the result will probably be meaningless. For example, a sample of lambs taken following a storm may reveal the starvation/exposure complex when an overall survey may indicate that dystocia is the main cause of lamb death.

Before a survey is undertaken, the clients should be well informed of their part in the exercise. This includes ensuring that all lambs are collected and delivered for necropsy at least twice a week during the main lambing season. Because lambs are sterile when born and have little body fat they may be held for several days without significant deterioration, provided they are kept in shade and protected from dogs.

Necropsy procedure

A full description of the necropsy procedure for lambs has been given by McFarlane (1965). The main points to note are as follows.

The lamb should be accurately weighed and then examined externally first for details of having walked, subcutaneous oedema, congenital abnormalities and signs of predation.

The lamb is then placed on its right side (for a right-handed operator) and the skin of the left side is reflected by an incision through the axilla (between the foreleg and the rib cage). This incision is continued down the left side, care being taken not to open the abdomen at this stage, but cutting the hind limb through the coxofemoral joint. Both limbs are still attached to the lamb by a significant flap of skin and some muscle. The lamb is now flipped over and the same procedure followed on the right side. The lamb is lying on its back and the partly severed limbs hold it in a secure position for necropsy examination.

The sternum is carefully opened by an incision which removes the breast bone (sternum) and continues down the abdominal muscles, allowing the thoracic and abdominal organs to be seen. The skin of the neck must be carefully reflected right up to the lower mandible so that the thyroid glands can be seen lateral to the trachea near the larynx. The thyroid glands should be removed and weighed on accurate scales that measure to 0.1 g and the thyroid weight (in grams) should be divided by the lamb bodyweight (in kilograms) to give a thyroid to bodyweight ratio (in g/kg).

For an extensive lamb mortality survey it would be advisable to design and print a postmortem protocol. A good example of such is that of Everett-Hincks and Duncan (2008), which is summarised in Table 5.2.

Pathology

The following summary sets out the significance of a number of features encountered during the lamb necropsy. Each of these should be looked for and recorded if present.

- **Decomposition** — indicates pre-partum death.
- **Weight** — optimal lamb birthweight range is 4.5–6.5 kg (allow for breed variations). Excessive weight suggests dystocia; underweight suggests pre-partum problem

Step	
1	Weigh lamb to nearest kg
2	Record lamb's sex
3	Examine lamb externally for abnormalities
4	Observe feet (walked or not)
5	Dissect lamb as described in autopsy procedure
6	Check for subcutaneous oedema of head (obvious with dystocia, see Figure 5.3). Also check the naval region for infection
7	Remove and weigh thyroid glands (see autopsy procedure)
8	Check lungs (breathed or not breathed)
9	Check carcass degradation (indicates either pre- or post-natal death)
10	Check liver for rupture or other lesions
11	Examine heart and kidneys and observe state of brown fat
12	Examine stomach for milk clot and intestines and lymphatics for signs of milk absorption
13	Diagnosis A confirmed, e.g. starvation. Diagnosis B not confirmed. Could include samples sent for lab examination or simply unknown cause
14	Congenital and inherited abnormalities

Table 5.2 Post-mortem examination procedure.

- (feed, infection), and is often associated with exposure.
- **Feet** — absence of 'slippers' over the hooves indicates that the lamb walked and death was post-partum.
- **Umbilical vessels** — a blood clot indicates that death was partum or post-partum.
- **Navel cord** — a shrivelled cord indicates post-partum death, a square end indicates partum and a tapered end indicates pre-partum death.
- **Brown fat reserves** — primarily surrounding the heart and kidneys, these change from normal white-pink to purple-brown gelatinous as they are metabolised. Absence indicates post-partum death (and starvation/hypothermia).
- **Presence of milk in stomach and intestinal lymphatics** — indicates post-partum death.
- **Lung aeration** — indicates partum or post-partum death. Lung aeration can be determined by placing a section of lung in a jar of water: if it floats, then the lung was aerated.
- **Marked subcutaneous oedema of distal legs/tail and head with a swollen and protruding tongue** — indicates dystocia. Mild oedema may be associated with hypothermia.
- **Hepatic rupture, thoracic, or abdominal haemorrhage** — indicates dystocia.
- **Abscessation of organs such as umbilicus, liver, lung, joints** — indicates post-partum infection.

Causes of perinatal lamb mortality

While infectious causes account for 10–30% of lamb deaths, many of the remaining dead lambs have birthweights that are below average or above average for the breed. Optimum lamb birthweight for best survival is 4.5–6.5 kg for singles and multiples. Small birth size contributes significantly to starvation/exposure and large birth size contributes significantly to dystocia.

Foetal undersize

Lamb birthweight is related to ewe nutrition during pregnancy and litter size.

Inadequate ewe nutrition

Nutrition of the pregnant ewe must be emphasised for the profound effect it has on the condition score of the ewe and the birthweight of the lamb and its subsequent survival. Also, pregnant ewes with low condition scores (≤2.0) leading into lambing are at risk of mortality as well as prejudicing the survival of their progeny. These points are emphasised in Figures 5.1 and 5.2.

While birthweight is an important aspect of lamb survival as demonstrated in these figures, it should also be noted that there appears to be an optimum birthweight for survival. In Figure 5.1 the survival of lambs of birthweight above 6 kg slowly declines, possibly as a result of an increase in dystocia losses.

The effects of ewe under-nutrition on foetal viability are as follows:

1. Nutritional effects on the placenta

Placental weight increases markedly until approximately 90 days of gestation, and the weight and size of the placenta seems to impose a limit on its capacity to transfer nutrients to the foetus. Foetuses with poor placental development show growth retardation, chronic hypoglycaemia and chronic hypoxaemia. Prenatal death is common in such foetuses. Underfeeding of the ewe before 80–90 days of gestation is known to impede placental development and in the longer term survival of the newborn lamb, especially multiples.

2. Nutritional effects on the foetus

Under field conditions the nutrient demands for foetal growth in late pregnancy exceed maternal dietary supply, especially when two or more foetuses are carried. The ewe is then obliged to mobilise its own tissue reserves to meet the deficit and hence become more susceptible to pregnancy toxaemia (hypoglycaemia) as pregnancy advances. The reduced availability of glucose to the foetus causes growth retardation, and affected foetuses are unable to sustain high rates of heat production for long periods after birth. Such animals are born with depleted energy reserves, especially brown fat, which makes them more susceptible to starvation/exposure.

3. Nutritional effects on the mammary glands

The udder develops throughout pregnancy but the greatest increase in ewe udder weight is seen in the 30 days before parturition. At birth the weight of udder tissue averages

30–40% of total lamb weight and the energy needed to develop new udder tissue is similar to that of foetal growth during the last 30 days of pregnancy.

Underfeeding affects both udder size and udder performance. Reduced udder growth occurs within 3–5 days of the onset of underfeeding and impedes the prenatal accumulation of colostrum, which delays the onset of copious milk production after birth. This makes the lamb more susceptible to starvation/exposure and also, if adequate colostrum intake is not achieved, to infection.

4. Nutritional effects on the newborn

Nutritional inadequacy before birth, whether this is caused by a small placenta, maternal underfeeding or both, results in below average birthweight which is a common feature of lambs that die in the perinatal area. Generally, however, it is not low birthweight itself that causes lamb death but instead various physiological impairments that accompany growth retardation. For instance, placental insufficiency restricts both nutrient and oxygen supply to the foetus and the chronic foetal hypoxaemia inhibits heat production for several hours after birth, thus threatening the survival of the newborn lamb.

In order to minimise the contribution of ewe undernutrition on lamb mortality, it is recommended that ewes are in good body condition at mating and that this body condition is maintained throughout pregnancy. Ewes should be set-stocked for lambing onto pasture covers of at least 1200 kg DM/ha (kilograms of dry matter per hectare) at such a rate that pasture cover is maintained or increases to around 1400 kg DM/ha over early lactation.

Large litter size

The birthweight of twins and triplets is lower than that for singles, and this renders them more susceptible to starvation/exposure. Also, when a ewe produces numerous lambs there is an increased likelihood of mismothering and inadequate colostrum intake or milk for one or some of the lambs. With the use in New Zealand of highly prolific sheep breeds (such as the Finn and the Booroola) or the use of vaccines against ovarian steroids, there is potential for associated increased lamb losses unless feeding and management regimens are in place to minimise these losses.

For full production advantage to be achieved and welfare

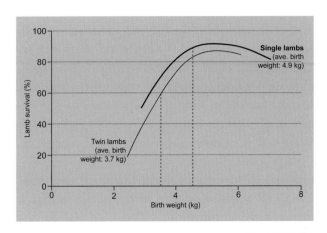

Figure 5.1 Survival of lambs at birthweight.

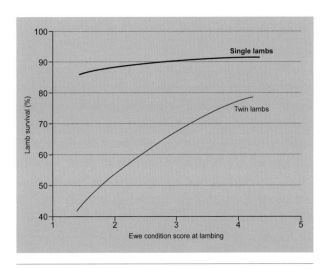

Figure 5.2 Condition score and lamb survival.

issues resulting from the increased numbers of multiple births occurring in New Zealand sheep flocks to be avoided, there is a challenging need for a better understanding of the breeding and husbandry of the high-performance ewe rearing multiple lambs. This may involve significant changes in breeding and selection, and greater attention to feeding and body condition and weight throughout the life of the ewe. Even the feeding of concentrate prior to lambing and the organisation of intensive lambing programmes, in some situations indoors, may be possibilities. It should be recognised that intensive indoor lambing systems have associated disease husbandry considerations and a high level of management is required. If supplements are to be fed, sheep need to be trained to eat them at least 6–8 weeks before lambing is due to start. For New Zealand pasture-fed sheep this can be a tedious procedure and requires patience.

Pre-lamb shearing

There is some evidence that shearing ewes 70 days after the mid-point of mating leads to an increase in both lamb birthweights and weaning weights. The increased lamb birthweight is also associated with higher survival rates to weaning in twin-born lambs. However, shearing ewes in winter can be associated with increased ewe losses, and if this technique is employed ewes should be shorn with a cover-comb and provided with adequate feed and shelter after shearing.

Dystocia

Dystocia is an important cause of parturient deaths and on some properties can contribute to very high percentages of lamb deaths. Large single lambs are the most likely to create problems and these are more common within some breeds or strains of sheep. However, dystocia may also be associated with smaller lambs, particularly in multiple births. Use of a large terminal sire breed of ram, particularly over hoggets, can also contribute. In some breeds of sheep overseas up to 50% of ewes may need assistance at lambing.

As long as early placental development is normal, starving or underfeeding ewes in late pregnancy is unlikely to influence the birthweight of the lamb but may lead to metabolic disease in the ewe, reduced foetal viability and reduced ewe milking ability. It has been suggested that excessively fat ewes have a higher incidence of dystocia (and vaginal prolapse) due to increased fat in the abdomen and pelvic canal. Thus it is recommended that ewe body condition score is maintained throughout pregnancy but that ewes do not become overfat, and that underfeeding of ewes in late pregnancy does not occur.

The criteria for assessing prolonged and difficult birth include:
- high lamb birthweights (up to 8 kg) — note that some small lambs also die from dystocia
- local subcutaneous oedema of the presenting position of the foetus
- abdominal haemorrhage derived from liver rupture or tearing of the liver capsule
- petechia and ecchymoses of the pleura, thymus and heart.

Central nervous system injury, haemorrhage and congestion in and around the cranial and spinal meninges have been reported as a particular feature occurring in a high percentage of parturient deaths (Haughey, 1973), although similar lesions have also been found in control lambs. Injuries to the central nervous system may cause failure to suck, depresses general viability, and may cause depressed growth of the lamb. Many lambs that survive a difficult birth will walk and feed but die subsequently.

The case history shown opposite of an investigation into a lamb mortality problem will help to emphasise the importance of a logical approach to the investigation of lamb deaths.

Trace-element deficiencies

Selenium deficiency/white muscle disease

In sheep, white muscle disease is now uncommon as the widespread use of selenium has largely prevented its occurrence. In goat kids it can be a significant disease on selenium-deficient country (see also Chapter 7).

White muscle disease may be responsible for perinatal deaths due to congenital white muscle disease. Such cases usually show heart lesions in particular, but skeletal

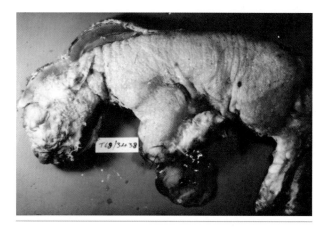

Figure 5.3 Dystocia caused by retention of forelegs. Note extensive oedema of neck and head.

muscles may also be affected. It has been reported in selenium-deficient areas post-docking. The clinical signs in these cases include:
- sudden onset of a flaccid or semi-flaccid paralysis
- muscle groups nevertheless are hard and stiff (necrosis and calcification)
- animals are frequently unable to walk or may only walk with difficulty and frequently may be seen dragging one leg
- difficulty in suckling, due to pharyngeal paralysis, is a frequent sign and lambs often appear starved; loss of appetite often precedes death by less than 48 hours
- difficulty in breathing may also be seen and this may be associated with an aspiration pneumonia.

Prevention of white muscle disease is attained by supplementing ewes at least 6 weeks pre-lambing with selenium and/or selenium and vitamin E.

Iodine deficiency

Goitre

Goitre is a potential cause of lamb mortality, particularly when feeding brassica crops during pregnancy as these contain the goitrogenic agents thiocyanate and thiouracil. Goats appear to have a higher requirement for iodine than other farmed species (see also Chapter 7).

The main features of goitre are the occasional birth of small woolless lambs and small kids that have an increased mortality rate. Overt goitre may be seen and the thyroid gland may be many times larger than normal. Sometimes goitre may lead to dystocia and subsequent lamb deaths.

CASE HISTORY

The farmer reported a large number of lambs which, although dead, showed no abnormal features. He was not assisting large numbers of ewes to lamb nor did he see ewes having difficulty lambing.
A summary of necropsy is as follows:

	Cause of death			
	Dystocia	Starvation	Pyelonephritis	Navel Infection
Male	16	2	1	1
Female	12	1		
Total number	28	3	1	1

Dystocia was obviously the predominant cause of lamb death.
A breakdown of weight for sex in these dystocia cases was:

Weight (kg)	3.0-3.5	3.6-4.0	4.1-4.5	4.6-5.0	5.1-5.5	5.6-6.0	6.1-6.5
Male	1	3	1	2	5	4	2
Female	1	2	4	1	2	0	0

Ram lambs were over-represented in this group and 50% of these weighed 5 kg or greater.

Subclinical iodine deficiency

Subclinical iodine deficiency may be a contributor to lamb mortality (see also Chapter 7). Affected lambs have a decreased metabolic rate, impaired brain development, reduced lung development and maturation and impaired suckling behaviour. Thus, depending on the weather conditions during lambing, many of these lambs may die from starvation/exposure.

Diagnosis of subclinical iodine deficiency is by postmortem examination of 15–20 dead lambs. As part of the routine necropsy procedure, lamb bodyweight and both thyroid glands should be weighed using accurate scales, and the thyroid to bodyweight ratio calculated. A mean ratio of greater than 0.4 g/kg is considered indicative of subclinical iodine deficiency, and ratios of over 0.7 g/kg are considered indicative of goitre.

Treatment

Lambs and kids that are over 3–5 days old should be given Lugol's iodine (a few drops in water) for 15 days. However, once established, only a slight reduction in the size of the goitre is likely following treatment.

Prevention of iodine deficiency

Goitre and subclinical iodine deficiency can be prevented by dosing ewes with 280 mg of potassium iodide 8 and 4 weeks prior to parturition, or by intramuscular injection of 1.5 ml of iodised oil (Depodine, Alleva Animal Health) prior to mating. The iodine in this product is bound to an oily adjuvant that provides a more regular and sustained supply of iodine to the ewe and developing foetus than does oral drenching.

Infectious causes

Infectious agents can contribute to lamb mortality directly, or indirectly by resulting in weak lambs that are slow to rise and suckle or follow the dam and as a consequence die from starvation/exposure.

Navel infection

A number of organisms cause navel infections and subsequent multi-organ abscessation, but the most common are *Fusobacterium necrophorum* and *Trueperella pyogenes* (*Arcanobacterium pyogenes*). Lambs born in wet, muddy, contaminated environments are likely to be more susceptible, as are those that do not receive adequate colostrum. In navel infection the following body and organ changes may be noted:

- gangrene of the ventral abdomen
- acute or subacute inflammatory changes in the umbilical-vesical membrane
- localised or diffuse serofibrinous or suppurative peritonitis
- liver or other organ abscesses, pleurisy, pericardial effusion and pericarditis are occasionally present.

Campylobacteriosis/toxoplasmosis/hairy shaker

These agents have been implicated as contributing to birth of weak lambs that are slow to rise and suckle and as a consequence commonly die of starvation/exposure (see Chapter 4).

Watery mouth (E. coli endotoxaemia)

This is an important cause of lamb mortality in Great Britain, but is less commonly diagnosed in New Zealand. It is, however, mentioned in *Surveillance* (Animal Health Laboratory) reports from time to time. In one such example, 50 of 1500 lambs died within two days of birth. The disease occurs in 1- to 3-day-old lambs and is thought to be due to the neutral pH of the abomasum (true stomach) during the first 24 hours of life allowing non-enterotoxigenic strains of *Escherichia coli* to pass into the intestine. The *E. coli* is lysed in the intestinal lumen and the subsequent endotoxin release leads to a generalised endotoxaemia. There is also gas production in the gastrointestinal tract causing abdominal distension and pain, and a septicaemia. Affected lambs are depressed with poor peripheral perfusion, congested mucous membranes, excessive salivation and distended abdomen. Eventually the lambs die of endotoxaemic shock or starvation/exposure.

Lambs ingest the organism from the dirty wool and udder of the dam during teat-searching, and thus cases are more likely to occur when environmental conditions are wet and muddy, pre-lamb crutching of the ewes has not been carried out or the ewe is producing little colostrum so teat-searching is protracted. Early colostrum intake prevents watery mouth and thus prevention is by lambing in a clean environment, pre-lamb crutching of ewes and ensuring adequate colostrum intake. In badly affected flocks, routine prophylactic treatment of lambs with oral antibiotics is sometimes undertaken. If treatment of watery mouth is undertaken, it should be instituted at an early stage of the disease. Affected lambs should be injected daily with antibiotics (amoxicillin or tetracyclines), fed three times daily by stomach tube with a glucose and electrolyte solution and be given a soapy enema to encourage gut movement. Non-steroidal anti-inflammatory drugs may also be useful.

Inherited and congenital conditions of sheep

A small percentage of lambs may show congenital defects at birth; others develop the signs of such defects later.

Table 5.3 contains a list of inherited and congenital conditions of sheep. Many are rare and not mentioned in this text, while others have, in their time, caused losses in the flocks in which they occurred. The latter conditions of importance are described in the context of their clinical and pathological presentation and will be found in the appropriate chapters of this book. For a detailed record of these diseases we are indebted to the extensive research and publications of Emeritus Professor RD Jolly (see Jolly RD, Blair HT, Johnstone AC, Genetic disorders of sheep in New Zealand: A review and perspective, *New Zealand Veterinary Journal* 52 (2), 52–64, 2004).

Starvation/exposure

Lamb losses due to starvation/exposure have been estimated at between 25% and 50% of the losses that occur in the first week of life, and these occur particularly 1–3 days after birth. Starvation and exposure are interlinked, as illustrated in Figure 5.4.

Starvation/exposure is a multifactorial syndrome and there are numerous predisposing factors such as:
- foetal undersize
- dystocia/birth injuries
- goitre or subclinical iodine deficiency
- unfavourable weather during lambing, particularly a combination of wind and rain
- steep or poorly sheltered lambing paddocks (lambing on steep topography increases the chances of lambs slipping down the hill away from the birth site and becoming mismothered)
- mastitis, hard udder or agalactia of the ewe
- poor mothering ability of the ewe (influenced by age, nutrition levels, litter size and individual variation between ewes — hoggets or two-tooths have lower lamb survival, underfed ewes will leave the birth site earlier to graze, large litters mean that the weaker lamb may be left behind)

Agenesis of cerebellar vermis (Dandy-Walker defect)
Amputated limbs in Southdown lambs
Atresia of the anus
Cataract
Cerebellar abiotrophy
Cerebellar cortical atrophy ('daft lamb' disease 1)
Chondrodysplasia of Texel sheep (dwarfing)
Cleft palate
Congenital deafness
Congenital dropsy of Southdown lambs
Ehlers-Danlos syndrome (skin fragility)
Entropion
Epidermolysis bullosa (skin and wool defect)
Familial episodic ataxia
Hereditary chondrodysplasia ('spider syndrome') of Suffolk sheep
Hypospadias
Hypothyroidism (congenital goitre)
Inherited rickets
Inherited taillessness
Intersexes (freemartins)
Inverdale streak ovary
Jaw defects (brachygnathia and prognathia)
Klinefelter syndrome
Lower motor neuron disease
Lustrous wool (Romney sheep)
Lysosmal storage disease
   (A) Glycogen storage disease (type 11)
   (B) GM1 gangliosidosis
   (C) Ceroid-lipofuscinosis
Mesangiocapillary glomerulonephritis in Finnish Landrace sheep
Microphthalmia
Neuroaxonal dystrophy
Osteogenesis imperfecta with skin fragility (multiple fractures of long bones and ribs)
Ovine spongiform leucoencephalopathy
Photosensitisation of Southdown sheep (hyperbilirubinaemia)
Polycystic kidneys
Short spine in Perendale sheep
Star gazing lambs ('daft lamb' disease 2)
Yellow fat

Table 5.3 Congenital and inherited defects.

- husbandry during the lambing period (this influences birth site location, bonding, mismothering, dystocia).

Thus, either as a combination of factors or in isolation, lambs that are weak at birth, inclement weather conditions, lambs that do not get adequate colostrum/milk and mismothering can result in starvation and/or exposure.

At necropsy, signs of starvation/exposure are:

Starvation

- General dehydration of the cadaver.
- Liver is small and less friable than usual.
- Stomach and small intestine are contracted and generally empty, may have fed and even have some chyle in lymph vessels. Meconium generally voided.
- Body fat is generally limited or completely absorbed.
- The lamb will usually have walked.

Exposure

If the lamb died soon after birth, there will be very few postmortem signs. The lamb may or may not have walked, fed or absorbed food, and there may have been only slight fat utilisation. At necropsy there may be:

- mild yellowish subcutaneous oedema of the extremities
- varying depletion of the brown adipose tissue
- haemorrhages in the meninges and occasionally in subcutaneous and periosteal tissues
- normal hydration of tissues
- empty gastrointestinal tract.

Because of New Zealand's outdoor lambing system and unpredictable weather, some degree of lamb loss from starvation/exposure is inevitable. However, losses can be minimised by reducing the predisposing factors. Thus:

- Ensure adequate ewe nutrition and general health throughout pregnancy and lactation.
- Avoid exacerbating dystocia by using large-breed rams over small ewes.
- If required, supplement with selenium and iodine and vaccinate for campylobacteriosis and toxoplasmosis.
- Ultrasound pregnancy scanning can be used to identify single and twin/triplet-bearing ewes. Ewes bearing multiples can then be preferentially fed and lambed in the more sheltered paddocks.
- Ideally, lambing paddocks should be of moderate topography and contain shelter.

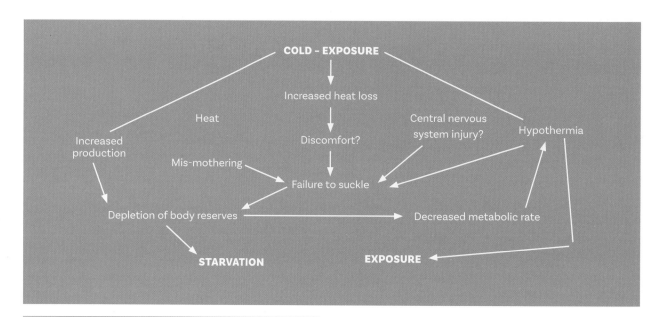

Figure 5.4 Starvation/exposure interactions (adapted from McCutcheon et al., 1981).

- Cull ewes with obvious udder defects.
- Most farmers cull mixed-age wet/dry ewes; many will identify and retain wet/dry hoggets/two-tooths.
- Ensure shepherding is of a high standard.

Lactation deaths

Nationally, losses in suckling lambs are usually minor but may be serious in individual flocks. Many of the causes are discussed elsewhere in this text but are listed at this stage to assist in the differential diagnosis.

Specific diseases that may cause lamb deaths between birth and lamb docking, and frequently later, are as follows:
- enterotoxaemia
- latent navel infections, particularly *Fusobacterium necrophorum*, *Trueperella pyogenes* and *Erysipelothrix rhusiopathiae*
- trace-element deficiencies:
    * Copper — swayback
    * Selenium/vitamin E — white muscle disease
    * Iodine — goitre
- many non-fatal diseases also appear at this time, e.g. scabby mouth, footrot, arthritis, pink eye, etc.
- bacterial and viral enteritides may be prevalent in intensive situations, e.g. indoor rearing

Immediately following lamb docking, the above diseases may still appear but the following are more likely to be important:
- tetanus 1–3 weeks from docking
- blackleg and malignant oedema 1–3 days after docking
- fatal haemorrhage (tail docking with knives) 1–2 days after docking

From lamb docking to weaning, any of the above diseases may occur but parasitic diseases now become more significant:
- coccidiosis — important under wet conditions and when lambs are overstocked
- nematode parasitism, particularly *Nematodirus* (South Island), *Haemonchus* and *Ostertagia*
- tick infestations (Northland and East Coast North Island in particular), although usually seen post-weaning

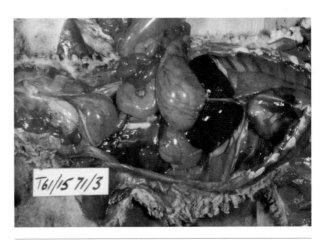

Figure 5.5 Starved lamb. Note the empty stomach and the metabolism of fat around the heart and kidney.

Predation

Occasionally lamb losses from predation may be severe. In New Zealand, predation is generally by feral pigs or uncontrolled dogs; on some New Zealand sheep stations considerable lamb losses have been suffered due to feral pig predation. Usually a particular boar or sow will become the main killer, even devouring lambs as they are born. Evidence of this is provided by detection of lamb carcasses in the gut contents of feral pigs at necropsy. Predation by foxes, dingoes, feral pigs and crows are common causes of perinatal lamb loss in Australia.

To confirm that the cause of death is due to predation (if the carcass is still available), there must be evidence of severe ante-mortem trauma and no other lesions that could have caused death. Carcasses need to be skinned so that the extent of the trauma can be properly ascertained.

General considerations

Dead lambs

Deaths are invariably concentrated in the first few days after birth, reflecting the problems of transition from an intra-uterine existence to a less dependent extra-uterine life.

Birthweight

Mortality is lowest at birthweights between 4.5 and 6.5 kg. Generally, below 3.5 kg there is an increase in starvation/exposure and above 6.5 kg increased dystocia problems are likely to occur.

Litter size

Mortality usually increases with litter size, mainly associated with decreased birthweight. Milk supply can also be a limiting factor affecting growth and survival (see above). This is especially of significance with highly fecund sheep such as the Booroola and Finnish Landrace, which invariably have multiple births.

Age and parity of ewes

Mortality can be very high in primiparas (exacerbated if ewes are lambed first as hoggets rather than as two-tooths). A major part of this is behavioural, but lambs born to two-tooths may be 15% lighter than those born to mixed-age ewes. The mortality rate is usually minimal over the next 4–5 pregnancies and then tends to rise again as the ewe becomes aged.

Breed

Some large breeds of sheep if mated with smaller ewes of another breed may cause dystocia problems. Differences also occur between strains of sheep within breeds. For example, in the Texel breed high levels of dystocia have been reported with some strains, while in others selection of easy lambing has resulted in dystocia not being a problem.

Slope	% of single-born lambs	% of twin-born lambs
0° to 24°	0	0
24° to 31°	4	12
31° to 44°	34	52

Table 5.4 Deaths (as percentage of lambs born) attributable to effects of slipping from birth site (Knight et al., 1983).

Sex

Male lambs have generally a slightly lower survival rate than females, although this may be complicated by dystocia.

Prevention of lamb losses

To prevent high lamb mortality occurring, management should aim at giving the lamb the best opportunity to survive. To this end the specific causes of loss such as disease, starvation, exposure and predation should, where possible, be minimised. The following factors should be considered in the advice that may be given to the farmer.

Nutrition during pregnancy

As discussed earlier in the chapter, nutrition of ewes is vital at all stages of pregnancy. In early pregnancy adequate nutrition is important for placental growth, while in late pregnancy it is necessary for foetal energy reserves, ewe mammary gland development and the prevention of pregnancy toxaemia.

The treatment of ewes according to litter size

The separation of single-bearing and multiple-bearing (multiple) ewes by ultrasound examination is of value. Because of the higher feed requirements of the twin-bearing ewes, these can be fed preferentially and thus reduce the risk of pregnancy toxaemia. This may be especially useful on farms with high stocking rates. Multiple-bearing ewes may also be lambed in the more sheltered paddocks.

General health of ewes

Good health of pregnant and lactating sheep is essential. This involves parasite control, attention to lameness (e.g. footrot), prophylactic vaccination with clostridial vaccines and in some cases Johne's disease control. Pre-lamb crutching is important for clearing the udder region of excess wool, enabling lambs to find teats and minimising bacterial ingestion, and this procedure is commonly combined with a clostridial booster vaccination and sometimes pre-lamb parasite control.

Selection of lambing paddocks and shelter

At times, ewes do not or cannot select a safe lambing site and will often lamb on the top of a slope or in an exposed area. Thus, selection of appropriate lambing paddocks is important for reducing lamb mortality. Ideally, the flatter paddocks should be selected for lambing as on steep slopes lambs will frequently roll away from the ewe (twin lambs in particular), become isolated and die of starvation (Table 5.4). Also, during the first few hours of life lambs on steep slopes have difficulty in rising and suckling.

Lambing paddocks should, where possible, be selected with some shelter against prevailing winds. The best shelter usually consists of trees or pampas grass planted as hedges. When shelter is being planned, ewes should be observed because they may select lambing areas irrespective of shelter (so plan shelter around where they choose to lamb). Shorn ewes tend to make better use of shelter than those that are unshorn.

For valuable or intensively managed flocks, commercial lamb covers are available. Commercially available sheets of synthetic material that can be attached to fences to act as a windbreak are also an option to increase shelter in exposed paddocks.

Stocking density, paddock size and feed quantity

Increased stocking density over lambing increases social stress, and mismothering of lambs increases disproportionately above 18 SU/ha. Paddocks should not be too large and water sources not too far apart, especially with multiple-bearing ewes, so that the risk of separation of ewe and lamb is minimised.

Poor pasture cover (less than 1000 kg DM/ha) may increase mismothering and lamb deaths, as poorly fed ewes move away from the birth site earlier and wander further to graze. It is recommended that lambing ewes are grazing pasture of at least 1200 kg DM/ha.

Husbandry

Depending on the situation of the sheep farm and the intensity of production, lambing systems can vary from easy or no care, minimal interference, intensive shepherding outdoors, drift lambing to indoor lambing.

Shepherding, unless done with care and by an experienced operator, can severely affect the ewes' behaviour and settling in a birth site. The birth site may be selected up to 3 days prior to lambing. Some breeds spend more time at the birth site than others. The Australian Merino will spend about 2 hours and the New Zealand Romney up to 6 hours at the birth site before lambing. Also young ewes (two-tooths) spend more time on the birth site than do older ewes that have lambed previously. Thus ewes in labour or about to enter labour can be upset if they are moved daily to new pasture or are frightened away from their selected birth site.

Time of lambing

To ensure a short lambing period, ewes should be mated at the time of optimum oestrous activity for a given geographical region. This also allows the best use of available pasture for the lactating ewe. Lambing dates can be established for several groups within a given flock by the use of crayons on tupping harnesses. The colour of the crayon is changed every 14–16 days during mating.

Selection and culling

Both the ewes' ability to rear lambs and lamb viability are heritable traits, although heritabilities may vary. Selection for high lambing may be helpful in raising lambing percentages, but it is a long-term process. Culling is generally made on the presence of a physical defect (mastitis, shearing damage to udder, etc.) or the inability to rear at least one lamb (except primiparous ewes). Rams should come from dams that have consistently reared live lambs.

Care of newborn lambs

Newborn lambs are susceptible to hypothermia and hypoglycaemia; thus, a source of warmth and glucose is required. Weak recumbent hypothermic lambs less than 5 hours old should be given a warmed 20% glucose injection at a rate of 10 ml/kg by the intraperitoneal route. Once the lamb can hold its head up it should be fed colostrum, either by bottle or by stomach tube.

To utilise maternal antibodies in colostrum, lambs need to ingest it within the first 12 hours and preferably within the first 6 hours of life. Ideally lambs should receive around 150–200 ml/kg of colostrum within the first 12 hours, but to avoid excess stomach distention only give around 50 ml/kg per feed.

Artificial rearing of lambs

Newborn lambs should be fed 2- to 4-hourly with colostrum for the first 12 hours. Then, up until 2–3 weeks of age they should ideally be fed about 3–4 feeds per day of warm milk. After this, 2 feeds a day of cold milk is sufficient. Most pet lambs are bottle-fed. There are a number of milk replacers available for lambs and these have a higher fat percentage than calf milk replacer, but many people still successfully rear lambs on calf milk replacer. Pasture and hay should be made available from 1 week of age to allow proper rumen development.

One of the main causes of death in artificially reared lambs is abomasal bloat. This appears to be a particular problem when lambs are fed milk replacer at variable temperatures at irregular intervals. Affected lambs have abdominal distension and show signs of colic including wide-base stance, vocalisation, kicking at the abdomen and lying down. Prevention is by consistent feeding with small volumes fed regularly. Yoghurtising the milk has also been reported to be effective, while research has suggested that injecting lambs with iron dextran may help reduce the incidence of abomasal bloat.

Fostering of lambs onto a ewe

A variety of techniques can be used, including:
- Rubbing on birth fluids at birth.
- Dunking the lamb in warm water and then letting the ewe lick it. Salt can also be used on the lamb to mislead the ewe into believing it is her lamb. A commercial spray may also be used.
- Confining the ewe and lamb in a pen with the ewe tied so that it does not consistently bunt the lamb and prevent it drinking. Careful management is required to maintain ewe welfare while it is tied up.
- Tying the skin of the dead lamb over the lamb to be fostered onto the ewe.
- Using oxytocin to increase milk let-down may also assist in fostering.

REFERENCES

Bray AR. Lamb survival research. *Proceedings of the Food Safety & Biosecurity, and Epidemiology & Animal Health Management Branches of the New Zealand Veterinary Association* 245, 181-5, 2005

Bull E, Binnie B. Artificial rearing of lambs; avoiding abomasal bloat. *Proceedings of the New Zealand Society of Animal Production*, 66, 386-9, 2006

Dennis SM. Hepatic rupture in the newborn lamb. *American Journal of Obstetrics and Gynecology* 106, 412-20, 1970

Eales A, Small J, Macaldowie C. *Practical lambing and lamb care* (3rd ed). Blackwell Publishing, Oxford UK, 2004

Everett-Hincks JM, Dodds KG. Management of maternal-offspring behaviour to improve lamb survival in easy care sheep systems. *Journal of Animal Science*, E259-70, 2007

Everett-Hincks JM, Duncan SJ. Lamb post-mortem protocol for use on farm: To diagnose primary cause of lamb death from birth to 3 days of age. *The Open Veterinary Science Journal* 2, 55-62, 2008

Fisher M. Lambing management in New Zealand: Ethics and welfare considerations. *Surveillance* 28, 16-17, 2001

Forest RH, Hickford JGH. Development of a gene-marker for cold tolerance in sheep. *Proceedings of the Society of Sheep and Beef Cattle Veterinarians, New Zealand Veterinary Association* 36, 141-50, 2006

Geenty K (Ed). *Making every mating count*. Beef and Lamb New Zealand, 2013

Gudex BW, Hickford JGH, Frampton CM. Sire-line differences in lamb losses from starvation-exposure. *Proceedings of the New Zealand Society of Animal Production* 65, 186-90, 2005

Gumbrell RC. Lamb autopsy technique. *Proceedings of the Society of Sheep and Beef Cattle Veterinarians, New Zealand Veterinary Association* 11, 1068, 1981

Hartley WJ, Boyes B. Incidence of ovine perinatal mortality in New Zealand with particular reference to intra-uterine infections. *New Zealand Veterinary Journal* 12, 336, 1964

Hartley WJ, Kater JC. Perinatal disease conditions of sheep in New Zealand. *New Zealand Veterinary Journal* 12, 49-57, 1964

Haughey KG, Hughes KL, Hartley WJ. The occurrence of congenital infections associated with perinatal mortality. *Australian Veterinary Journal* 43, 413-20, 1967

Haughey KG. Cold injury in newborn lambs. *Australian Veterinary Journal* 49, 554-63, 1973

Haughey KG. Vascular abnormalities in the central nervous system associated with perinatal lamb mortality. 1. Pathology. *Australian Veterinary Journal* 49, 1-8, 1973

Haughey KG. Vascular abnormalities in the central nervous system associated with perinatal lamb mortality. 2. Association of the abnormalities with recognised lesions. *Australian Veterinary Journal* 49, 9-15, 1973

Haughey KG. Birth injury and cold exposure as components of perinatal lamb mortality. *Proceedings of the Society of Sheep and Beef Cattle Veterinarians, New Zealand Veterinary Association* 5, 79-88, 1975

Hughes KL, Haughey KG, Hartley WJ. Perinatal lamb mortality: Infections occurring among lambs dying after parturition. *Australian Veterinary Journal* 47, 472-6, 1971

Jolly RD, Blair HT, Johnstone AC. Genetic disorders of sheep in New Zealand: A review and perspective. *New Zealand Veterinary Journal* 52, 52-64, 2004

Kenyon PR, Morris ST, Corner RA, Stafford KJ, Jenkinson CMC, West DM. Manipulating triplet lamb survival. *Proceedings of the Society of Sheep and Beef Cattle Veterinarians, New Zealand Veterinary Association* 35, 83-90, 2005

Kenyon PR, Revell DK, Morris ST. Mid-pregnancy shearing can increase birthweight and survivial to weaning of multiple-born lambs under commercial conditions. *Australian Journal of Experimental Agriculture* 46, 821-5, 2006

Kerslake JI, Everett-Hincks JM, Campbell AW. Lamb survival: A new examination of an old problem. *Proceedings of the New Zealand Society of Animal Production* 65, 13-18, 2005

Knight TW, McMillan WH, Kilgour R. Effects of slope on lamb survival. *Annual Report, Agricultural Research Division, NZMAF, 1982-1983*, pp143-4. Ministry of Agriculture and Fisheries, Wellington, New Zealand, 1983

Lashley VD, Roe WD, Kenyon PR, Thompson KG. Perinatal lamb mortality: An assessment of gross, histological and immunohistochemical changes in the central nervous system. *New Zealand Veterinary Journal* 62, 160-6, 2014

Lynch JJ, Alexander G. Sheltering behaviour of lambing merino sheep in relation to grass hedges and artificial windbreaks. *Australian Journal of Agricultural Research* 28, 691-701, 1977

McCutcheon SN, Holmes CW, McDonald MF. The starvation-exposure syndrome and neonatal lamb mortality: A review. *Proceedings of the New Zealand Society of Animal Production* 41, 209-17, 1981

McDonald IW. Ewe fertility and neonatal lamb mortality. *New Zealand Veterinary Journal* 10, 45-53, 1962

McFarlane D. Neonatal lamb mortality in the Gisborne area. *Proceedings of the New Zealand Society of Animal Production* 15, 104-19, 1955

McFarlane D. Perinatal lamb losses. *Australian Veterinary Journal* 37, 105-9, 1961

McFarlane D. Perinatal lamb losses. I. An autopsy method for the investigation of perinatal losses. *New Zealand Veterinary Journal* 13, 116-35, 1965

Morel PCH, Morris ST, Kenyon PR. Effects of birth weight on survival in twin born lambs. *Proceedings of the New Zealand Society of Animal Production* 69, 75-9, 2009

Muir PD, Thomson BC, Knight TW. Factors affecting lamb survival. *Proceedings of the Society of Sheep and Beef Cattle Veterinarians, New Zealand Veterinary Association* 35, 73-82, 2005

Nicoll GB, Dodds KG, Alderton MJ. Field data analysis of lamb survival and mortality rates occurring between pregnancy scanning and weaning. *New Zealand Society of Animal Production* 59, 98-100, 1999

Orr M. Watery mouth — a growing problem. *Vetscript* XII, 8, 1999

Sargison ND. Lamb mortality — conception to weaning. *Proceedings of the Society of Sheep and Beef Cattle Veterinarians, New Zealand Veterinary Association* 27, 73-85, 1997

Sargison ND, West DM. Iodine deficiency: An emerging problem in New Zealand sheep flocks? *Proceedings of the New Zealand Society of Animal Production* 58, 202-4, 1998

Smart JA. Watery mouth in lambs: Report of a survey in South Otago and Southland. *Proceedings of the Society of Sheep and Beef Cattle Veterinarians, New Zealand Veterinary Association* 33, 189-94, 2003

Stamp JT. Perinatal loss in lambs with particular reference to diagnosis. *Veterinary Record* 81, 530-4, 1967

Stevens DR. Ewe nutrition: Decisions to be made with scanning information. *Proceedings of the New Zealand Society of Animal Production* 59, 93-4, 1999

Sargison ND, West DM, Parton KH, Hunter JE, Lumsden JS. A case of 'watery mouth' in a New Zealand Romney lamb. *New Zealand Veterinary Journal* 45, 67-8, 1997

Surveillance

(1994) 21(1): 3   Congenital micropthalmia in lambs

(1995) 22(1): 4   Watery mouth in newborn lambs

(1995) 22(1): 4   Polycystic kidneys in newborn lambs

(1995) 22(4): 4   Lethal osteogenesis imperfecta and skin fragility

(1995) 21(1): 3   Eye abnormalities in newborn lambs

Sykes AR. The shelter requirements of the newborn lamb. *Proceedings of the New Zealand Society of Animal Production* 42, 1982

Vatn S, Torsteinbo WO. Effects of iron dextran injections on the incidence of abomasal bloat, clinical pathology and growth rates in lambs. *Veterinary Record* 146, 462-5, 2000

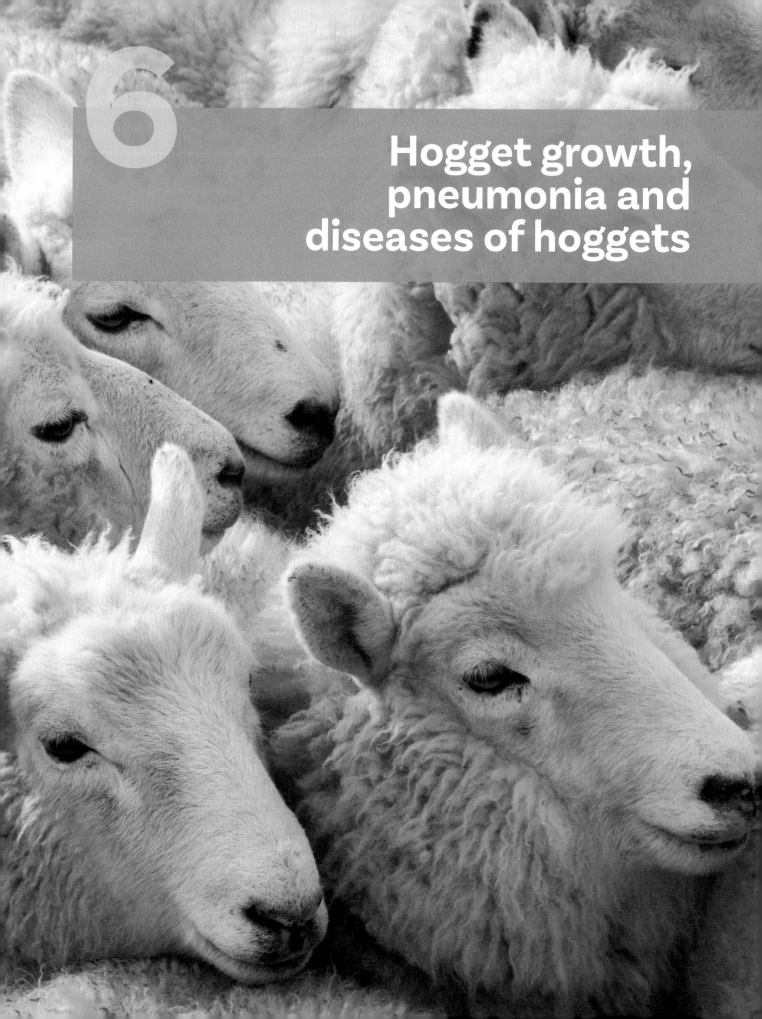

6 Hogget growth, pneumonia and diseases of hoggets

Historical

With the increase in sheep numbers in New Zealand in the several decades following World War II there was also a marked increase in diseases that affected the thrift of young sheep and their ultimate performance as adults. In the 1950s, hogget losses and wastage became so severe in some areas that a government inquiry into hogget ill thrift was commissioned by the then Minister of Agriculture. Since those times there has been a considerable advance in therapeutic products (trace elements, anthelmintics and vaccines) available to combat the diseases that were responsible for some of the earlier losses. In addition, a more objective approach has been taken to the raising of young stock and there are now many realistic farmers who are mindful of the importance of having target weights for grazing sheep. With increasing numbers of farmers electing to breed from their ewe hoggets, excellent health and nutrition of these animals is essential to ensure they achieve satisfactory mating weights and then grow to optimal adult weights. Sheep veterinarians have a very significant role to play in assisting farmers to achieve excellence in hogget health and growth.

The performance of the weaned lamb right through to the two-tooth stage is a critical predictive indicator of farm performance. For many years the sheep industry in New Zealand was impaired by the low reproductive performance of many two-tooth ewes, particularly those grazing North Island hill country. The main contributing factor to this was the poor growth achieved by hoggets. For example it was noted by Coop (1964) that despite apparent good health, many hill-country ewe lambs (replacement sheep) gained little weight from weaning until the following spring. Because of the close relationship between liveweight and fertility, the reason for poor two-tooth performance was clear but changing 'the system' has been a difficult task.

So, frequently, autumn overstocking of sheep farms with unsold wether lambs and even unsold cull ewes has been the key to disaster for the oncoming crop of replacement ewe hoggets. This repetitive management mistake has been a major factor that has produced feed shortages, assisted parasite burdens to increase and fostered the wastage diseases that affect growing sheep.

The growth of hoggets and target liveweights

The ultimate size of the adult sheep is dependent on good nutrition at all stages of its development. The importance of maternal nutrition and the size of the lamb at birth has been emphasised in Chapter 5. It is also important to provide ewes with adequate nutrition during lactation to aid milk production to ensure good lamb growth during that period and thus peak weaning weights. Lambs that have good weaning weights are more likely to reach good two-tooth weights than those that are light.

The importance of early growth rates is shown in Table 6.1.

Liveweight gain birth to weaning (g/day)	Liveweight at 10 weeks (kg), assuming a birthweight of 4.5 kg
200	18.5
250	22.0
300	25.5
350	29.0
400	32.5

Table 6.1 Effect of different growth rates on liveweight at 10 weeks of age.

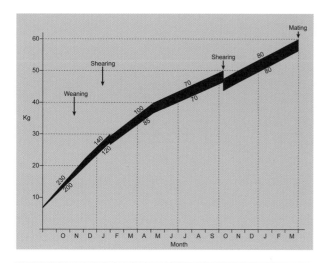

Figure 6.1 Target liveweights for unmated replacement ewes based on a ewe with a mature liveweight of 55–60 kg.

It is important that hoggets are fed so that they achieve target liveweights, demonstrated in Figure 6.1. If hoggets are to be mated, they should be at the very top end of this range to achieve a 40 kg mating weight. It should be noted that some of the composite breeds, such as the Finn and East Friesian crosses, may reach liveweights of up to 70 kg.

Two-tooth ewes growing at the top and bottom of this range would reach pre-tupping weights of 55–60 kg. Even this difference, 5 kg between tupping weights, may mean an 8–10% difference in lambing performance. Or, put another way, for every kilogram increase in mating weights, lambing performance may increase by 1–2%.

Following weaning, the growth of hoggets has often been disappointing, especially during autumn and winter. Feed quantity and quality are both important factors in post-weaning growth, as is disease such as gastrointestinal parasitism. The importance of feed quality for growing hoggets is illustrated in Figure 6.2.

Pasture availability, quality, growth rate and ill thrift

The main factors that affect the growth rate of pasture-raised hoggets are the availability and quality of pasture, internal parasitism, trace-element deficiencies, ingestion of fungal toxins and pneumonia. For lambs, these health issues have been shown to contribute to poor liveweight gain in 60% of incidences. The significance of internal parasitism and trace elements on ill thrift in growing and adult sheep is explained in Chapters 7 and 8. However, a major contributing factor to poor hogget growth (ill thrift) is the availability of good-quality pasture.

The various components of pasture differ markedly in quality. Green leaf and stalk has a higher quality than dead matter, and within the green material there are several species of plants — clover (and herb) leaf and stem, and grass leaf and stem. The quality of clover leaf changes little with age, but grass quality declines significantly as it ages. With this decrease in pasture quality there is also a notable decrease in metabolisable energy (ME)[1]. The ME available in pasture can vary significantly, depending on the pasture

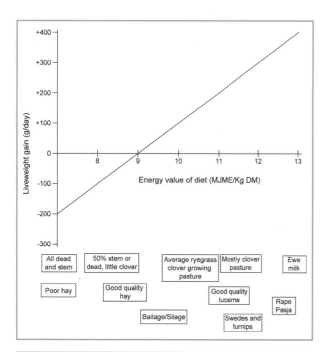

Figure 6.2 Liveweight gain of a 30 kg lamb and the energy value of the diet (from Kerr, 2000).
Source: *400 plus — A guide to improved lamb growth*, edited by P Kerr and Beef and Lamb New Zealand (2000).

---

1 Metabolisable energy is the amount of energy in ingested feed left for maintenance and production after losses in faeces, urine and methane. Values for pasture range from 8 to 12 MJ ME/kg DM.

components, age of the herbage, season and geographical location.

As a guide, the following are approximate working levels of ME:
- Clover leaf has an ME of about 11.8 MJ/kg DM (megajoules per kilogram of dry matter).
- Young grass leaf has an ME of about 11.5, which declines at about 0.03 MJ/kg DM/day.
- Dead matter has an ME of 8.0 MJ/kg DM or less.

The rapid growth of lambs through the summer period often coincides with a decline in pasture quality. Pasture grown in cooler, compared with hotter, times of the year is of inherently higher quality (see Figure 6.3). However, summer pastures are mainly grass-dominant and have a low clover content and an increasing dead matter content, especially in moister regions. Hence, matching animal demand to pasture growth can prove difficult. Further regional differences in pasture quality need to be taken into account. Figure 6.3 also shows the regional differences in measured pasture quality, the effect being most marked in Waikato and least marked in Southland. This also demonstrates the higher potential for summer–autumn stock performance in cooler regions compared with warmer regions.

Before turning to the practical procedures involved in achieving good hogget growth, attention must be drawn to the overriding importance of adequate nutrition, Tables 6.2 and 6.3.

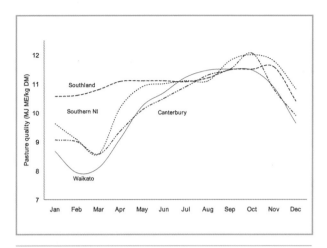

Figure 6.3 Measured pasture quality (MJ ME/kg DM) for four regions across New Zealand (Lambert and Litherland, 2005).

Growth rate (g/day)	Residual dry matter (kg DM/ha)
0	500
50	800
100	1000
150	1200-1400

Table 6.2 The effects of residual pasture mass on the growth rate of lambs.

Table 6.3 The expected growth (g/day) for lambs/hoggets throughout the year grazed on pasture with good residual dry matter levels.

Period	Growth rate (g/day)	Residual green herbage (kg DM/ha)	
		Rotational grazing	Set stocking
10 January–31 March	150	1200	1200
1 April–1 May	90	1400	1400
1 June–31 August	72	800	1100
1–30 September	100	1000	1000
1 October–10 December	130	1700	1200

More information on lamb growth can be found in *400 plus – A guide to improved lamb growth*.

Achieving target weights

The veterinarian who is involved in helping the farmer improve stock performance must emphasise two aspects of hogget growth. Firstly, the regular recording of bodyweight from weaning to first mating; and secondly, the monitoring of animal health and feed requirements.

Guessing the thrift and weight of ewe lambs and hoggets is not reliable; many a farmer who claims to have a 'good eye' for stock has been astonished when confronted with the 'hard data' of weighed sheep. Weighing sheep produces a permanent record against which we can measure progress, watch for lack of progress and diagnose the cause. It also demonstrates to the farmer the wide variation in liveweight inherent in any flock of sheep and creates a spirit of achievement and interest.

There is a large range of sheep-weighing systems available, ranging from basic cage models to sophisticated electronic auto-drafting systems. Weighing devices are available that have the ability to collect a large amount of data that can be downloaded for analysis. This can be done at the mob level or, if sheep are individually identified with electronic ear-tags, at the individual animal level.

Weighing is not a laborious procedure and can usually be carried out in association with some other yarding purpose, i.e. drenching, crutching or shearing.

Body condition scoring of sheep

Unlike cattle, sheep cannot be body condition scored 'by eye' because of the confounding effect of the fleece. Instead they should be packed tightly into a race or crush and condition scored by pressing the thumb onto the spinous processes and the fingers onto the transverse processes of the lumbar vertebrae as shown in Figure 6.4. Condition scoring is a skill requiring experience. It assesses the amount of muscle or fat cover of these regions and is scored on a 1 to 5 system (Figure 6.5). A condition score above 2.5 is usually considered satisfactory.

The clinical approach to hogget health and disease

While achieving target weights has been emphasised as the key to good animal health and hence good financial returns to the farmer, the veterinarian must be able to successfully and quickly diagnose any degree of ill health or poor feeding which is impairing this attainment.

Dealing with such an investigation is essentially similar to any other clinical examination.

History

Specific areas to cover may include:
- time of lambing and weaning
- feed supply at lambing and through lactation
- lambing spread and lambing percentage
- age of docking
- grazing management of ewes and lambs
- drenching with anthelmintics (times and materials used)
- use of trace elements
- records from previous years (often these are anecdotal and not reliable)
- topdressing programme and any soil or pasture analyses done
- stocking rate. Any investigation into hogget ill thrift should always include a clear picture of the overall farm stocking rate, cattle/sheep ratios and whether store animals are being held which normally should

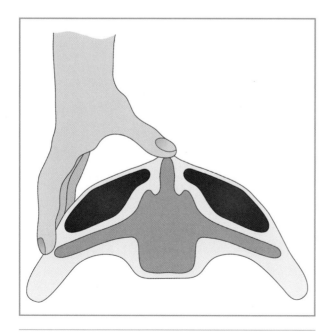

Figure 6.4 Hand position for condition scoring.

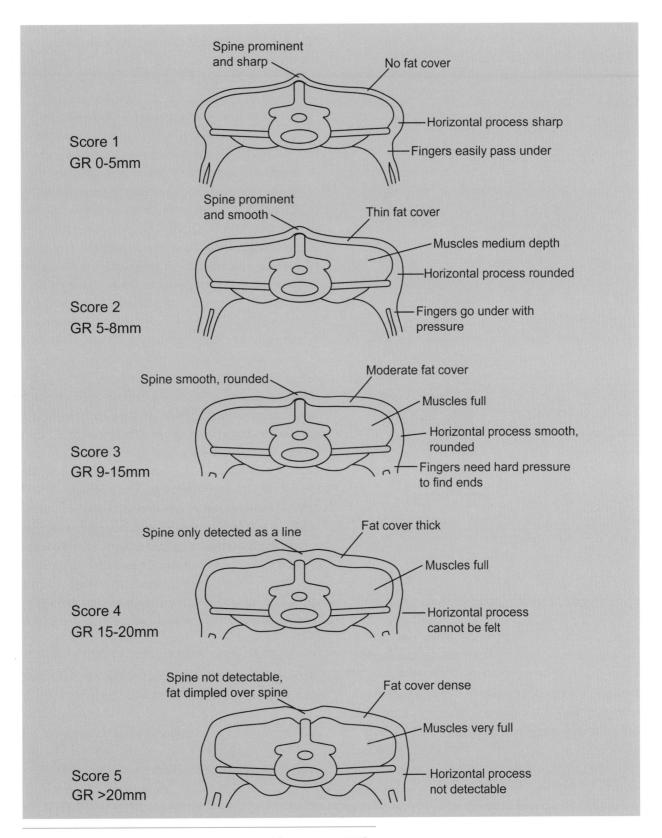

Figure 6.5 Body condition scoring of sheep (adapted from Geenty, 1997).

have been sold. Experience will show that many farmers are 'high stockers' while others like to have feed reserves available and stock their farms more conservatively.

Clinical examination

With sheep problems it is very important to become a good observer and be able to readily recognise signs of health and ill health. Features to observe within a flock for example include:

- Size variations, weight and body condition.
- Fleece — look for evidence of flystrike and any defects such as dermatophilosis, lice and the quality of the fleece.
- Lameness — look for evidence of footrot, scald and, occasionally, rickets.
- Coughing — coughing is common in hoggets but the cause is often hard to diagnose without the necropsy of several selected cases. Enzootic pneumonia is always a consideration. Note particularly if sheep cough when first moved.
- Scouring/diarrhoea — in most cases this is due to parasitism.
- Available feed — veterinarians should be able to estimate available dry matter (DM) for a given pasture. This can be done visually (Table 6.4) or by the use of a measuring plate. The quality of the available feed is also important. Look carefully at the paddock the hoggets have recently come from and the feed they are going to. If hay is being fed, the quantities and quality are also important.

Following a visual appraisal at a distance, it may be appropriate to examine a small selection of the worst affected, or poorest, animals in greater detail. For example, to examine for anaemia (haemonchosis), coughing, dyspnoea (pneumonia), photosensitisation and jaundice (facial eczema). In addition, necropsy of some of the

Pasture height (cm)	Summer (1/1-28/2)	Autumn (1/3-31/5)	Winter (1/6-31/8)	Spring (1/9-31/10)	Late spring (1/11-31/12)
15	3800	3500	3300	2980	3750
14	3670	3410	3150	2850	3600
13	3540	3310	3000	2720	3450
12	3400	3180	2850	2590	3300
11	3250	3040	2690	2460	3150
10	3100	2880	2505	2330	3000
9	2950	2700	2330	2200	2840
8	2800	2500	2150	2070	2680
7	2640	2300	1950	1930	2520
6	2450	2100	1740	1790	2360
5	2250	1900	1520	1640	2200
4	1950	1680	1290	1480	2000
3	1650	1460	1060	1300	1800
2	1300	1180	810	1080	1560
1	900	860	560	800	1280

Source: *400 Plus — A guide to improved lamb growth.*

Table 6.4 Assessing approximate pasture dry matter (kg DM/ha) by measuring pasture height.

worst cases (3–6) will often yield valuable information that can confirm a diagnosis and allow remedial action to be recommended with confidence. Samples can also be collected for additional tests, such as blood and liver for trace-element analysis, gut contents for total worm counts, and faecal samples for faecal egg counts.

Response trials

It may be necessary on occasion to include a response trial in the clinical investigation, although the need for these is less than previously because of improved methods for diagnosis, particularly for trace-element requirements.

Within these general comments about the approach to investigating hogget thrift problems the veterinarian must also be aware of what particular diseases are likely to be important. Many of these are dealt with in other sections of this text, but the following are often more pertinent to hogget health.

Very important	Relatively unimportant
Parasitism — internal	Rickets
— external	Bowie
Trace-element deficiencies	Yersiniosis
(cobalt, selenium)	Eperythrozoonosis
Pneumonia	
Facial eczema	
Foot diseases	
Ryegrass staggers	

Table 6.5 Diseases likely to affect hogget thrift.

Enzootic pneumonia

Enzootic pneumonia is a common disease of sheep, particularly hoggets. In New Zealand, outbreaks have been recorded over many years with the disease first reported by Gilruth in 1900, who noted suppurative pneumonia and pleurisy in sheep slaughtered in an abattoir. It is generally agreed that the disease seen in this country in sheep occurs in two main clinical and pathological forms: acute fibrinous pneumonia in sheep of all ages (but particularly hoggets) and chronic non-progressive pneumonia in lambs or hoggets between 3 and 10 months of age. Early reports by Downey (1957) and Salisbury (1957) referred to an acute pneumonia of ewes in particular. The disease commonly occurred in heavy ewes in October to December in Southland and Otago, and hence became known as 'Southland pneumonia'. In appearance and aetiology it is an acute fibrinous pneumonia similar to that described in lambs and hoggets in the North Island.

The inter-relationship between these forms of the disease is unclear. It is believed by some that the chronic and subacute lesions arise from the progression of mild forms of acute pneumonia which develop into a residual form of the disease. Alternatively it is likely that the acute pneumonias of the 'Pasteurella-type' develop from pre-existing, chronic non-progressive pneumonia in circumstances when the animal's respiratory system is stressed or when super-infection occurs with more-virulent strains of organism. Losses to individual farmers from sudden deaths resulting from acute pneumonia may be quite severe. In turn the loss to the meat industry through rejection and downgrading at slaughter of carcasses that have lesions of chronic pneumonia and/or pleurisy is nationally a very important problem. A third and important aspect of hogget pneumonia is its detrimental effect on weight gain in affected animals.

Aetiology and pathogenesis of pneumonia in hoggets

Pneumonia in young sheep is a disease of complex aetiology, involving interactions between a range of different micro-organisms and the immunological and physiological responses of the host. Pasteurellosis, a term often used to describe the disease (pneumonia) in sheep, is mainly associated with bacteria of the family *Pasteurellaceae* which is now classified in the genera *Pasteurella*, *Manneheimia* and *Bibersteinia*. The micro-organisms associated with pneumonia in sheep are listed in Table 6.7. Of these, *Manneheimia (Pasteurella) haemolytica* is considered to be the main bacterium responsible for lung injury in both forms of pneumonia, although *Pasteurella multocida* is also emerging as a common isolate in some areas. Parainfluenza virus type 3 and adenoviruses have been implicated in causing damage and initiating bacterial invasion, but the role of the other viruses is unclear. In

Bacteria	*Manneheimia (Pasteurella) haemolytica* *Pasteurella multocida* *Bibersteinia (Pasteurella) trehalosi* *Bordetella parapertussis*
Mycoplasmas	*Mycoplasma ovipneumoniae* *Mycoplasma arganini*
Viruses	Parainfluenza virus type 3 Respiratory syncytial virus Ovine adenovirus type 6 Bovine adenovirus type 7 Unidentified cell-associated agent

Table 6.6 Micro-organisms associated with pneumonia in lambs in New Zealand.

chronic non-progressive pneumonia, colonisation of the lung with mixed strains of *Mycoplasma ovipneumoniae* may result in ciliostasis, allowing colonisation of the lung with other bacteria. *Bordetella parapertussis* may play a role in initiating or prolonging chronic non-progressive pneumonia.

Experimental work conducted by Davies et al. at Wallaceville Central Animal Health laboratory emphasised the complexity of the disease but also showed some experimental developments that are similar to the disease as seen in the field. When viruses and pasteurellae are inoculated sequentially or mycoplasmas and pasteurellae are inoculated together, the full pathogenic potential of these organisms is realised and extensive pneumonic lesions develop in the sheep thus challenged. However, not all infections, even under ideal experimental conditions, result in the development of pneumonia, indicating the complexity of the disease. It is only when the antibacterial defences of the lung are overwhelmed and bacterial proliferation occurs that pneumonia develops. The nature of the pneumonic lesions is determined by the bacterial proliferation. At restrained levels of inoculation, a purulent lesion develops which may resolve rapidly if the inciting organism is overcome by the body's defences. At high levels of micro-organisms in the inoculum, necrosis of the lung parenchyma occurs and in some cases escape of bacteria from the lesion leads to death of the lamb from septicaemia.

In some cases the infection is confined to the lung and thoracic cavity, and an acute necrotising pneumonia and pleurisy result. The latter lesions never resolve completely and permanent fibrous scars are left in the lung and pleura. These acute necrotising pneumonias are common in New Zealand in January to March, and are similar to experimentally induced pneumonias in pathogen-free lambs inoculated with viruses or mycoplasmas and *M. haemolytica*.

The subacute and chronic pneumonias are seen throughout New Zealand in all seasons in apparently healthy lambs sent for slaughter. These, like the acute pneumonias, tend to be more common in late summer/autumn to early winter. Experimentally, these subacute and chronic lesions are seen in lambs following the inoculation of suspensions of pneumonic lung and sometimes following the inoculation of viruses and *M. haemolytica*.

Epidemiology

There are several reports that give the morbidity and mortality rates associated with outbreaks of acute fibrinous pneumonia. Losses of 2–8% are usual but Sorensen (1976) reported 600 deaths out of 2850 hoggets with 353 animals downgraded at slaughter from the 2238 surviving animals. The case example opposite outlines a case of 62 deaths from a mob of 850 lambs (7.3% mortality).

In contrast to the losses from acute fibrinous pneumonia, the insidious nature of chronic non-progressive pneumonia is often not appreciated and its course may often be several months in duration. Despite this, resolution invariably occurs during the winter months. Both the morbidity and the severity of the disease vary considerably between farms, with a mean of about 30% of slaughtered lambs affected in the March/April period (Manawatu district) and a range of 5–70%. In one epidemiological study (Goodwin et al., 2001), marked regional differences in prevalence were reported. Pneumonia prevalence averaged 22% in Southland lambs, 49% in King Country lambs and 58% in Northland lambs. Overall, 46% of the total number of lambs investigated had pneumonic lesions but 69% of these had less than 5% of the lung surface area affected. Figure 6.6 shows the prevalence of pneumonia as reflected in pleurisy reported from lambs slaughtered between December and May in three different regions.

In one North Island survey the very high prevalence of 90% of subclinical enzootic pneumonia in slaughtered

CASE EXAMPLE

The flock affected consisted of 850 Perendale ewe hoggets aged 8 months. They were shorn in mid-January and because of dry weather were fed only sufficient pasture for maintenance during the March/April period. Poor stockmanship certainly contributed to this outbreak. It was dry summer weather and on 20 March the lambs were mustered from the back of the farm and driven hard to the stockyards at the front of the property, and held for 2-3 days with little food and water. In previous years mustering and driving the lambs this distance would have been done over 2 days. A week after this muster, 24 hoggets were found dead and the 4 that were necropsied had lesions of acute fibrinous pleuropneumonia with heavy growth of *M. haemolytica* from the lungs. Over the following 2 weeks a further 28 lambs died. The lambs were then yarded again on 26 April and a further 7 died of fibrinous pleuropneumonia in the days following.

From this case the following epidemiological points are worth noting:

1. A mild to moderate level of chronic non-progressive pneumonia was present in the flock in mid-March, prior to the mortalities commencing.
2. 60% of the total losses (36 lambs) occurred in the first 10 days of the outbreak. These animals had an acute fibrinous pleuropneumonia.
3. A further 25% of the total losses occurred over the next 2 weeks. These sheep had fibrinopurulent lesions or an organising fibrinous pleurisy and pericarditis.
4. Sporadic deaths in apparently healthy animals continued during the early winter following periods of stress (e.g. drenching, facial eczema). These animals had incompletely resolved pulmonary abscesses and extensive areas of chronic pleuritis.

At hogget shearing in September the mean bodyweight of this flock was 33 kg (well below target weight). In subsequent years, following the installation of sprinklers to allay the dust in the yards and a more careful mustering of the sheep, only sporadic losses from pneumonia occurred on this property, although high levels of chronic non-progressive pneumonia and pleurisy were sometimes recorded in lambs sent to slaughter.

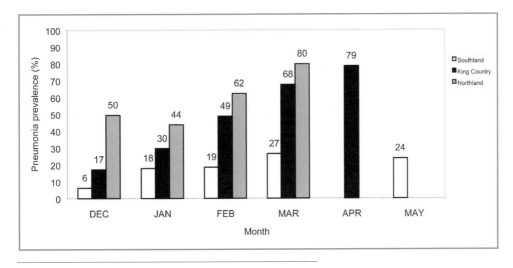

Figure 6.6 Pneumonia prevalence of lambs identified at slaughter, by region and time (Goodwin et al., 2001).

lambs has been reported. It is assumed that the majority of pleural lesions reported from slaughter surveys are a consequence of subclinical pneumonia; however, the prevalence of subclinical pneumonia decreases as lambs grow. In contrast, the prevalence of pleurisy increases until, on a national basis, more than 16% of lambs slaughtered at 1 year of age are affected.

Economic effects of enzootic pneumonia

The economic losses both nationally and to the farmer as a result of enzootic pneumonia are hard to assess, but there are four main areas involved.

1. Direct losses of stock on the farm. These may be very high under some circumstances. Further, the presence of enzootic pneumonia in a flock of young sheep frequently makes normal management such as stock movements and drenching difficult.
2. From the example case history given above it can be seen that prolonged sporadic losses due to flare-ups of pulmonary and pleural abscesses during autumn and winter may occur.
3. Reduced weight gain and wool production have been recorded from some trials both in New Zealand and overseas. An extensive trial in New Zealand highlighted the detrimental effect of pneumonia on the liveweight gain of lambs. When over 20% of lung surface area was affected (lung consolidated with red or grey/red lesions), the weight gain of the affected lambs was 50% lower than unaffected lambs. Thus for a lamb weighing 25 kg at the end of January a 50% reduction in average daily growth would increase the time needed to reach a slaughter weight of 30 kg from 37 days to 63 days.
4. Condemnation and downgrading of carcasses in stock sent for slaughter. There are several excellent reports of the seriousness of this loss to the New Zealand meat industry. The prevalence of pleural lesions shows a marked seasonal and geographical variation. Much higher prevalences are shown in the North Island than the South Island.

As far as the loss to the meat industry is concerned, this is not only through the condemnation or partial condemnation that occurs but also through the extra work involved in trimming even very small pleural lesions before marketing is possible. This involves double handling and double meat inspection, adding to the already high expense of the killing process.

Predisposing factors for enzootic pneumonia

Both acute fibrinous pneumonia in sheep of all ages and subclinical chronic progressive pneumonia in lambs and hoggets occur throughout New Zealand. Outbreaks of acute fibrinous pneumonia associated with the death of some lambs and coughing in the group as a whole is of concern to many farmers. Such outbreaks are almost invariably associated with a period of stress involving mustering and yarding, often in dry, dusty conditions. It is presumed that chronic non-progressive pneumonia is also present in these flocks and that pathogens such as *M. haemolytica* are also present in the upper respiratory tract and possibly the lung itself. It is presumed that the panting and mouth-breathing associated with mustering and yarding in hot, dusty conditions aids the establishment and proliferation of pathogens such as *M. haemolytica* in the lung, especially if the lung defences have already been compromised by viral and/or mycoplasma infections.

It should be remembered that open-mouth panting in sheep is a sign of heat stress and is a cooling mechanism by which the sheep uses its respiratory system to lower elevated body temperature. Heat stress is common on New Zealand sheep farms, and exercise-induced heat stress occurring during mustering and droving is probably the major predisposing factor of pneumonia seen so frequently on our farms. Heat stress may also be exacerbated by the pyretic effect of ergovaline in high-endophyte grasses present during summer and autumn.

Heat stress has also been attributed as the main predisposing factor in the deaths due to pneumonia that have occurred during the transport of sheep to the Middle East for the live sheep trade. The live sheep trade was indeed curtailed because of both the losses due to pneumonia on board ships and the stressful conditions encountered in the feedlots following disembarkation.

A case study of 316 farms by Goodwin et al. (2004) emphasised three important risk factors of husbandry that were associated with pneumonia in lambs and hoggets. These were:
- Shearing lambs on the day of weaning, which possibly

increased heat stress and brought animals into closer contact for the transmission of contagious micro-organisms.
- Breeding ewe replacements on-farm.
- Increased average slaughter age of lambs. Both this and the previous factor increased farm stocking rate and density when available feed was often becoming limited.

Other situations that may be associated with pneumonia (non-enzootic)

Climatic changes

After shearing and stress from handling, particularly when animals are hungry, pneumonia may be a sequel to the stressed/starvation syndrome. There are many reports of losses of hoggets, lambs and ewes from cold shock following shearing, with lingering deaths occurring for a time afterwards. This is reported in severe snow seasons, particularly from the South Island.

Dipping

Outbreaks of pneumonia have occurred following both shower- and plunge-dipping. Deaths from post-dipping pneumonia usually commence 4–7 days from dipping. Parainfluenza type 3 virus, mycoplasmas and *Pasteurella* spp have been isolated from sheep that die after dipping; thus, the dipping may be regarded as a precipitating factor of clinical pneumonia. But as with other proposed precipitating factors, the role of dipping in causing pneumonia is uncertain.

Lungworm

Lungworm has been incriminated as a possible factor due to the irritation these parasites may cause. Large numbers of *Dictyocaulus filaria* can cause blockage of the bronchi and death. However, lungworms usually affect the diaphragmatic or caudal lobes, whereas enzootic pneumonia is mainly confined to the anterior, ventral lobes.

Facial eczema

Facial eczema has been seen in groups of hoggets suffering from pneumonia losses and it is possible that it is a contributing stress factor.

Shipment of sheep

Pneumonia is one of the main causes of deaths associated with shipments of live sheep, especially in young animals. These losses mainly occur when the ventilation system of the sheep is either inefficient or breaks down. Presumably heat stress, the accumulation of ammonia and other toxic gases plays a role as a precipitating agent.

Clinical findings

As just described, in nearly all occurrences of enzootic or acute pneumonia there is some predisposing factor that

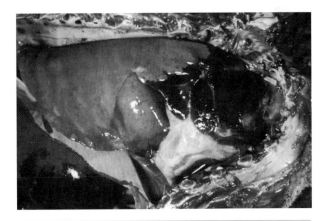

Figure 6.7 Acute pneumonia; note the hepatisation of the anterior lung lobes, and the sheets of fibrin over these lobes and over the heart.

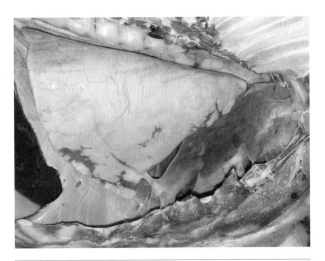

Figure 6.8 Chronic non-progressive pneumonia with hepatisation, predominantly of the anterior lung.

has preceded the outbreak. In acute cases sheep may just be found dead. A common prodromal sign is coughing. In most mobs of lambs where pneumonia is occurring there will be a significant number of sheep that will cough, particularly when driven, even over a short distance.

Before death, severely affected cases will lag behind the mob, display extreme respiratory distress and usually lie down. In some outbreaks, lambs will continue to die for 4–6 weeks or even longer. Some animals will become chronically unthrifty due to lesions of pleurisy or lung abscesses that may develop.

Pathology

In acute pneumonia there is usually a severe fibrinous pleurisy with adhesions between the parietal and visceral pleura. There are large volumes of fibrinous exudate in the pleural cavity and frequently in the pericardium. The lungs are dark red and solid. The main lesions are usually seen in the anteroventral lobes of the lungs, but other areas become affected depending on the severity of the case.

In so-called chronic or non-progressive pneumonia there is grey hepatisation of the anteroventral portions of the lungs, sometimes with focal fibrinous pleurisy and pericarditis. Focal necrosis and abscessation of the lung parenchyma with a more severe pleurisy is seen in some cases with a superimposed pyogenic infection.

Treatment

The treatment of individual lambs, hoggets or ewes with various antibiotics has generally proven unsatisfactory, although long-acting tetracyclines may be useful in some cases. Earlier reports on the treatment of 'Southland pneumonia' with sulphamezathine and penicillin were encouraging. In general, most cases are only detected in the terminal phase when chemotherapy is too late.

Prevention

An important way of reducing the occurrence of pneumonia is to minimise the predisposing factors by avoiding unnecessary stress to the lambs or hoggets. Thus, yarding and close confinement of stock under hot, dusty conditions should be avoided or kept to a minimum. However, this may conflict with the necessity of yarding for parasite or facial eczema control. Therefore, sheep should be mustered in the early morning when the weather is cooler and mustering should not be unduly hasty. Planning a grazing rotation so that yarding coincides with times when sheep are closer to the shed is encouraged to minimise droving distances.

Many farmers in pneumonia risk areas have sprinkler systems in their sheep yards which can be used to dampen down dust before the mob is yarded. In some cases extra temporary or permanent yards may need to be erected to avoid long periods of droving, or portable yards may also be used. Control of dogs when not working, particularly huntaways, is also important. These are frequently left to disturb sheep unnecessarily, particularly when yarded. Otherwise, maintaining good stock health during the risk period is important. This particularly involves drenching for parasite control and keeping good feed available for young stock.

In the past a vaccine was available, but its efficacy was limited and it has since been withdrawn from the market.

'Bowie' or 'bent leg'

Bowie, an osteodystrophic disease of sheep, is a disease of hoggets and younger lambs that has been reported in New Zealand but is now of little importance. It is characterised by the bowing inwards of the forelimbs and occasionally the hind limbs, causing the affected animal to walk with difficulty. The disease has been reported in Scotland and is pathologically distinct from rickets. The most comprehensive report of the disease in New Zealand is that written by Fitch (1954).

Incidence and epidemiology

Bowie has had a fairly widespread distribution in the South Island occurring in Marlborough, Kaikoura, North and South Canterbury. It has rarely been seen in the North Island. It was mainly studied in the Marlborough county.

Pastures on which bowie occurred were mainly danthonia and browntop. It was also observed that where pastures were topdressed with superphosphate and sown with English grasses the disease did not appear.

The incidence of bowie varied from year to year and there did not appear to be any correlation between its occurrence and climatic conditions. In the past, up to 40% of a line of lambs were affected in one season and some (about half) so severely affected that they had to be culled. Fitch quoted as many as 200 and 400 lambs culled annually on the larger sheep stations, although no total numbers of the flock sizes were given. All breeds of sheep that grazed the areas were affected including Merinos, Romneys, Corriedales, Lincolns, halfbreds and Southdown crosses. In a 1999 report, 160 of 400 4-month-old Merino lambs in the central South Island developed bowie. The land they were grazing had not been topdressed for 8 years.

In Australia a similar condition has been reported in lambs in Northern New South Wales and Southern Queensland. In these areas it is suggested that the condition is associated with the grazing of white parsnip (*Trachymene glaucifolia*).

Clinical features

The disease is sometimes seen in lambs as young as 3–4 weeks of age, but the number of animals affected and the severity of the lesions progress until weaning, by which time they have usually attained their maximum severity. In the early stages there may be some tenderness of the feet and a very slight tendency for the legs to bend out at the knees.

As the disease worsens the forelimbs, in particular, bow outwards, in some animals more severely than in others. Some animals show a bowing of the hind limbs also. The bowing may be so severe that the front feet may actually cross when walking. The toes are turned in and there is a tendency for the weight to be borne on the lateral side of the outer hoof so that the coronet on that side is sometimes damaged by contact with the ground. The hooves become excessively long.

Many bowie lambs do not seem to be lame, while others show marked lameness. In general, chronic, old-established cases will not be lame. By weaning time, affected lambs are showing obvious ill thrift.

Pathology

Macroscopically, the most striking lesions are seen in the radius and metacarpal bones. The distal extremity in both cases is bent medially. This deformity is the result of two factors: an inward bending of the lower end of the shaft and a partial collapse medially of the epiphysis into the expanded end of the diaphysis.

The long bones are well developed and not unduly porotic. The epiphyseal cartilages may be greatly thickened in parts, but are usually supported by fairly dense spongy bone.

The ribs are usually of normal strength and fractures are rare. The distal extremities may show a sudden expansion to about twice their normal width at the costochondral junction.

Histologically the disease is distinct from rickets. In the latter, cartilage cells persist at the sites of endochondral ossification. In bowie, although the zone of mature cartilage cells is greatly increased there is no gross failure of calcification as in rickets.

Treatment and prevention

There is no treatment for this disease and it appears that it can be prevented by superphosphate topdressing and moving susceptible stock onto improved pasture. There are few reports of this disease at present.

Cud staining and ill thrift in lambs

Cud staining down one or both sides of the mouth is seen in a small proportion of lambs from many flocks. It does not always appear to affect the thrift of some animals, but in some cases it is associated with ill thrift. In older sheep such as stud rams, it is aesthetically unacceptable and may also be associated with oral lesions.

Cud staining of sheep is likely to have multiple causes, including injuries to the mouth from drenching guns, dental problems of the molar teeth and injuries from other causes. The pain associated with these lesions is likely to restrict grazing and rumination, resulting in ill thrift and cud staining.

Rickets in hoggets

In recent decades rickets has become a relatively uncommon disease in sheep in New Zealand, although there are still occasional reports of its occurrence in Southland. It is essentially a disease of growing animals in which there is defective calcification of growing bone. The poorly mineralised bones are subject to distortion, producing lameness and permanent limb defects.

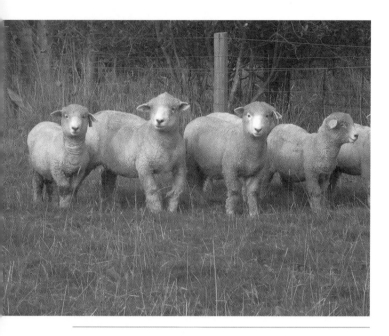

Figure 6.9 Lambs affected with rickets.

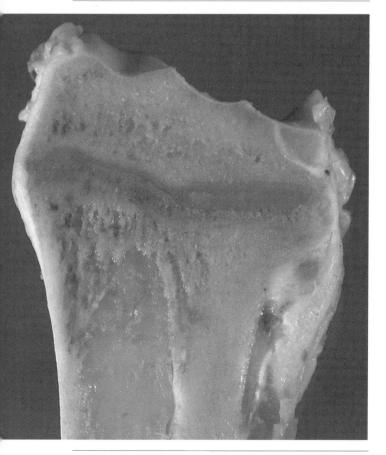

Figure 6.10 Widening of the growth plate of the proximal radius. (Photographs courtesy KG Thompson)

Aetiology

In New Zealand most cases of rickets in lambs have been associated with the grazing of soft green crops, such as green-feed oats and even some crops of ryegrass. It is believed that the main cause is a lack of vitamin D at crucial periods of the year (mid-winter), which affects the metabolism of calcium and phosphorus from the diet. Other factors such as the high carotene levels (vitamin A) in lush green-feed may also have an antagonistic effect on the availability of vitamin D. Congenital rickets has also been reported in lambs born to ewes that had been grazed on a fodder beef crop during pregnancy, most likely due to low phosphorus levels in the crop.

A genetic form of rickets has been reported in New Zealand Corriedale sheep in the Marlborough district. It occurred in a low annual incidence of up to 20 lambs from 1600 purebred Corriedale ewes. The lambs were normal at birth but became lame and unthrifty during the first 2 months of life; the most severely affected lambs died early, but some survived to breeding age. The skeletal pathology was typical of rickets and it was concluded that the likely cause was a defect in end-organ responsiveness to 1,25-dihydroxyvitamin D.

In addition, heavy parasite burdens may have influenced the calcium uptake of the growing animals. Hence, the generally better parasite control in lambs and hoggets that is now achieved may have contributed to the decrease of this disease.

Clinical findings

The disease is usually seen in hoggets in late winter and early spring. It is characterised by poor growth and a very apparent lameness. The limb joints are frequently enlarged and sometimes a distinct swelling can be palpated at the costochondral junction of the ribs. The bones of the limbs frequently become twisted and rib bones bend easily. Congenital rickets has been reported in newborn lambs.

Defects of the jaws and teeth have also been reported in rickets and include swollen mandible, irregular tooth eruption, enamel hypoplasia and malocclusion.

Pathology and diagnosis

At autopsy most carcasses are in very poor condition but the main findings are restricted to abnormal bones and teeth. The bone shafts are larger in diameter due to the subperiosteal deposition of osteoid tissue. The joints are enlarged and the epiphyseal cartilage can be seen to be thicker than usual.

To confirm a diagnosis of rickets it may be necessary to send affected bones to a diagnostic laboratory for histological examination of the metaphyseal region or to radiograph affected limbs.

An estimation of the ratio of ash to organic matter is also a valuable diagnostic aid. Normally the ratio is 3 parts of ash to 2 parts of organic matter, but in a rachitic bone this may be depressed to 1 : 2 or even 1 : 3 in extreme cases.

Treatment and control

Severely affected sheep if left untreated will usually become more unthrifty and eventually die. Mild cases may respond if dosed with vitamin D as cod liver oil. The disease can be prevented in areas where it is likely to occur by taking precautions to ensure that if crops such as green-feed oats are used, they are not the only diet. In addition, well before the shortest day of the year (low ultraviolet light period) susceptible lambs should be dosed with calciferol or a suitable vitamin D substitute.

In addition to the above, good parasite control should be maintained.

Eperythrozoonosis

Mycoplasma ovis, formerly known as *Eperythrozoon ovis*, is an epi-erythrocytic blood parasite of sheep that produces anaemia and ill thrift, particularly in young sheep.

Aetiology and transmission

Mycoplasma ovis has been transmitted experimentally by inoculating infected blood into susceptible animals. The natural mode of transmission is not fully understood but it is believed that the biting fly *Stomoxys calcitrans* could be a vector. Other biting insects such as *Melophagus ovinus* and *Linognathus ovillus* may be involved but good evidence of this is lacking.

However, the weight of circumstantial evidence supports the hypothesis that infection is spread by insects, since all diagnosed spontaneous cases of ovine eperythrozoonosis have occurred in summer and autumn, which suggests a biting insect as the vector. In addition, in Australia and South Africa the infection mainly occurs in areas with higher rainfall, again favourable for insect vectors. Transmission could also be via contaminated inoculation equipment. It may also be associated with mulesing of sheep — extensive areas of bare and bleeding tissue are created and it is believed that biting flies may assist in transmission.

Incubation period and development of parasitaemia

Little information is available on the incubation period of the disease following natural transmission. It is believed that the rate of infection is dependent on the density of the sheep population and the number of insects present. It has also been noted that after the organisms are first noted in the blood following infection they increase rapidly for 5–10 days, becoming 25–100 times as numerous as the erythrocytes. This rapid phase of multiplication may continue until about the time the anaemia appears. At this stage a sudden decrease in numbers of organisms occurs, so that when the anaemia is most marked there may be few or no organisms to be seen; an important point to be noted in the diagnosis of the disease.

As the parasitaemia diminishes, the haemoglobin levels return to normal. Reappearance of the parasite in blood smears, after being apparently free from infection, has also been recorded.

Clinical features

Some spontaneously infected sheep with only a slight parasitaemia develop no clinical signs. It is believed that the severity of the anaemia is related directly to the intensity of the parasitaemia. One of the first clinical signs recorded is a fever, and a febrile reaction as high as 41.5°C has been observed to be intermittent or continuous for 3–4 days.

Tetany and haemoglobinuria are also seen in rare cases and are indicative of rapid erythrocyte destruction. Other clinical signs are referable to the severity of the anaemia and include dullness, anorexia, loss of condition, debility, weak pulse and rapid respiration.

In South Africa loss of bodyweight has been recorded in lambs 1–3 weeks after the organisms have been seen in the blood. However, this weight loss is usually only temporary. In some cases there have been deaths associated with the disease, but these are usually few in number. It is believed that the Merino breed may be more susceptible to the effects of the disease than other breeds. However, this may be linked to the mulesing operation.

In New Zealand, eperythrozoonosis in sheep is uncommon but occasional outbreaks occur in Merino lambs each year. For example, in one case reported in Merino lambs in Ranfurly, over 100 lambs from a flock of 1000 died within a few weeks. Affected lambs showed jaundice and anaemia and *E. ovis* organisms were demonstrated in the blood of affected animals.

The association of the parasite with outbreaks of ill thrift in lambs and hoggets has been difficult to establish, but in New South Wales, South Australia, Victoria and Western Australia most researchers have considered a close association between the ill thrift and the presence of *E. ovis*. Other factors, nutritive, immunological or otherwise, may increase the susceptibility of sheep to *E. ovis*.

Pathology

Generalised signs of anaemia and jaundice are the main features of the autopsy. There may also be haemoglobinuria and most animals will show signs of anorexia. *Eperythrozoon ovis* can be demonstrated in blood smears from infected animals. The smears need to be stained with one of the Romanovosky stains. The organisms are pleomorphic and may be ring-shaped, filamentous, 'wispy', ovoid or triangular and are seen in clear association with the erythrocytes.

Treatment

Most animals recover spontaneously. However, tetracyclines have been found to be effective in the treatment of eperythrozoonosis in other species and may be of use with valuable sheep.

Yersiniosis of sheep

Yersiniosis in farmed livestock in New Zealand is usually associated with red deer. In that species sporadic outbreaks of the disease attributable to *Yersinia pseudotuberculosis* are usually observed in the winter and are thought to be precipitated by nutritional stress. In New Zealand sheep the disease is uncommon and may be associated with several strains of *Yersinia* including *Y. enterocolitica* and *Y. pseudotuberculosis*. It is, however, a relatively common disease of young sheep in Australia, causing diarrhoea primarily in the winter and spring months.

Clinical features and aetiology

In sheep, most reported outbreaks of yersiniosis have been in hoggets and associated with periods of feed shortage, usually in the winter. There may or may not be an associated high parasite burden. In most cases there is severe diarrhoea associated with often foul-smelling watery faeces which may be blood tinged. Animals may become terminally dehydrated and moribund. Morbidity rates estimated at a third of the flock have been reported, but mortality rates have seldom been higher than 3%. In most cases the course of the epidemic is about 2 weeks and animals often recover spontaneously when moved to better feed. It has been suggested that some biotypes of *Y. enterocolitica* can cause scouring in lambs with little effect on weight gain. It should be noted that isolation of *Yersinia* spp from the gastrointestinal tract or faeces is not diagnostic in itself, as sheep may carry and shed the organism without developing clinically significant signs.

In an unusual case, 10% of 335 lambs were found at slaughter to have abscessation of the mesenteric lymph nodes from which *Y. enterocolitica* was isolated. *Yersinia* spp occasionally cause abortion in pregnant ewes.

From field cases in New Zealand *Y. enterocolitica* and *Y. pseudotuberculosis* have both been isolated. However, abattoir samples have also shown the presence of other *Yersinia* spp in lambs, including *Y. intermedia* and *Y. frederiksenii*.

Pathology

The main postmortem features usually include an emaciated and dehydrated carcass with varying degrees of gastroenteritis. Faeces are often blood-tinged and foul-smelling.

Treatment

Treatment of affected animals with long-acting tetracyclines and isolation from the rest of the flock appear to assist recovery.

REFERENCES

ENZOOTIC PNEUMONIA

Alley MR. The bacterial flora of the respiratory tract of normal and pneumonic sheep. *New Zealand Veterinary Journal* 23, 113-8, 1975

Alley MR. The effect of chronic non-progressive pneumonia on weight gain of pasture-fed lambs. *New Zealand Veterinary Journal* 35, 163-6, 1987

Alley MR. Pneumonia in sheep in New Zealand: An overview. *New Zealand Veterinary Journal* 50 (Suppl.), 99-101, 2002

Alley MR, Clarke JK. The influence of micro-organisms on the severity of lesions in chronic ovine pneumonia. *New Zealand Veterinary Journal* 25, 200-2, 1977

Alley MR, Clarke JK. The experimental transmission of ovine chronic non-progressive pneumonia. *New Zealand Veterinary Journal* 27, 217-20, 1979

Alley MR, Clarke JK. The effect of chemotherapeutic agents on the transmission of ovine non-progressive pneumonia. *New Zealand Veterinary Journal* 28, 77-80, 1980

Alley MR, Quinlan JR, Clarke JK. The prevalence of *Mycoplasma ovipneumoniae* and *Mycoplasma arginini* in the respiratory tract of sheep. *New Zealand Veterinary Journal* 23, 137-41, 1975

Alley MR, Ionas G, Clarke JK. Chronic non-progressive pneumonia of sheep in New Zealand — a review of the role of *Mycoplasma ovipneumoniae*. *New Zealand Veterinary Journal* 47, 155-60, 1999

Beckett F. Growth of young sheep on North Island hill country. *Proceedings of the 2nd Annual Seminar of the Sheep Society of the New Zealand Veterinary Association*, 103-7, 1972

Black H. *Pasteurella* isolates from sheep pneumonia cases in New Zealand. *Surveillance* 24, 5-8, 1997

Black H, Alley MR, Goodwin-Ray KA. Heat stress as a manageable risk factor to mitigate pneumonia in lambs. *New Zealand Veterinary Journal* 53, 91-2, 2005

Carter ME, Hunter R. Isolation of parainfluenza type 3 virus from sheep in New Zealand. *New Zealand Veterinary Journal* 23, 113-18, 1970

Davies DH, Jones S. Serological evidence of respiratory syncytial virus infection in lambs. *New Zealand Veterinary Journal* 33, 155-6, 1985

Davies DH. Isolation of parainfluenza virus type 3 from pneumonic lambs. *New Zealand Veterinary Journal* 28, 148-53, 1980

Davies DH. Aetiology of pneumonias of young sheep. *Progress in Veterinary Microbiology and Immunology* 1, 229-48, 1985

Davies DH, Davis GB, Price MC. A longitudinal survey of respiratory virus infection in lambs. *New Zealand Veterinary Journal* 28, 125-7, 1980

Davies DH, Dungworth DC, Humphries S, Johnson AJ. Concurrent infection of lambs with parainfluenza virus type 3 and *Pasteurella haemolytica*. *New Zealand Veterinary Journal* 25, 263-5, 1977

Davies DH, Herceg M, Thurley DC. Experimental infection of lambs with an adenovirus followed by *Pasteurella haemolytica*. *Veterinary Microbiology* 7, 369-81, 1982

Davis GB. A sheep mortality survey in Hawke's Bay. *New Zealand Veterinary Journal* 22, 39-42, 1974

Davies DH. The aetiology and pathogenesis of pneumonia in lambs. *Proceedings of 17th Seminar of the Sheep and Beef Cattle Society, New Zealand Veterinary Association*, 150-5, 1987

Donachie W. The prevention of pasteurellosis. *British Veterinary Journal* 148, 93-5, 1992

Downey NE. A preliminary investigation into the aetiology of enzootic pneumonia of sheep ('Southland pneumonia'). *New Zealand Veterinary Journal* 5, 128-33, 1957

Goodwin KA, Jackson R, Brown C, Davies PR, Morris RS, Perkins NR. Enzootic pneumonia of lambs in New Zealand: Patterns of prevalence and effects on production. *Proceedings of the 31st Seminar of the Society of Sheep and Beef Cattle Veterinarians, New Zealand Veterinary Association*, 1-6, 2001

Goodwin KA, Jackson R, Brown C, Davies PR, Morris RS, Perkins NR. Pneumonic lesions in lambs in New Zealand: Patterns of prevalence and effects on production. *New Zealand Veterinary Journal* 52, 175-9, 2004

Goodwin KA, Heuer C, Davies PR. Case-control study of pneumonia in growing lambs in New Zealand. *Proceedings of the 34th Seminar of the Society of Sheep and Beef Cattle Veterinarians, New Zealand Veterinary Association*, 173-9, 2004

Goodwin-Ray KA, Stevenson MA, Heuer C. Effect of vaccinating lambs against pneumonic pasteurellosis under New Zealand field conditions on their weight gain and pneumonic lung lesions at slaughter. *Veterinary Record* 169, 9-11, 2008

Goodwin-Ray KA, Stevenson MA, Heuer C, Cogger N. Economic effect of pneumonia and pleurisy in lambs in New Zealand. *New Zealand Veterinary Journal* 56, 107-14, 2008

Herceg M, Thurley DC, Davies DH. Oat cells in the pathology of ovine pneumonia-pleurisy. *New Zealand Veterinary Journal* 30, 170-3, 1982

Hicks J. Sudden deaths in mixed age ewes — an outbreak of *Pasteurella trephalosi* septicaemia. *The Sheep and Beef Cattle Veterinarians Newsletter* No. 28, 15-18, 2005

Jones GE, Donachie W, Gilmour JS, Rae AG. Attempt to prevent the effects of experimental chronic pneumonia in sheep by vaccination against *Pasteurella haemolytica*. *British Veterinary Journal* 142, 189-94, 1986

Jones GE, Field AC, Gilmour JS, Rae AG, Nettleton PF, McLauchlan M. Effects of experimental chronic pneumonia on bodyweight, feed intake and carcase composition. *Veterinary Record* 110, 168-73, 1982

Kirton AH, O'Hara PJ, Shortridge EA, Cordes DO. Seasonal incidence of enzootic pneumonia and its effect on the growth of lambs. *New Zealand Veterinary Journal* 24, 59-64, 1976

Kirton AH, O'Hara PJ, Shortridge EH, Cordes DO. Pneumonia in sheep: Does it affect weight gain? *New Zealand Veterinary Journal* 25, 195-6, 1977

Lambert G, Litherland A. Pasture quality and ill thrift in young sheep and cattle. *Proceedings of the 35th Seminar of the Society of Sheep and Beef Cattle Veterinarians, New Zealand Veterinary Association*, 121-7, 2005

McGowan B, Thurley DC, McSporran KD, Pfeffer AT. Enzootic pneumonia-pleurisy complex in sheep and lambs. *New Zealand Veterinary Journal* 26, 169-72, 1978

Pfeffer A, Thurley DC, Boyes BW, Davies DH, Davis GB, Price MC. The prevalence and microbiology of pneumonia in a flock of lambs. *New Zealand Veterinary Journal* 31, 196-202, 1983

Pyke BN. Sheep mortality in the King Country. *New Zealand Veterinary Journal* 22, 196-7, 1974

Salisbury RM. Enzootic pneumonia of sheep in New Zealand. *New Zealand Veterinary Journal* 5, 124-7, 1957

Sorenson NN. Epidemiology of enzootic pneumonia in sheep as observed in Central North Island Practice. *Proceedings of the 6th Annual Seminar of the Sheep Society of the New Zealand Veterinary Association*, 101-4, 1976

Thurley DC, Boyes BW, Davies DH, Wilkins MJ, O'Connell E, Humphreys S. Subclinical pneumonia in lambs. *New Zealand Veterinary Journal* 25, 173-6, 1977

BOWIE

Fitch LW. Osteodystrophic diseases of sheep in New Zealand II 'Bowie' or 'Bent-leg'. *New Zealand Veterinary Journal* 2, 118-27, 1954

Philbey AW. *Trachymene glaucifolia* associated with bentleg in lambs. *Australian Veterinary Journal* 67, 468, 1990

Surveillance

(1999) 26: 16   Bowie in Merino lambs

CUD STAINING

Ridler AL, West DM, Johnstone AC. An investigation into cud-staining and ill-thrift in lambs. *Proceedings of the 33rd Seminar of the Society of Sheep and Beef Cattle Veterinarians, New Zealand Veterinary Association*, 101-3, 2003

RICKETS

Dittmer KE, Morley RE, Smith RL. Skeletal deformities associated with nutritional congenital rickets in newborn lambs. *New Zealand Veterinary Journal* 65, 51-5, 2017

Thompson KG. Skeletal diseases of sheep. *Small Ruminant Research* 76, 112-19, 2008

Thompson KG, Dittmer KE, Blair HT, Fairley RA, Sim DFW. An outbreak of rickets in Corriedale sheep: Evidence for a genetic aetiology. *New Zealand Veterinary Journal* 55, 137-42, 2007

EPERYTHROZOONOSIS

Sutton RH. *Eperythrozoon ovis* — a blood parasite of sheep. *New Zealand Veterinary Journal* 18, 156-64, 1970

Sutton RH, Jolly RD. Experimental *Eperythrozoon ovis* infection of sheep. *New Zealand Veterinary Journal* 21, 160-6, 1973

Surveillance

(1988) 15(2): 27   Eperythrozoonosis
(1990) 17(4): 15   An *Eperythrozoon ovis* outbreak in Merino lambs
(2000) 27(2): 23   Review of diagnostic cases

YERSINOSIS

Bullians J. Yersinia species infection of lambs and cull cows at an abattoir. *New Zealand Veterinary Journal* 35, 65-7, 1987

Gill J. Yersiniosis of farm animals in New Zealand. *Surveillance* 23, 24-6, 1996

Hodges RT, Carman MG, Mortimer WJ. Serotypes of *Yersinia pseudotuberculosis* recovered from domestic livestock. *New Zealand Veterinary Journal* 32, 11-13, 1984

McSporran KD, Hansen LM, Saunders BW, Damsteegt A. An outbreak of diarrhoea in hoggets associated with infection by *Yersinia enterocolitica*. *New Zealand Veterinary Journal* 32, 38-9, 1984

Slee KJ, Button C. Enteritis in sheep and goats due to *Yersinia enterocolitica* infection. *Australian Veterinary Journal* 6, 396-8, 1990

Surveillance

(1989) 16(4): 3   Review of diagnostic cases
(1994) 21(4): 3   Review of diagnostic cases
(2001) 28(2): 17   Review of diagnositic cases

Yang R, Ryan U, Gardner G, Carmichael I, Campbell A, Jacobson C. Prevalence, faecal shedding and genetic characterisation of Yersinia spp. in sheep across four states of Australia. *Australian Veterinary Journal* 94, 129-37, 2016

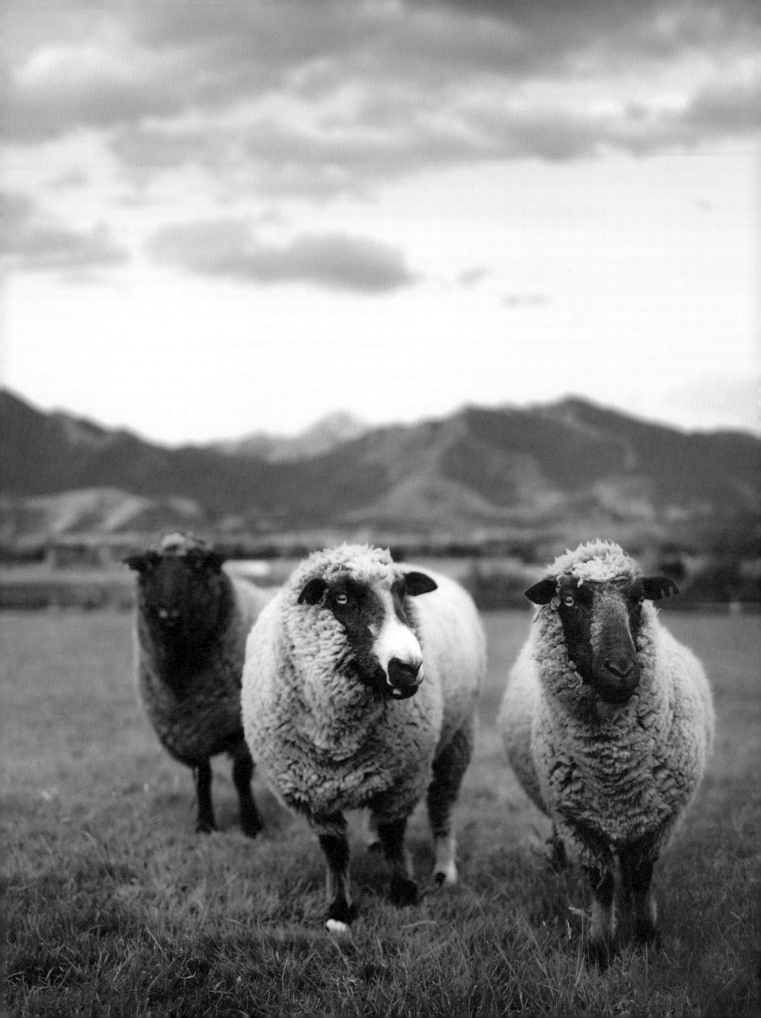

7 Clinical aspects of trace-element requirements of grazing ruminants with particular reference to sheep and cattle

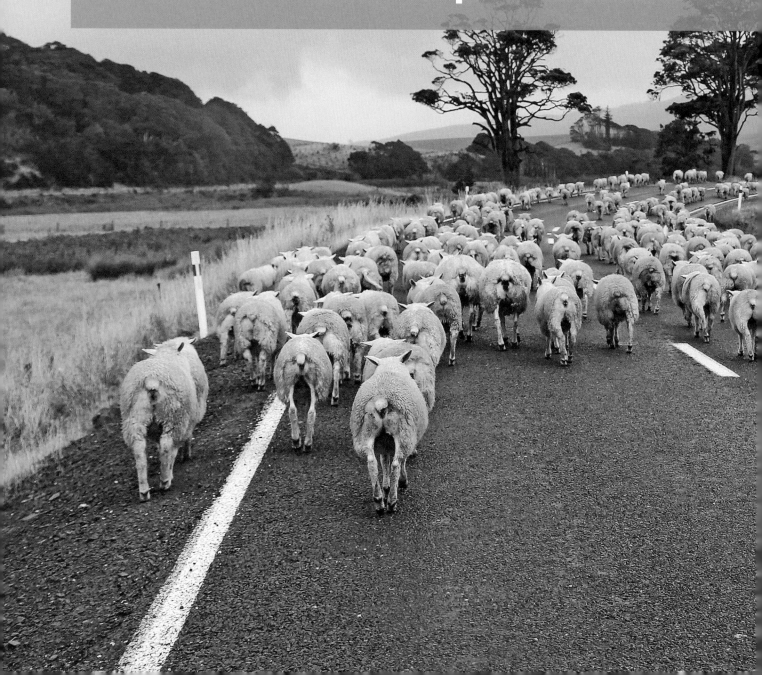

Introduction

In any discussion of trace elements, the requirements of both sheep and cattle must be considered because of their close association on most New Zealand sheep farms. Veterinarians are frequently faced with determining the trace-element status of farm animals; this is of particular importance because of the common occurrence of deficiencies of selenium, copper, cobalt and occasionally iodine. New Zealand farmers are conscious of the impact of trace-element deficiencies on production. Bush sickness or cobalt deficiency once made the raising of sheep and cattle almost impossible in certain areas, particularly the pumice country in central North Island. White muscle disease and selenium-responsive ill thrift in lambs were widespread in Canterbury and other areas of New Zealand until, in the 1950s, selenium supplementation was shown to prevent these conditions. Copper deficiency, especially in calves on peat land, has been recognised for many years.

Despite its small size, New Zealand has an extremely varied geology because it is situated on the interface of two of the world's tectonic plates. When two plates meet, the heavier plate is forced under the lighter plate with the lighter material being forced up into mountain chains such as the Southern Alps. The volcanic ash from which some soils are derived is geologically very recent and the mineral content of these soils is dependent on both the type of material that has erupted from the volcanoes in the area and the subsequent effects of weathering. Soils from older ash showers are usually higher in trace-element content because they have had more time for weathering to release minerals.

It is essential that veterinarians have a sound understanding of the diagnosis of trace-element sufficiency/deficiency and are able to prescribe the most effective supplementation. To a farmer confounded by poor thrift in young animals or a poor lambing performance from the ewes, the 'magic of minerals' offers an easy but frequently wasteful and ineffective answer to the problem. The tendency over the years to 'shotgun'-treat animals with mineral mixes has often been wasteful and in some instances quite ineffective or even unnecessary. It must be emphasised that excellent diagnostic tests for trace elements in animals are available and there is no need for the indiscriminate use of mineral supplements.

Another significant trend in the development of good animal health is the move towards the diagnosis of sufficiency and ensuring that animals have adequate supplies and reserves, rather than concentrating solely on the diagnosis of deficiency. Except perhaps for selenium and iodine, most animals, if fed an adequate diet, will absorb the required levels of essential minerals in their foraging. This fact is frequently overlooked and it is not always appreciated that most supplementation supplies only minor quantities of the required mineral relative to the quantities available in the diet.

From the extensive research and the mass of clinical data and experience that are available, the diagnosis of trace-element sufficiency/deficiency is not difficult. Most tests can be conducted on animal tissue, fodder or soil at low cost. The tests are accurate and offer a professional approach to determining the mineral status of a property and its animals. In the development of any animal health programme it is essential that the veterinarian soon presents the farmer with a clear picture of the farm's trace-element levels and requirements. From this information a logical programme of mineral supplementation can be developed and applied on a regular basis.

If such a procedure is followed, the occasional monitoring of trace-element levels from the tissues of target animals will allow adjustment to the supplementation to be made as required. In most cases the sampling of the mineral levels, once the programme is up and going, will give the farmer the assurance that the animals are acquiring all the essential minerals needed to maintain full health and production.

It is with this approach in mind that the following section is presented — sufficiency for good health rather than deficiency and supplementation when the health of the animals is seriously affected and their production reduced.

Selenium

Selenium was first identified as an element in 1817 and was named from the Greek word *selene*, meaning the moon. Early interest in selenium was on its toxic properties when in 1930 it was shown to be the agent that caused 'alkali disease' or 'blind staggers' in cattle and horses in North America. It was not until 1957 that selenium was shown to be an essential trace element for animals, when it was discovered that selenium could prevent liver necrosis in rats. Soon after, work in the United States and New Zealand showed that white muscle disease in sheep and cattle could be prevented by selenium therapy. Growth rate responses in lambs to selenium were identified throughout much of the eastern South Island and on the coarse pumice soils and some coastal sands of the North Island.

Curiously, many of the diseases that selenium was effective in preventing could also be prevented by vitamin E or slowed by sulphur-containing amino acids, but by the late 1960s the essential nature of selenium even in the presence of vitamin E had been firmly established. However, the discovery of a biochemical role for selenium and an explanation for its intriguing relationship with vitamin E was not made until 1973. Until the discovery of the prophylactic effect of selenium in the animal myopathies (white muscle disease) that became apparent in New Zealand during the 1950s, dosing lambs and calves with vitamin E was used to prevent such diseases developing.

It is now known that the most important function of both selenium and vitamin E is the protection of biological membranes. Peroxides and oxygen radicals are serious cellular toxins that can destroy connective tissue, damage biological membranes, oxidise sulphydryl groups, inactivate enzymes and cause peroxidative damage of nucleic acids. Lipid peroxides are produced particularly during the breakdown of polyunsaturated fatty acids. The functional combination of selenium and vitamin E helps to prevent the damage. Vitamin E is localised in the cell membranes as a biological antioxidant and inhibits the formation of lipid peroxides. Selenium is an essential part of glutathione peroxidase (GSH-px), which catalyses the reduction of peroxides to less harmful hydroxyacids in the cytoplasm. If this protective function of selenium and vitamin E fails, the increased quantities of lipid peroxides may trigger a chain reaction that causes further peroxides and free radicals to be formed, and may eventually lead to the damage of biological membranes and cell death.

Selenium and vitamin E are also important for the maintenance of resistance to infectious disease. Reactive oxygen metabolites produced by granulocytes and macrophages are eliminated by selenium and vitamin E. Various functions of the immune system are inhibited by selenium and vitamin E deficiency, including the migration of leucocytes and phagocytosis. This is particularly important in dairy cows, where it has been found that mammary polymorphonuclear leucocytes from selenium-deficient cows can destroy micro-organisms less efficiently than those from selenium-adequate cows. In the male, adequate selenium levels are necessary for normal sperm development.

While the most important function of selenium is in the protection of biological membranes, a range of other functions have been suggested such as a role in the arachidonic cascade, production of prostaglandin F2α, cell-mediated and humoral immunity and conversion of thyroid hormone thyroxine (T4) to the active tri-iodothyronine (T3) form.

Deficiencies of selenium

The selenium concentration in blood is very responsive to and dependent on the level of selenium in the diet. New Zealand has a low selenium status compared with other countries. When visitors from UK or USA come to New Zealand their blood levels of selenium fall to those of New Zealand's population and vice versa. However, there has been a significant increase in the selenium status of New Zealand humans since 1988; it is not known whether this is due to increased supplementation of livestock or importation of food such as grain from overseas.

Earlier liveweight gain trials conducted on lambs in New Zealand showed selenium responsiveness to be area-dependent, and the responsive areas corresponded closely to regions of low soil selenium content.

A number of factors influence pasture and animal selenium levels, but ultimately the selenium level in plants is highly related to soil levels. Some plants are selenium selectors and concentrate the element many times in their foliage. Such plants do not occur naturally in New Zealand but are present in parts of Queensland, Australia.

Other factors influencing selenium uptake by stock are rainfall and pasture composition. In general, legumes tend to be lower in selenium compared with grasses, particularly low-quality species such as browntop. The pH of the soil is also important in the availability of selenium to plants. Alkalinity encourages the absorption of selenium, as seen in 'alkali disease' in horses. Fertiliser application, particularly the sulphur in superphosphate, may compete for absorption sites with selenium in both plants and animals.

There is also seasonal variation in the selenium content of pasture, the content being generally lowest in spring when rainfall is heaviest. Seasonal variations in cattle blood have ranged as much as from a low mean concentration of 10 µg/l selenium to 20 µg/l selenium, with similar variations recorded in sheep as well.

Other factors are associated with variations in the blood levels of selenium. Marked differences are also seen between animal species.

There may be a relationship between low copper levels

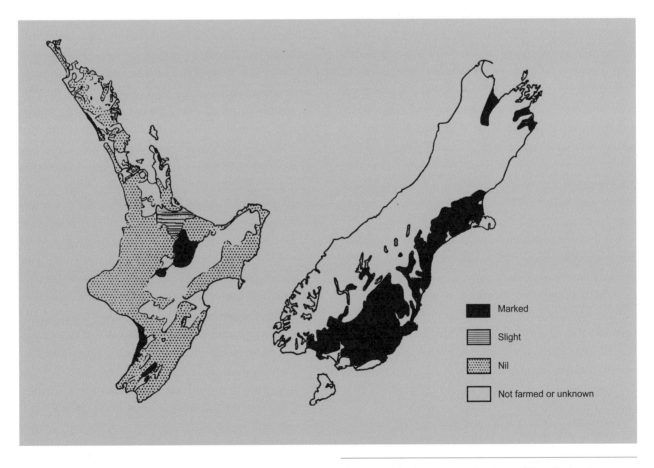

Figure 7.1 Selenium-responsive areas of New Zealand as determined by lamb growth trials (adapted from Andrews et al., 1968).

in sheep and a selenium-deficient diet. The dosing of selenium-deficient sheep with selenium not only raises the selenium level of the animals but may also increase copper storage and retention.

There does not appear to be an age influence on selenium levels in blood of various species, and any variations between sex and breed are minor compared with the dominating influence of dietary selenium levels.

Between 3 million and 5 million hectares of New Zealand are considered to have selenium-deficient soil; these are shown in Figure 7.1. However, it is wise to be cautious about too rigorous an extrapolation from Figure 7.1 to individual farms. In many instances, quite noticeable selenium deficiencies have been recorded in areas considered marginal or even to have normal soil levels of selenium. This may indicate small regional differences or seasonal variations.

A deficiency of selenium can occur when the total level in soil is below 0.03 ppm, and unthriftiness is likely when selenium levels in pasture are less than 0.02 ppm. It is not seen in pastures with above 0.03 ppm of selenium.

One of the most economically important effects of selenium deficiency occurs in sheep and cattle up to approximately 15 months of age and is manifest as slow growth and poor production. It is likely that deer can also be affected. Young cattle may show faded coats with delayed shedding of the winter coat. These signs are non-specific and must be differentiated from under-nutrition, parasitism and other deficiencies.

Weight responses of lambs to dosing with selenium salts have occurred widely in New Zealand. In most instances these responses, some quite remarkable, have been related to areas that could be described as severely selenium-deficient as judged by soil analysis. Extensive trials conducted in 1974–1975 emphasised the importance of the marginally deficient situation. In some of these trials, weight gain responses were achieved when the mean soil selenium levels were 0.56ppm (below 0.5ppm is likely to produce unthriftiness).

The challenge facing the veterinarian is the diagnosis of marginal deficiencies where selenium-responsive ill thrift may go unrecognised by the farmer. Many areas of New Zealand come into this category. No accurate estimate of the economic losses that accrue from uncorrected selenium-responsive unthriftiness can be made, but even on farms where expected weight responses may be small the low cost of supplementation would be more than offset by extra returns as a result of improved animal health.

Myopathy (white muscle disease)

The first reports of white muscle disease in lambs in New Zealand were in 1953. The following year, severe losses from the disease occurred in newborn lambs and lambs a few weeks of age; the main losses reported were from Canterbury and the pumice land of the North Island. Losses of 500 out of 900 and 850 out of 1650 lambs born were recorded by one of the authors on two properties in North Canterbury. These examples were not unique. Because of the differing age occurrence of the deficiency in lambs and calves, the names congenital and delayed white muscle disease were given.

1. **Congenital white muscle disease** has been reported in lambs, calves and kids. Lambs are often born dead or die suddenly soon after birth. In some cases, lambs die of starvation as they are unable to suckle and lesions of the lingual muscles are not uncommon. At necropsy affected lambs usually show distinct white necrotic lesions on the myocardium, which may be streaked with calcified deposits. Animals that have survived for a few days may also have symmetrical myonecrosis, especially of the hind limbs. The muscles take on the appearance of 'cooked chicken flesh'.

2. **Delayed white muscle disease** may occur in lambs from a few days to even several months of age, but is usually seen at about 2–6 weeks of age. It may be precipitated by some procedure such as moving lambs and ewes or yarding for docking. Lambs may walk with a stiff gait and hunched back. They may be unable to suckle. Frequently they are unable to walk at all and will just become recumbent and rather unresponsive. In some cases they will be found dead having died from respiratory failure. At necropsy the familiar lesions of myonecrosis may be seen in skeletal muscles. Frequently such lesions are glistening with streaks of calcified tissue.

White muscle disease can be a cause of death in goat kids between birth and 3 months of age. Losses are usually below 10%, but in some flocks over 50% of kids have died. Affected kids are often found dead but others show signs of dyspnoea, depression, stiffness and nervous signs for 1–2 days prior to death. It has also been reported in calves and deer fawns. The features seen at necropsy are largely the result of right-sided heart failure. There is a variable amount of clear fluid containing fibrin in the thoracic and peritoneal cavities, enlarged liver and typical lesions in the heart and possibly skeletal muscle. Because severely selenium-deficient areas of New Zealand are now recognised and appropriate supplementation is undertaken, it is rare to see clinical white muscle disease. The subclinical effects of selenium deficiency are more common.

Impaired reproduction

Early New Zealand studies on selenium deficiency and reproduction in sheep indicated that it did not affect conception rates but had a significant effect on embryonic survival. This early work described infertility in ewes with lambing percentages as low as 25% because of embryonic death at about 3–4 weeks from conception. Some affected ewes did conceive a second time and appeared as late lambers, but in most cases became dry/dry ewes for that season. This work was later confirmed at Wallaceville Animal Research Centre in 1983. Although there was no appreciable difference in conception rate between the control group of ewes and a group dosed with selenium before mating, and all embryos in both groups were alive up to 23 days after mating, by 30 days no embryos were alive in the selenium-deficient ewes. This contrasted markedly with the selenium-dosed flockmates in which all embryos remained alive over the same period.

An extensive South Island study of the reproductive performance of Merino ewes dosed with 5 mg of sodium selenate 17 days prior to mating showed a 12% reduction in barren ewes compared with those in the control flock. In the same study there was an 8% reduction in barren ewes in a flock grazed on selenium-topdressed pasture. Presumably the effect was also due to a reduction in foetal/embryonic death. A report from the UK in 2009 described the effect of selenium supplementation in marginal/selenium-deficient flocks, on fertility, prolificacy and lambing performance of hill-country sheep.

The above information has shown that in some marginal/selenium-deficient flocks supplementation may have a positive effect on lambing performance. As a result,

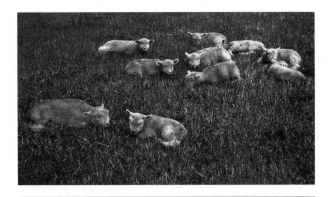

Figure 7.2 Lambs suffering from delayed white muscle disease, North Canterbury, 1955. Note recumbency and pinched faces due to jaw muscle dystrophy.

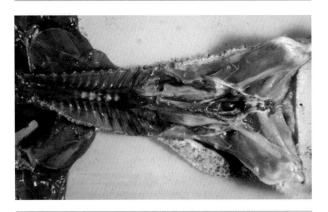

Figure 7.3 Delayed white muscle disease. Note the pale colour of the skeletal muscles.

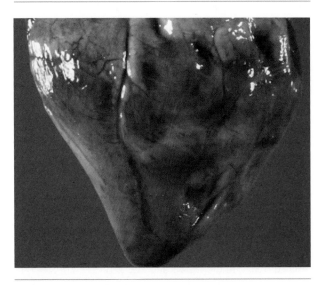

Figure 7.4 Congenital white muscle disease causing scarring of the heart.

some New Zealand sheep farmers, somewhat empirically, dose their ewes with selenium prior to mating, believing that lambing performance will improve. The benefits of this practice would be difficult to assess and consultant veterinarians should deal with each situation as presented, bearing in mind the selenium status of the farm and its animals.

There are reports that have associated low selenium levels with reduced fertility in cows. In Taranaki, Tasker et al. (1987) indicated reduced submission rates and conception rates in unsupplemented dairy cattle when mean glutathione peroxidase levels were below 1 KIU/l.

Selenium deficiency has also been implicated in contributing to retained foetal membranes of dairy cows overseas, although it should be recognised that this condition has multiple causes.

Inflammation and immunity

Selenium deficiency has been shown to inhibit (a) resistance to microbial infections, (b) neutrophil functions, (c) antibody production, (d) proliferation of lymphocytes in response to mitogens, and (e) cyto-destruction by lymphocytes. There is evidence that the effects of selenium on disease resistance may operate at levels higher than those found to be necessary to prevent traditional disease syndromes. Hence there is a need to be aware of these other roles for the element, and there is also a need for further studies to be conducted to investigate the role of selenium in disease resistance under New Zealand conditions. The need for trials to be conducted under New Zealand conditions is paramount because selenium plays a part in only one of a number of antioxidant systems that protect against various types and levels of oxidant challenge.

The antioxidant properties of the selenium-containing enzyme glutathione peroxidase, and the closely related enzyme phospholipid glutathione peroxidase, explain the role of the element in many of the diseases of domestic livestock, where it acts along with membrane-bound vitamin E (α-tocopherol) and other antioxidants to protect cells from oxidant injury. At a cellular level, selenium is involved in three major types of activity. The role of selenium in inflammation and the immune response is thought to be related to the protection of sensitive cellular membranes and enzymes from oxidant attack and also to selenium's involvement in eicosanoid metabolism. The latter has recently been implicated in transmembrane signalling in T lymphocytes.

There have been few field reports linking low selenium to an increased susceptibility to disease. A small number of research trials have been published assessing the relationship between the selenium status of dairy cows and somatic cell counts in milk, and the morbidity of feedlot cattle. These have given mixed results.

Reduced milk production

A number of research trials have investigated milk volume production in response to selenium supplementation. These indicate that economically significant milk production increases with selenium supplementation are unlikely at mean blood selenium levels greater than 250 nmol/l or GSH-px levels greater than 2 KIU/l. At selenium levels below this, responses are variable but there is a tendency for the magnitude of the response to increase with decreasing blood levels (Ellison, 1992; Wichtel et al., 1998).

Other species

Selenium deficiency and vitamin E deficiency have been associated with hepatosis diatetica and mulberry heart disease in pigs; myopathy and exudative diathesis in poultry; and myopathy and steatitis in horses, cats, dogs and ferrets.

Diagnosis of selenium deficiency

A diagnosis of selenium status can be made by one or a combination of three methods:

1. On-farm assessment — previous experience

The history of the farm, including previous experience with clinical manifestations of selenium deficiency, selenium supplementation, knowledge of other farms in the same district and results of previous chemical analysis, should be considered.

Other relevant factors would include the clinical signs, age, species, pasture species, stage of growth and management. The usefulness of this approach is limited by how much is known about the area and the vague nature of the clinical manifestations of marginal selenium deficiency.

2. Chemical analysis

As previously discussed, selenium levels in soil, plants and animals in the same location show a very close relationship. Thus, if the soil is known to be deficient in selenium the likelihood of livestock problems occurring is very high. However, tissue samples from animals, often young animals, are preferred as they give the best indication of the selenium absorbed. As there is usually little between-animal variation in selenium levels in samples taken from the same farm, the number of samples required is small and usually 3–5 samples will suffice. Soil and plant levels may be useful in forecasting the possibility of future selenium deficiency, for example on an unstocked farm or land being converted to livestock from cropping or horticulture.

Selenium is present in all tissues, but the liver and kidney normally have the highest selenium concentrations. Liver is the organ normally used for selenium assay and liver biopsies may be taken serially from an individual animal.

Selenium levels can be determined from either serum or whole-blood samples. Alternatively, blood glutathione peroxidase (GSH-px) levels may be used. If the latter are used it must be remembered that there is a delay in the response of erythrocyte GSH-px activity to changes in selenium status. Erythrocyte GSH-px activity depends on the selenium availability during erythropoiesis and as erythrocytes remain in circulation for some months, sudden changes in selenium status will not immediately be reflected in erythrocyte GSH-px activity.

The type of sample selected will differ depending upon the objective of testing, as indicated by Table 7.1 (adapted from Clark and Ellison, 1993).

Reference ranges

Reference ranges may vary with different laboratories; the one to consult is that from the laboratory performing the analysis in question.

The interpretation of analytical results requires careful consideration and experience by the advising veterinarian. In some cases a decision may be made to supplement animals even though the likelihood of a production response is uncertain. Always remember that sufficiency throughout the year is required for good animal health, and therefore for preventative animal health the focus should be on ensuring sufficiency rather than diagnosing deficiency.

Reason for sampling	Time to sample	Species and age	Sample type	Sample #	Interpretation
Poor performance	At the time of the problem	Affected animals	EDTA blood	3	Means
Farm deficiencies	Seasonal variation minor. Could be any time, esp. late spring/early summer	Unsupplemented adults or young stock	EDTA blood	3	Means
Adequate reserves	Late winter/early spring	Unsupplemented adults or young stock	EDTA blood	3	Means
		If supplemented:	Serum/liver	Pref. 10	Individual values
Supplementation	Half-way point between planned supplementations	Animals being supplemented	Serum or liver best	Pref. 10	Individual values

Table 7.1 Sampling for selenium depending upon the reason for sampling.

	Low	Marginal	Adequate
Glutathione peroxidase — whole blood (KIU/l); sheep	<1	1–3	>3
Glutathione peroxidase — whole blood (KIU/l); cattle	<0.5	0.5–2	>2
Blood selenium — nmol/l	<130	130–250	>250
Liver selenium — nmol/kg (sheep)	<250	250–450	>450
Liver selenium — nmol/kg (cattle)	<600	600–850	>850
Serum selenium — nmol/l (cattle)	<85	85–140	>140

Table 7.2 Example of reference ranges for selenium in sheep and cattle.

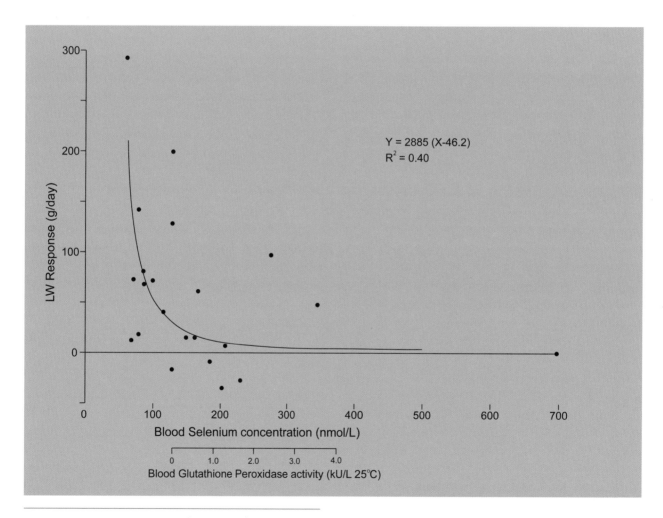

Figure 7.5 The average blood selenium concentrations of flocks of unsupplemented control lambs and the observed liveweight responses of their selenium-supplemented cohorts. Each point represents a controlled selenium supplementation trial (modified from Ellison, 1992).

In dairy cows, selenium levels have sometimes been recommended much in excess of those outlined above. However, the justification for this is largely based on research undertaken overseas and care should be taken in extrapolating such data.

Clear growth rate responses to selenium supplementation have been demonstrated, as shown in Figure 7.5.

3. Controlled trials

Due to increased sophistication of analytical methods it is no longer necessary or desirable to conduct controlled treatment trials to diagnose selenium deficiency. The clinical manifestations of selenium deficiency are varied, and marginal deficiencies are difficult to confirm using controlled trials because of seasonal variations in selenium uptake, the vague nature of some of the signs of deficiency, farmer reluctance to leave animals unsupplemented and the cost and time involved in conducting trials. However, where the reference ranges are uncertain there is a need for carefully conducted response trials.

Prevention of selenium deficiency

Following a decision to supplement, advice is given on which animals should be supplemented, by what method, how much and how often. These decisions are made on the basis of the clinical findings, past local experience, appropriate research findings and economics. It is often wise to monitor the effect of a programme and modify it accordingly, because the degree of deficiency varies markedly from farm to farm and supplementation programmes vary also. Young stock in particular are usually supplemented, and in addition ewes before tupping and lambing and cows before calving may be treated. In many instances all animals may require treatment. The lactating dairy cow is a special case, not considered in this text, but such animals may be at high risk of selenium deficiency in many parts of New Zealand.

It should be noted that with the increased awareness of New Zealand's marginal selenium status and the availability of a range of supplements, animals are in danger of being supplemented unnecessarily without tissue selenium analysis to justify the decision. Selenium is extremely toxic in overdose and supplements should be used with caution. For more information on selenium toxicosis, refer to Parton et al. (2006).

Methods of supplementation

Drench

As a cheap and safe method of supplying selenium to sheep, drenching is effective provided it is done at the appropriate times of the year and periodic monitoring of animals is undertaken. A single dose of selenium usually provides adequate supplementation for 5–6 weeks. Virtually all oral anthelmintic drenches in New Zealand are selenised, and as such lambs and hoggets, in most cases, receive quite adequate selenium supplementation by this method during the summer–autumn period because of routine monthly drenching programmes to control internal parasites (see Chapter 8). In the case of older sheep, if selenium supplementation is required then both ewes and rams should be dosed at least 1–2 months before joining and the pregnant ewes may need to be dosed once or twice during pregnancy. Further dosing may be necessary after lambing depending on the degree of deficiency.

Because of better bioavailability of selenium, sodium selenate is the usual oral form of selenium used and is available pre-mixed as a supplement for oral dosing. Care should be taken to ensure the appropriate dose rate is used.

Intra-ruminal bolus

Intra-ruminal boluses, frequently containing a combination of trace elements, have been shown to be effective for 6–12 months. Additionally, long-acting anthelmintic capsules that are sometimes given to ewes prior to lambing frequently contain selenium.

Subcutaneous injection

Sodium selenate is available for animal use in injectable form, sometimes also combined with vitamin B12. Selenium may also be included in some clostridial vaccines or injectable anthelmintics. However, the 'safety factor' with these injectable forms of selenium is considerably less than selenium given orally, so extreme caution should be applied in their use. There are numerous reports of selenium toxicity following the use of injectable forms, particularly when selenised clostridial vaccines are given to lambs at docking. The period of efficacy of these short-acting injections is approximately 4–7 weeks.

Several long-acting selenium injections, sometimes combined with vitamin B12, are available; these contain barium selenate. Because release is slow, the risk of toxicity is reduced. These injections give a supply of selenium for 6–18 months depending on the dose rate and class of livestock in which they are used. Selenium crosses the placenta, so an injection given to a ewe pre-mating will also raise her lamb's selenium levels through to about weaning. Tissue reactions may occur, so care in choosing the site of injection is essential.

Selenium pour-on

Selenium can be absorbed dermally and a pour-on formulation is available for use in cattle and deer.

Topdressing with selenium prills

The annual application of slow-release selenium prills is effective in preventing deficiency for approximately 12 months and is a relatively economical method of providing supplementation.

Selenium topdressing, even when used in strips rather than as a blanket treatment, will raise blood levels of selenium in sheep and cattle several times. Further, these levels are maintained for several months and in most cases remain elevated for up to a year. Following topdressing, blood selenium rises rapidly to a maximum after 2–3 months (as measured by GSH-px in blood) and then decreases at a slightly slower rate, usually reaching pre-topdressing levels in 12 months.

When sodium selenate is used as a topdressing, 15% of the selenium is absorbed into foliage within 24 hours to increase the concentration to perhaps 100 times. Thereafter it decreases rapidly and exponentially with a half-life of only 3–4 weeks, so that after 2–3 months the pasture concentration is only 10% of the peak. The soil absorbs some selenium very rapidly and most of the remainder is reduced to selenite within a week. Slow-release selenium prills incorporate barium selenate and provide a longer period of supplementation.

Even under conditions of very high rainfall, such as encountered in south Westland, the use of selenium topdressing to supplement animals' selenium has proven highly successful. An annual rainfall in that area of 4000–5000 mm per annum is regularly recorded, and sheep grazing topdressed areas maintained more than adequate selenium levels for 12 months.

Cobalt

Cobalt deficiency in ruminants is primarily a wasting disease characterised by anorexia, ill thrift, cachexia, anaemia and in some cases death of the affected animals. It is important to recognise that there is an 'order' of sensitivity to the disease among grazing animals. The most sensitive are young sheep; then, in order, mature sheep, calves in the 6- to 18-month age group and, least sensitive of all, adult cattle. Horses are not affected.

Historical

'Bush sickness' is a term seldom heard nowadays, yet up until the early 1930s it signified a mysterious deficiency that had taken out of production vast areas of land on which stock sickened and died. In the first report of the New Zealand Department of Agriculture, dated 1893, E Clifton, Stock Inspector for the Auckland district, reported that excessively high losses of sheep caused by a condition known locally as 'Tauranga disease' had stopped all progress and settlement in that district. In other areas the disease acquired further regional names such as 'Morton Mains disease' in Southland and 'Mairoa dopiness' in the Mairoa region of the King Country.

Until the early 1930s, New Zealand investigations were based on the theory that bush sickness was due to a deficiency of iron. In 1933, Australian workers established that it was not the iron in ilmenite that cured 'coast disease' and 'wasting disease' — instead, cobalt, a trace constituent of the crude material, was the key dietary element. The connection between bush sickness and cobalt deficiency was soon made in New Zealand also.

The fact that cobalt deficiency was in reality vitamin B12 deficiency was not recognised until after the isolation of vitamin B12 by American and British workers in 1948. Research workers in New Zealand, of whom Andrews was the most prominent, developed an intense interest in cobalt deficiency, its diagnosis via tissue vitamin B12 levels, and its control. By 1940, areas of deficiency had been mapped in broad outline, diagnostic criteria had been established, and methods of controlling the disease, based largely on the use of cobaltised superphosphate, had been established.

In New Zealand the regular use of cobalt on farms with severely deficient soils has resulted in the virtual disappearance of cobalt deficiency as a major disease in cattle and to a large extent in mature sheep. However, in young sheep cobalt deficiency remains a problem and the clinical syndrome is often far from clear-cut, a point to be emphasised. The main losses in production from cobalt deficiency are now in those areas where deficiency is marginal, and a low grade or 'subclinical' disease is produced where poor performance of stock may be unrecognised or accepted as normal. A further contributing factor to the re-emergence of cobalt deficiency has been a fall in the use of cobalt in fertiliser on deficient or marginally deficient areas.

In addition to the classical form of cobalt deficiency, animal B12 status has been linked to a variety of conditions such as polioencephalomalacia in sheep, white liver disease of lambs, infertility and metabolic disease of cattle, and depressed milk production in cows. Also suggested are a variety of lesions of the brain, spinal cord and peripheral nerves, myocardium and skeletal muscle. Cobalt deficiency has also been linked with Phalaris staggers and ragwort toxicity.

Function and metabolism of cobalt

Cobalt is the essential constituent of true vitamin B12. The term vitamin B12 is loosely applied to a group of four metabolically active cobalamines which may be present in animal tissue. The term vitamin B12 should correctly be given only to one of these, cyanocobalamin, which is in fact about the rarest of the tissue cobalamines. Microbial production of cobalamin and cobalamin analogues in the rumen is dependent on cobalt and the organic substrates that the organisms have.

Absorption of true vitamin B12 is considered to occur mainly from the small intestine and appears to be enhanced by slower rates of passage of ingesta through the intestine. The intestinal absorption of vitamin B12 may vary from about 3% up to 33%. The principal storage depot for vitamin B12 is the liver, although true storage for a water-soluble vitamin has been debated. Serum vitamin B12 levels tend to reflect dietary cobalt and to a lesser extent liver vitamin B12 status.

The primary metabolic defect in vitamin B12 deficiency is a block in the utilisation of propionic acid, one of the essential volatile fatty acids produced in the rumen and a main source of blood glucose.

Propionate is produced as a result of the fermentation of

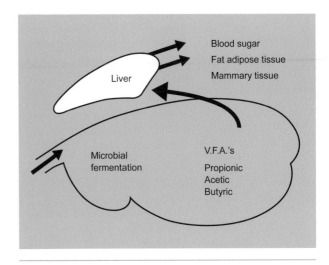

Figure 7.6 Ruminant carbohydrate metabolism.

soluble carbohydrate either directly or through succinate (see Figure 7.7).

From Figure 7.7 it can be seen that the main pathway of propionate metabolism is via methyl malonate to succinate, in which form it enters the Krebs cycle and can function as a source of glucose. The transformation of malonate to succinate is dependent on the methyl malonyl coenzyme A isomerase enzyme system, which is dependent on vitamin B12. Hence, the failure of this system is the basis of the starvation aspect of cobalt deficiency. In deficient sheep there is a marked increase in methyl malonic acid and propionic acid in the blood, with a concurrent increase in methyl malonic acid in the urine.

Deficiencies of vitamin B12 in sheep also interfere with the metabolism of folic acid, because vitamin B12 is required for the metabolism of methionine, which facilitates the transport of folic acid into liver cells. The fatty infiltration of the liver is considered to be secondary to a deficiency of methionine. Methionine is also essential for optimum wool growth.

Cobalt requirements

It is believed that pastures containing 0.11 mg Co/kg DM or greater are adequate to meet the cobalt requirements of sheep and cattle. Weaned lambs have a vitamin B12 requirement of 11 µg/day. Vitamin B12 is present in milk at 10.3 µg/l in cobalt-supplemented sheep and may fall to

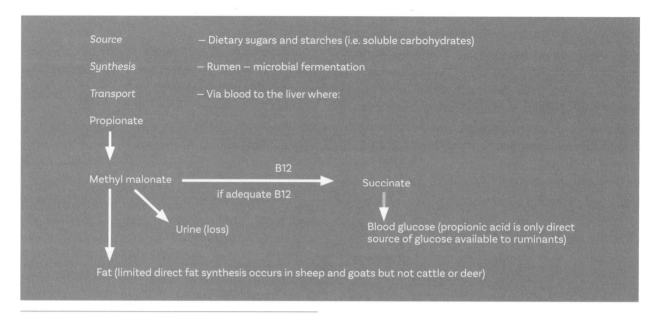

Figure 7.7 Ruminant metabolism of propionic acid.

Plant	Cobalt (mg/kg DM)
Timothy	0.09
Cocksfoot	0.11
Meadow fescue	0.12
Short-rotation ryegrass	0.13
Perennial ryegrass	0.16
Red clover	0.23
White clover	0.24

Table 7.3 Cobalt contents in different pasture plants grown under the same conditions (Andrews, 1971).

2.5 µg/l in ewes grazing cobalt-deficient pasture.

In some soils the cobalt level *per se* is adequate for animal requirements but is not fully available in their diet. In New Zealand, one area of classical cobalt deficiency is the Morton Mains region of Southland which has relatively high total soil cobalt levels, 3.3–4.8 mg/kg. The development of deficiency depends largely on the extractable cobalt available. Where animal deficiencies occur, cobalt concentrations are usually less than 2 mg/kg and the extractable cobalt is below 0.25 mg/kg.

Acid soils such as granite generally lack cobalt, while basaltic soils are usually adequate. Sedimentary and volcanic soils often reflect the cobalt content of the parent rock. For example, the central plateau of the North Island has ash soils from volcanic eruption and is recognised as a cobalt-deficient area.

The cobalt content in soil can be decreased by weathering, leaching and repetitive cropping. Plants growing in waterlogged soils appear to have cobalt levels many times higher than the same soil types with good drainage. Other minerals such as manganese, iron and nickel can reduce cobalt uptake. Liming, by reducing soil acidity, also reduces cobalt uptake by plants. The legumes tend to have a greater uptake of cobalt than grasses, but the differences between plants become negligible when the soil cobalt is very low.

There are also seasonal variations in pasture cobalt concentrations in deficient and marginally deficient regions. Pasture levels are generally lower in spring and summer and higher in autumn and winter. In New Zealand, cobalt deficiency appears to be associated with lush spring growth although the severe clinical signs may not become evident until summer.

The ingestion of cobalt from soil is important in deficient areas, so that in marginally deficient pasture a low grazing intensity is more likely to induce deficiency than heavy grazing. Because liver reserves of vitamin B12 can be adequate for 3–4 months, the signs of deficiency do not necessarily coincide with the time of lowest intake.

Clinical features of cobalt deficiency

Young growing sheep, particularly weaned lambs, are the most sensitive of all animals to cobalt deficiency and it is this class of stock that veterinarians are most likely to use to assess the adequacy of cobalt status. The next group that may be affected are adult sheep, then calves 6–18 months of age and mature cattle, in that order. If the weaner lambs are healthy, cobalt deficiency is unlikely in other classes of animal.

The sensitivity of deer to cobalt deficiency is largely unknown. A surveillance report (*Surveillance* 2, 29, 2004) described a large mob of yearling deer that had lost condition and were unthrifty. Trace-element testing of 10 animals picked at random showed that vitamin B12 concentrations were below <57 pmol/l, surprisingly low. The animals were injected with vitamin B12 and a dramatic response was reported. Although this is a circumstantial report, it does suggest that deer may also be sensitive to cobalt deficiency. However, it is suggested that deer are less susceptible to cobalt deficiency than sheep, and the vitamin B12 reference ranges used for sheep should not be used to diagnose deficiency in deer.

Cobalt deficiency is characterised by loss of appetite producing poor growth and hence is essentially a simple starvation, although animals are usually grazing on adequate feed. In sheep, a watery discharge from the eyes may be present and the wool is white or washy and has a reduced growth rate. A normocytic normochromic anaemia may develop later in the disease. A fatty liver may be present on necropsy.

These classical signs of cobalt deficiency may still be seen, but more commonly one would expect to be confronted mainly with a problem of impaired weight gain in lambs around or after weaning. Because inappetence is also an important clinical sign of nematode parasitism, assessing the cobalt status is one aspect of a comprehensive approach to investigating hogget and lamb ill thrift. It should be noted that in young lambs, during the transition phase from monogastric to ruminant, there is little change in their trace-element status. Hence, on deficient or marginal properties, monitoring lamb vitamin B12 levels at docking is justified.

A number of diseases have also been linked with low vitamin B12 status: in sheep, polioencephalomalacia, ovine white liver disease and Phalaris staggers; in cattle, infertility, metabolic disease and depressed milk production. Experimental work in sheep in Scotland has linked cobalt deficiency in ewes with fewer lambs, more stillbirths and neonatal mortalities (Fisher and MacPherson, 1990).

Diagnosis of cobalt status

A full range of diagnostic criteria should be used when assessing cobalt status.

1. Geographical position of the farm

It is important to consider the location of the property in relation to soil maps of New Zealand (see Figure 7.8). Most cobalt-deficient and marginally deficient areas have been well defined. In addition, it is important to consider the history of the property with regard to topdressing, pasture species, season and any previous investigations into ill thrift in young sheep. In some cases the results of previous analyses of animal tissue may be available for consideration.

2. Clinical signs

Clinical signs themselves are obviously not diagnostic of cobalt deficiency, but the weighing of a representative sample of hoggets or lambs and comparing the data with targets may convince the farmer just how depressed the animals have become. Observant farmers will usually notice flock anorexia, which is always an important feature of cobalt deficiency.

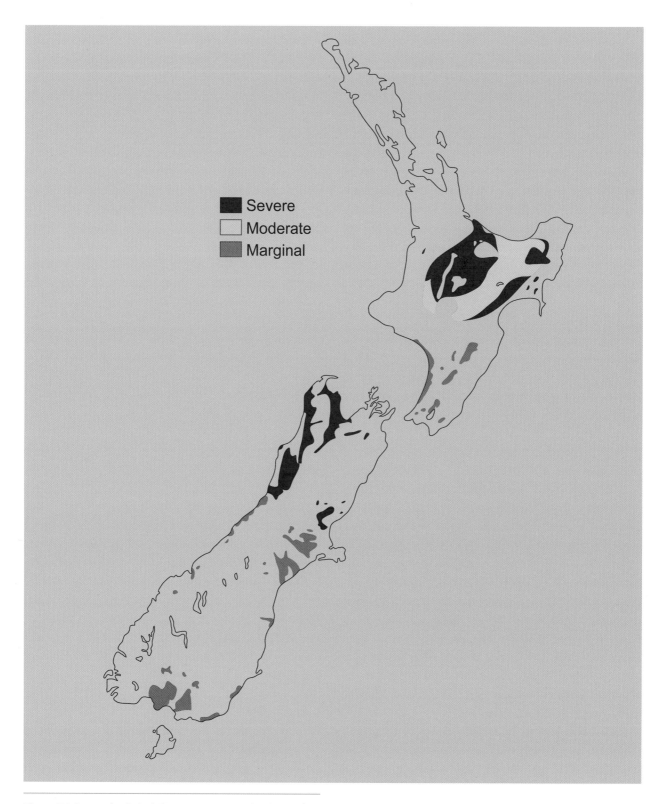

Figure 7.8 Areas of cobalt deficiency in New Zealand.

3. Chemical analysis of tissues and blood
Liver and serum vitamin B12

The liver appears to be the essential site where vitamin B12 is utilised. Thus, liver vitamin B12 levels measure reserves and responsiveness and are considered one of the more accurate ways of assessing cobalt status. While the reference range for sheep has been derived from a number of response trials, there is relatively little reliable data for cattle, and levels must be interpreted with caution. At least three liver samples and preferably more are required.

Serum vitamin B12 levels reflect cobalt intake, but when liver reserves are low and sheep are grazing pasture of low cobalt content then the serum vitamin B12 also indicates responsiveness.

Approximately 10 serum samples are required. Serum vitamin B12 levels must be interpreted with caution as levels may be elevated if liver damage is present, if sheep have been yarded for even short periods or if sheep have grazed cobalt-sufficient pasture for a few days before being sampled. The time of sampling and the type of samples collected is likely to vary depending on the objective of testing, as demonstrated by Table 7.4.

In areas classified as marginally cobalt-deficient, year-to-year variations are likely to occur in the incidence of deficiency in lambs. In these areas it is advisable to sample unsupplemented lambs at docking or weaning, especially in seasons with lush spring growth.

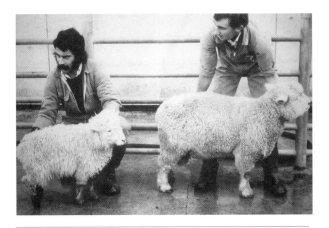

Figure 7.9 A severely cobalt-deficient hogget (left) compared with a normal hogget of the same age and breed.

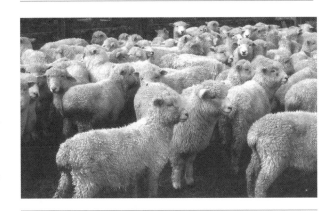

Figure 7.10 A group of ewe hoggets with cobalt deficiency. In May, the average weight of these hoggets was 22 kg.

Reason	Time to sample	Species and age	Sample type	Sample number	Interpretation
Poor performance	Time of problem	Affected animals	Serum or liver	10 serum, 3 liver	Means only
Farm deficiencies	NI: Nov-Feb SI: Feb-Mar	Weaned lambs	Liver	3	Means only
Adequate reserves	Late spring/early summer	Weaned lambs	Liver	3	Means only
Supplementation	Halfway through expected period of insufficiency	Animals being supplemented	Liver best or serum	At least 3 liver or 10 serum	Means only

NI: North Island; SI: South Island.

Table 7.4 Sampling for cobalt depending on the reason for sampling (adapted from Clark and Ellison, 1993).

	Sheep Vitamin B12 Serum (pmol/l)	Sheep Vitamin B12 Liver (nmol/kg)	Cattle Vitamin B12 Liver (nmol/kg)
Responsive	<336	<280	<75
Marginal	336–500	280–375	75–220
Adequate	>500	>375	>220

Table 7.5 Example of reference ranges for vitamin B12.

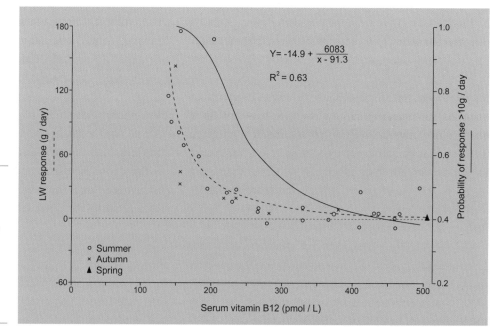

Figure 7.11 Serum vitamin B12 levels related to weight gain response and probability of a weight gain response of >10 g/day in response to vitamin B12 treatment for data closest to the middle of January (from Clark, 1989).

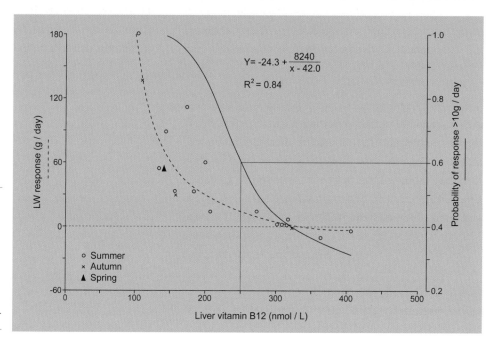

Figure 7.12 Liver vitamin B12 levels related to weight gain response and probability of a weight gain response of >10 g/day in response to vitamin B12 treatment for data closest to the middle of January (from Clark, 1989).

Interpretation of laboratory results

It is important to recognise that the probability of achieving a growth rate response to supplementation decreases as the serum or liver vitamin B12 levels increase. Thus, even lambs with levels in the 'responsive' range may not show a significant growth response to supplementation in every case. This is best illustrated by Figures 7.11 and 7.12.

The interpretation of these graphs is as follows:
1. The individual open circles, crosses and triangles (o, x, ▲) relate to individual experiments investigating cobalt deficiency.
2. The dotted line (- - -) shows the linear regression best fit curve of the liveweight response (g/day) for these experiments.
3. The solid line (—) represents the probability of obtaining a weight gain response of >10 g/day at various serum or liver vitamin B12 levels.

It can be seen from these graphs that, for example, lambs in January with mean liver vitamin B12 levels of 250 nmol/kg (in the 'responsive' range) have an approximately 60% probability of achieving an economically significant growth rate response to supplementation. It would be prudent to supplement these lambs, but a response is not guaranteed.

It has been suggested that the reference range for vitamin B12 in sheep should vary for different age groups. Thus the cut-off values for ewes should be lower than that for hoggets, which should be lower than that for lambs (Clark, 1998).

Other diagnostic tests

Urinary methylmalonic acid and/or formiminoglutamic acid are possible diagnostic tests, as both these metabolites are elevated in cobalt deficiency. They are not currently offered by diagnostic laboratories as they are more costly than liver and serum vitamin B12 tests and, while they confirm the presence of deficiency, they are not as useful in predicting the likelihood of a response. However, it should be noted that serum methylmalonic acid (MMA) is claimed to give a more precise indication of responsiveness to vitamin B12 or cobalt supplementation. Field trials have shown that neither low serum vitamin B12 nor elevated MMA concentrations were necessarily indicative of responsiveness to supplementation in suckling lambs, but they may indicate an impending response.

Pasture analysis for cobalt levels are of limited value in assessing the cobalt status of animals unless they are performed on a regular basis (probably monthly). This is because animals can survive for considerable periods on low pasture cobalt due to a liver storage of vitamin B12. Soil analysis may give an indication of deficiency but many factors influence the level of cobalt in the soil that is available to the animal.

4. Controlled response trials

Controlled response trials have been used extensively in the past to diagnose cobalt deficiency; while they are a definitive test, they may fail to diagnose marginal deficiencies in certain years or instances where the trial is not conducted at the correct time. Chemical analysis should always be conducted in conjunction with these trials.

The most commonly used trial is a weight gain response in weaned lambs using approximately 50 control lambs and 50 lambs treated with an injection of vitamin B12. Regular weighing is required and the lambs must be individually identified with an ear tag.

Treatment and prevention of cobalt deficiency

Topdressing

Following the discovery of cobalt deficiency as the cause of 'bush sickness', topdressing pastures with cobaltised superphosphate at a rate of 350 g of cobalt sulphate/ha per annum became a standard practice in deficient areas of New Zealand. Although only between 1% and 4% of cobalt is taken up by plants and utilised by animals, this practice proved to be effective, simple and economical. On pumice soils where cobalt has been applied regularly for 10 years or more, cobalt levels have remained satisfactory for three or four years following cessation of topdressing, and as a result it was recommended that the rate of application on these farms be reduced to 175 g/ha of cobalt sulphate every 3 years. The current recommendation is 70 g Co/ha per annum, applied in spring. In some instances, even lower rates have been applied and cobalt deficiency has occurred as a result. In cobalt-deficient areas, cobalt topdressing gives good protection of young lambs for up to 7 months, which in most cases should take them through the danger period. It should be applied before lambs are weaned, because of the short-term nature of cobalt sulphate in raising cobalt levels. On soils with a high manganese content, cobalt topdressing may be less effective. Although a valuable and effective way of supplementing cobalt to animals, the relatively high cost of cobalt has diminished the attractiveness of topdressing as the sole means of supplementation. In areas where deficiency is infrequent, direct supplementation of lambs with vitamin B12 is likely to be a more cost-effective method of supplementation.

Oral dosing

Because animals require a regular dietary intake of cobalt, drenching is not a practical form of treatment. Even though there are a number of oral supplements on the market, weekly dosing is required to ensure sufficient intake and this is not feasible for most farmers.

The recommended oral dose for lambs is 7 mg cobalt (35 mg $CoSO_4.7H_2O$) per week or 35 mg cobalt (175 mg $CoSO_4.7H_2O$) for cattle per week. Monthly dosing with 300 mg cobalt has been used to reduce death rates in severely deficient country, but does not prevent suboptimal growth. Virtually all oral anthelmintics available in New Zealand are mineralised and contain about 2–3 mg of cobalt/10 ml, but these are not a sufficient form of supplementation.

Vitamin B12 injections

Vitamin B12 injections are widely used in many areas of New Zealand to protect lambs against cobalt deficiency and may be combined with injectable anthelmintics or vaccines. The period of protection given by vitamin B12 injections depends on the liver reserves of the animal and the level of cobalt deficiency in the pasture. In New Zealand two types of vitamin B12 injections are available. Water-soluble formulations will boost levels of the vitamin for a period of about a month. A long-acting product incorporating vitamin B12 in a lactide/glycolide polymer is also available and may also incorporate selenium. This product has been reported to raise liver and serum vitamin B12 levels for 6–8 months and may be given to lambs in cobalt-deficient areas at docking or weaning time. Long-acting injections are generally more expensive, and so on some properties may be reserved for replacement ewe lambs while slaughter lambs would receive the cheaper, short-acting injections.

Intra-ruminal capsules

Intra-ruminal capsules containing a range of trace elements including cobalt are available in New Zealand and give a period of protection for up to a year. Care must be taken in dosing to avoid damage to the larynx or pharynx. Anthelmintic capsules frequently include mineral additives including cobalt.

Supplementation of ewes with cobalt capsules, given early in pregnancy, have been shown to protect the growth performance of lambs for up to 90 days of age and also influence the subsequent serum vitamin B12 response in the lamb to vitamin B12 injections.

Pasture foliar spraying

Boom spraying of pasture with 0.14 kg $CoSo_4$ per hectare is a supplementation method that may be utilised on flat or rolling country. The mixture should be sprayed onto actively growing pasture 2–3 weeks pre-grazing to allow suitable uptake by the grass before it is grazed.

Other methods of supplying cobalt include the use of $CoSo_4$ in drinking water and cobalt in stock licks, but neither of these methods is particularly satisfactory in ensuring that animals ingest adequate levels of cobalt. This is especially the case for sheep, who drink relatively little water.

Copper

Copper is an essential element required by a number of enzymes involved in specific oxidase-type reactions in the animal's body. Copper is derived by grazing animals from plants, which in turn have drawn their copper from the soil. Under many grazing situations the copper in soil and plants is not easily available for absorption by the animal because of interference by other elements. Large areas of New Zealand have soils that are either low in available copper or have elements that interfere with copper uptake so that the copper requirements of many animals, particularly cattle, are inadequate.

Copper deficiency, both clinical and subclinical, is common and always represents a challenge to the veterinarian in diagnosis and effective therapy. If this is not conducted carefully, ineffective therapy may result. In some cases copper poisoning may occur, particularly in sheep.

Copper in soil

New Zealand soils commonly contain about 17 ppm of copper. Some New Zealand soils have levels as low as 2 ppm, but most rarely exceed 25 ppm of copper. The availability of copper in soils to plants and animals is extremely complex. Copper may be bound in the soil, in water-soluble form, as exchangeable ions, as organic complexes, or in association with iron, aluminium and manganese and other mineral complexes.

The mobility and availability of copper is related to soil texture, drainage, redox potential, pH and organic matter. Up to 99% of copper in soil may be complexed with organic matter. Wet soils are usually anaerobic and tend to convert copper to various insoluble sulphides. If the soil is low in organic matter, the soluble copper compounds are leached out.

Increasing soil pH with lime generally decreases the mobility of copper in soil by increasing the adsorption of Cu^{++} ions onto iron and manganese oxides and clay lattices. Over-liming can render copper largely unavailable from soil. Lime topdressing raises the soil pH and increases the availability of molybdenum. This has been associated with copper deficiency in New Zealand and is also an important cause of copper deficiency on Scottish hill country.

Because of these complicating factors, the diagnosis of copper deficiency in animals by the measurement of copper in soil over which they graze is of little value.

Copper in plants

Plant tissues normally contain 5–20 ppm dry matter of copper. Copper deficiency usually occurs when the concentration falls below 4 ppm, while toxicity occurs when levels rise above 20 ppm. In New Zealand very few areas grow pastures that contain more than 13 ppm of copper. The young shoots of plants contain the highest amounts of copper, but levels decrease as the plant matures.

Legumes have a higher affinity for copper than do grasses, especially when they are growing in soils of high copper content. Similarly, some of the newer forages fed to livestock, such as chicory and plantain, contain higher levels of copper than grasses. The application of copper fertilisers to copper-deficient soils will increase the copper content of plants growing in that soil, but nitrogenous fertilisers that promote plant growth tend to reduce the pasture copper content. The copper content of plants, along with molybdenum, sulphur and iron levels, are frequently measured during the investigation of the copper levels in animals as they are important factors in deciding the most appropriate form of therapy.

Copper absorption and storage

Animals obtain copper mainly from plants but also from ingested soil. Copper is absorbed from the intestinal tract, transported in the blood loosely bound to albumin, and most is stored in the liver, which may contain between 40% and 70% of the total body copper.

By the twelfth week of gestation, the lamb foetus is beginning to accumulate copper in its liver. This coincides with a concurrent decrease in the ewe's liver stores. The newborn lamb absorbs copper very efficiently. Immediately after birth, almost 100% of the lamb's copper intake is absorbed but this decreases to 10% by weaning.

Adult sheep absorb less than 10% of dietary copper and only about 5% of this intake is stored in the liver. The absorption of copper is partially controlled by the sheep, as during lactation there is a temporary increase in the efficiency of absorption. A similar situation is also found in sheep with hypocupraemia. The efficiency with which copper is assimilated from the diet depends on the solubility of the copper, which in turn is dependent on pH. In the rumen, most of the copper is present in an insoluble form while abomasal absorption is minimal, but with the rising pH of the ingesta distally, copper is freed and absorbed in the ileum and large intestine.

The differences in the absorption rate and in the excretion rate of copper between species may affect the copper requirements of the animal. Sheep are more susceptible than other domestic ruminants to copper accumulation and toxicity. The reason for this is that they have less control over intestinal homeostasis, a limited capacity to excrete copper from the liver and their lysosomes are unable to sequester large amounts of copper.

Factors influencing copper absorption and metabolism

1. Age

Newborn lambs have a higher total copper concentration than their dams; up to 50% of their copper being present in the liver. However, their plasma copper levels are lower than those of their dam as the foetus is unable to synthesise caeruloplasmin. Plasma copper levels rise rapidly to adult levels 7 days after birth. Young lambs are able to absorb copper very efficiently while they are on a liquid diet. This is due to the high absorption capacity of the large intestine and the lack of interference by sulphide in the rumen. The efficiency of absorption falls with age as the rumen becomes functional and only 2–10% of ingested copper is then absorbed.

2. Pasture composition

The amount of copper absorbed from pasture varies considerably, depending on the species of plant and the season. The copper contained in stored fodder such as hay or silage may be absorbed at a higher rate than that of pasture. However, silage can have very low available copper, which may be related to the amount of soil (and thus iron and molybdenum) that contaminates the silage when it is being made. The absorption of copper from various feeds is shown in Table 7.6.

3. Genetic influence

There is considerable variation between breeds and strains of sheep in their ability to absorb copper.
- Sheep on the island of Orkney would normally eat a considerable amount of seaweed, which interferes with copper availability. By a process of natural selection they have become very efficient at absorbing copper from their diet and when shifted to mainland Britain, sheep died of copper poisoning once seaweed was absent from their diet.
- Wiener in Scotland has demonstrated the genetic influence affecting the occurrence of swayback in lambs. Not only was the incidence of swayback variable between breeds, but he was also able to select sheep for high and low copper absorption rates based on serum copper levels from within a population. The occurrence of swayback in different sheep breeds run on the same pasture is shown below (Wiener, 1966). Orkney, Texel and Welsh Mountain

Scottish Blackface	40%
Welsh Mountain	0%
Cheviot	11%
S. Blackface x Cheviot	20%
S. Blackface x Welsh Mountain	15%
Cheviot x Welsh Mountain	5%

sheep are very efficient at absorbing copper and are less likely to show signs of copper deficiency than some other breeds. They are, however, more susceptible to copper poisoning. In New Zealand sheep breeds, the Texel is efficient at absorbing copper and is more susceptible to copper toxicity than other breeds. In contrast, the Finnish Landrace is more susceptible to copper deficiency and has similar copper requirements to cattle.

The absorption differences for copper shown between breeds of sheep diminishes as the molybdenum content of the diet is increased. It is also believed that the genetic variation is due to differences in absorption of copper rather than in its utilisation and excretion.

4. Gastrointestinal parasitism

It has been suggested that gastrointestinal parasitism may reduce copper absorption. This is probably similar to the parasitic effects shown in the absorption of macro-elements such as calcium and phosphorus.

5. Molybdenum and sulphur

Molybdenum is present naturally in some soils, and in others it has been used as a fertiliser to stimulate legume growth. Sulphur is applied in fertiliser as in superphosphate, gypsum or elemental sulphur and may

Feed	% absorption
Summer pasture	2.3
Autumn pasture	1.2
Hay	7.2
Silage	4.9
Leafy brassicas	12.8
Root brassicas	6.7

Table 7.6 Copper absorption from various feeds (Suttle, 1981).

reach quite high levels, particularly on dairy farm pastures (sheep farms 0.1–0.25%; dairy farms 0.3–0.4%). Pasture molybdenum levels increase during spring and along with sulphur form insoluble thiomolybdates in the rumen which then combine with copper, forming insoluble copper thiomolybdates. In addition to the interference of copper absorption in the gut, tetrathiomolybdate has a post-absorptive effect on systemic copper metabolism by increasing copper excretion in the bile and thus reducing liver copper reserves.

Depending on the species, cattle or sheep, and the relative levels of molybdenum and sulphur present, it is possible to predict, at least roughly, whether a given diet is likely to be copper-deficient.

It must be emphasised that plant analysis should not be used alone to establish the copper status of a farm and its animals. It must be remembered that:
- Animals (particularly sheep) can store considerable reserves of copper which can be mobilised during periods when dietary supply is inadequate.
- Copper, molybdenum and sulphur concentrations in herbage vary throughout the year.
- The concentrations of the three elements vary between plant species and considerable variation is possible within a single paddock. As a result, care must be taken when collecting pasture samples to ensure that they are representative of what the animals are eating.

Naturally high soil molybdenum occurs in few places in the world, e.g. the 'Teart' areas of Somerset, England. In New Zealand a few Northland soils give pastures with > 3 ppm Mo. Some of the Kaipara site soils and some peats may also approach this level, as may the Balmoral soils in a small area of North Canterbury.

The heavy use of molybdic fertilisers and lime altered the Cu : Mo ratio in herbage on many farms in the 1960s and 1970s, causing a spring rise in molybdenum levels to > 5 ppm. The excessive use of these fertilisers was believed to have been responsible for the first copper deficiency diseases in Northland in the same period (post-parturient haemoglobinuria). Since then, the disorders have been largely controlled because of more-informed fertiliser usage and copper supplementation.

As a rule of thumb, Cu : Mo ratios of 2 : 1 in the feed of housed sheep lead to copper deficiency, but in pasture-fed animals, because of high levels of sulphur, higher ratios of Cu : Mo may be dangerous and molybdenum levels as low as 2 ppm in pasture may induce copper deficiency in cattle.

6. Iron

Iron is a major component of soil, and high levels of soil ingestion are common in New Zealand stock. In some circumstances up to 30% of total dry matter ingested may be soil.

Dietary iron intake can have a marked inhibitory effect on the utilisation of dietary copper. Levels as low as 250 mg iron/kg diet are sufficient to reduce hepatic copper reserves of calves. Concentrations of iron in soils are frequently approximately 20,000 mg/kg. If soil ingestion accounts for 10% of an animal's dry matter intake and if only 25% of iron were released, iron would be equivalent to 500 mg/kg, which would significantly reduce the utilisation of dietary copper.

Researchers at the Rowett Institute in Aberdeen found that 800 mg iron/kg diet had the same effect on copper status as did 5 mg molybdenum/kg diet. Unfortunately, little is known of the mechanisms whereby iron disturbs copper metabolism.

In New Zealand there are several reports where iron appears to have been the main element associated with severe copper deficiency syndromes. In the Waipipi iron sand area of South Taranaki, classical cases of copper deficiency were reported in cattle in 1980–1982. In the animals examined, the liver reserves of copper were very low, but the pasture levels of copper, molybdenum and sulphur were such that a severe copper deficiency should not have existed (Table 7.7). The iron levels, however, were extraordinarily high (range 2000–29,299 mg/kg/DM). Such high levels of iron were due to soil contamination of the fodder, which it is believed led to the severely depressed copper status of the grazing cattle.

Many New Zealand soils have a naturally high iron content and other factors may have to contribute before a serious effect on copper uptake occurs, as cited above. High levels of iron are found in some ground-waters and particularly bore water may be seriously contaminated. An aspect that warrants further investigation in New Zealand is drinking water as a source of iron, particularly for dairy cows. Many dairy sheds have water supplies heavily contaminated with iron. Similarly, waterlogged soils tend

| | | Pasture analysis | | | |
Sample number	Liver Cu (mg/kg)	Cu (mg/kg)	Mo (mg/kg)	S (%)	Fe (mg/kg)
1	24.0	12.0	0.20	0.24	10,740
2	6.3	13.0	0.10	0.30	3260
3	16.0	9.0	0.20	0.23	2060
4	6.0	12.0	0.20	0.31	4280
5	4.2	18.0	0.09	0.24	29,200

Iron levels:
Mean pasture levels — 9908 mg/kg
Range — 2060–29,200 mg/kg
Normal   legumes — 200–300 mg/kg
             lucerne — 700–800 mg/kg
             grass — 100–200 mg/kg

Table 7.7 Animal tissue and pasture analysis from a Taranaki farm with severe iron induced hypocuprosis in cattle (Bruère, 1982).

to support plants with high available iron and a positive relationship has been established between waterlogging and hypocuprosis.

A more general association of hypocuprosis with waterlogging has been observed at times on the Hauraki Plains and is combined with a low pasture copper. The high ingestion rates of soil by some stock, particularly over the winter period, in this area is also associated with qualitative differences between soil types in the extractability of their mineral elements in rumen liquor. Iron in the Hauraki Plains clay loam appears to be more soluble in rumen liquor than in other soils. This solubility is also retained in duodenal liquor, which is a major site of iron absorption.

7. Other metals

Other metals that may affect the uptake and/or utilisation of copper by grazing ruminants include zinc, cadmium, silver and mercury. Zinc is regularly used in facial eczema prevention in New Zealand and could be a contributing factor to hypocuprosis, particularly in dairy cattle, which may be dosed with zinc drenches each day for several weeks. Concern has also been expressed about the levels of cadmium in some lines of superphosphate, which could also contribute to inducing copper deficiency.

The role of copper and its metabolism

After intestinal absorption, much of the copper is rapidly deposited in the liver hepatocytes: the distribution being 20% in the nuclear fraction, 10% in microsomes and 20% in the large granules of mitochondria and lysosomes. The remainder is stored in the cytosol as either copper-dependent enzymes or metallothionein. As the liver becomes saturated with copper the kidneys become the secondary site of copper deposition.

The main transport of copper is by the globulin caeruloplasmin. Caeruloplasmin is synthesised in the liver and its rate of formation depends on the hepatic copper concentration. Blood actually contains copper in five separate fractions: in erythrocytic superoxide dismutase (60% of erythrocyte copper), in an erythrocyte copper complex, in plasma caeruloplasmin (60–95% of plasma copper), in albumin copper and bound to plasma amino acids. The total copper content of the erythrocyte does not fluctuate in spite of variations in the copper status of the animal and erythrocytes are not involved in copper transport.

Copper is incorporated into the molecular structure of five major enzymes and several less important ones, as well as being part of several proteins and amino acids. The main copper-dependent enzymes are listed in Table 7.8.

Caeruloplasmin (ferroxidase I) is an oxidative enzyme involved in releasing iron into plasma from stores during erythropoiesis. Thus, copper is essential for the normal functioning of iron in the living organism. Some copper is also essential in erythrocytes, where it is found in the same concentration as plasma; when deficient, the life span of the red cell is reduced. A deficiency of copper can thus lead to anaemia resulting from shortened red cell life span, and from limited capacity of the bone marrow to produce red cells.

Cytochrome oxidase is the terminal enzyme in the oxidative phosphorylation process. Young animals appear to be more severely affected by deficiency than older stock, probably because faulty oxidation interferes with the development of growing tissues. Loss of cytochrome oxidase activity is associated with a reduction in the formation of myelin lipids, as seen in the central nervous system of swayback-affected lambs.

The enzyme lysyl oxidase (amine oxidase) is involved in elastin and collagen synthesis. These give strength and elasticity to connective tissue and cartilage, and a deficiency may lead to skeletal defects, abnormal gait and fragility of blood vessels (aorta). In sheep and cattle grazing copper-deficient pastures, spontaneous fractures have often been observed.

Tyrosinase, an oxidase important in the keratinisation of fibres, is also required for the conversion of tyrosine to melanin, needed for pigmentation. In this respect the wool of black sheep has been found to contain twice as much copper as that of white sheep.

Copper requirements of sheep and cattle

If the copper associated with the liver is excluded, a fully fleeced sheep contains about 60 mg of copper; each kilogram of bodyweight containing 0.8 mg of copper and each kilogram of wool 6–8 mg of copper. A newborn lamb contains a total of 10 mg of copper. The net requirements for maintenance rarely exceed 4 µg of copper per kilogram of bodyweight per day and show no relationship to metabolic rate. Growth requires approximately 1.1 mg of copper per kilogram of bodyweight increase and the lactating ewe requires an extra 0.3 mg of copper for each litre of milk produced.

The amounts of copper associated with the endogenous loss, growth, pregnancy and lactation in sheep and cattle are shown in Tables 7.9, 7.10 and 7.11 (Grace, 1983).

Enzyme	Activity	Source	Function
Caeruloplasmin	Ferroxidase	Plasma	Iron transport
Cytochrome oxidase	Terminal oxidase	Mitochondria	Energy metabolism and phosphorylation
Lysyl oxidase (amine oxidase)	Peptide cross-linkage	Aorta and cartilage	Collagen and elastin formation
Tyrosinase (polyphenol oxidase)	Oxidase	Melanocytes	Tyrosine to melanin
Superoxide dismutase	Dismutase	All aerobic cells	$O_2 + O_2 + H_2O$ $6H_2O_2 + O_2$ (antioxidant)
Dopamine-B-hydroxylase	Oxygenase	Adrenal gland	Dopamine to norepinephrine
Peptidyglycine α-amidating monooxygenase	Elaboration of numerous biogenic molecules		Appetite effect

Table 7.8 Essential copper-containing enzymes and their functions.

	Sheep	Cattle
Endogenous loss (inevitable loss)	4 µg Cu/kg liveweight/day	7.1 µg Cu/kg liveweight/day
Growth	1.1 mg Cu/kg gain	1.0 mg Cu/kg gain
Lactation	0.32 mg Cu/kg milk (early) 0.22 mg Cu/kg milk (late)	0.1 mg Cu/kg milk
Pregnancy (daily increment in conceptus)		
— early	0.015 mg Cu/day	0.60 mg Cu/day
— mid	0.085 mg Cu/day	1.63 mg Cu/day
— late	0.186 mg Cu/day	2.07 mg Cu/day
Wool	7 mg Cu/kg	

Table 7.9 The amounts of copper associated with the endogenous loss, growth, pregnancy and lactation in sheep and cattle.

	Liveweight (kg)	Weight gain (g/day), stage of pregnancy or milk yield	Dietary req. mg Cu/day	mg/kg DM
Growing lamb	5	150	0.21	1.0
	10	150	0.40	1.0
	20	150	1.2	1.8
	30	150	3.7	2.9
	40	75	2.7	2.1
		150	3.7	2.2
		300	5.6	2.7
Adult ewe				
— maintenance	55		4.8	5.0
— late pregnancy	55	single	6.6	5.0
		twins	10.0	5.9
— lactation	55	1 kg milk/day	10.0	4.4
		2 kg milk/day	15.5	5.2

Table 7.10 Estimated dietary copper requirements of sheep.

	Liveweight (kg)	Weight gain (kg/day), stage of pregnancy or milk yield	Dietary req. mg Cu/day	mg/kg DM
Pre-ruminant calf	40	0.5	1.2	-
Growing calf	100	0.5	25	10
		1.0	35	10
	200	0.5	39	9
		1.0	48	8
	300	0.5	54	9
		1.0	65	8
Dairy cow — maintenance	380		54	10
— late pregnancy	380	9 months	95	10
— lactation	380	10 kg milk/day	74	8
		20 kg milk/day	94	7
		30 kg milk/day	114	7
Beef cow — lactation	450	10 kg milk/day	84	10

Table 7.11 Estimated dietary requirements of cattle.

Clinical features

In general cattle and deer are more susceptible to copper deficiency than sheep, so in a mixed-farming enterprise clinical signs of deficiency usually develop in these species first.

Cattle

One of the earliest signs to develop in cattle is loss of coat colour, followed in order by diarrhoea and unthriftiness, skeletal defects and anaemia. It is important to recognise that these are relatively non-specific signs and similar signs would be seen with other causes of ill thrift such as internal parasitism.

1. Growth rate

The effect of copper most frequently responsible for economic loss is the decline in growth rate occurring in calves and yearlings when deficiency becomes established. The reason why this effect arises and why it is often such a variable characteristic between individual animals exposed to the same dietary circumstances is not known. Research has shown that the small intestine of animals undergoing copper depletion suffers marked cellular damage that is probably of sufficient severity to affect absorptive function, and this may underlie the marked decline in efficiency of food utilisation that has been shown to accompany the early development of copper deficiency induced experimentally.

2. Diarrhoea

Marked persistent diarrhoea occurs in many cases of secondary copper deficiency induced by hypermolybdenosis (peat scours and teart), providing further evidence of a key role for copper in the maintenance of normal function of the gastrointestinal tract.

3. Skeletal defects

These are relatively uncommon in cattle in New Zealand, but when they do occur it is mainly in young, rapidly growing animals. Affected animals commonly have a stilted gait and show ataxia during movement, but they may recover temporarily after rest. Boney changes include marked reduction in the thickness of the shaft wall, and thickened epiphyses at the fetlock of calves causing them to become stiff and swollen. Spontaneous fractures of ribs and limbs may also be seen when hypocuprosis is severe.

4. Coat colour changes

Copper is involved in the production of hair pigment, so in a deficiency there is a lightening of the coat colour. Black areas have a brown-grey tint (Angus cattle) and red areas become yellow-sandy (Hereford cattle). In black cattle, 'spectacles', patches of grey hair, often develop around the eyes.

5. Poor reproductive performance

The direct effects of copper deficiency on reproduction are still debated. Reproductive performance may suffer when animals are exposed to pastures of high molybdenum concentration because molybdenum inhibits the activity of reproductive hormones, and responses to copper may arise secondarily because it acts as an antidote to molybdenum.

6. Depressed milk yield

It is thought that copper deficiency can have an adverse effect on milk yield, but there have been few published experiments detailing the milk yield response of dairy cows to copper supplementation. In these experiments the response to supplementation was variable.

7. Anaemia and post-parturient haemoglobinuria

In Northland, New Zealand, a relationship was found to exist in cattle between low copper status and the incidence of post-parturient haemoglobinuria. In addition the occurrence of post-parturient haemoglobinuria in a herd can also indicate the presence of an anaemic state that usually affects the majority of the herd.

The copper deficiency is usually associated with the excessive application of molybdenum fertiliser and lime to pastures. However, other factors such as the excessive excretion of phosphorus play an important role in the cause of this disease.

8. Cardiovascular disorders

These have been reported in Western Australia and involve slow degeneration of the myocardium with replacement fibrosis. Occasionally cattle die of acute heart failure or 'falling disease'.

Deer

Enzootic ataxia

The most common manifestation of copper deficiency in deer has been enzootic ataxia, which occurs mainly in deer over 9 months of age. It occurs most commonly in spring. There is the gradual onset of incoordination, especially of the hind limbs, and, on necropsy, demyelination of the spinal cord. The reason for the age difference between deer and sheep in the onset of enzootic ataxia has not been explained. Bone disorders such as bone fragility and osteochondrosis (Figure 7.14) have been reported. Reduced growth rates may also occur in deer with copper deficiency. It appears that copper levels need to be very low before economic growth responses will occur, but further research is required.

Sheep

In New Zealand, visible signs of copper deficiency are seldom seen in adult crossbred sheep even when there is a marked depletion of liver copper. However, a wide variety of clinical abnormalities of grazing sheep have been attributed to a dietary deficiency of copper. These include loss of wool crimp, loss of pigment, anaemia,

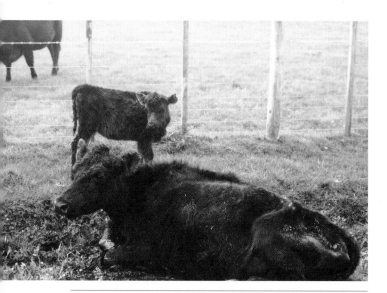

Figure 7.13 Severely copper-deficient cow and her calf.

loss of condition, bone disorders, impaired reproductive performance and neonatal ataxia (swayback).

In Britain, the commonest manifestation is swayback in lambs, while in Australia wool abnormalities and anaemia are seen. In New Zealand, probably bone fragility of lambs and hoggets and occasional cases of swayback are most commonly reported.

1. Swayback — enzootic ataxia

This condition is characterised by hypomyelinogenesis of the central nervous system so the lambs are unable to stand or have incoordination of the hind limbs. It may be congenital, which involves hypomyelinogenesis largely of the cerebrum; or delayed, in which the lambs are apparently normal at birth but become affected in the first few weeks of life. This is due mainly to hypomyelinogenesis of the spinal cord.

It is thought that there are two peak periods during which myelination of nervous tissue takes place in the sheep's development: one period around 20 days prior to birth, the other 10–20 days after birth.

2. Bone fragility, osteoporosis

Bone fragility, particularly of the long bones (humerus and femur) is recorded in New Zealand as a result of copper deficiency. This may be seen at docking time as an increased occurrence of fractured bones when lambs are released from the docking cradle, or it may occur in hoggets during autumn and winter and is usually associated with yarding or stock movements (Figure 7.15).

3. Wool abnormalities

In black sheep in New Zealand, copper deficiency has been shown to be associated with loss of pigmentation, the wool becoming a gingery-brown colour. However, as black sheep age their fleece often becomes a gingery-brown to grey colour so that differentiation of the normal from the deficient is difficult.

Loss of crimp has been reported mainly in Merino sheep in Australia, but rarely in New Zealand. Colloquially it was called steely wool because of its reduced lustre.

4. Fertility (ewes)

Copper deficiency has been associated with infertility in ewes, but mainly on an experimental basis. The feeding of

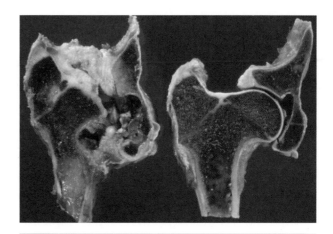

Figure 7.14 Osteochondrosis of the femoral head of a copper-deficient deer calf (left) compared with a femur from a normal deer calf.

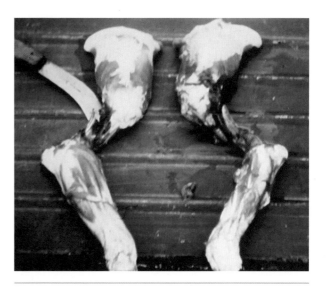

Figure 7.15 Bilateral spontaneous fractures of the humeri of a hogget due to copper deficiency. This problem was induced following topdressing with molybdenum.

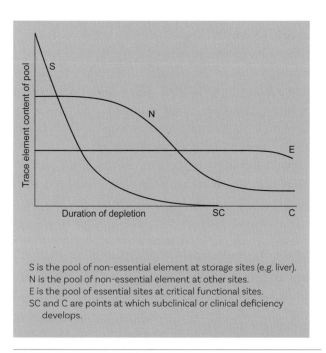

Figure 7.16 Schematic illustration of relationships in the development of copper deficiency (from Suttle, 1976).

high levels of molybdenum and sulphur were thought to have increased foetal loss and a decrease in the number of lambs born. However, ewes must be exceedingly copper-deficient before fertility suffers.

5. Fertility (rams)

After a year living on an experimentally induced copper-deficient diet, South African Mutton Merino rams produced semen ejaculates of low volume, low sperm concentration and poor sperm motility and morphology. Histologically the testes of such rams showed poor development of the seminiferous tubules and Sertoli cells, which were also inactive. Such changes were reversible when the copper deficiency was corrected.

Diagnosis of copper status

When the clinical signs of hypocuprosis appear, copper reserves in the animal are very severely depleted and it is likely also that other members of the herd or flock are in a precarious health position. Therefore veterinarians should be concerned with adequacy rather than deficiency. Further, there is much clinical data clearly indicating that animals with low but adequate levels of blood copper may within a very short time fall into the danger area of hypocuprosis. In other words, levels of adequacy must not be taken too rigidly when interpreting diagnostic material but must be used with full consideration of the health status of the flock, time of year and feed supplies available.

The schematic illustration of Suttle (1976) demonstrates the relationship between clinical signs and copper depletion. It is the objective of good animal health advice to ensure that a herd or flock of valuable animals does not deplete the so-called nonessential Cu pool putting animals at risk of clinical hypocuprosis.

It can be seen that the storage sites (S) are depleted first, followed by other non-essential sites (N). Only when these two pools are depleted do the amounts in essential sites decline and deficiency signs develop. Thus, examining either or both non-essential sites (blood or liver) does not estimate the essential sites and hence the degree of deficiency.

It is therefore essential to follow the routine clinical procedure when attempting to determine copper status of a farm and its animals and to consider all the factors involved, such as the following:

- age, species and breed of animals
- feed type
- concentrations of copper, molybdenum, sulphur and iron in feed
- the length of time animals have been on that feed
- clinical features
- previous copper supplementation
- tissue levels.

Liver and blood copper measurement

When the supply of copper from the diet declines, copper stored in the liver is mobilised for use, and maintains blood levels. When liver levels become depleted, blood levels also fall and clinical signs appear. Thus the measurement of liver copper gives a direct and reasonably accurate means of diagnosing copper status. It can also be used to predict the likelihood of supplementation being required in the next few months, given a knowledge of likely copper nutrition. There can be considerable variation in the liver copper levels between individuals within a herd, and laboratories recommend that up to 16 liver samples are collected for analysis. However, cost becomes an issue if this number of samples is analysed so more commonly 4–7 samples are used to give an indication of whether levels are deficient, marginal or adequate. For more precise estimates, a larger number of samples are needed and more-frequent sampling intervals may be required. As a generalisation, the within-herd variation is most marked when the mean level is in the mid-range, and reduces at low and high ranges.

While giving a useful measure of copper reserves, liver analysis will not indicate whether the reserves are increasing, static or declining. Furthermore, liver reserves may fall from normal values to very low levels before plasma copper declines. Also, a severe copper deficiency induced by excess molybdenum in the diet could cause signs such as diarrhoea before liver reserves are diminished if liver copper cannot be mobilised fast enough.

Blood levels are more easily collected and are usually low at the time of deficiency. Either serum copper or serum ferroxidase can be measured; these tests give similar information. However, during blood clotting the copper concentration in serum is reduced and it is now recommended that copper in plasma should be measured in preference to serum. In cattle and probably deer, measuring blood or serum copper from approximately 7–10 animals can confirm a diagnosis of copper deficiency but is of little value in predicting the need for supplementation in the future if levels are normal. In sheep, blood copper levels fall late in the development of a deficiency and, while they are of value in controlled experiments, are considered too insensitive an indicator for field use; in sheep, therefore, liver copper levels are the more appropriate indicator of copper status.

As with other trace elements, the samples collected depend on the objective of testing, as illustrated by Table 7.12.

It must be remembered that copper deficiency is a dynamic condition within a flock or herd, and at the time of sampling the status of individuals within the group may be improving or declining depending on recent diet. Therefore, in checking with reference ranges (Table 7.13) the clinician should be mindful of the appended note that these levels refer to deficiency risk and not to a projected adequate level for the maintenance of good health. This latter is a very important point and cannot be overemphasised.

There is limited information on which to develop

Reason	Time to sample	Species and age	Sample type	Sample number	Interpretation
Poor performance	Time of problem	Affected animals	Serum (or liver)	7–10 serum	Means only
Farm deficiencies	Late winter/ spring	Cattle – late pregnancy/early lactation or fast growing cattle >6 months	Liver	At least 4, preferably more	Mainly means, take notice of individuals
Adequate reserves	Early winter	Cattle	Liver	At least 4, preferably more	Mainly means, take notice of individuals
Supplementation	Halfway through expected period of insufficiency	Animals being supplemented	Liver	At least 4, preferably more	Compare individual animals with previous samples

Table 7.12 Sampling for copper depending upon the reason for sampling (Clark and Ellison, 1993).

reference values for deer, although it has been suggested by Wilson and Grace (2001) that for this species liver levels <60 µmol/kg or serum levels <5 µmol/l are considered 'deficient' and liver levels of 60–100 µmol/kg are considered 'marginal'.

Soil or feed analysis

The concentration of copper in soil or animal feeds is of limited value in assessing the necessity of copper supplementation of the animal. This is because most copper deficiencies are caused by the interaction of other elements such as molybdenum, iron or sulphur and are not related to the actual levels of copper in the plant or soil. If copper deficiency occurs in stock, however, soil or feed analysis may help in determining why the deficiency has occurred.

Treatment and prevention of copper deficiency

Clearly, the number of complicating factors affecting copper uptake and usage by animals demands a wide knowledge of the copper status not only of the flock or herd but also of the farm and its pasture before copper therapy is instituted. Unfortunately, in many cases the approach to copper therapy on many New Zealand properties can at best be described as empirical and has not been based on sound analytical facts that are, in most cases, easy to obtain.

Oral administration of copper

1. Drenching

Where antagonistic factors are low, oral drenching with copper sulphate or copper oxide may supply adequate copper levels for some weeks, but the traditional recommendation has been the weekly administration of copper. Drenching at this frequency is impractical for sheep, and may be practical for dairy cattle where the daily copper requirements may not be easily met from feed or other means of supplementation. Anthelmintics with mineral additives do not contain sufficient copper for effective supplementation.

2. Copperised salt licks and copper added to drinking water

Copperised salt licks under nearly all circumstances should be discouraged as a source of copper for grazing animals. Some people have prepared their own salt licks with dangerously high levels of copper salts (5%). Further, the grazier has no control of the dose of copper ingested by individual animals and some sheep have an affinity for licks and ingest a toxic dose of copper quite readily. Similar comments may be made about copper in drinking water unless it is controlled by a dispensing device that delivers an accurate amount of copper to a given volume of drinking water. The latter are used successfully in some areas of New Zealand, particularly for dairy cattle.

		Low	Marginal	Adequate
Cattle	Liver (µmol/kg*)	<45	45–95	>95
	Serum (µmol/l*)	<4.5	4.5–8.0	>8.0
	Ferroxidase (U/l)	<7	7–14	>14
Sheep	Liver (µmol/kg)	<65	65–300	>300

Table 7.13 Reference range for copper levels in sheep and cattle.

* Copper levels have been measured in New Zealand diagnostic laboratories in standard units since 1982. Unfortunately the majority of the international literature still records levels as weight, e.g. mg/kg DM or ppm (parts per million). To convert weight units mg/kg to molecular units, multiply by 15.7. Conversely, divide by 15.7.

Note: These levels are guidelines for the diagnosis of deficiency and not for the need for supplementation. For instance, it is recommended that to ensure adequate copper status, breeding cows should have liver copper levels over 300 µmol/kg at the onset of winter.

3. Copper oxide capsules (needles)
Copper oxide capsules are small particles of copper oxide wire that are designed to lodge in the reticulorumen and dislodge slowly to dissolve in the abomasum. This provides a source of copper for months and possibly up to a year. Data available for both cattle and deer support that this form of therapy may effectively raise copper storage levels in animals for 5–12 months depending on the species and the circumstances in which they are used. They also have a minimal risk of toxicity.

4. Slow-release rumen bullets
A balanced trace-element sustained-release bolus (All-trace Trace Element Bolus; Vetpak NZ) is available that provides copper, cobalt, selenium, manganese, zinc, iodine, sulphur and vitamins A, D and E.

5. Topdressing
Topdressing of pastures with 1.5–3 kg of copper/ha (usually as copper sulphate) has been a traditional method of preventing copper deficiency. However, cost may be a limiting factor on more extensive areas. The copper is usually applied in autumn or spring, often in conjunction with superphosphate, and should not be grazed for at least 3 weeks or until heavy rain has washed all traces of fertiliser away in case copper poisoning occurs. For animal supplementation purposes, copper is normally applied annually.

The length of time that copper is available following topdressing is variable. It is difficult to increase the copper content of herbage since most plants have mechanisms to prevent the uptake of heavy metals. Suttle (1981) claimed that copper topdressing was generally disappointing and the effect on pasture is largely gone in 6 months. Experiments have been undertaken grazing bulls (West et al., 1997) and deer (Grace et al., 2001) on copper-topdressed pasture. For the first 100–200 days the liver copper levels of animals grazed on topdressed pasture declined in a similar way to those of control animals, but levels then slowly increased and were significantly different from controls to day 300–350. The reason for this apparent delay between topdressing and increasing liver copper levels is unknown. More research is required to evaluate the use of copper topdressing as an animal supplement for copper deficiency.

Where low copper levels caused by induced copper deficiency (e.g. high molybdenum and/or sulphur) occur in animals, then directly supplementing the animal may be more effective than copper topdressing. Plant analysis for copper, together with other interfering elements, will be necessary in deciding the benefits of copper topdressing in such situations. The possibility of topdressing hay paddocks, particularly lucerne, from which hay can be fed out during the next winter has not been explored but may be a useful recommendation.

Parenteral administration
There are a variety of products that have been developed for the parenteral treatment of copper deficiency. Apart from economic factors, the parenteral administration of copper is therapeutically sound since it bypasses the inhibition of copper absorption in the gut. Its main disadvantages are that at a given injection only a limited amount of copper can be given because of toxic implications which have been recorded regularly in New Zealand. Injection-site lesions may occur.

1. Copper calcium edetate
This is an injectable form of copper based on ethylene diamine tetra-acetic acid (EDTA). This is a chelating agent which it is able to form a very stable ring structure with metallic ions. In association with copper it is readily absorbed from the injection site, thus minimising the risk of local reactions. It also allows non-ionised copper to circulate, which under normal circumstances makes it non-toxic. There is usually a small local reaction at the site of injection that quickly subsides.

2. Copper glycinate
This is usually a depot formulation that ensures slow release of copper into the circulation and uptake by the liver. Products contain 60 mg elemental copper per ml. These products should only be given subcutaneously and care must be taken to ensure that intramuscular injection does not occur.

Precautions with copper therapy
Copper toxicity can occur through chronic poisoning or an acute toxicity. In cattle, the 'safe range' for liver concentrations is around 95–1500 µmol/kg fresh tissue and

chronic toxicity has been associated with concentrations in the range 2500–9000 µmol/kg. Death through overdosing with copper is distinct from chronic copper poisoning and does not usually involve a haemolytic crisis. The lesions of acute liver damage are characteristic, with speckled dark areas in a usually pale liver. Sub-endocardial and epicardial haemorrhages and accumulation of fluid in serous cavities are also seen. Liver copper levels are not markedly elevated.

Copper toxicity is frequently reported in sheep and cattle. However, sheep generally are more susceptible to copper toxicity than cattle, and there is often little difference between normal blood levels of copper and those associated with toxicity. The situation of parenteral administration of copper to sheep is also exacerbated by the fact that the transplacental transfer of copper to the foetus by the ewe is poor; thus, in order to give sufficient copper to the foetus, the dose given to the ewe has a small therapeutic index. It must also be borne in mind that there is generally a great deal of variation in bodyweight within a flock of ewes all being given a standard dose of copper. Superimposed on this are the genetic differences in sheep and their ability to metabolise copper.

The warnings associated with injectable copper use should be clearly stated to the user and include:
- Confirmation of a deficient copper status before administration.
- Taking care when administering copper to young and debilitated animals, particularly where liver damage is suspected.
- The simultaneous administration of other compounds is contraindicated.
- Injections must be subcutaneous.
- Avoiding prolonged yarding periods and other stress.
- Using feed supplements with caution. Some supplements, such as palm kernel, contain high levels of copper, often greater than 20 ppm of dry matter.

Frequency of copper therapy

The frequency of copper administration cannot be accurately predicted for each situation. As already described, many factors affect the ultimate absorption and retention of copper by individual animals, and the degree of deficiency varies markedly from farm to farm and at different times of the year. The general approach is therefore somewhat empirical but, nevertheless, should be based on regular monitoring to assess the adequacy of therapy on a particular farm.

The following is given as a guideline and should be used with caution.
- For sheep, one annual dose of copper may be adequate to control copper deficiency. Injecting prior to mating should be sufficient to reduce the incidence of swayback and prevent spontaneous bone fracture.
- In beef cattle, it is generally suggested that three doses of copper are needed in young animals and thereafter twice-yearly dosing. Frequency of dosing may have to be increased in adults if they show signs of copper deficiency or if liver biopsy samples reveal very low levels.
- In dairy cattle, copper requirements are usually higher and more regular supplementation may be needed.
- Molybdenum levels in pasture are highest and copper levels lowest during late winter/early spring. Therefore, monitoring copper reserves before winter is useful in predicting whether supplementation is required.

Molybdenum and copper deficiency

In many parts of New Zealand the excessive use of molybdenum on pastures has precipitated a copper-deficiency problem in animals grazing these pastures. On some farms in the past, molybdenised superphosphate was used as frequently as once a year and at very high levels. Trials conducted at Wallaceville research station showed that the regular application of molybdate each year to light, stony soils raised pasture concentrations of molybdenum to dangerous levels, which rose even higher during spring. These coincided with clinical signs of lameness and loss of mobility in young stock grazing the pastures. It was concluded that there are few soils in New Zealand that would require amounts of molybdate in excess of 200 g/ha every 4–5 years.

Copper deficiency in cattle and not sheep on the same property

In Table 7.14, a number of properties are shown where copper deficiency has been clinically diagnosed and confirmed in cattle but not in sheep. Analysis of liver material from six of these properties demonstrated that a serious deficiency of copper may have existed in some cattle while sheep on the same property had adequate copper stores which were unlikely to be depleted. These observations should not necessarily be taken to infer that the clinical signs of copper deficiency would always appear in cattle before sheep. On some properties, cattle have apparently thrived while young sheep showed swayback and osteoporosis.

Conclusion

In any animal health investigation or programme, the monitoring of the copper status of a property should be a routine procedure. The application of history, clinical signs, and the chemical analysis of animal tissues and blood are essential. Pasture samples from several areas of the property should also be monitored for copper, molybdenum, sulphur and iron and sometimes levels of other elements such as zinc and manganese. This full diagnostic routine is required before sound professional advice can be given on the use of any of the several forms of copper therapy available.

Property	No.	Mean	Range
A	10 cattle	91.8	38.0 – 282.6
	10 sheep	476.0	94.2 – 1884.0
B	5 cattle	56.5	18.8 – 152.0
	3 sheep	1051.9	736.0 – 1381.6
C	5 cattle	251.2	12.5 – 540.0
	3 sheep	1476.0	1256.0 – 1876.0
D	7 cattle	252.0	31.4 – 262.0
	6 sheep	845.0	628.0 – 1099.0
E	3 cattle	105.0	26.7 – 177.0
	6 sheep	1868.0	785.0 – 3768.0
F	6 cattle	75.36	28.2 – 208.8
	3 sheep	1582.6	850.9 – 2088.0
Total	Cattle	114.6	7.8 – 540.0
	Sheep	1213.6	204.0 – 3768.0

Table 7.14 Liver copper levels (µmol/kg) in cattle and sheep.

Iodine

Introduction

The occurrence of goitre in lambs and calves in New Zealand was first noted by Gilruth in 1901. However, it was not until 1925 that iodine deficiency was documented as the cause of goitre in human and animal populations in this country. The latter discovery led to the widespread use of dietary iodised salt in the 1930s and a consequent decline in the prevalence of goitre in humans.

Although a dietary deficiency of iodine has commonly been regarded as a cause of goitre, goitrogens that occur in many animal fodders (particularly brassica crops) are also an important cause of the disease. In sheep, congenital goitre occurs when the iodine concentration of herbage falls into the range 0.09–0.18 mg/kg DM. Goats appear most susceptible to iodine deficiency, followed by sheep. Occasional cases of goitre have been reported in calves and newborn deer.

Metabolism and function of iodine

In adult sheep iodine is effectively trapped in the thyroid gland, which contains approximately 80% of the body's iodine. These reserves may give adult sheep sufficient iodine for adequate thyroid hormone secretion for many months after iodine intake decreases. This situation is different in the developing foetal lamb. The lamb's thyroid gland develops independently from that of the ewe, and production of adequate levels of thyroid hormone for foetal development and maturation depends on sufficient amounts of iodine, derived from its mother's daily intake, being transported across the placenta. Therefore the lamb cannot use its mother's reserves and for this reason subclinical iodine deficiency usually affects lamb health and production.

The only known role of iodine in animals is in the synthesis of the thyroid hormones, thyroxine (T4) and tri-iodothyronine (T3) in the thyroid gland. Thyroid hormones are important for energy metabolism and protein synthesis of cells. Tri-iodothyronine stimulates the production of enzymes involved in energy metabolism and is thus closely related to heat production and oxygen usage. Thyroid hormones are essential for the development of foetal brain, lungs, heart, and wool follicles. Along with cortisol the thyroid hormones are important in stimulating the maturation of the cells lining the lung alveoli and can stimulate the production of surfactant, which is important in lung maturation and necessary for the survival of the newborn lamb.

In ruminants, iodine is mainly absorbed in the rumen. Some endogenous iodine is secreted into the abomasum but is reabsorbed in the small intestine. Iodine is ingested and absorbed more readily than most other elements.

Dietary iodine, as well as iodine produced by degradation of thyroid hormones, is trapped in the thyroid gland where it combines with tyrosine to form a range of iodinated amino acids. The main one is thyroxine, which is stored, in combination with protein, as thyroglobulin. Iodine is released from the thyroglobulin in the thyroid gland as thyroxine, which is bound to globulin, prealbumin and albumin and as such is transported in the blood. Typical plasma concentrations of thyroxine in adult and foetal sheep are 40–70 and 100–120 mmol/l, respectively.

Thyroxine is reduced to tri-iodothyronine, which is the active form of the hormone, chiefly in the thyroid and pituitary glands, liver and kidneys. Tri-iodothyronine is almost non-detectable in foetal blood, while in normal healthy sheep plasma tri-iodothyronine levels are 1.8–2.2 mmol/l. During tissue metabolism tri-iodothyronine is degraded to inorganic iodine, most of which is again trapped by the thyroid gland. A small amount is excreted in the urine.

The requirements for iodine

The presence of goitrogens in feed is a major factor affecting iodine requirements. Only one of the two types of goitrogen (thiouracil-type and thyiocyanate-type) has been detected in vegetation in New Zealand. The thiocyanate-type goitrogens found in New Zealand vegetation block the uptake of inorganic iodide by the thyroid gland and hence reduce thyroxine synthesis. The thiouracil-type goitrogens found overseas in tropical legumes block the conversion of thyroxine to tri-iodothyronine. Plants of the *Brassica* species, which include the forage kales, cabbages, Brussels sprouts and broccoli, contain glucosinolates that are broken down during cudding to form inorganic thiocyanate ions. Swedes and turnips do not produce thiocyanate to any significant extent, but the forage sorghums yield hydrocyanic acid on chewing which combines with sulphur in the rumen to produce thiocyanate. New Zealand cultivars of clover also contain high levels of thiocyanate, as this confers resistance to slug predation.

Fortunately the goitrogenic properties of inorganic thiocyanate can readily be prevented by iodine supplementation. The thiocyanate ion can also readily cross the placenta, as can inorganic iodide; hence, iodine supplementation of pregnant ewes consuming a goitrogenic diet is especially important to ensure that the developing foetus, which is particularly vulnerable to iodine deficiency, obtains adequate levels of iodine.

The ingestion of soil caused by high stocking rates is said to reduce the incidence of goitre. However, as a practical point, the effects of overstocking can be deleterious in other ways so this does not really offer a realistic alternative to the prevention of goitre. Similarly, anecdotal information suggests that iodine deficiency is more common during dry seasons and this may be related to lower levels of soil intake compared with wet seasons.

Iodine requirements are increased in high-producing animals where energy intake, heat production and protein synthesis are all high. This includes pregnant ewes, lactating ewes and cows, and rapidly growing animals.

Occurrence of iodine deficiency

Iodine deficiency may occur in high-rainfall areas such as Westland or inland areas such as Otago, Canterbury and Manawatu. In New Zealand, most occurrences of goitre seem to have been associated with goitrogens in feed.

While goitre-producing areas of New Zealand have been identified for sheep in the past, the occurrence of goitre in goat kids on farms where sheep have been run without ever having exhibited signs of goitre suggests that goats may be more susceptible to iodine deficiency. The main goitre-producing areas in New Zealand are shown in Figure 7.17. It should be noted that these are also the regions where brassica crops, the main contributing goitrogenic feeds, are grown in New Zealand. However, the possibility of subclinical iodine deficiency occurring outside of these areas cannot be discounted.

The iodine concentration has been found to be much higher in perennial ryegrass and white clover than in browntop and *Poa* spp. Seasonal trends are also likely, with the highest concentrations occurring in the improved species during winter, corresponding to their lowest rates of DM production. In contrast, highest concentrations in the unimproved species are seen during spring and summer; see Table 7.15.

The content of iodine in forage kale is consistently lower than that of ryegrass/clover pasture sampled over autumn and winter. Hence, kale is not only goitrogenic but can be iodine-deficient as well. Likewise, the bulbs of swedes (*Brassica napus*), which are frequently fed to pregnant ewes, have a very low iodine content, often <0.05 mg/kg. Within each type of forage, considerable variation occurs from year to year which is reflected in the severity and incidence of neonatal goitre of lambs born of ewes grazing such forage. Plant concentrations of iodine are affected by the locality in which they are grown. For example, in one series of data the iodine concentration in ryegrass/clover grown on Manawatu hill country was 5–7 times higher than equivalent pasture grown at Invermay.

Clinical findings

Enlargement of the thyroid glands of lambs (goitre) is the most obvious sign of iodine deficiency and is seen more commonly when the ewe has eaten either iodine-deficient or goitrogenic fodder during the last half of pregnancy. In addition, neonatal mortality may be severely increased and has been reported as high as 60% where ewes have been grazed on kale. Gestation lengths may be slightly reduced (3–7 days), and in severe cases lambs are born with little wool and pink bare skin. Lack of iodine may also impair brain development and reduce lung development

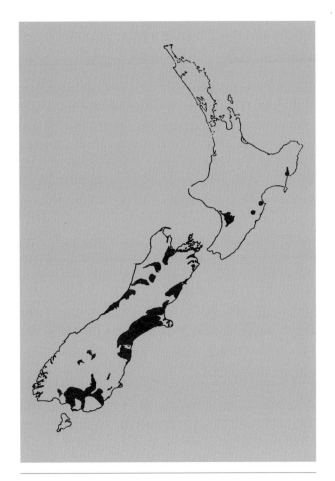

Figure 7.17 Goitre-producing areas in New Zealand.

Pasture species	Season				Mean annual concentration
	Autumn	Winter	Spring	Summer	
Perennial ryegrass	1.35	1.86	1.30	1.30	1.45
White clover	0.77	1.23	0.80	0.83	0.91
Browntop	0.19	0.18	0.22	0.30	0.22
Poa annula	0.08	0.09	0.08	0.19	0.11
Poa trivialis	0.09	0.08	0.28	0.19	0.16

Table 7.15 Mean iodine concentrations (mg/kg DM) in pasture species sampled at 3-monthly intervals (Manawatu hill country) (Johnson and Butler, 1957).

and maturation. These factors contribute to making the weak newborn lamb highly susceptible to cold stress.

Subclinical iodine deficiency is associated with an increased perinatal lamb mortality rate (see also Chapter 5). In some experiments, iodine supplementation resulted in an increase in mean litter sizes in treated compared with untreated ewes. It has been suggested that small depressions in wool production and milk production may also occur. There is one report of a weight-gain response in hoggets on improved native tussock in the South Island.

Diagnosis

In comparison with the other trace elements, the iodine status of ruminants is perhaps the most difficult to define for the practising veterinarian.

Clinical goitre may be detected by palpation of the thyroid gland, by determining the thyroid to bodyweight ratio, and by histopathology. Goitrous lambs usually have a thyroid to bodyweight ratio greater than 0.7 g/kg or a total weight of more than 2 g for both thyroid glands. In many cases the goitre is obvious, but mild individual cases may be harder to detect in the live lamb. A mean thyroid to bodyweight ratio of greater than 0.4 g/kg from necropsy examination of 10–20 newborn lambs, in conjunction with a high perinatal mortality rate, is considered highly suggestive of subclinical iodine deficiency. Both thyroid glands should be carefully dissected and weighed accurately and the weight in grams compared with the weight of the lamb in kilograms. Histologically, thyroids from goitrous animals have follicles depleted of colloid and lined with columnar epithelium.

At present the most reliable way to diagnose iodine deficiency is examination of the thyroid glands of 10–20 lambs (or more) that die at or soon after birth. However, this only provides retrospective information. Knowles and Grace (2007) suggest the following practical approach to deciding whether supplementation is required.
- If feeding brassica crops, then supplement ewes.
- If overt goitre has been recorded previously and any thyroid-weight : birthweight ratio is >0.8 g/kg, then supplement ewes.
- If all or most thyroid-weight : birthweight ratios are <0.4 g/kg, there is probably no need to supplement ewes as the probability of benefit is low.
- If many thyroid-weight : birthweight ratios fall between 0.4 and 0.8 g/kg, then the iodine status of the flock is unclear. Supplement ewes if other evidence is persuasive, such as iodine deficiency in the district.

Serum and urine tests

Serum total iodine concentrations have been used to assess the effects of iodine supplementation, and showed that they were sensitive to the effects of iodine supplementation at a level proportional to the dose rate. Lambs from supplemented ewes also showed raised iodine concentrations using this test. However, there are no clear reference ranges that indicate the level at which goitre might occur or a diagnosis of subclinical iodine deficiency can be made. Goitre did not occur in lambs when the mean iodine concentration of the ewes exceeded 43 mg/l but did occur when the concentrations fell below 30 mg/l.

In a controlled trial conducted on a single farm (Kelly et al., 2009), no response to iodine supplementation was found despite ewe serum and urine iodine concentrations being in the 'deficient' laboratory reference range in July (mid-pregnancy) and September (late pregnancy).

Determination of serum or plasma thyroxine and tri-iodothyronine concentrations can be undertaken, but there are no reference ranges for these values and their use is limited. It has been suggested that a better assessment of iodine status is obtained from measuring milk iodine concentration. Milk iodine concentrations less than 80 mg/l indicate inadequate iodine intake by the ewe. Milk iodine concentrations are sensitive to daily changes in dietary intake, and this may limit the usefulness of single milk samples to assess iodine intake. Another limitation is due to the critical period being before the lamb is born and the ewe is lactating. Herbage iodine levels are of limited use.

Treatment

Some affected lambs, kids and calves with moderate to severe goitre will survive if treated with iodine, either as a drench of potassium iodide (20 mg per lamb) or an injection of an iodised oil preparation.

It should be noted that selenium is essential for normal thyroid hormone metabolism, for instance the conversion of T4 to T3, but it is not directly implemented in the development of goitre. Nevertheless, attention to the selenium status of the flock is important.

Prevention

The routine procedure to prevent iodine deficiency in ewes grazing goitrogenic or iodine-deficient pasture is either of the following:

1. Inject ewes with iodised oil given by intramuscular injection. Doses of 1.5 ml are required for ewes and does. This should be given 1 month before mating or not less than 2 months before the start of lambing. It is recommended to treat stock at least 2 months prior to the feeding of goitrogenic crops. This provides a long-term depot of iodine in the muscle, which is released slowly. Annual re-treatment is recommended.
2. Drench ewes with 280 mg potassium iodide 8 and 4 weeks prior to parturition. Given that some experiments have found that treated ewes have an increased mean litter size, it may also be prudent to dose ewes prior to mating.

Although iodine supplements have been incorporated in the past into licks, intake is variable and there is extensive loss of iodine by oxidation, volatilisation and leaching.

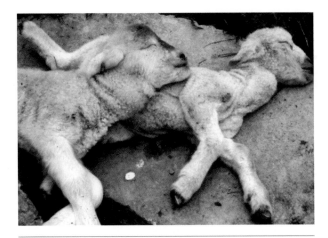

Figure 7.18 Goitre in lambs. Note the swollen thyroid glands of the neck.

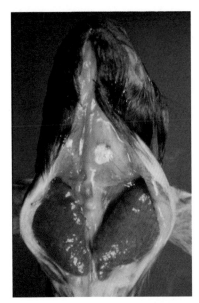

Figure 7.19 Severely enlarged thyroid glands.

Liver biopsy

Trace-element monitoring, particularly of copper and to a lesser extent vitamin B12 levels, is best done by analysis of liver. Liver can either be collected from animals at slaughter or can be obtained from the live animal by liver biopsy. Liver biopsy is a relatively straightforward technique which, if done correctly, results in very few if any complications. The general procedure can be used for sheep, cattle and deer.

Preparation

Animals should be biopsied straight off pasture, as the full rumen keeps the liver in a consistent position. Adequate restraint is essential. For cattle, restraint is best achieved in a cattle crush and head bail that allows access to the right-hand side of the animal. Sheep should be held in left lateral recumbency on a table or similar. Deer should be sedated and restrained in left lateral recumbency.

Procedure

On the right-hand side of the animal an area should be clipped and surgically prepared, centred over the eleventh intercostal space (second-to-last intercostal space) at approximately one-quarter of the distance between the thoracic vertebrae and the sternum. Inject local anaesthetic (2% lignocaine) into the biopsy site, both subcutaneously and into the muscle. Once the local anaesthetic has become effective, make a small stab incision of approximately 1 cm in length into the biopsy site using a scalpel blade.

A 4 mm x 230 mm stainless steel trochar and cannula is used to make the liver biopsy. This should be introduced into the stab incision perpendicular to the body wall. It must be advanced through the body wall, pleural cavity and diaphragm before entering the liver. Therefore, there should be two distinct feelings of 'popping' through tissue — once through the body wall and once through the diaphragm. Once through the diaphragm, the trochar should be removed and the cannula twisted as it is advanced through the liver. Advancing the cannula through the liver gives a gritty or grating feel (similar to coring an apple), which is particularly apparent with cattle and less so for sheep and deer. If necessary the biopsy cannula may be withdrawn slightly and redirected one or two more times to ensure adequate sampling. The cannula is advanced through the liver for a distance of 2–3 cm and then a 5 ml syringe is attached to the end of it and the plunger withdrawn 2–3 ml to provide sufficient negative pressure to retain a core of liver in the cannula. Maintaining this negative pressure, the cannula should be quickly withdrawn.

A core of liver of approximately 1 cm in length is required for each analyte. This should be put onto blotting paper to remove excess blood and then transferred to a plain vacutainer tube or clean pottle for transport to the laboratory. The skin incision at the biopsy site may be left unsutured, sutured or closed with a Michel clip depending on personal preference and the size of the incision. The trochar and cannula should be immersed in aqueous Hibitane (chlorhexidine digluconate) solution before use on the next animal. Parenteral antibiotics may be used if it is thought necessary, but are not used routinely.

Using this technique, with increasing experience 6–12 animals per hour can be sampled with a success rate of greater than 90% even in fractious animals. If no liver sample is obtained on the first attempt the animal should be passed. Complications following liver biopsy are rare. Results from studies assessing pain-related behaviour in cattle following liver biopsy have been mixed, but suggest that cows experience no or only mild inflammatory pain from liver biopsy and that administration of non-steroidal anti-inflammatory drugs at the time of the procedure has little effect.

REFERENCES

SELENIUM

Andrews ED, Hartley WJ, Grant AB. Selenium-responsive diseases of animals in New Zealand. *New Zealand Veterinary Journal* 16, 3–17, 1968

Andrews ED, Hogan KG, Sheppard AD. Selenium in soils, pasture and animal tissues in relation to the growth of young sheep on marginally selenium-deficient areas. *New Zealand Veterinary Journal* 24, 111–16, 1976

Bourne N, Laven R, Wathes DC, Martinez T, McGowan M. A meta-analysis of the effects of vitamin E supplementation on the incidence of retained foetal membranes of dairy cows. *Theriogenology* 67, 494–501, 2007

Braun U, Forrer R, Fürer W, Lutz H. Selenium and vitamin E in blood sera of cows from farms with increased incidence of disease. *Veterinary Record* 128, 543–7, 1991

Clark RG, Ellison RS. Mineral testing — the approach depends on what you want to find out. *New Zealand Veterinary Journal* 41, 98–100, 1993

Cooper BS. Sheep toxicoses from selenium supplementation. *Proceedings No. 103, Veterinary Clinical Toxicology, University of Sydney, Post-Graduate Committee in Veterinary Science*, 175–86, 1987

Cusack P, McMeniman N, Rabiee A, Lean I. Assessment of the effects of supplementation with vitamin E on health and production of feedlot cattle using meta-analysis. *Preventive Veterinary Medicine* 88, 229–46, 2009

Drake C, Grant AB, Hartley WJ. Selenium and animal health: The effect of selenium on unthrifty weaned lambs. *New Zealand Veterinary Journal* 8, 7–10, 1960

Ellison RS. A review of copper and selenium reference ranges in cattle and sheep. *Proceedings of the 22nd Seminar of the Society of Sheep and Beef Cattle Veterinarians, New Zealand Veterinary Association*, 3–26, 1992

Ellison RS. Major trace elements limiting livestock performance in New Zealand. *New Zealand Veterinary Journal* 50 (Suppl.), 35–40, 2002

Grace ND, Knowles SO. Trace element supplementation of livestock in New Zealand: Meeting the challenges of free-range grazing systems. *Veterinary Medicine International*, doi: 10.1155/2012/639472, 2012

Grant AB, Sheppard AD. Selenium in New Zealand pastures. *New Zealand Veterinary Journal* 31, 131–6, 1983

Hill MK, Walker SD, Taylor AG. Effects of 'marginal' deficiencies of copper and selenium on growth and productivity of sheep. *New Zealand Journal of Agricultural Research* 12, 261–70, 1969

Jolly, RD. A preliminary experiment on the effect of selenium on the growth rate of calves. *New Zealand Veterinary Journal* 8, 13, 1960

Jolly RD. A preliminary experiment to investigate the optimum dose rate and frequency of administration of selenium to unthrifty lambs. *New Zealand Veterinary Journal* 8, 11-12, 1960

McLean JW, Thomson GG, Claxton JH. Growth responses to selenium in lambs. *New Zealand Veterinary Journal* 7, 47-52, 1959

McLean JW, Thomson GG, Lawson BM. A selenium responsive syndrome in lactating cows. *New Zealand Veterinary Journal* 11, 59-60, 1963

McSporran K. Selenium and its role in disease resistance. *Surveillance* 19, 39-40, 1992

Millar KR, Meads WJ, Albyt AT, Sheppard AD, Scahill BG. The effect of copper on the response of lambs to selenium supplementation when grazing selenium deficient pasture. *New Zealand Veterinary Journal* 36, 59-62, 1988

Munoz C, Carson AF, McCoy MA, Dawson LER, Irwin D, Kilpatrick DJ. Effect of supplementation with barium selenate on the fertility, prolificacy and lambing performance of hill sheep. *Veterinary Record* 164, 265-71, 2009

Parton K, Bruère AN, Chambers JP. *Veterinary Clinical Toxicology*, 3rd Ed. Publication No. 249, Veterinary Continuing Education, Massey University, Palmerston North, New Zealand, 2006

Rammell CG. Vitamin E status of cattle and sheep 1: A background review. *New Zealand Veterinary Journal* 31, 179-81, 1983

Sanson RL. Selenium supplementation of sheep by topdressing pastures under high rainfall conditions. *New Zealand Veterinary Journal* 38, 1-3, 1990

Sheppard AD, Blom L, Grant AB. Levels of selenium in blood and tissues associated with some selenium deficiency disorders in New Zealand sheep. *New Zealand Veterinary Journal* 32, 91-5, 1984

Sheppard AD, Blom L, Grant AB. Selenium levels in miscellaneous materials. *New Zealand Veterinary Journal* 32, 97-8, 1984

Sheppard AD, Millar KR. Stability of glutathione peroxidase in ovine blood samples under various storage conditions and the response of this enzyme to different methods of selenium supplementation. *New Zealand Veterinary Journal* 29, 77-80, 1981

Shortridge EH, O'Hara PJ, Marshall PM. Acute selenium poisoning of cattle. *New Zealand Veterinary Journal* 19, 47-50, 1971

Sissons CH, Watkinson JH, Byford MJ. Selenium deficiency, the drug metabolising enzymes and mycotoxicoses in sheep. *New Zealand Veterinary Journal* 30, 9-12, 1982

Stephenson JB, Grant AB. Selenium residues in meat. *New Zealand Veterinary Journal* 27, 232, 1979

Surveillance

(1975) 2: 18		Deficiencies, statistics on diagnosis
(1976) 3: 18		Selenium and/or vitamin E deficiency
(1982) 9 (Special issue)		Laboratory diagnosis of trace element deficiency disease
(1999) 26(4): 17		Selenium deficiency — retained foetal membranes in cattle
(2004) 3: 23		Selenium and copper deficiency in calves
(2005) 2: 29		Selenium deficiency in deer
(2008) 2: 30		White muscle disease in deer

Tasker JB, Bewick TD, Clark RG, Fraser AJ. Selenium responses in dairy cattle. *New Zealand Veterinary Journal* 35, 139-40, 1987

Thompson JC, Thornton RN, Bruère SN, Ellison RS. Selenium reference ranges in New Zealand. *New Zealand Veterinary Journal* 46, 65-7, 1998

Thompson KG, Fraser AJ, Harrop BM, Kirk JA, Bullians J, Cordes DO. Glutathione peroxidase activity and selenium concentration in bovine blood and liver as indicators of dietary selenium intake. *New Zealand Veterinary Journal* 29, 3-6, 1981

Thomson GG, Lawson BM. Copper and selenium interaction in sheep. *New Zealand Veterinary Journal* 18, 79-82, 1970

Watkinson JH. Prevention of selenium deficiency in grazing animals by annual topdressing of pasture with sodium selenate. *New Zealand Veterinary Journal* 31, 78-85, 1983

Wichtel JJ. A review of selenium deficiency in grazing ruminants: Part 1: New roles for selenium in ruminant metabolism. *New Zealand Veterinary Journal* 46, 47-53, 1998

Wichtel JJ. A review of selenium deficiency in grazing ruminants: Part 2: Towards a more rational approach to diagnosis and control. *New Zealand Veterinary Journal* 46, 54-8, 1998

COBALT

Andrews ED. Cobalt deficiency. *New Zealand Journal of Agriculture* 92, 239-44, 1956

Andrews ED. Cobalt poisoning in sheep. *New Zealand Veterinary Journal* 13, 101-3, 1965

Andrews ED, Anderson JP. The effect of cobalt topdressing in preventing cobalt deficiency disease of lambs in Southland. *New Zealand Veterinary Journal* 3, 78-9, 1955

Andrews ED, Hogan KG. Methylmalonic acid excretion and incipient cobalt deficiency disease in sheep. *New Zealand Veterinary Journal* 20, 33-8, 1972

Andrews ED, Stephenson BJ, Anderson JP, Faithful WC. The effect of length of pastures on cobalt deficiency disease of lambs. *New Zealand Journal of Agricultural Research* 1, 125-39, 1957

Andrews ED, Stephenson BJ, Isaacs CE, Register RH. The effects of large doses of soluble and insoluble forms of cobalt given at monthly intervals on cobalt deficiency disease in lambs. *New Zealand Veterinary Journal* 14, 191-6, 1966

Bruère AN. Low lamb performance: A case study. *Proceedings of the 12th Annual Seminar of the Society of Sheep and Beef Cattle Veterinarians, New Zealand Veterinary Association*, 222-35, 1982

Clark RG. Cobalt deficiency — diagnosis, treatment control and soil factors. *Proceeding of the 25th Annual Seminar of the Society of Sheep and Beef Cattle Veterinarians, New Zealand Veterinary Association*, 99-110, 1995

Clark RG. Cobalt/vitamin B12 deficiency from lamb to adult ewe. *Proceedings of the 28th Annual Seminar of the Society of Sheep and Beef Cattle Veterinarians, New Zealand Veterinary Association*, 105-22, 1998

Clark RG, Ellison RS. Mineral testing — the approach depends on what you want to find out. *New Zealand Veterinary Journal* 41, 98-100, 1993

Clark RG, Wright DF. Cobalt deficiency in sheep and diagnostic reference ranges. *New Zealand Veterinary Journal* 53, 265-6, 2005

Clark RG, Cornforth IS, Jones BAH, McKnight LJ, Oliver J. A condition resembling ovine white liver disease in lambs on irrigated pasture in South Canterbury. *New Zealand Veterinary Journal* 26, 316, 1978

Clark RG, Wright DF, Millar KR. A proposed new approach and protocol to defining mineral deficiencies using reference curves. Cobalt deficiency in young sheep is used as a model. *New Zealand Veterinary Journal* 33, 1-5, 1985

Clark RG, Mantleman L, Verkerk GA. Failure to obtain a weight gain response to vitamin B12 treatment in young goats grazing pasture that was cobalt deficient for sheep. *New Zealand Veterinary Journal* 35, 38-9, 1987

Clark RG, Duganzich DM, Mortleman L, Fraser AJ. The effect of sporidesmin toxicity on ovine serum vitamin B12 levels. *New Zealand Veterinary Journal* 36, 51-2, 1988

Clark RG, Wright DF, Millar KR, Rowland JD. Reference curves to diagnose cobalt deficiency in sheep using liver and serum vitamin B12 levels. *New Zealand Veterinary Journal* 37, 7-11, 1989

Ellison RS. Major trace elements limiting livestock performance in New Zealand. *New Zealand Veterinary Journal* 50 (Suppl.), 35-40, 2002

Fisher GEJ, MacPherson A. Effect of cobalt deficiency in the pregnant ewe on reproductive performance and lamb viability. *Research in Veterinary Science* 50, 319-27, 1990

Grace ND. Effect of ingestion of soil on the iodine, copper, cobalt (vitamin B12) and selenium status of grazing sheep. *New Zealand Veterinary Journal* 54, 44-7, 2006

Grace ND, Lewis DH. An evaluation of the efficacy of injectable microencapsulated vitamin B12 in increasing and maintaining the serum and liver vitamin B12 concentrations in lambs. *New Zealand Veterinary Journal* 47, 3-7, 1999

Grace ND, West DM. Effect of an injectable microencapsulated vitamin B12 on serum and liver vitamin B12 concentrations in calves. *New Zealand Veterinary Journal* 48, 70-3, 2000

Grace ND, Knowles SO, Sinclair GR, Lee J. Growth response to increasing doses of microencapsulated vitamin B12 and related changes in tissue vitamin B12 concentrations in cobalt-deficient lambs. *New Zealand Veterinary Journal* 51, 89-92, 2003

Grace ND, Knowles SO, Sinclair GR, Lee J. Re: Growth response to increasing doses of microencapsulated vitamin B12 and related changes in tissue vitamin B12 concentrations in cobalt-deficient lambs. *New Zealand Veterinary Journal* 52, 51, 2004

Grace ND, Knowles SO, West DM. Dose response effects of long-acting injectable vitamin B12 plus selenium (Se) on the vitamin B12 and Se status of ewes and their lambs. *New Zealand Veterinary Journal* 54, 67-72, 2006

Grace ND, Knowles SO. Trace element supplementation of livestock in New Zealand: Meeting the challenges of free-range grazing systems. *Veterinary Medicine International*, doi: 10.1155/2012/639472, 2012

Gruner TM, Sedcole JR, Furlong JM, Grace ND, Williams SD, Sinclair G, Sykes AR. Changes in serum concentrations of methylmalonic acid and vitamin B12 in cobalt-supplemented ewes and their lambs on two cobalt-deficient properties. *New Zealand Veterinary Journal* 52, 117-28, 2004

Gruner TM, Sedcole JR, Furlong JM, Grace ND, Williams SD, Sinclair G, Hicks JD, Sykes AR. Concurrent changes in serum vitamin B12 and methylmalonic acid during cobalt or vitamin B12 supplementation of lambs while suckling and after weaning on properties in the South Island of New Zealand considered to be cobalt-deficient. *New Zealand Veterinary Journal* 52, 129-36, 2004

Gruner TM, Sedcole JR, Furlong JM, Sykes AR. A critical evaluation of serum methylmalonic acid and vitamin B12 for the assessment of cobalt deficiency of growing lambs in New Zealand. *New Zealand Veterinary Journal* 52, 137-44, 2004

Hannah RJ, Judson GJ, Reuter DJ, McLaren LD, McFarlane JD. Effect of vitamin B12 injections on the growth of young Merino sheep. *Australian Journal of Agricultural Research* 31, 347-55, 1980

Hartley WJ, Kater J, Andrews ED. An outbreak of polio-encephalomalacia in cobalt deficient sheep. *New Zealand Veterinary Journal* 10, 118-20, 1962

Knowles SO, Grace ND. The vitamin B12 and Se status of lambs during their transition from milk-fed monogastric to grazing herbivore. *New Zealand Veterinary Journal* 65, 113-18, 2017

MacPherson A, Moon FE, Voss RC. Biochemical aspects of cobalt deficiency in sheep with special reference to vitamin status and a possible involvement in the etiology of cerebro-cortical necrosis. *British Veterinary Journal* 132, 294-308, 1976

Millar KR, Albyt AT. A comparison of vitamin B12 levels in the liver and serum of sheep receiving treatments used to correct cobalt deficiency. *New Zealand Veterinary Journal* 32, 105-8, 1984

Millar KR, Lorentz PP. Urinary methylmalonic acid as an indicator of vitamin B12 status of grazing sheep. *New Zealand Veterinary Journal* 27, 90-2, 1979

O'Connor MB. Copper and cobalt topdressing. *Proceedings of the 22nd Annual Seminar of the Society of Sheep and Beef Cattle Veterinarians, New Zealand Veterinary Association*, 121-4, 1992

Smart JA. Cobalt deficiency in sheep. A review of available therapies. *Proceedings of the 28th Annual Seminar of the Society of Sheep and Beef Cattle Veterinarians, New Zealand Veterinary Association*, 123-35, 1998

Surveillance

(1976) 4: 23		Cobalt deficiency
(1977) 3: 22		Cobalt deficiency (mapping)
(1987) 3: 21		White liver disease in goats
(1998) 25(1): 11		Cobalt deficiency in lambs
(2004) 2: 29		Cobalt deficiency in deer

Sutherland RJ, Cordes DO, Carthew GC. Ovine white liver disease — an hepatic dysfunction associated with vitamin B12 deficiency in sheep. *New Zealand Veterinary Journal* 27, 227-32, 1979

Wilson PR, Grace ND. A review of tissue reference values used to assess the trace element status of farmed red deer (*Cervus elaphus*). *New Zealand Veterinary Journal* 49, 126-32, 2001

COPPER

Bingley JB, Anderson N. Clinically silent hypocuprosis and the effect of molybdenum loading on beef calves in Gippsland, Victoria. *Australian Journal of Agricultural Research* 23, 885-904, 1972

Bruère AN. The clinical diagnosis of copper deficiency/sufficiency. *Proceedings of 11th Annual Seminar of the Sheep and Beef Cattle Cattle Veterinarians, New Zealand Veterinary Association*, 15-23, 1981

Bruère AN. Advances in the diagnosis of copper deficiency — iron induced hypocuprosis. *Proceedings of 12th Annual Seminar of the Sheep and Beef Cattle Veterinarians, New Zealand Veterinary Association*, 374-83, 1982

Campbell AG, Coup MR, Bishop WH, Wright DE. Effect of elevated iron intake on copper status of grazing cattle. *New Zealand Journal of Agricultural Research* 17, 393-9, 1974

Cunningham IJ. The toxicity of copper to bovines. *New Zealand Journal of Science and Technology* 27A, 372-6, 1946

Cunningham IJ. Parenteral administration of copper to sheep. *New Zealand Veterinary Journal* 7, 15-17, 1959

Cunningham IJ, Hogan KG, Lawson BM. The effect of sulphate and molybdenum on copper metabolism in cattle. *New Zealand Journal of Agricultural Research* 2, 145-52, 1959

Cunningham IJ, Perrin DD. Copper compounds as fertilisers for pastures deficient in copper. *New Zealand Journal of Science and Technology* 28A, 252-65, 1946

Dick AT. Influence of organic sulphate on the copper-molybdenum interrelationship in sheep. *Nature* 172, 637-8, 1953

Ellison RS. A review of copper and selenium reference ranges in cattle and sheep. *Proceedings of the 22nd Annual Seminar of the Society of Sheep and Beef Cattle Veterinarians, New Zealand Veterinary Association*, 3-26, 1992

Ellison RS. Major trace elements limiting livestock performance in New Zealand. *New Zealand Veterinary Journal* 50 (Suppl.), 35-40, 2002

Farquarson BC. Some aspects of copper toxicity in sheep grazing New Zealand pastures. *PhD Thesis*, Massey University Library, Palmerston North, 1984

Grace ND. Copper. *New Zealand Society of Animal Production*. Occasional publication No. 9. Mineral requirements of grazing animals, 56-66, 1983

Grace ND, Wilson PR, Thomas WJ. Effect of topdressing pasture with copper on the copper status of young red deer (*Cervus elaphus*). *Proceedings of a Deer Course for Veterinarians, Deer Branch of the New Zealand Veterinary Association* 18, 117-21, 2001

Grace ND, Knowles SO, West DM, Lee J. Copper oxide needles administered during early pregnancy improves the copper status of ewes and their lambs. *New Zealand Veterinary Journal* 52, 189-92, 2004

Grace ND, Wilson PR, Quinn AK. The effect of copper-amended fertiliser and copper oxide wire particles on the copper status of farmed red deer (*Cervus elaphus*) and their progeny. *New Zealand Veterinary Journal* 53, 31-8, 2005

Grace ND, Wilson PR, Quinn AK. Impact of molybdenum on the copper status of red deer (*Cervus elaphus*). *New Zealand Veterinary Journal* 53, 137-41, 2005

Grace ND, Knowles SO. Trace element supplementation of livestock in New Zealand: Meeting the challenges of free-range grazing systems. *Veterinary Medicine International*, doi: 10.1155/2012/639472, 2012

Harrington KC, Thatcher A, Kemp PD. Mineral composition and nutritive value of some common pasture weeds. *New Zealand Plant Protection* 59, 261-5, 2006

Hogan KG, Money DFL, White DA, Walker R. Weight responses of young sheep to copper and connective tissue lesions associated with the grazing of pastures of high molybdenum content. *New Zealand Journal of Agricultural Research* 14, 687-701, 1971

Knowles SO, Grace ND. A recent assessment of the elemental composition of New Zealand pastures in relation to meeting the dietary requirements of livestock. *Journal of Animal Science* 92, 303-10, 2014

Laven RA, Lawrence KE, Livesey CT. The assessment of blood copper status in cattle: A comparison of measurements of caeruloplasmin and elemental copper in serum and plasma. *New Zealand Veterinary Journal* 55, 171-6, 2007

Laven RA, Smith SL. Copper deficiency in sheep: An assessment of the relationship between concentrations of copper in serum and plasma. *New Zealand Veterinary Journal* 56, 334-8, 2008

Lorentz PP, Gibb FM. Caeruloplasmin activity as an indication of plasma copper levels in sheep. *New Zealand Veterinary Journal* 23, 1-3, 1975

Osborn PJ, Bond GC, Millar KR. The distribution of copper, vitamin B12 and zinc in the livers of sheep. *New Zealand Veterinary Journal* 31, 144-5, 1983

Sharman JR. The laboratory confirmation of acute copper poisoning. *New Zealand Veterinary Journal* 17, 67-9, 1969

Smith B. Copper and molybdenum imbalance in relationship to post-parturient haemoglobinuria in cattle. *New Zealand Veterinary Journal* 21, 240, 1973

Smith B. I. The effects of copper supplementation on stock health and production. *New Zealand Veterinary Journal* 23, 73-7, 1975

Smith B, Coup MR. Hypocuprosis: A clinical investigation of dairy herds in Northland. *New Zealand Veterinary Journal* 21, 252-8, 1973

Smith B, Moon GH. Hypocuprosis: The effects of administration of copper sulphate to cattle through water supply. *New Zealand Veterinary Journal* 24, 132-4, 1976

Smith B, Woodhouse DA, Fraser AJ. II. The effects of copper supplementation on stock health and production. *New Zealand Veterinary Journal* 24, 132-4, 1975

Sommerville GF, Mason JB. Copper overdosage in sheep. *New Zealand Veterinary Journal* 33, 98-9, 1985

Surveillance

(1986) 1: 11	Deer liver and serum copper levels
(1978) 4: 22	Paresis in deer
(1978) 5: 19	Copper deficiency and ovine enzootic ataxia
(1978) 5: 22	Enzootic ataxia in deer
(1980) 5: 10-11	Hypocupraemia: What does it mean
(1981) 1: 11	Parasitically induced copper deficiency in cattle
(1975) 4: 19	Low copper and sudden death
(2005): 2: 29	Copper and selenium deficiency in deer
(2007): 1: 15	Enzootic ataxia in lambs
(2008): 3: 20	Copper toxicity and palm kernel feed

Suttle NF. The treatment and prevention of copper deficiency in ruminants. *Proceedings of the 11th Annual Seminar of the Society of Sheep and Beef Cattle Veterinarians, New Zealand Veterinary Association*, 24-33, 1981

Suttle NF, McLauchlan M. Predicting the effects of dietary molybdenum and sulphur on the availability of copper to ruminants. *Proceedings of the Nutrition Society* 35, 22A, 1976

Suttle NF, Alloway BJ, Thornton I. An effect of soil ingestion on utilisation of dietary copper by sheep. *Journal of Agricultural Science, Cambridge* 84, 249-54, 1975

Suttle N. Chapter 11 — Copper. *Mineral nutrition of livestock*, 4th Edition, pp 255-305. CAB International, Oxfordshire, UK, 2010

Thompson KG, Audige L, Arthur DG, Julian AF, Orr MB, McSporran KD, Wilson PR. Osteochondrosis associated with copper deficiency in young farmed red deer and wapiti red deer hybrids. *New Zealand Veterinary Journal* 42, 137-47, 1994

Towers NR, Young PW, Wright DE. Effect of zinc supplementation on bovine plasma copper. *New Zealand Veterinary Journal* 29, 113-14, 1981

Vermunt JJ, West DM. Predicting copper status in beef cattle using serum copper concentrations. *New Zealand Veterinary Journal* 42, 194-5, 1994

Wiener G. Genetic and other factors in the occurrence of swayback in sheep. *Journal of Comparative Pathology* 76, 435-47, 1966

Wells N. Soil studies using sweet vernal to assess element availability. Part 3: Copper in New Zealand soil sequences. *New Zealand Journal of Science and Technology* 380, 884-902, 1957

Wilson PR. Enzootic ataxia in red deer. *New Zealand Veterinary Journal* 27, 252-4, 1979

Wilson PR. Bodyweight and serum copper concentrations of farmed red deer stags following oral copper administration. *New Zealand Veterinary Journal* 37, 94-7, 1989

Wilson PR, Grace ND. A review of tissue reference values used to assess the trace element status of farmed red deer (*Cervus elaphus*). *New Zealand Veterinary Journal* 49, 126-32, 2001

IODINE

Bruere S, Smart J. Long acting iodine injections in sheep — what happens? *Proceedings of the Sheep and Beef Cattle Veterinarians of the NZVA and Cervetec*, 77-82, 2015

Clark RG. Thyroid histological changes in lambs from iodine-supplemented and untreated ewes. *New Zealand Veterinary Journal* 46, 223-5, 1998

Clark RG, Sargison ND, West DM, Littlejohn RP. Recent information on iodine deficiency in New Zealand sheep flocks. *New Zealand Veterinary Journal* 46, 216-22, 1998

Contreras PA, Wittwer F, Matamoros R, Mayorga IM, van Schaik G. Effect of grazing pasture with a low selenium content on the concentrations of triiodothyronine and thyroxine in serum, and GSH-Px activity in erythrocytes in cows in Chile. *New Zealand Veterinary Journal* 53, 77-80, 2005

Davis GBm, Stevenson BJ, Price MC. Inherited goitre in sheep. *New Zealand Veterinary Journal* 27, 126-7, 1979

Davis GH, Barry TN. Responses to supplementation in high fecundity Booroola Merino x Romney ewes. *Proceedings of the Nutrition Society of New Zealand* 8, 110, 1983

Grace ND. Effect of ingestion of soil on iodine, copper, cobalt (vitamin B12) and selenium status of grazing sheep. *New Zealand Veterinary Journal* 54, 44-7, 2006

Grace ND, Knowles SO. A practical approach to managing the risks of iodine deficiency in flocks using thyroid-weight : birthweight ratios of lambs. *New Zealand Veterinary Journal* 55, 314-18, 2007

Grace ND, Knowles SO, Sinclair GR. Effect of premating iodine supplementation of ewes fed pasture or a brassica crop prelambing on the incidence of goitre in newborn lambs. *Proceedings of the New Zealand Society of Animal Production* 61, 164-7, 2001

Johnson JM, Butler GW. Iodine content of pasture plants. Method of determination and preliminary investigation of species and strain differences. *Physiologia Plantarium* 10, 100-11, 1957

Kelly K, Bryan M, Roe A. How long can we go? An update on iodine — laboratory testing and production responses. *Proceedings of the 39th Annual Seminar of the Society of Sheep and Beef Cattle Veterinarians, New Zealand Veterinary Association*, 129-39, 2009

Knowles SO, ND Grace. A practical approach to managing the risks of iodine deficiency in flocks using thyroid-weight : birthweight ratios of lambs. *New Zealand Veterinary Journal* 55, 314-18, 2007

Knowles SO, Grace ND. Serum total iodine concentrations in pasture-fed pregnant ewes and newborn lambs challenged by iodine supplementation and goitrogenic kale. *Journal of Animal Science* 93, 425-32, 2015

Mulvaney CJ. The role of iodine in Merino sheep — is there a subclinical condition affecting lamb survival? *Proceedings of the 27th Annual Seminar of the Society of Sheep and Beef Cattle Veterinarians, New Zealand Veterinary Association*, 117-24, 1997

Sargison ND, West DM, Clark RG. An investigation of the possible effects of subclinical iodine deficiency on ewe fertility and perinatal lamb mortality. *New Zealand Veterinary Journal* 45, 208-11, 1997

Sargison ND, West DM, Clark RG. The effects of iodine deficiency on ewe fertility and perinatal lamb mortality. *New Zealand Veterinary Journal* 46, 72-5, 1998

Scott D, Maunsell LA, Willis BH. Lack of weight gain of sheep following iodine supplementation in inland regions of the South Island. *New Zealand Veterinary Journal* 31, 120-2, 1983

Sinclair DP, Andrews ED. Goitre in newborn lambs. *New Zealand Veterinary Journal* 2, 72-9, 1954

Sinclair DP, Andrews ED. Prevention of goitre in newborn lambs from kale-fed ewes. *New Zealand Veterinary Journal* 6, 87-95, 1958

Sinclair DP, Andrews ED. Failure of mild goitre to influence growth rates in kale-fed weaned lambs. *New Zealand Veterinary Journal* 7, 39-41, 1959

Sinclair DP, Andrews ED. Deaths due to goitre in newborn lambs prevented by iodised poppy-seed oil. *New Zealand Veterinary Journal* 9, 96-100, 1961

Surveillance

(1976) 1: 19	Congenital goitre in a calf
(1982) 1: 23	Goitre in kids
(1990) 4: 10-11	The effect of iodine supplementation

LIVER BIOPSY

Barratt LA, Beausoleil NJ, Benschop J, Stafford KJ. Pain-related behaviour was not observed in dairy cattle in the days after liver biopsy, regardless of whether NSAIDs were administered. *Research in Veterinary Science* 104, 195-9, 2016

Beausoleil NJ, Stafford KJ. Is a non-steroidal anti-inflammatory drug required to alleviate pain behavious associated with liver biopsy in cattle? *Journal of Veterinary Behaviour* 7, 245-51, 2012

West DM, Vermunt JJ. Liver biopsy in cattle. *Proceedings of the 25th Annual Seminar of the Society of Sheep and Beef Cattle Veterinarians, New Zealand Veterinary Association*, 206-7, 1995

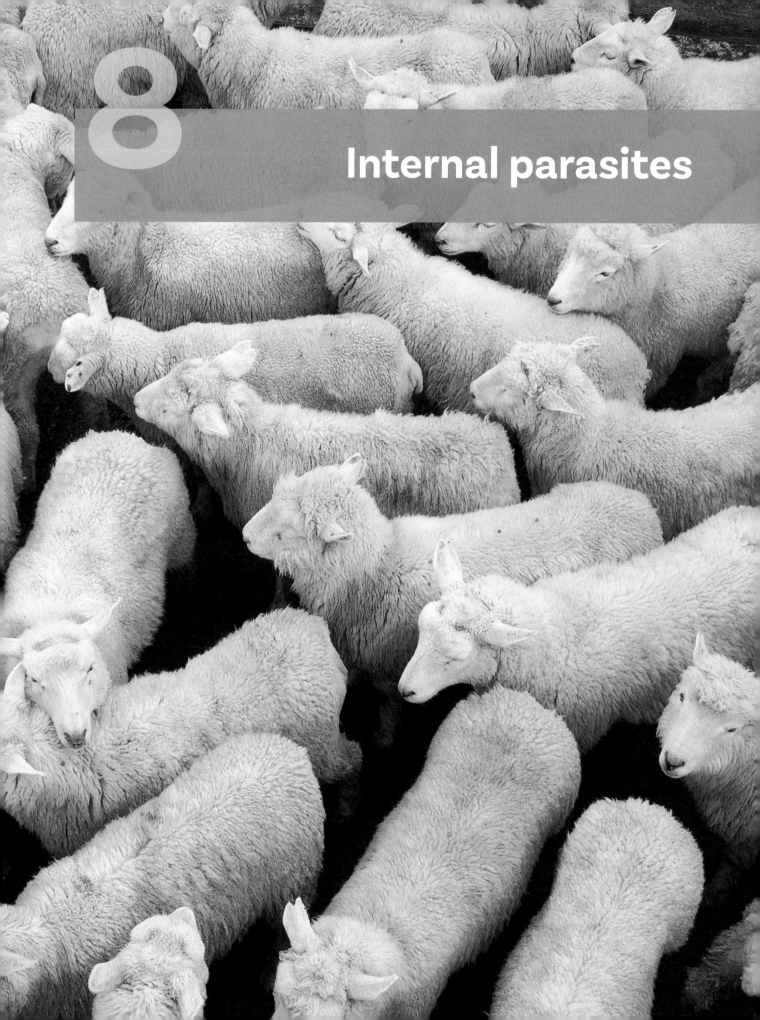

8 Internal parasites

Gastrointestinal nematode parasites

Gastrointestinal nematode parasitism is probably the most important production-limiting disease of sheep in New Zealand, especially on farms with high sheep stocking rates. In some cases the loss of production may go unnoticed as it is associated with subtle decreases in weight gain (subclinical parasitism). In other cases the problem will be obvious with ill-thrifty, scouring stock that lose weight (clinical parasitism).

Adequate control of internal parasites is essential for optimal production, but emerging drench resistance, as well as concerns about the levels of chemical use, have led to debate about the sustainability of many parasite control practices. It is important to remember that parasitism is a dynamic condition that relies on the interaction between the agent (the parasite), the environment and the host (the sheep). Changes in any of these variables (e.g. emergence of anthelmintic-resistant worms, rainfall, or lowering of host immunity due to under-nutrition) will affect the parasite status of the farm. While general guidelines regarding control can be made, variations on these will be required for individual farms.

Aetiology

Sheep harbour a number of different nematode species, but only the more important species will be dealt with here. The abomasal parasites *Haemonchus*, *Teladorsagia (Ostertagia)* and *Trichostrongylus* and the small-intestinal species of *Trichostrongylus*, *Nematodirus* and to some extent *Cooperia* are most commonly associated with production loss and clinical disease. Occasionally, relatively high burdens of *Bunostomum* or *Chabertia* are found in adult sheep and may contribute to ill thrift.

Note: Parasitologists consider that the correct name for what we have traditionally called *Ostertagia* in sheep is now *Teladorsagia*. However, it should be noted that many veterinarians and farmers may still use the name *Ostertagia*.

In general terms these nematodes are found throughout the country, but there are regional differences. Because *Haemonchus* requires a higher range of temperatures for larval development than other genera, worm burdens of this species reach higher levels in sheep in the North Island compared with the South Island. Species of *Nematodirus* are common throughout the country, but because of their ability to survive cold winters may develop in large numbers in the spring, and become pathogenic, especially in areas such as Canterbury, Otago and Southland.

Life cycle of important parasites

With the exception of *Nematodirus* the important gastrointestinal nematodes of sheep have similar life cycles. This basic trichostrongylid life cycle is summarised in Figure 8.1. Typically it takes about 21 days from the ingestion of worm larvae to the appearance of worm eggs in the faeces. This is called the pre-patent period.

For some genera, such as *Haemonchus*, this period may be slightly shorter. The pre-patent period is important because it enables the efficacy of a drench on-farm to be tested by estimating faecal egg counts both before and during the period from 5–14 days after drenching — during this period, for an effective product the egg counts should be zero or very close to zero. In addition, the pre-patent period means that regular drenching of lambs (every 28 days) not only removes the parasites from the host but also reduces pasture contamination while still allowing some eggs to pass to contribute to refugia.

The essential difference with *Nematodirus* species

is that development to the third infective stage occurs entirely within the egg, allowing the larval stage within the egg to survive extremely low temperatures and in general to develop at a much slower rate. Therefore in colder areas, these eggs may overwinter on pasture and be available to infect lambs in the spring.

Development of larvae on pasture

New Zealand's moist moderate climate is particularly favourable for the development and survival of the free-living stages on pasture. The eggs and pre-infection stages require warm, moist conditions to develop successfully. Provided there is adequate moisture, optimum development occurs between 15°C and 30°C but some development can occur within the temperature range 4–35°C. Below 10°C (generally May to October), development rates are lower. Under optimum conditions provided in a laboratory infective L3 larvae can develop in 5–7 days, but under field conditions this varies considerably and it usually takes 2–3 weeks or more. Maximum numbers of infective larvae on pasture may not develop for 3–6 weeks.

In general, eggs that fail to hatch within the first week

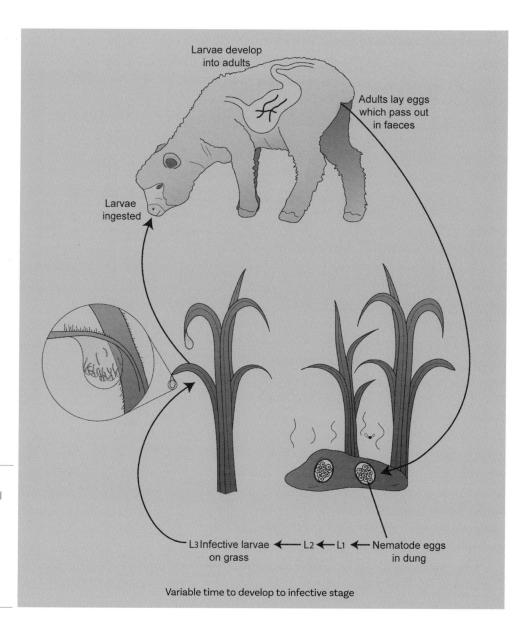

Figure 8.1 The basic life cycle of gastrointestinal nematode parasites of sheep. Pre-patent period (the time from larvae ingestion to egg production) is approximately 3 weeks.

or so normally fail to develop further. First- and second-stage larvae are active feeding stages and are vulnerable to desiccation. However, once the infective third stage is reached, larvae can survive for considerable periods as this stage can withstand some desiccation due to the retention of the cuticle from the second stage. In the summer, larvae may survive up to 10–12 weeks depending on the degree of exposure to sunlight or desiccation. Some open-sward pasture species provide a less suitable environment for larval survival than those such as browntop that have a dense thatch that retains moisture. In dry areas, desiccation is a major limiting factor to larval survival. Survival rates in autumn are greater. Larvae commonly survive 3–6 months, with smaller numbers surviving up to 12 months and in the case of *Nematodirus* for over 18 months. Once pasture is contaminated it takes at least 2–3 months for larval numbers to decline significantly. In winter this may be considerably longer as, contrary to popular belief, infective L3 larvae can survive frosts, and cool conditions actually enhance the potential for survival. However, development rates are reduced. Infective larvae of *Haemonchus* are less resilient under cold conditions than those of *Telodorsagia* or *Trichostrongylus* and most *Haemonchus* larvae do not survive on pasture over winter.

The percentage of eggs that develop to infective L3 larvae is very variable and often <1%. Under favourable moist, warm conditions, which often occur in late summer and early autumn, >10% of eggs can successfully reach the infective stage.

Seasonal availability of infective larvae

Despite knowing many of the factors that affect larval development, it has not been possible to reliably predict potential outbreaks of parasitism from weather patterns alone. Nevertheless, seasonal patterns of larval availability usually occur with a minor peak in late spring/early summer and a major peak in late summer/autumn — see Figure 8.2.

The magnitude of these larval peaks can vary markedly from year to year, and data from Dargaville, Ruakura, Wallaceville, Winchmore and Woodlands over 3 years confirm a broadly similar pattern (see Figure 8.3). However, it must be appreciated that these extraordinarily high rates of pasture larval contamination resulted from the grazing of undrenched lambs. Under these circumstances, numbers of infective L3 larvae on pasture often exceeded 10,000 per kg herbage. This is in contrast to the pasture larval counts considered necessary to maintain adequate parasite control. Levels of below 100 L3/kg herbage have been suggested as being necessary and one can appreciate how easily this can be exceeded given the high fecundity of worms (*Haemonchus* lay up to 10,000 eggs per day) and the regular occurrence of favourable larval development conditions in sheep-raising districts of New Zealand.

Distribution of larvae on pasture

Larvae tend to be clumped around the faecal dung areas. In set stocking grazing systems, sheep camp in specific areas, which concentrates faeces, but with rotational grazing faeces and infective larvae are distributed more evenly.

Larvae are concentrated at the base of the sward, including the root mat and soil (see Figure 8.4). Therefore, the practice of intensive grazing exposes sheep to much higher levels of larval intake than that experienced by sheep lightly grazing the same pasture.

Population dynamics

The relationships between pasture contamination, the availability of infective larvae and the build-up of infections in young sheep were studied extensively by Brunsdon and Vlassoff at Wallaceville Animal Research

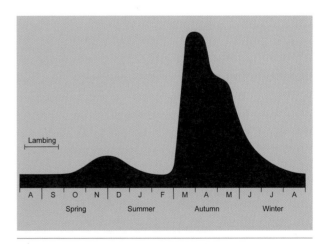

Figure 8.2 Seasonal pattern of larvae on pasture (from Vlassoff, 1982).

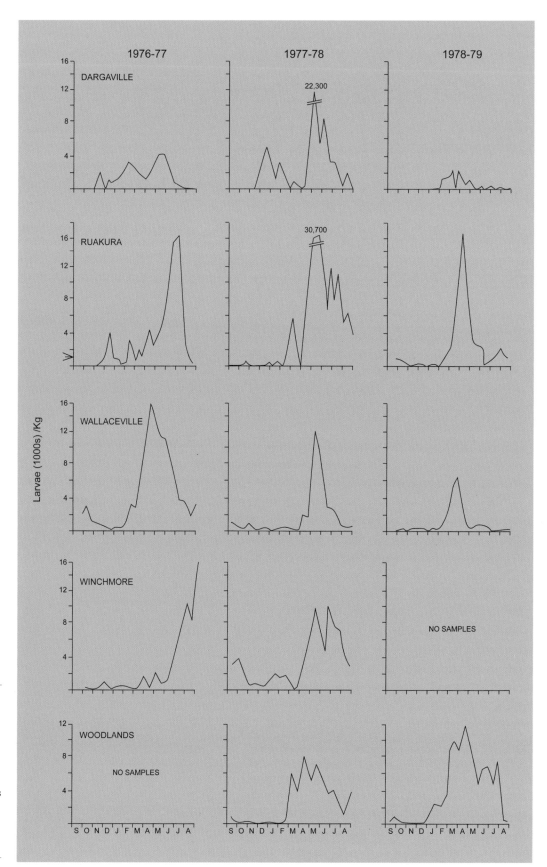

Figure 8.3 The seasonal pattern of infective nematode larvae on pasture at selected geographical sites in New Zealand (from Vlassoff, 1982).

Centre and elsewhere. The following is a summary of their findings (see Figure 8.5).

1. The spring rise of larvae on pasture is contributed from two main sources:
   a. the periparturient rise in faecal egg count of ewes
   b. overwintered larvae
2. Larvae from these sources result in the first generation of worms, which accumulate in the lambs during summer.
3. Eggs deposited by lambs in February and March are the source of the large autumn peak of infective larvae on pasture.
4. These larvae produce the second generation of worms in lambs — that which causes clinical disease in autumn and winter. A proportion of these larvae also overwinter on pasture to provide a source of infection for ewes and lambs in the spring.
5. Many of the eggs deposited in the autumn (from the second-generation worms) fail to develop because of progressively declining temperature.

An important exception to this regular sequence is *Nematodirus filicollis* which, due to its slow development, differs from the other parasites in that infection is transmitted directly (via the pasture) from one season's lambs to the next. *Nematodirus spathiger* will to some extent behave as other trichostrongylids.

In general, lambs ingest larvae from the moment they begin eating grass, with the peak period of challenge occurring in the autumn. There are basically only two generations of parasites annually, the first being derived from overwintered larvae and those that have developed from the periparturient rise of the ewe, and the second being derived from the contamination of the lambs themselves. *Nematodirus*, particularly *N. filicollis*, is an exception and only involves one generation from the lambs in one season to those of the next.

The foregoing sequence of events represents only an average picture; the level of larval contamination and the timing of peaks in population vary between years and in different localities. The predominant species changes from *Nematodirus* in spring, *Telodorsagia* in spring and summer, *Haemonchus* in summer and autumn to *Trichostrongylus* in autumn and winter. Furthermore, the superimposing of a drench programme and rotational grazing may alter the

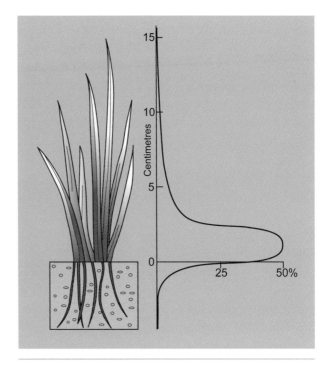

Figure 8.4 The distribution of infective nematode larvae on pasture (from Vlassoff, 1982).

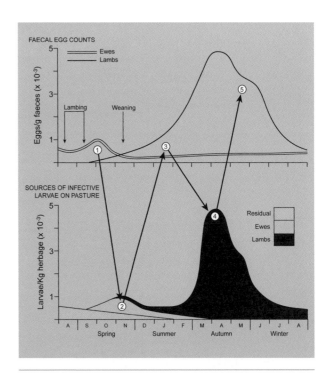

Figure 8.5 The sequential inter-relationship between pasture contamination by ewes and lambs and the population of infective larvae on pasture (from Vlassoff, 1982).

pattern or relative source of contamination considerably. For instance, if lambs are drenched regularly every 4 weeks from weaning time, there will be a considerable reduction in the number of larvae on the pasture in autumn. Of the larvae that are present then, a much greater proportion would be derived from contamination passed either by mixed-age ewes or hoggets (which become two-tooths over this period).

Contamination of pasture by older sheep

As mentioned previously, the periparturient rise in faecal egg output by ewes has been regarded as the main contribution by older sheep to the pasture larval nematode population to which young sheep are exposed. Under New Zealand pastoral conditions, the importance of the periparturient rise as the sole source of contamination has been questioned. In some flocks, high levels of faecal egg counts have been observed in both 18-month-old ewes (two-tooths) and mixed-age ewes during the autumn and winter periods.

In general, contamination from lambs and hoggets is the major source of pasture contamination on sheep farms because their faecal egg counts can reach high levels if the sheep are not drenched. However, if young sheep are drenched regularly at intervals close to the pre-patent period, their contribution to pasture larval contamination is reduced markedly and ewes (two-tooth and mixed-age) may then be an important source of pasture contamination relative to the young sheep.

The faecal egg output of the ewe falls abruptly in the later stages of lactation to very low levels, and generally from then on the ewe adds very little to the pasture contamination — in fact, because the ewes are resistant, they eat and destroy far more larvae than they contribute to the total contamination. However, a review of faecal egg output by adult sheep on farms in the Manawatu district (Stafford et al., 1993) indicates that during spring and late summer to autumn, ewes (especially two-tooth ewes) may be an important source of pasture contamination under normal management conditions where lambs are drenched regularly (see Figure 8.6).

In the South Island, Familton and others working with sheep on irrigated pastures found that ewes (in particular the younger ewes) showed consistently elevated faecal egg counts over the autumn and winter period. When this contamination was calculated on an annual basis it was found that adults contributed between 65% and 70% of the total parasite egg contamination on the pasture, depending on the type of drenching programme being used. The work of Beckett and Hutchings on nine dryland farms on the east coast of the North Island indicate that this phenomenon described by Familton is not just an aberration of the effect of irrigation on parasite status. The results from dryland are very similar to those seen in the South Island irrigation areas. However, in general, grazing ewes on the same area of the farm as lambs can help reduce the worm challenge to the lambs.

The effects of nematodes on sheep

Clinical parasitism

Nematodes damage their hosts in a variety of ways. Species such as *Haemonchus* suck blood, while others alter the metabolism and performance of sheep. In general, nematodes reduce appetite, skeletal growth, haemopoiesis, protein and mineral metabolism. These effects result in the classical clinical signs associated with nematode parasitism of loss of appetite, weight loss, dark-coloured diarrhoea and, in the case of *Haemonchus*, anaemia.

Diarrhoea is a particular feature of severe *Trichostrongylus* infection, which is seen particularly in

Flock	Date	Mean faecal EPG
1	February	1350
2	February	785
3	March	2730
4	March	460
5	March	1310
6	March	3880
7	June	260
8	June	750
9	October	1020
10	December	600

Table 8.1 Examples of higher than expected ewe faecal egg counts (from West, 1982).

the late autumn and early winter and can sometimes result in rapid death. Similarly, acute *Nematodirus* infection of young lambs can result in a profuse watery diarrhoea with a sticky mucous appearance. In severe outbreaks of haemonchosis, the sudden death of either ewes or lambs is frequently the first recognised sign.

Subclinical parasitism

While losses from clinical parasitism are still commonly seen, the losses associated with exposure to low levels of infective larvae on pasture are of much greater economic significance. Much of our understanding of the effect on the host of regular exposure to low levels of infective larvae has come from the work at the Moredun Research Institute in Scotland. Pair-fed control sheep were used to differentiate between the effects of parasites on appetite and their effects on efficiency of feed conversion. Exposing sheep to a daily intake of either 4000 *Telodorsagia circumcincta* larvae or 2500 *Trichostrongylus colubriformis* larvae more than halved the liveweight gain of exposed lambs compared with control sheep fed *ad libitum* (see Tables 8.2 and 8.3). Approximately half of this reduced gain was due to a reduction in appetite, and half due to reduced efficiency of feed conversion. In addition to having a marked effect on weight gain, low-level infections of either *T. colubriformis* or *T. vitrinus* produced a most striking effect on calcium and phosphorus retention. Complete cessation of skeletal mineral deposition occurred when lambs were continuously dosed with only 2500 larvae of either species per day.

The challenge doses used in these experiments are similar to those that may be experienced by sheep grazing New Zealand pasture. As mentioned previously, pasture larval counts can exceed 10,000 larvae/kg herbage and often range from 1000 to 5000. As lambs consume between 5 and 10 kg of herbage per day, their larval intake may exceed 50,000 L3 per day.

In addition to these effects on growth, wool production is similarly affected by continuous exposure to low levels of larvae on pasture. Depression in wool growth in the order of 16–26% has been shown to occur in sheep exposed to infection but in which faecal egg counts were zero because of previously acquired host resistance preventing larval development. It is assumed that the reduced wool production reflects the 'cost' of maintaining host

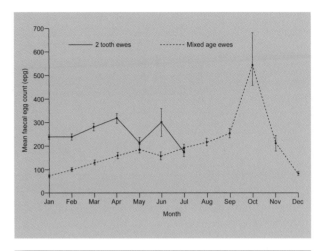

Figure 8.6 Monthly mean faecal egg counts (± standard error) from ewe flocks in the Manawatu district (total 4100 faecal egg counts) (from Stafford et al., 1993).

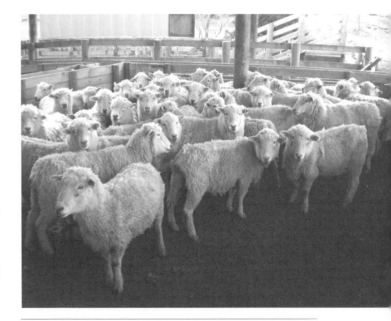

Figure 8.7 Older sheep likely clinically affected by parasitism.

	ALC[1]	ALI[2]	PF[3]
Liveweight gain	100	48	80
Fat deposition	100	58	84
Protein deposition	100	49	66
Ca deposition	100	36	75

ALC[1]	=	Controls fed *ad libitum*
ALI[2]	=	Infected sheep fed *ad libitum*
PF[3]	=	Controls pair-fed to AL1

Table 8.2 The effect of chronic infection (4000 larvae/day for 100 days) with *Telodorsagia circumcincta* on the body composition of growing lambs. Values are expressed as a percentage of those obtained in controls fed *ad libitum* (Sykes et.al., 1977).

	ALC[1]	ALI[2]	PF[3]
Liveweight gain	100	38	74
Fat deposition	100	50	72
Protein deposition	100	23	83
Ca deposition	100	1	110

ALC[1]	=	Controls fed *ad libitum*
ALI[2]	=	Infected sheep fed *ad libitum*
PF[3]	=	Controls pair-fed to AL1

Table 8.3 The effect of chronic infection (2500 larvae/day for 100 days) with *Trichostrongylus colubriformis* on the body composition of growing lambs. Values are expressed as a percentage of those obtained in controls fed *ad libitum* (Sykes et.al., 1979).

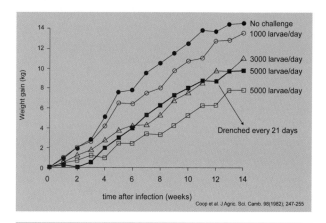

Figure 8.8 Effect of intake of larvae and anthelmintic on growth of young lambs (modified from Sykes, 1982).

resistance to the larval challenge.

Once pastures become contaminated with infective larvae it is difficult to prevent production losses occurring in sheep (especially young sheep) that graze them. Although frequent anthelmintic drenching improves animal performance in these circumstances, it does not remove all the effects of continuous infection. Coop and co-workers at Moredun, Scotland, infected sheep daily with 5000 *Telodorsagia circumcincta* larvae and this reduced growth rates to half that of control sheep (see Figure 8.8). Drenching at 21-day intervals suppressed egg counts but only restored 20% of the loss in growth rate.

Diagnosis

The diagnosis of clinical parasitism is relatively straight-forward and usually follows a history of inadequate worm control and the progression of typical signs of listlessness, inappetence, ill thrift and scouring. If *Haemonchus* is the predominant species, anaemia may also be present and scouring is not a feature. In fact, sheep can have high burdens of *Haemonchus* and still have pelleted faeces. In acute haemonchosis, sudden death may be the first sign of infection.

Faecal egg counts (FECs) provide a very useful means of estimating the level of the worm burdens, and worm counts on slaughtered sheep provide valuable information as to the number and composition of the burden present. The demonstration of parasite burdens by field necropsy is a valuable veterinarian/client exercise and will often help in emphasising how numerous internal parasites may be. In the abomasum, female *Haemonchus* can be seen as large red-and-white-striped worms (barber's pole; Figure 8.9). The smaller, brown-coloured *Telodorsagia* worms can also be seen by careful inspection of the abomasal mucosa.

McKenna (1982) demonstrated that apart from *Nematodirus* there was a good association between faecal egg counts and the level of strongyle infection in young sheep if arbitrarily defined levels of low, medium and high worm burdens and faecal egg counts were used (see Table 8.4).

The worm burdens and faecal egg counts defined as 'low' by McKenna may still impair sheep performance and it is generally agreed that gastrointestinal parasitism has a more marked effect on the metabolism and performance of sheep than has been recognised previously.

In general, the effect of worm burdens on sheep is

Egg counts	Total worm counts		
	'Low' (up to 4000)	'Moderate' (4000–10,000)	'High' (>10,000)
'Low' (up to 500 epg), n = 110	106	4	0
'Moderate' (600–2000 epg), n = 36	17	14	5
'High' (>2000 epg), n = 44	4	6	34

Table 8.4 Numbers of young sheep falling into three classes of egg and worm counts (n = 190) (from McKenna, 1982). Note: These are arbitrarily defined levels.

influenced to a large extent by the numbers of worms and the pathogenicity of the species present. Australian researchers have suggested that a pathogenic index be used to take account of the variety of species present in most sheep. The worm counts that can be regarded as being significant in causing clinical disease as a sole pathogen in lambs are given in Table 8.5. Where a mixed burden is present, an approximate assessment of its significance can be obtained by adding the appropriate fractions of the pathogenic index.

Because of individual variation in susceptibility it is preferable to perform worm counts on at least three or four sheep if a reasonable assessment of the infection level in a mob is to be obtained, along with faecal egg counts from at least 10 sheep. Larval cultures can be used to identify the genera of worms involved. Other diagnostic procedures such as measuring plasma pepsinogen levels have proved to be less reliable and are seldom used.

In contrast to the clinical condition, low-level parasitism can be more difficult to assess. Production losses can be significant even when faecal egg counts are below 400 or 500 eggs per gram. In addition, lambs are often being drenched regularly, close to the time of the pre-patent period, and under these circumstances worm egg counts and total worm burdens give little indication of the larval challenge experienced by the lambs. Histopathological examination of stained sections of the gut, looking for worms and the damage they cause, can prove useful in such cases.

To date, pasture larval counts are far from precise, are costly and are technically demanding to perform. For these reasons they have not been available for routine diagnosis.

Because the correlation between FEC and worm burden

Genus	No. of worms	Pathogenic index
Haemonchus	500	1
Telodorsagia	5000	1
Trichostrongylus	5000	1
Nematodirus	2000	1
Cooperia	10,000	1
Bunostomum	150	1
Oesophagostomum	500	1
Chabertia	200	1

Table 8.5 Worm counts regarded as sufficient to cause clinical disease when present as a sole pathogen (modified from McKenna, 1981).

is poorer in adult ewes than it is in lambs, and eggs shed by adult ewes may sometimes be from less pathogenic worms such as *Cooperia*, FECs are less frequently used in ewes than they are in lambs. They can, however, still be of benefit in adult ewes provided that they are interpreted with caution.

The control of gastrointestinal nematode parasites of sheep

Effective control of gastrointestinal parasites of sheep must be based on limiting their exposure to infective larvae on pasture. This can be achieved by reducing the contamination of pasture by worm eggs and restricting the exposure of susceptible stock to infective larvae. In addition, host responses are enhanced by good nutrition and the overall level of feeding, including the adequate availability of trace elements. Pastures with low levels of

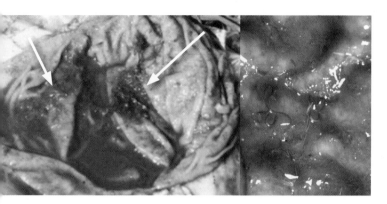

Figure 8.9 Large clusters of *Haemonchus contortus* worms (arrows) on the mucosa of an opened abomasum. Right: close-up view of *Haemonchus contortus* on the abomasal mucosa. Note the distinctive red and white stripes leading to the common name of 'barber's pole worm'.

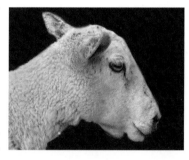

Figure 8.10 Submandibular swelling ('bottle jaw') of a ewe with a heavy mixed gastrointestinal nematode parasite burden which included *Haemonchus contortus*.

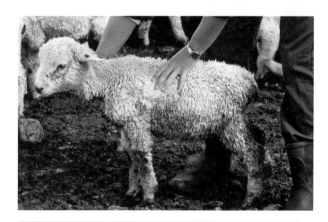

Figure 8.11 A poorly grown hogget with a heavy gastrointestinal nematode parasite burden, illustrating the effects that internal parasitism can have on the growth and health of sheep.

infective larvae, perhaps as low as 100 or 200 infective L3/kg herbage, are considered 'safe' and the objective of parasite control is to achieve 'safe' pasture.

The control of internal parasitism should be thought of in terms of an integration of management (grazing systems, 'dilution' with resistant stock, alternate species grazing) and strategic anthelmintic use. It is important to recognise that every farm is different, with a different mix of stock (species, and age-groups within species), different micro-climates and different grazing systems. While general guidelines about parasite control can be given, a parasite control programme for each individual property should be developed over time based on general principles, monitoring and experience.

Wormwise (www.wormwise.co.nz) is an online resource developed by veterinarians, parasitologists and the livestock industries and provides valuable free resources for veterinarians and farmers. They have suggested a number of principles that should be considered fundamental to parasite control:

- Healthy animals harbour worms and always will — eradication is neither an appropriate goal nor achievable.
- Well-fed animals are less affected by worms than those under nutritional stress.
- Older animals are generally less susceptible to worms than younger ones and, at times, can be used to reduce the number of infective larvae on pastures.
- Animals vary in their susceptibility to parasites (genetic variability).
- Animals can be selectively bred for resistance or resilience to roundworms.
- Each farm is unique and effective worm management may be different from farm to farm.
- When breeding for a characteristic, increased selection pressure will result in more-rapid change being made (applies both to livestock and parasites).
- Breeding for a single trait leads to more-rapid change than breeding for a combination of traits.
- Most of the year there are more worms, in the various life stages, on pasture than inside the animals.
- Anthelmintics are a finite resource. The way in which you use drenches and manage parasites can change the rate at which you select for resistant worms.
- Long-acting drench formulations may hasten

development of drench resistance. Once present on a farm, resistance to anthelmintics can be considered permanent.
- Anthelmintics used in combination can delay the onset of resistance.
- A population of un-drenched worms should be maintained on farm.

Source: Wormwise New Zealand (www.wormwise.co.nz).

The provision of safe pasture by grazing and pasture management

At the outset it must be emphasised that management and grazing procedures have implications for the entire farm and it may not be practical to alter grazing systems just to control parasites. In many situations the reverse is the case: the parasite control programme is designed to cope with the problems that arise because of the production system. Nevertheless, it is increasingly important to use pasture management to help cope with parasite problems, especially as the efficacy of drenches may be reduced by drench resistance. In addition, the desire of farmers to reduce the number of drenches used, and in some instances to not use them at all, means that more attention must be given to control by pasture management.

The following management strategies may be used:

Pasture resting and rotational grazing

Fodder crops, new pasture, hay and silage aftermaths all initially provide safe pasture. However, in most sheep farms only a limited area of land, if any, is used for these purposes.

Rotational grazing was once thought to offer a useful means of reducing pasture infectivity, but the periods of resting required are unacceptably long (4–5 months in autumn and winter, 2–3 months in spring and summer). Furthermore, under some circumstances rotational grazing may return animals to a much higher, rather than a reduced, level of pasture infestation. For instance, maximum larval development after a period of intensive grazing of pasture may take approximately 3–6 weeks. If sheep are grazed as a single species around a series of paddocks at an interval close to that for maximum larval development, the sheep are regularly exposed to maximum numbers of larvae on pasture.

Mixed grazing to reduce parasite challenge

Pasture contamination can be reduced by either decreasing the stocking rate or by mixed species/age-group grazing. In both situations there should be a reduction of infective parasite larva on the pasture. In general, parasite challenge increases with increased stocking rates, particularly of the same age groups and the same species of animal. However, the relationship is not necessarily linear. One of the consequences of increasing the sheep stocking rate is the persistent losses caused by parasitism, especially if cattle numbers are not increased proportionally. In the past, various livestock retention schemes have encouraged farmers to maintain high sheep numbers, the effect of which was to increase parasite burdens. Some farmers even went so far as to remove cattle completely, placing a heavy reliance on the use of anthelmintics to control parasite levels. Such management was unsatisfactory and in some cases unsustainable.

It is possible to reduce the parasite challenge to susceptible animals by mixed grazing with resistant stock, either cattle or, in some cases, adult sheep, with younger animals. This concept is exemplified by the rearing of

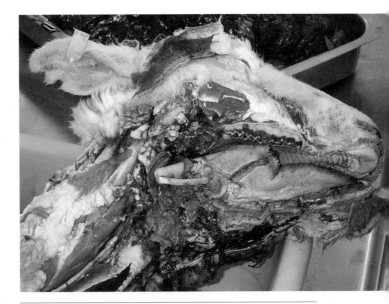

Figure 8.12 Care must be taken when administering intra-ruminal boluses such as anthelmintic capsules to ensure that damage to the larynx, pharynx or oesophagus does not occur, as demonstrated by this postmortem finding.

Cattle	Sheep and goats
—	Haemonchus contortus
Ostertagia ostertagi	—
O. leptospicularis	—
—	Telodorsagia circumcincta
Trichostrongylus axei	Trichostrongylus axei
—	T. colubriformis
—	T. vitrinus
—	T. capricola*
—	—
Cooperia oncophora	Cooperia curticei
—	—
Nematodirus helvetianus	Nematodirus spathiger#
—	N. filicollis#
—	Bunostomum trigonocephalum
Trichuris ovis	Trichuris ovis
Oesophagostomum radiatum	—
—	Oesophagostomum venulosum
—	Chabertia ovina
Dictyocaulus viviparous	—
—	Dictyocaulus filaria
—	Muellerius capillaris

* rarely found in sheep.
\# rarely found in goats.

Table 8.6 Nematode species normally found in natural infections of cattle, sheep and goats (Bisset, Vlassoff and Pulford, 1991).

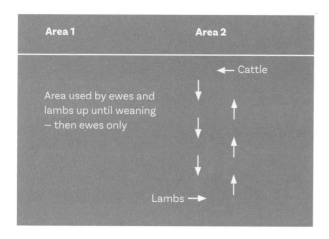

Figure 8.13 Plan of sheep and cattle grazing as a sole means of controlling parasitism.

dairy cattle replacements set stocked at one or two calves in each paddock of the farm. For sheep farmers, the mixed grazing of cattle, particularly with young sheep, is now recognised practice to reduce both parasite burdens and give better pasture control.

Perhaps one of the most under-utilised way of achieving reduced pasture contamination is by reducing the proportion of young to adult sheep on the farm. Lambs and hoggets display the most obvious and serious effects of parasites and are usually the main contributor to pasture contamination. Therefore parasitic disease may be reduced simply by reducing the proportion of these most vulnerable animals in the flock. Many farmers keep male lambs for too long and overwinter all their ewe lambs rather than selecting replacements at an earlier age. It is ironic that lambs are often retained for these longer periods because of the difficulty of growing them to prime condition for slaughter, a situation contributed to by the effects of parasitism.

Alternate grazing by hosts of different species

Alternate grazing of sheep and cattle can provide good control of gastrointestinal nematode parasites. This is because they share very few of the same species of worm (Table 8.6).

Some cross-transmission can take place, especially with *T. axei*, but the majority of ingested larvae do not establish in the heterologous host. To be fully effective for both sheep and cattle they should occupy a similar proportion of the grazing area. Morley (1980) claimed that to provide safe grazing for 2000 ewes at lambing, the cattle enterprise should consist of at least 350–400 cattle.

Using the principles of sheep and cattle alternation it has been possible to raise sheep without the use of anthelmintics (Niezen et al., 1991). The experimental unit, which consisted of 44 ha carrying 200 mixed-age ewes and replacements, finished the balance of lambs and in addition 75 store lambs were purchased and finished. Sixty-four weaner cattle were grazed and 15 ha of crop grown. The stocking rate of 15.2 SU/hectare was projected to increase to 19 SU/hectare, the district average on similar soil types.

To achieve adequate control, grazing management must be planned carefully. Basically the grazing area is divided in two (Figure 8.13).

On the first area, the ewes are grazed from lambing time until weaning. At weaning the ewes remain in that area but the lambs are shifted to area 2, which has been prepared by cattle. The lambs are put on each feed break for 10 days during periods of rapid larval development, and 14 days otherwise. Following grazing by lambs, the feed break is rested for approximately 30 days and then grazed by cattle, again for 10–14 days. Following grazing by cattle, a further spell of 30 days is required before the lambs are introduced again. Thus the interval between lamb grazing is approximately 70 days with a grazing by cattle midway. Each year, lambing is alternated between area 1 and area 2 and lambs after weaning do not graze pasture that was grazed by lambs the previous autumn.

Using this grazing system it is possible to maintain the level of pasture infectivity below 200 L3/kg herbage. Deer could be used to complement the effect of cattle in preparing clean pasture for sheep. However, it should be emphasised that drenching animals and moving them to 'clean' pasture with low larval contamination is selective for anthelmintic resistance, so care must be taken to incorporate refugia into such systems (see below).

Alternate grazing by hosts of the same species

Older sheep are generally more resistant to helminths than lambs and, because they usually reject a higher proportion of ingested larvae and have lower levels of worm egg output in faeces, alternate grazing with ewes should reduce the level of exposure of lambs. This effect has been demonstrated in carefully conducted field trials (Leathwick et al., 2008), and even where parasite control in the lambs is not highly effective, for instance in the presence of anthelmintic resistance, grazing ewes can be used to suppress the growth of parasite populations.

However, while these effects occur in sheep they are much less reliable than in cattle, and in some circumstances adult sheep can contaminate pastures significantly, especially with species such as *H. contortus*. In addition, the production of the ewes, especially wool production, is compromised if they are regularly exposed to high larval counts.

Integrated control

By late November/early December, high levels of pasture infectivity usually arise on areas where ewes and lambs have grazed. This contamination is derived from ewes during the post-parturient period and to some extent from the lambs themselves. Thus, one of the first aims of a farmer attempting to control parasites by grazing management should be to provide 'safe' pasture onto which the lambs can be moved following weaning, in late November/early December. Drenching at the time of the move will slow the contamination of the 'safe' area, but increases the risk of anthelmintic resistance (see later). However, with the sheep-to-cattle ratios used in New Zealand it is often difficult to provide sufficient safe pasture at this critical time. The area grazed by ewes and lambs is usually highly contaminated, which only leaves those areas grazed by replacement hoggets or cattle. It cannot be assumed that hoggets will automatically provide safe pasture for weaned lambs, as they can be a significant source of contamination. In addition, the hoggets are usually grazed on an area not considered suitable for lambing ewes, especially on hill-country farms. Such areas often have poor-quality pasture species that may not be suitable for weaned lambs.

The second requirement of an integrated control programme is drenching and movement of the lambs in late February/early March to pasture that has not been grazed by lambs since weaning. This is usually more easily achieved than the weaning time move but still requires careful planning by the farmer.

The initial concept of integrated control only contained these two strategic shifts combined with drenching (November/December and February/March). However, there have been problems in implementing this scheme and additional treatments 4 weeks after each move has been recommended. Thus, a total of four drenches are given.

The production of safe pasture by means of anthelmintic treatment

Realistically, on most New Zealand sheep farms the use of anthelmintics at strategic times is necessary to achieve adequate parasite control. On many farms, management of grazing is limited by relatively high sheep stocking rates with small numbers of cattle, so that the control of parasites depends to a large extent on the use of anthelmintics. In addition, multiple dosing has some clear attractions as it requires little change in the farmer's traditional management. However, it must be emphasised that the grazing practices referred to earlier are not excluded, nor should they be ignored; and there is a need for increased use of control by management if

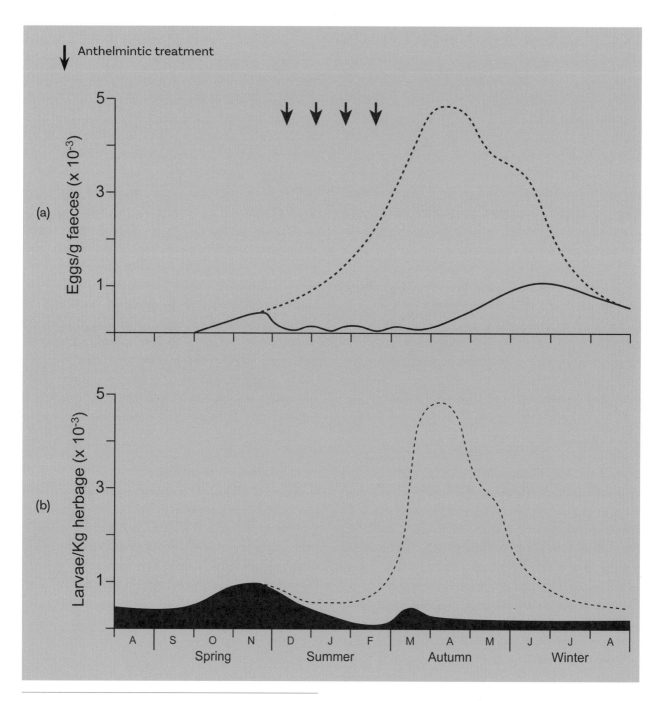

Figure 8.14 The effect of four monthly drenches from weaning on **(a)** the faecal egg output of lambs (—) and **(b)** the pattern of larval availability on pasture, compared with the expected levels if drenching is not done (----) (Brunsdon, 1981).

the useful life of anthelmintics is not to be limited by the development of anthelmintic resistance.

From studies of the population dynamics referred to earlier it is evident that the bulk of the autumn rise in larval numbers on pasture comes from eggs deposited by lambs earlier in the season. Thus a preventative drenching programme has been developed. This involves drenching lambs during the summer/autumn period at 28-day intervals, with the objective of reducing the

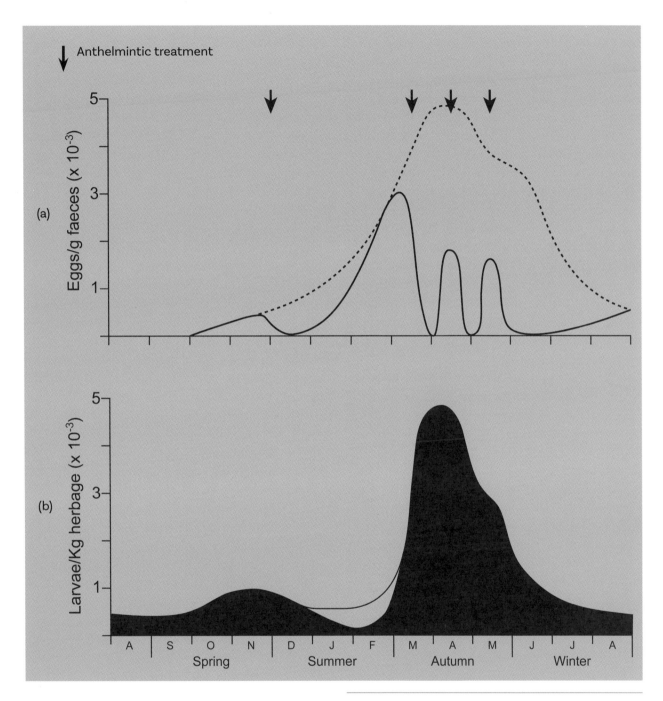

Figure 8.15 The effect of a weaning drench and three autumn drenches on **(a)** the faecal egg output (—) and **(b)** the pattern of larval availability on the pasture, compared with the expected levels if drenching is not done (- - - -) (Brunsdon, 1981).

shedding of eggs onto pasture.

Soon after the introduction of the broad-spectrum drenches in the early 1960s, farmers developed control programmes based on monthly drenching of lambs. This has since become the basis of worm control on most sheep farms. Initial work by Brunsdon at Wallaceville suggested that four drenches be given at 28-day intervals (Figure 8.14), but this recommendation has since been modified to 4–5 'routine' drenches at intervals of not more than 28 days.

Generally the first drench is given to lambs at weaning time, but in warmer areas of the country lambs may already have significant worm burdens at this time and the first drench may need to be given prior to weaning. This programme means that on most farms the last drench is given sometime in March/April. However, while this preventive drenching programme has been found to give good control of parasitism during the period of treatment, it may not prevent parasite build-up in April, May and June. It is suggested that this failure may be due to contamination from ewes, especially two-tooth ewes which can have substantial rises in faecal egg counts in autumn. This problem can be overcome by additional drenches given in April, May and June if there is a rise in lamb faecal egg counts. As larval development in winter is progressively inhibited by cold, the interval between drenches can probably be extended to 6 weeks or more at this time. Faecal egg count monitoring is a useful aid in making these decisions.

In contrast, if lambs are drenched at weaning but then not drenched again until the autumn, the contribution of these animals to the pasture larval contamination during the intervening period can be considerable (Figure 8.15).

Anthelmintics
Broad-spectrum anthelmintics
Broad-spectrum anthelmintics have activity against numerous parasite species and began with the discovery of phenothiazine in 1940. This has been replaced by newer, safer anthelmintics developed between 1960 and 1980, during which time three successful classes of compound, the benzimidazoles, levamisole and the macrocyclic lactones, each with distinct modes of action, became available. Most of the current anthelmintics on the market belong to one of these classes, or combinations of them.

Benzimidazoles (BZs, 'white drenches')
Benzimidazole drenches were the first of the 'modern' anthelmintics to be used in New Zealand. These drenches work by binding to tubulin and interfering with the polymerisation and formation of microtubules in cells. Microtubules form a component of the intracellular skeleton and are important for a number of normal cellular functions including cell division. They form the mitotic spindles during mitosis.

Specific drugs within the family include oxfendazole, fenbendazole, rycobendazole and albendazole. At higher dose rates some of these drugs have efficacy against tapeworm and mature liver fluke. There is a large amount of parasite resistance to these drenches, particularly by the *Nematodirus* genera, but also most other genera found in sheep. Triclabendazole is a benzimidazole anthelmintic specific for liver fluke (see later). It should be noted that this family of anthelmintics are called 'white' drenches because they have an opaque appearance when formulated. However, many of them are not white and may be other colours such as blue.

Levamisole and morantel ('clear drenches')
These drugs are cholinergic agonists of nematodes, which result in paralysis. They have efficacy against nematode parasites only. The safety margin is relatively small and care should be used to avoid gross overdosing. For example, they are not used in horses because the margin between therapeutic and toxic doses is too close. In sheep this ratio is quoted as between three- and sevenfold.

Macrocyclic lactones (avermectins/milbemycins, endectocides)
These drugs work by binding to glutamate-gated chloride-ion channels on nerves, which allows chloride ions into the nerve. This results in hyperpolarisation of the nerve so that an action potential cannot be generated, resulting in paralysis. In sheep, specific drugs within the family include abamectin, ivermectin, moxidectin and doramectin. Additionally in cattle, the drug eprinomectin is also used. These drugs have efficacy against nematode parasites. Some products available in injectable and pour on/spot on form also have efficacy against ectoparasites such as cattle lice, and mites.

Combination drenches
Combinations of the above three action families are also available in commercial formulations. These include benzimidazole/levamisole combinations, levamisole/macrocyclic lactone combinations and combinations of all three of these action families.

Amino-acetonitrile derivatives (AADs)
These drugs are relatively new synthetic compounds that have been demonstrated to have a unique mode

of action; one of these, monepantel, is available in New Zealand combined with abamectin. AADs appear to be well tolerated by sheep and are effective against various parasitic nematode species that may be resistant to other drenches. They also have a high safety level.

Spiroindoles

A new semi-synthetic spiroindole, the drug derquantel has been developed and was available in New Zealand in combination with abamectin, but is currently unavailable.

Narrow-spectrum anthelmintics

These drugs are specific to only a few parasite genera. An example is closantel, which is effective against *Haemonchus contortus* and liver fluke. Praziquantel, a drug effective against *Moniezia expansa*, is often combined with broad-spectrum products to create a nematode and tapeworm anthelmintic.

Persistent activity of anthelmintics

Some anthelmintics, in particular moxidectin, display persistent activity, which means that as well as killing adult worms any ingested larvae are killed for a certain period of time. This persistent activity comes about because moxidectin is highly lipophilic and the chemical is absorbed into fat depots and released over time. It is important to note that the persistent activity is effective against some parasite genera and not others, and this also varies depending on formulation (oral vs injection). For example, oral moxidectin has a persistent activity label claim against *Haemonchus contortus* of 35 days and against *Telodorsagia circumcincta* for 21 days, but has no label claim against other important parasites such as *Trichostrongylus* and *Nematodirus*. Moxidectin is sometimes used at an increased drenching interval in lambs, but there is the risk that this allows high pasture contamination with *Trichostrongylus*. In addition, long-acting depot injections of moxidectin are available for sheep with even longer claims of persistency, but these also have extended meat withholding periods.

Parasite control in adult sheep

The control of parasitism in adult sheep is also important, but there is a dilemma in that undrenched ewes can help delay the emergence of anthelmintic resistance (see later). Increased production of wool and lamb may be achieved by the appropriate drenching of adult sheep. However, the slavish drenching of ewes pre-tupping and at other times, without due consideration being given to bodyweights, faecal egg counts and available feed, could be expensive and is likely to help the development of anthelmintic resistance. On the other hand, there are situations where drenching ewes may be desirable. It is in these situations that veterinarians should direct their skills to diagnosis and advice in drenching management. In addition, not all ewes in a mob may need to be treated and treating only the lighter ewes may be more appropriate.

Anthelmintic treatment pre-tupping

Lewis in 1975 reviewed 81 trials in New Zealand involving 62,000 ewes and reported a mean increase of 3.6% lambs produced by drenched ewes, but the response was extremely variable ranging from –11% to +20%. The effect was one of increased twinning, but the level of barrenness was not affected. While both liveweight increase between drenching and mating and the reduction in the faecal egg count are important preconditions for the expression of a fertility response, their effects appear to act independently. It should be noted that these studies are now very dated and there have been many changes in New Zealand sheep-farming systems since then, so extrapolation of these data may not be appropriate. It is generally considered that routine pre-tupping anthelmintic treatment of all ewes should not be necessary, but it may be appropriate to target-treat at-risk, thin or young ewes.

Anthelmintic treatments of ewes pre- and post-lambing

There have been a number of studies that have examined the benefits of drenching ewes before and/or after lambing. Many of these trials have failed to measure a full range of production benefits. The more-recent trials have largely focused on the use of long-acting anthelmintic treatments in ewes prior to lambing.

Anthelmintic treatment of ewes before lambing with a short-acting anthelmintic usually fails to control the periparturient rise in faecal egg counts, although drenching ewes 3–4 weeks after lambing can control the periparturient rise to some extent and has been shown to increase the production of both ewes and lambs. However, the most practical time to drench ewes after lambing is at docking time, at which time many ewes have lambed more than 3–4 weeks previously. In recent studies, drenching ewes with a short-acting anthelmintic at docking time has not improved ewe or lamb weaning weights.

The most commonly used anthelmintic treatments for ewes pre-lambing are controlled-release capsules (containing ivermectin, albendazole or albendazole/abamectin combinations) or long-acting injectable moxidectin. The injectable product can also be combined with clostridial (5 in 1) vaccines. A small number of studies have assessed the production responses from the use of long-acting pre-lamb anthelmintic treatments in ewes on commercial farms, including lamb weaning weight, weight of lamb weaned per ewe, ewe weaning and pre-mating weights, and ewe dag score. Perhaps unsurprisingly the results have been mixed, with variation between farms and between years, suggesting that routine blanket use of these treatments will not give consistent production benefits. Further, it has been established that these treatments select for anthelmintic resistance. Hence it is recommended that where possible, farmers should avoid treating all the ewes and if they wish to treat at all, consider selectively treating those most at risk — likely to be pregnant ewe hoggets, lighter ewes, or ewes scanned as having multiple lambs.

Farmers and veterinarians are confronted with a dilemma regarding the drenching of ewes. While clinical parasitism requires prompt remedial action, routine drenching of all ewes appears likely to accelerate the development of resistance to anthelmintics. For this reason, monitoring of faecal egg counts to limit drenching to when it is most appropriate, or restricting treatments to ewes most at risk, is recommended. In addition, consideration should be given to modifying pasture management and in some situations increasing the cattle-to-sheep ratios to help reduce pasture contamination.

Conclusion

While the nematode control principles that have been outlined can be applied to many areas in New Zealand, the temptation to assume that what has already been discovered is of universal application must be resisted. The details of control programmes must be worked out by the veterinarian and the farmer with due regard for the farming system, different species of parasite and climatic conditions that prevail.

Selecting sheep for resistance (immunity) to gastrointestinal nematodes

A method for control of internal parasites that is receiving increasing attention is breeding sheep that have improved natural resistance to the parasites. To some extent there may be natural selection taking place, but the intensive drenching programmes practised on some stud farms probably negate any progress.

The method used has been based on faecal egg counts following a period of untreated worm challenge, giving an indirect assessment of resistance to worm establishment. Lambs with below-average faecal egg counts are considered to have increased resistance. An antibody test on saliva is also available.

Heritability estimates for faecal egg counts have been shown to be moderate, ranging from around 0.23 when based on a single faecal egg count taken in January/February, to 0.35 when based on the average of two faecal egg counts from two separate challenge periods. This indicates that breeding for increased resistance will improve the immunity of the flock to parasitism, although the long-term production benefits have not been quantified.

The relationship between low faecal egg counts and other productive traits has not been clearly established and there is the possibility that resistance may incur a cost of reduced production. While some progress has been made in identifying genetic markers for resistant sheep, further research is needed for this to have a significant impact.

Other control options

Research into developing other methods of nematode control is ongoing. A vaccine against *Haemonchus contortus* is available overseas. Other areas investigated include the utilisation of nematophagic fungi in faeces to kill nematode larvae, and immunomodulation strategies to down-regulate the deleterious components of the host immune system.

Anthelmintic resistance

Anthelmintic resistance is a serious issue in most sheep-raising countries, including New Zealand, and it is a topic that attracts considerable discussion and debate. However, it must be remembered that the primary issue is not anthelmintic resistance but parasite control, and that the development of anthelmintic resistance will merely make this objective more difficult and expensive to achieve. It should also be remembered that the development of resistance by internal parasites is an inevitable consequence of using anthelmintics, just as development of resistance by bacteria is an inevitable consequence of antimicrobial usage.

Clearly, the frequent use of anthelmintics is likely to enhance the development of resistance because of the high degree of exposure of the parasite to these drugs. However, a fundamental dilemma of parasite control is that the better the parasite control, the lower the level of pasture larval challenge, but this is nearly always accompanied by increased selection for anthelmintic resistance. This is because if sheep are drenched and put onto 'clean' (low larval contamination) pasture, the only eggs shed and therefore larvae developing will be from resistant worms, and the frequency of the resistant gene in the population increases. In contrast, if a large number of larvae with the susceptible genotype are also present on the pasture, this will effectively 'dilute' the resistant genes and result in a lower frequency of the resistant gene in the population.

The resistance of nematode worms to drenches was first reported in New Zealand by Vlassoff and Kettle in 1980. Since then resistance has been recorded in many of the common gastrointestinal nematode genera of sheep and goats, including *Haemonchus*, *Telodorsagia*, *Trichostrongylus* and *Nematodirus*. National and regional surveys have identified the decline in drench efficacy over time. Resistance to 'triple combinations' (benzimidazole/levamisole/macrocyclic lactone) has been reported, as has resistance to the newer drug, monepantel, in goat flocks.

What is anthelmintic resistance?

Anthelmintic resistance is a change in the genetic make-up of a parasite that allows it to survive exposure to a dose of chemical that would normally be fatal. The resistant parasites that survive continue to contaminate pasture with their eggs, which carry the genes for resistance — thus, over time, an increasing proportion of the population becomes resistant. If the same anthelmintic continues to be used, it becomes increasingly ineffective and clinical signs of parasitism become evident in treated sheep.

The development of resistance by different worm genera is complex and not completely understood. The characteristics of the anthelmintic used may also influence the rate of resistance development. Two aspects of the drench are considered most important are: the therapeutic efficacy and the persistent activity. An ideal drug will have a high efficacy, removing as many parasites as possible including those with genotypes that may be developing partial resistance. By killing these, the resistant genes will not be passed to the next generation. This is often referred to as 'head selection'. 'Tail selection', on the other hand, refers to the persistent activity of the drug and reproductive advantage given to resistant and partially resistant worms that can infect the sheep earlier after drenching, mate and pass their genes on to the next generation. In effect, the declining concentration of drug in the host screens the incoming worm population, giving preference to those with resistant genotypes which, when they establish, can only mate with other resistant worms. Often there are opposing selective forces that apply to the use of a certain drench. For instance, the increased potency achieved by the persistent presence of a drug such as moxidectin has to be balanced by the tendency of the 'tail' to allow resistant parasites to establish during the protection period.

Resistance to a drug within an action family eventually confers resistance to all drugs within that action family. For example, resistance to oxfendazole, a benzimidazole drench, will also eventually confer resistance to other benzimidazoles such as fenbendazole, albendazole, etc. This is sometimes called 'side resistance'.

The following situations may arise on a farm:
- Individual worms being resistant to two or more action families (**multiple resistance**).
- Sheep harbouring more than one genera of parasite resistant to one action family (some authors call this **multigeneric resistance**).
- Sheep harbouring one genera of worms resistant to one action family and another genera resistant to a different action family.

The diagnosis of anthelmintic resistance

From a farmer's point of view, it is important to determine the efficacy of drenches on the farm, and this is an important step in determining what further action might be appropriate to slow the development of resistance.

It is not simply a matter of deciding whether resistance is present or not; the resistant genotypes are widespread and it is likely that most farms will have some genera of worms present with genes conferring resistance to one of the anthelmintic classes. It is highly recommended that, at the very least, all farmers carry out a drench check in lambs (see below) at least once per year to give a crude guide as to the likely efficacy of the currently used anthelmintic. To more accurately assess drench efficacy, a variety of different procedures have been advocated, but the most commonly used is a faecal egg count reduction test (FECRT). In spite of this being labour-intensive and relatively insensitive, it is currently the only practical means of detecting anthelmintic resistance and it is the best indicator available at present until molecular tests to identify resistance markers in the parasites themselves are developed. Ideally farms should carry out a full FECRT every 2–3 years and do annual drench checks in-between times; however, the time and cost associated with FECRTs mean they are rarely undertaken at this frequency.

1. Drench check

A drench check is simply a check 5–10 days (usually 7) after drenching that the egg counts from 10 randomly collected faecal samples are all zero or near to zero. For this purpose, collecting fresh (warm) faecal samples off the ground after the lambs have been held in a corner for a few minutes will suffice. The assumption is made that adult egg-laying worms were present before drenching but because pre-treatment egg counts were not performed, a percentage reduction cannot be calculated. Even low numbers of eggs remaining after drenching should be interpreted with suspicion and, if there is doubt, an FECRT undertaken.

2. Faecal egg count reduction test (FECRT)

Faecal egg count reduction tests measure the number of eggs present before and after drenching and calculate the percentage reduction. It is important to recognise that this test gives an indication of the approximate efficacy of an anthelmintic on a property, but resistant genes can be present at low levels within a parasite population for a long period of time before 'resistance' is detected by this method. The following is a suggested minimum that can be done to provide a result in which one may have reasonable confidence.

- **For testing a single drench:** Preferably use lambs or hoggets that are passing at least 200 eggs per gram of faeces and preferably more. Lambs that have not been drenched for at least 4 weeks are usually suitable. A minimum of 10 are required, but since at least 10 faecal samples are required at the second sampling, selecting 12–15 lambs is preferable. At day 0, rectal faecal samples are collected from each animal, which is marked with raddle, weighed and dosed with the recommended dose of the drench to be tested. Either a syringe or a carefully calibrated drenching gun may be used. Seven to 10 days after drenching the group of 12–15 lambs is re-sampled to ensure that a minimum of 10 rectal samples are obtained. The arithmetic mean egg count of all samples from day 0 is compared with the mean egg count at re-sampling. In general terms a reduction of less than 95% indicates resistance, but it should be recognised that this is not absolute and should be interpreted cautiously. Larval cultures should be used on pre-treatment and post-treatment samples to identify the genera of worms subjected to the test and to calculate the percentage reduction of each genera. Some operators also include a control group of 12–15 lambs which is left undrenched.

- **For testing more than one drench:** A similar procedure to the above is followed except that for each drench to be tested, a group of 12–15 sheep is used. Each group should be identified using different-coloured raddle. Individual sheep identification is not usually necessary but can be an advantage. At day 0, faecal samples are collected from the sheep that are to be dosed with the drench whose efficacy is suspect. Post-treatment samples are collected from all groups and compared with the pre-treatment counts. In some cases it is prudent to collect samples from all groups pre-treatment but this adds to the cost.

Timing of the drench test is important if all the main sheep parasite genera are to be tested. From December until March most genera are likely to be present, but from late March to May *Trichostrongylus* spp tend to dominate and there may be insufficient numbers of *Telodorsagia* present to provide a satisfactory test for this genus. The worm burden of ewes may be quite different in composition from lambs over this period, and lambs should be used for the test if possible (Table 8.7).

Considerable useful information can be obtained from a well-conducted FECRT. The efficacy of each of the drenches tested can be assessed for each of the genera adequately represented in the pre-drench samples. From this information, decisions can be made about the appropriate anthelmintics to use and whether modifications to management are indicated.

Nematodirus species are relatively poor egg-producers and FECRTs may be unreliable in detecting resistance to this parasite. Consideration should be given to dosing and slaughtering a number of sheep (up to 5) to provide additional and more-direct evidence if this genus is thought to be of concern.

3. Larval culture

With the exception of *Nematodirus*, which has a morphologically distinctive egg, it is difficult to differentiate the other nematode genera from egg counts. However, the larvae of these genera can be differentiated, and cultivating larvae from post-treatment egg counts usually provides an assessment of which genera of worm is resistant. Comparing the proportion of larvae both pre- and post-treatment improves this assessment.

Knowing which genera of parasite is developing resistance to specific drenches is important in the management of resistance.

4. Worm counts

Slaughtering sheep 5–10 days after drenching provides direct evidence of the presence of resistant worms and the species involved. Because of costs, worm counts are not used routinely but in the case of *Nematodirus* they can provide valuable information.

5. Laboratory tests

A number of laboratory tests have been used to test for anthelmintic resistance, generally under experimental conditions. The most commonly used test is a larval development assay, where eggs are grown through to the infective L3 stage under varying concentrations of benzimidazole, levamisole or ivermectin. It is best validated for the former two. Another commonly used test is the egg hatch assay, in which eggs of a single species

	% larval cultures	
	Lambs	Ewes
Haemonchus	47	2
Telodorsagia	46	20
Trichostrongylus	7	4
Cooperia	-	4
Chabertia/Oesophagostamum	-	70

Table 8.7 Composition of the worm burden of ewes and lambs in January grazing on the same farm as assessed by larval cultures.

of nematode suspected of benzimidazole resistance are incubated in various concentrations of thiabendazole. The hatching percentages are compared with those of known benzimidazole-susceptible strains. Neither of the assays has been offered for commercial use in New Zealand.

Delaying the development of anthelmintic resistance

Anthelmintics will remain the cornerstone of gastrointestinal nematode control in sheep and cattle for the foreseeable future, but to ensure their continued effectiveness farmers and veterinarians should be aware of the need to maintain adequate reservoirs of unselected worms (worms in refugia) to minimise the increase of the resistant population. Leathwick (2008) defines refugia as 'deliberately retaining a gene pool of susceptibility by allowing some parasites to reproduce without exposing them to anthelmintic'. It is important to appreciate that this relates only to the worms that are ingested by sheep, mate and produce eggs that contribute to subsequent generations. A common misconception is that it simply means parasite larvae on pasture (those that successfully reproduce), but it also includes the parasites in sheep on the property that are not treated with anthelmintic. While the issue is about retaining susceptible genotypes, realistically this means parasites that have not been exposed to an anthelmintic. There are different ways of achieving a worm population not exposed to drenching, and a number of higher-risk practices have been identified from surveys comparing management practices on farms where resistance was common with farms where it was not. However, the following are considered high-risk farm practices.

1. Purchasing sheep without a quarantine drench
A New Zealand national survey identified purchasing of sheep as a risk factor for the presence of anthelmintic-resistant genotypes. This can be readily prevented by adopting a quarantine procedure at the time of introduction. Ideally this would involve administering a highly efficacious or novel drench or drenches and holding the sheep for up to 24–48 hours in yards or holding paddocks, providing food and water. If the sheep have been transported some distance and yarding is considered undesirable, then drenching (as above) and putting the sheep in a paddock likely to be heavily contaminated should reduce the risk.

2. Drenching and moving onto 'clean' pasture
On New Zealand sheep farms, pastures with low levels of infective larvae are not readily available. Areas of new grass following cropping, hay aftermath or where cattle have been grazing exclusively for some months are all examples of 'clean' pasture. If lambs are drenched and then introduced to these areas, there is an increased risk of selecting for resistant parasites; this risk can be reduced either by leaving a proportion of the lambs untreated or by grazing undrenched ewes after the lambs. The proportion that need to be left untreated depends on the efficacy of the drench; the higher the drench efficacy, the fewer animals that need to be left untreated to dilute out the resistant genotypes. Most trials have left from 2% to 10% untreated; realistically, on commercial farms leaving a relatively low proportion of lambs untreated (1–5%) is likely to be more acceptable, and will be most effective if a highly efficacious drench is being used. While leaving some lambs undrenched is likely to result in increased levels of pasture contamination, this should have minimal impact on production if the pasture larval numbers were low to begin with. Farmers have to balance the need to control nematode parasites with selection for anthelmintic resistance.

3. Treating adult ewes pre-lambing
Treating adult ewes before lambing with long-acting products such as drench capsules or injectable moxidectin has been associated with the development of drench resistance. Farmers should consider targeting these treatments to those ewes most at risk from parasitism, for example young ewes (pregnant ewe hoggets, two-tooths), multiple-bearing ewes (triplets, twins) or ewes in poor body condition. However, there is limited research into the effectiveness or otherwise of target-treating such animals. They should also ensure that some untreated animals remain in each mob. Use of an 'exit' drench, a highly efficacious short-acting anthelmintic given at the end of the protective period, has been advocated by some experts.

4. Preventive drenching of lambs
As mentioned previously, drenching lambs every 28 days from weaning for five or six treatments has been found to be an effective way of controlling worm burdens and preventing much of the autumn contamination of pasture that would otherwise have occurred. Although this procedure will select to some degree for anthelmintic resistance, the risk can be mitigated to some extent by maintaining refugia, for example by (a) rotationally grazing undrenched ewes after the lambs; (b) if considered necessary, leaving a small proportion of lambs undrenched; and (c) not drenching at too short an interval, thus allowing some unselected worms to complete their life cycle in the lambs. It is considered that 28-day intervals are a useful compromise, but those farmers with access to regular faecal egg counting may wish to extend this interval. However, this needs careful monitoring as egg counts can rise rapidly and within a week reach high levels, thus negating the benefits of the preventive drenching programme.

5. Using single active versus combination drenches
Studies have indicated that using anthelmintics in combination will delay the emergence of resistant genotypes because parasites that are developing resistance to one active ingredient will be killed by another drug and so the resistant genes cannot be passed on. The best time to use combinations to extend drench efficacy is before resistance has developed to any of the individual active drugs.

6. Under-dosing
Farmers and veterinarians should regularly check the drenching equipment used on the farm to ensure that the

correct dose is delivered. Weighing sheep regularly also ensures that the correct dose is given. While under-dosing has been used as a means of selecting resistant worms in laboratories, its role in the development of anthelmintic resistance on farms is less clear. It has been suggested that because goats often metabolise anthelmintics quickly, the rapid emergence of resistance in this species reflects under-dosing. However, *Telodorsagia circumcinta* was fully susceptible to a half-dose of ivermectin, yet despite this it has become the dominant species to develop resistance to the macrocyclic lactones. Irrespective, farmers should use the correct dose and dosing technique.

7. Drench rotation

In the past, the annual rotation of the anthelmintic family was advocated as a way of slowing the onset of resistance. However, there has been no evidence that this strategy necessarily influences the onset of resistance. While some farmers may still use drench rotation, it is important to ensure that it does not mask the presence of resistance.

'Knockout' drenching involves the substitution of one routine lamb drench with a novel anthelmintic (e.g. monepantel), and computer modelling has suggested it will delay the onset of resistance to the existing routine anthelmintics being used on-farm. The greatest benefit is likely to occur if it is used when climatic conditions are at their most favourable for larval survival and development on pasture. This is likely to vary between locations and from year to year, but in general will usually be in early autumn.

Conclusions

The control of gastrointestinal parasitism in grazing livestock is a most important aspect of animal husbandry and the attainment of high productivity. Anthelmintics play a key role in the control of parasites in livestock and this is likely to remain so in the foreseeable future. A range of effective anthelmintics is available to deal with this problem but because of the development of parasite resistance, their use must be carefully monitored. In addition, good husbandry (feeding and stock management) must be used with the drench programmes to obtain the most effective result.

The following is a checklist of the important features of internal parasite control for grazing livestock:

- Have a parasite management plan for the farm. For most farms this will include a preventive drenching programme for the lambs.
- Sell surplus stock, i.e. cull ewes and lambs as soon as possible. Retaining unwanted stock frequently leads to feed shortages and parasite problems as summer/autumn feed becomes limited in dry seasons.
- Where possible ensure that stocking rates of sheep are limited to the feed available. Maintain adequate nutrition for all stock throughout the year and ensure supplementary feed stores for dry periods as well as winter.
- In spite of a wide range of otherwise very effective nematode anthelmintics, parasite resistance to these has become a significant problem. Hence their use requires greater discretion than previously to limit the spread of resistant parasites.
- Know the effectiveness of drenches against the important nematode genera on the farm. Where practical, use combination drenches administered accurately.
- Understand and use the concept of refugia to help dilute resistant genotypes of worms.
- While controlling parasitism in ewes is important on many farms, limit the treatment of ewes to when it is most appropriate. The decision on whether to treat each group of ewes should be based on faecal egg counts and/or a consideration of condition score, age or pregnancy rank. Consider treating only part of a flock.
- Have a quarantine programme for all bought-in stock.
- Integrate adult sheep and cattle with the grazing area of lambs.
- Be alert for sudden occurrences of haemonchosis over the summer/autumn period. Sudden death of outwardly thrifty lambs or two-tooths may be the first sign of haemonchosis.
- Lay readers of this text are advised to consult your veterinarian regularly as diagnostic procedures and new information on anthelmintics and parasite control are ongoing.

Trematodes — fascioliasis

Liver fluke is a reasonably common parasite of adult sheep in New Zealand. It also occurs in cattle and goats, but rarely in horses and deer. Fascioliasis has been found in nearly all sheep-raising areas of the North Island. In the South Island it has been reported mainly in the West Coast, Nelson and Marlborough but has been seen in Central Otago, Southland and Canterbury.

Aetiology and life cycle

The adult liver fluke, *Fasciola hepatica*, is found in bile ducts of sheep, causing hepatic fibrosis and severe interference with liver function.

Infection occurs when metacercariae encysted on pasture are ingested. When these hatch in the host, the young flukes migrate via the intestinal wall and peritoneal cavity to the liver. The migration to the liver takes only 24–28 hours, but the young flukes may then migrate at random through the liver for 4–6 weeks before settling in the bile ducts. Mature flukes in the bile ducts produce eggs from about 8 weeks onwards. Egg laying is extremely prolific.

The voided eggs hatch under warm, moist conditions to produce the miracidium, the free-living stage, which, if it survives, will swim until it finds a snail host to invade. Eventually, each miracidium develops into hundreds of cercariae, which leave the dying snail host to encyst on blades of grass as the metacercariae. In New Zealand there are three snails known to act as intermediate hosts: *Pseudosuccinea (Lymnaea) columella*, *Lymnaea (Austropeplea) tomentosa* and *Galba (Lymnaea) truncatula*.

Pseudosuccinea columella is the main snail host; it is widespread throughout the North Island and has been reported in several locations of the South Island. It is an American species and was first identified in New Zealand in 1969. *Lymnaea tomentosa* is an Australian species and was assumed to be the principal host in the 'traditional' fluke areas of New Zealand prior to 1950. However, *P. columella* is now also found extensively in these areas and appears to have become the major host, while *G. truncatula* has apparently shown little tendency to spread and exists in only a few places.

Snail habitat

Both *P. columella* and *L. tomentosa* inhabit ponds and marshes, but appear to differ in their suitability to the two types of habitat. They may also be found on irrigation pasture, but avoid fast-flowing water. Neither species is able to persist in areas that dry out in the summer, and the most suitable habitats are areas that are permanently wet from seepages and springs. Both species are found submerged in or on the surface of the water.

The suitability of the snail habitat can be altered by the effects of animals, particularly cattle, trampling through them. The exclusion of cattle may reduce snail populations markedly.

Populations of snails drop to low numbers during winter with rapid repopulation in early summer.

Epidemiology in New Zealand

Epidemiological investigations in New Zealand have proved complicated because of the three snail hosts. In addition, acute fascioliasis has seldom been recorded so that time of acquisition of infections cannot be determined from disease outbreaks, as in some countries.

It would appear that most infections begin with the early to mid-summer uptake of metacercariae and cease 6–7 months later in about mid-winter. The absence of overwintering infections is attributed to the high snail mortality in winter. The period over which infection is available appears constant from year to year, but there is a tendency for larger infections to be acquired when mid-summer rainfall is low. In dry summers, animals are forced to graze the permanent snail habitats more than they would if enough grass was available elsewhere. In wet summers such areas are avoided by stock, especially sheep. Sheep do not develop resistance to liver fluke, and infections may accumulate over months or years.

Clinical features

Chronic fascioliasis is mainly seen in adult sheep during the autumn/winter period. As the flukes feed on the bile duct lining there is inflammation and eventually fibrosis of the duct walls. The flukes ingest blood, and further blood is lost from the damaged bile duct epithelium. Further, there is leakage of plasma proteins through the biliary mucosa and these factors lead to anaemia and hypoalbuminaemia. Thus chronic fascioliasis is characterised by ill thrift, anorexia and anaemia. In advanced cases, ascites may be seen and in some sheep a submandibular oedema (bottle jaw) develops. When such signs develop, death is inevitable.

Acute fluke disease causing sudden death is seldom seen in New Zealand. It is caused by uncomplicated massive hepatic damage associated with migrating immature flukes. Sudden death in sheep due to *Clostridium novyi B* (black disease — see Chapter 15) may also be attributed to liver damage caused by migrating flukes.

Pathology

In the acute form of the disease the liver is enlarged and mottled with haemorrhagic tracts and subcapsular haemorrhages. There is blood-stained fluid in the peritoneal cavity and an acute fibrinous peritonitis.

In the chronic form, which is most commonly recorded, varying degrees of hepatic fibrous and bile-duct thickening are seen. Varying degrees of compensatory hypertrophy may be seen, giving the liver a knobbly appearance. Mature flukes may be found within the bile ducts. Other features include anaemia, ascites and general body oedema.

Chemical	Comments
Closantel	Immature and mature flukes
Triclabendazole	Immature and mature flukes
Oxyclozanide	Mature flukes
Albendazole	Mature flukes, ovicidal
Oxfendazole	Mature flukes
Ricobendazole	Mature flukes, ovicidal

Table 8.8 Fasciolicides available in New Zealand.

Diagnosis

A diagnosis of fascioliasis may be confirmed at necropsy. The characteristic pathology described above and the demonstration of adult flukes in the bile ducts is adequate in most cases. Liver fluke eggs may also be demonstrated in faeces, although the faecal egg counting method used to detect fluke eggs differs from that used to detect nematode eggs. Routine haematology may reveal anaemia, hypoproteinaemia and an eosinophilia, although these changes are not specific to liver fluke infection. A serological ELISA test is also available.

Treatment and control

There are a number of fasciolicides available for treating both adult and immature flukes. These are listed in Table 8.8.

In selecting the most appropriate fasciolicide consideration needs to be given to the severity of the fluke challenge and other parasite control programmes. A number of the drugs available, notably the benzimidazoles, are not effective against immature flukes, and with some the dose is higher than recommended for routine nematode treatment. Drugs such as triclabendazole are extremely effective and if used regularly may even result in eradication of fluke from a farm. However, resistance to triclabendazole has been reported overseas and may also be developing in New Zealand.

The drugs are usually given over the period of maximum risk for grazing animals; this is in autumn and early winter. Treatment in autumn will reduce stock losses from chronic fascioliasis in winter and may improve animal health as well. Anthelmintic treatment in late winter/early spring may help to reduce the release of *Fasciola* eggs in spring and early summer, thus reducing infection rates in the new generation of snails.

In the endemic fluke areas where sheep are at risk from black disease, vaccination with *Cl. novyi B* is necessary before the young flukes begin migration in summer (see Chapter 15).

Control of the intermediate host may also be an important aspect of fluke control. This may prove difficult in many New Zealand situations. However, the draining of snail habitats or fencing these off from grazing stock at danger periods may be helpful. In European countries, molluscicides such as copper sulphate have been used against the snail host. These have proved of limited value in New Zealand but may still be considered under some circumstances. Overseas, research is being undertaken into the use of vaccines to control liver fluke.

Cestodes

Tapeworms of sheep (*Moniezia expansa*)

The tapeworm, *Moniezia expansa*, occurs world-wide in the small intestine of sheep and some other ruminants, and segments are often seen in the faeces of young animals. There is still some debate about the economic relevance of tapeworm on lamb productivity, with most trials showing no response to treatment while another showed a significant liveweight response to treatment. Many farmers believe that tapeworm infection results in increased dagginess and increases the risk of flystrike. The balance of evidence indicates that *M. expansa* infestations are generally harmless even when tapeworms are present in large numbers in young lambs. This raises doubts about the treatment of sheep for *M. expansa* on the basis of any likely benefit to health or improved production.

Life cycle and general factors
The mature tapeworm found in the young sheep originates from ingested cysticercoids produced by the intermediate host, a free-living oribatid mite. The mites live mostly in scattered colonies of high local concentration. High numbers are mainly found on old-established pasture, which may remain infective for up to 22 months.

Moniezia expansa in lambs killed immediately after removal from pasture are found mainly in the anterior half of the small intestine, whereas in animals deprived of food for some hours prior to slaughter the tapeworms are located predominantly in the posterior half.

The prevalence of infection varies with the season, the age of the host and its previous experience of the parasite, and the availability of the host mite. Lambs that become infected in spring spontaneously lose their infection over 4–5 months and generally become resistant to re-infection.

Treatment
Most of the benzimidazole drenches encompass *M. expansa* in their range of activity, but there is some evidence that drench resistance does occur occasionally. Praziquantel is a drug used specifically for tapeworm control, usually combined with another broad-spectrum drench for nematode control.

Echinococcus granulosus, Taenia ovis, Taenia hydatigena
These three tapeworms are carried by dogs, but the intermediate stages, the hydatid cyst *Cysticercus ovis* and *Cysticercus tenuicollis*, are found in sheep. Because of their importance to human health (hydatids) and to downgrading of carcass meat and/or livers (*C. ovis* and *C. tenuicollis*), the control of these tapeworms in dogs became compulsory under the Hydatids Act 1982. Under the Biosecurity Act 1993, regulatory control of tapeworms was removed and control was left to individual farmers. An education programme, Ovis Management, financed by meat-processing companies, was undertaken to encourage farmers to maintain control efforts. The last recorded case of *E. granulosus* cysts in sheep was in 1996 on Arapawa Island in the Marlborough Sounds, and it is now almost certainly eradicated from New Zealand. In 2002 the Ministry of Agriculture & Forestry declared New Zealand hydatids-free (Pharo, 2002). However, *C. ovis* lesions in sheep meat are still of major concern to the meat industry. Although the sheep plays a vital role in the perpetuation of these diseases they are not discussed here, as they are not significant in affecting sheep health as discussed in this text.

Protozoal diseases

Coccidiosis
In New Zealand acute coccidiosis is mainly seen in young lambs less than 4 months of age. It is characterised by acute diarrhoea, ill thrift and sometimes death.

Aetiology
Coccidiosis of sheep is usually due to a mixed infection of *Coccidia*, although one species may predominate. *Coccidia* are highly host-specific and there is no transfer of infection between different host species. In New Zealand sheep, 11 coccidial species have been recognised but only *Eimeria ovinoidalis* and *E. crandallis* are considered to be pathogenic.

Life cycle and general factors
The life cycle of *Eimeria* species is complicated. Basically, thousands of oocysts are shed in the faeces of an infected animal. The shed oocysts sporulate, and if ingested by a susceptible animal liberate sporozoites that invade the gut endothelium and undergo two generations of schizogony. Eventually, gametocyte formation occurs and the microgametes fertilise the macrogametes to form a zygote. The zygote becomes the oocyst, which is eventually shed from the gut cell and is passed into the faeces.

The survival of the oocysts depends on many

factors including soil type, exposure to direct sunlight or otherwise, the amount of humus in the soil and in particular soil moisture.

Coccidial infections are self-limiting. Even under natural conditions, where repeated infection occurs, most animals develop immunity so that the life cycle is progressively inhibited. Lambs develop immunity from 6–8 weeks of age.

Predisposing factors

As mentioned above, young animals are most susceptible; outbreaks are usually associated with a high stocking rate, which increases contamination and concentration of the oocysts. Warm, moist conditions are optimal for rapid sporulation. The disease is often associated with poor nutrition, resulting in decreased resistance as well as forcing animals to graze low and ingest more oocysts. It is most likely to be associated with indoor-rearing of lambs, such as on sheep dairy farms or artificial rearing of orphan lambs. Subclinical infection of earlier-born lambs leads to environmental contamination and clinical infection in later-born lambs.

Clinical signs

Affected lambs are generally undersized and unthrifty. The appearance of acute diarrhoea in numbers of such lambs is suggestive of coccidiosis. In some animals the diarrhoea may contain blood. Anorexia is common, and affected animals become very dehydrated. Left untreated, severe cases may die; others may recover slowly but may remain unthrifty for some time.

Diagnosis

The diagnosis is based on the clinical signs and confirmation by the presence of large numbers of oocysts in the faeces. However, it is important to remember that young lambs may have large numbers of oocysts present in faeces without any clinical signs. At necropsy a severe enteritis may be seen. In acute cases very high numbers of oocysts may be recorded. However, even in some animals with diarrhoea, oocyst numbers may have declined as the resistance of the animal has increased. To confirm a diagnosis, histology of fixed sections of the small intestine are valuable as well as the examination of gut smears for oocysts.

Treatment

As well as drug therapy it is important to remove affected lambs to new and better grazing and a clean water source. It is also important to simultaneously check for the presence of nematode infestation.

A variety of drugs may be used against *Coccidia*; these include sulphonamides and the coccidiocides, toltrazuril and amprolium. Sulphonamides are variable in their effect against different species of *Coccidia* given at different stages of infection. Treatment needs to be given over several days. Amprolium and toltrazuril, licensed mainly for the treatment of avian coccidioses, are both effective in mammals. Toltrazuril has the added advantage of being effective following a single dose.

Cryptosporidiosis

Cryptosporidiosis is a disease caused by a non-host-specific and very small coccidian (*Cryptosporidium parvum*), which attaches to the epithelial surface of the small-intestine villi. It affects a variety of species including lambs. Mainly very young lambs are affected, but it may occur in adult sheep as well. It has not been reported as causing disease in lambs in New Zealand, although it is probably present within the national flock.

Overseas, outbreaks have been quite severe. The clinical signs may include acute diarrhoea, usually without death resulting. Frequently, cryptosporidia may be present without causing clinical signs at all. Diagnosis may be confirmed by the examination of fixed sections of small intestine, for changes to the villae and the presence of sporulated oocysts. Usually the disease resolves without treatment. It should be noted that cryptosporidiosis is zoonotic.

Sarcocystosis

Infections with *Sarcocystis* spp are apparently common, but disease is rare. In sheep, myositis, abortion, malaise, anaemia and ill thrift have been reported overseas.

Toxoplasmosis

This protozoal disease is dealt with in Chapter 4.

REFERENCES

GASTROINTESTINAL NEMATODE PARASITES

Bisset SA, Vlassoff A, Pulford H. Rotational grazing/grazing interchange systems. *Proceedings of the 21st Annual Seminar of the Society of Sheep and Beef Cattle Veterinarians, New Zealand Veterinary Association,* 47-54, 1991

Bisset SA, Vlassoff A, West CJ. Breeding for resistance/tolerance to internal parasites. *Proceedings of the 21st Annual Seminar of the Society of Sheep and Beef Cattle Veterinarians, New Zealand Veterinary Association,* 83-92, 1991

Bisset SA, Morris CA, McEwen JC, Vlassoff A. Breeding sheep in New Zealand that are less reliant on anthelmintics to maintain health and productivity. *New Zealand Veterinary Journal* 49, 236-46, 2001

Brunsdon RV. Importance of the ewe as a source of trichostrongyle infection for lambs: Control of the spring-rise phenomenon by a single post-lambing anthelmintic treatment. *New Zealand Veterinary Journal* 14, 118-25, 1996

Brunsdon RV. Control of internal parasites — the present state of play. *Proceedings of the Ruakura Farmers Conference,* 115-23, 1981

Brunsdon RV, Vlassoff A. Parasite control — a revised approach. *Internal Parasites of Sheep,* pp 53-64, edited by Ross AD. Lincoln University, 1982

Brunsdon RV, Vlassoff A. Long-term parasitological consequences and production responses in ewes and lambs after a single post-parturient anthelmintic treatment of ewes. *New Zealand Journal of Experimental Agriculture* 13, 135-40, 1985

Brunsdon RV, Vlassoff A, West CJ. Effects of natural trichostrongylid larval challenge on breeding ewes. *New Zealand Journal of Experimental Agriculture* 14, 37-41, 1986

Charleston WAG, McKenna PB. Nematodes and liver fluke in New Zealand. *New Zealand Veterinary Journal* 50 (Suppl.), 41-7, 2002

Cook T. Long-term approach to a serious drench resistance issue. *Proceedings of the 38th Annual Seminar of the Society of Sheep and Beef Cattle Veterinarians, New Zealand Veterinary Association,* 93-6, 2008

Coop RL, Angus KW, Sykes AR. Chronic infection with *Trichostrongylus vitrinus* in sheep. Pathological changes in the small intestine. *Research in Veterinary Science* 26, 363-71, 1979

Familton AS, Nicol AM, Mcaulty R. Epidemiology of internal parasitism of sheep on irrigated pasture and the possible control measures. *Proceedings of the 16th Annual Seminar of the Society of Sheep and Beef Cattle Veterinarians, New Zealand Veterinary Association,* 210-19, 1986

Hein WR, Shoemaker CB, Heath ACG. Future technologies for control of nematodes in sheep. *New Zealand Veterinary Journal* 49, 247-51, 2001

Hoskin, SO. Alternative forages for parasite control in ruminant livestock. *Proceedings of the 36th Annual Seminar of the Society of Sheep and Beef Cattle Veterinarians, New Zealand Veterinary Association,* 11-19, 2006

Hughes PL, Dowling AF, Callinan APL. Resistance to macrocyclic lactone anthelmintics and associated risk factors on sheep farms in the lower North Island of New Zealand. *New Zealand Veterinary Journal* 55, 177-83, 2007

Hughes PL, McKenna PB. Confirmation of resistance to ivermectin by *Cooperia curticei* in sheep. *New Zealand Veterinary Journal* 53, 344-6, 2005

Hughes PL, McKenna PB, Dowling AF. A survey of the prevalence of emerging macrocyclic lactone resistance and of benzimidazole resistance in sheep nematodes in the lower North Island of New Zealand. *New Zealand Veterinary Journal* 53, 87-90, 2005

Johnstone IL. The integration of beef cattle with sheep in parasite control. *Proceedings of the 9th Annual Seminar of the Society of Sheep and Beef Cattle Veterinarians, New Zealand Veterinary Association,* 19-30, 1979

Lawrence KE, Leathwick DM, Rhodes AP, Jackson R, Heuer C, Pomroy WE, West DM, Waghorn TS, Moffat JR. Management of gastrointestinal nematode parasites on sheep farms in New Zealand. *New Zealand Veterinary Journal* 55, 228-34, 2007

Lawrence KE, Rhodes AP, Jackson R, Leathwick DM, Heuer C, Pomroy WE, West DM, Waghorn TS, Moffat JR. Farm management practices associated with macrocyclic lactone resistance on sheep farms in New Zealand. *New Zealand Veterinary Journal* 54, 283-8, 2006

Leathwick DM. Refugia — why, how and how much? *Proceedings of the Society of Sheep and Beef Cattle Veterinarians, New Zealand Veterinary Association,* 85-9, 2008

Leathwick DM, Hosking BC. Managing anthelmintic resistance: Modelling strategic use of a new anthelmintic class to slow the development of resistance to existing classes. *New Zealand Veterinary Journal* 57, 203-7, 2009

Leathwick DM, Hosking BC, Bisset SA, McKay CH. Managing anthelmintic resistance: Is it feasible in New Zealand to delay the emergence of resistance to a new anthelmintic class? *New Zealand Veterinary Journal* 57, 181-92, 2009

Leathwick DM, Miller CM, Atkinson DS, Haack NA, Waghorn TS, Oliver AM. Management of anthelmintic resistance: Untreated adult ewes as a source of unselected parasites, and their role in reducing parasite populations. *New Zealand Veterinary Journal* 56, 184-95, 2008

Leathwick DM, Miller CM, Atkinson DS, Haack NA, Alexander RA, Oliver A-M, Waghorn TS, Potter JF, Sutherland IA. Drenching adult ewes: Implications of anthelmintic treatments pre- and post-lambing on the development of anthelmintic resistance. *New Zealand Veterinary Journal* 54, 297-304, 2006

Leathwick DM, Waghorn TS, Miller CM, Atkinson DS, Haack NA, Oliver A-M. Selective and on-demand drenching of lambs: Impact on parasite populations and performance of lambs. *New Zealand Veterinary Journal* 54, 305-12, 2006

Lewis KHC. Ewe fertility response to pre-mating anthelmintic drenching. *New Zealand Journal of Experimental Agriculture* 3, 43-7, 1975

Mason PC, Hosking BC, Nottingham RM, Cole DJW, Seewald W, McKay CH, Griffiths TM, Kaye-Smith BG, Chamberlain B. A large-scale clinical field study to evaluate the efficacy and safety of an oral formulation of the amino-acetonitrile derivative (AAD), monepantel, in sheep in New Zealand. *New Zealand Veterinary Journal* 57, 3-9, 2009

McKenna PB. The diagnosis of gastrointestinal parasitism in cattle and sheep. *Proceedings of the 11th Annual Seminar of the Society of Sheep and Beef Cattle Veterinarians, New Zealand Veterinary Association*, 95-103, 1981

McKenna PB. Diagnosis of gastro-intestinal parasitism in young sheep flocks: The contribution of animal health laboratories. *Proceedings of the 12th Annual Seminar of the Society of Sheep and Beef Cattle Veterinarians, New Zealand Veterinary Association*, 108-29, 1982

McKenna PB. A comparison of faecal egg count reduction test procedures. *New Zealand Veterinary Journal* 54, 202-3, 2006

McKenna PB. Further comparison of faecal egg count reduction test procedures: Sensitivity and specificity. *New Zealand Veterinary Journal* 54, 365-6, 2006

McKenna PB. How do you mean? The case for composite faecal egg counts in testing for drench resistance. *New Zealand Veterinary Journal* 55, 100-1, 2007

McKenna PB. An examination of the relative reliability of laboratory case submissions in determining the prevalence of anthelmintic resistance in sheep nematodes in New Zealand, and the possible influence of test analysis methodology on such data. *New Zealand Veterinary Journal* 56, 155-9, 2008

McEwan J. Managing the risk — utilizing resistant sheep to manage anthelmintic resistance. *Proceedings of the 36th Annual Seminar of the Society of Sheep and Beef Cattle Veterinarians, New Zealand Veterinary Association*, 29-35, 2006

Miller CM, Waghorn TS, Leathwick DM, Gilmour ML. How repeatable is a faecal egg count reduction test? *New Zealand Veterinary Journal* 54, 323-8, 2006

Miller CM, Ganesh S, Garland CB, Leathwick DM. Production benefits from pre- and post-lambing anthelmintic treatment of ewes on commercial farms in the southern North Island of New Zealand. *New Zealand Veterinary Journal* 63, 211-19, 2015

Morley FHW, Donald AD. Farm management and systems of Helminth control. *Veterinary Parasitology* 6, 105-34, 1980

Morris CA. Host genetics and internal parasitism. *Proceedings of the 32nd Annual Seminar of the Society of Sheep and Beef Cattle Veterinarians, New Zealand Veterinary Association*, 99-104, 2002

Niezen JH, Stiefel W, Ransom J, MacKay AD. Controlling internal parasitism on an organic sheep and beef unit. *Proceedings of the 21st Annual Seminar of the Society of Sheep and Beef Cattle Veterinarians, New Zealand Veterinary Association*, 65-72, 1991

Pomroy WE. An overview of the consequences of drenching adult ewes pre and post lambing. *Proceedings of the 28th Annual Seminar of the Society of Sheep and Beef Cattle Veterinarians, New Zealand Veterinary Association*, 63-71, 1998

Pomroy WE. Anthelmintic resistance in New Zealand: A perspective on recent findings and options for the future. *New Zealand Veterinary Journal* 54, 265-70, 2006

Rhodes AP, Leathwick DM, Pomroy WE. Best practice parasite management: An approach to working with farmers to best manage multiple anthelmintic resistance. *Proceedings of the Society of Sheep and Beef Cattle Veterinarians, New Zealand Veterinary Association*, 2.16.1-2.16.8, 2011

Stafford KJ, West DM, Pomroy WE. Nematode worm egg output in ewes. *New Zealand Veterinary Journal* 42, 30-2, 1994

Sutherland IA. Recent developments in the management of anthelmintic resistance in small ruminants — an Australasian perspective. *New Zealand Veterinary Journal* 63, 183-7, 2015

Sykes AR, Coop RL, Angus KW. The influence of chronic *Ostertagia circumcincta* infection on the skeleton of growing sheep. *Journal of Comparative Pathology* 87, 521-9, 1977

Sykes AR, Coop RL, Angus KW. Chronic infection with *Trichostrongylus vitrinus* in sheep. Some effects on food utilisation, skeletal growth and certain serum constituents. *Research in Veterinary Science* 26, 372-7, 1979

Sykes AR, Coop RL. Interactions between nutrition and gastrointestinal parasitism in sheep. *New Zealand Veterinary Journal* 49, 222-6, 2001

Vlassoff A. Seasonal incidence of infective trichostrongyle larvae on pasture grazed by lambs. *New Zealand Journal of Experimental Agriculture* 1, 293-301, 1973

Vlassoff A. Biology and population dynamics of the free-living stages of gastrointestinal nematodes of sheep. *Internal Parasites of Sheep*, edited by Ross AD. Lincoln University, 1982

Vlassoff A, Leathwick DM, Heath ACG. The epidemiology of nematode infections in sheep. *New Zealand Veterinary Journal* 49, 213-21, 2001

Waghorn TS, Leathwick DM, Miller CM, Atkinson DS. Brave or gullible: Testing the concept that leaving susceptible parasites in refugia will slow the development of anthelmintic resistance. *New Zealand Veterinary Journal* 56, 158-63, 2008

Waghorn TS, Leathwick DM, Rhodes AP, Lawrence KE, Jackson R, Pomroy WE, West DM, Moffat JR. Prevalence of anthelmintic resistance on sheep farms in New Zealand. *New Zealand Veterinary Journal* 54, 271-7, 2006

Waghorn TS, Leathwick DM, Skipp RA, Chen LY. Nematophagous fungi: A New Zealand perspective. *Proceedings of the 36th Annual Seminar of the Society of Sheep and Beef Cattle Veterinarians, New Zealand Veterinary Association*, 21-8, 2006

West DM. Gastrointestinal parasitism of adult sheep. *Proceedings of the 12th Annual Seminar of the Society of Sheep and Beef Cattle Veterinarians, New Zealand Veterinary Association*, 236-45, 1982

West DM, Pomroy WE, Kenyon PR, Morris ST, Smith SL, Burnham DL. The effect of subclinical parasitism on a ewe flock. *Proceedings of the 38th Annual Seminar of the Society of Sheep and Beef Cattle Veterinarians, New Zealand Veterinary Association*, 97-102, 2008

Wilson L. Wormwise — your challenge your opportunity. *Proceedings of the 37th Annual Seminar of the Society of Sheep and Beef Cattle Veterinarians, New Zealand Veterinary Association*, 155-8, 2007

Wrigley J, McArthur M, McKenna PB, Mariadass B. Resistance to a triple combination of broad-spectrum anthelmintics in naturally-acquired *Ostertagia circumcincta* infections in sheep. *New Zealand Veterinary Journal* 54, 47-9, 2006

TAPEWORMS OF SHEEP

Davidson RM. Control and eradication of animal diseases in New Zealand. *New Zealand Veterinary Journal* 50 (Suppl.), 6-12, 2002

Elliot DC. Tapeworm (*Moniezia expansa*) and its effect on sheep production: The evidence reviewed. *New Zealand Veterinary Journal* 34, 61-5, 1986

Mason P, Moffat J, Cole D. Tapeworm in sheep revisited. *Proceedings of the 32nd Annual Seminar of the Society of Sheep and Beef Cattle Veterinarians, New Zealand Veterinary Association*, 147-51, 2002

Pharo H. *VetScript* XV, 9, 8-9, 2002

Southworth J, Harvey C, Larsen S. Use of praziquantel for the control of Moniezia expansa in lambs. *New Zealand Veterinary Journal* 44, 112-5, 1996

COCCIDIOSIS

Gregory M, Catchpole J. Ovine coccidiosis: Heavy infection in young lambs increases resistance without causing disease. *Veterinary Record* 124, 458, 1989

Mason PC. Coccidiosis. *Proceedings of the 18th Annual Seminar of the Society of Sheep and Beef Cattle Veterinarians, New Zealand Veterinary Association*, 86-98, 1988

Ridler AL. Disease threats to sheep associated with intensification of pastoral farming. *New Zealand Veterinary Journal* 56, 270-3, 2008

Stafford KJ, West DM, Vermunt JJ, Pomroy W, Adlington BA, Calder SM. The effect of repeated doses of toltrazuril on coccidial oocyst output and weight gain in suckling lambs. *New Zealand Veterinary Journal* 42, 117-19, 1994

Taylor M. Diagnosis and control of coccidiosis in sheep. *In Practice* April, 172-7, 1995

CRYPTOSPORIDIOSIS

Foreyt WJ. Coccidiosis and cryptosporidiosis in sheep and goats. *Veterinary Clinics of North America: Food Animal Practice* 6, 655-70, 1990

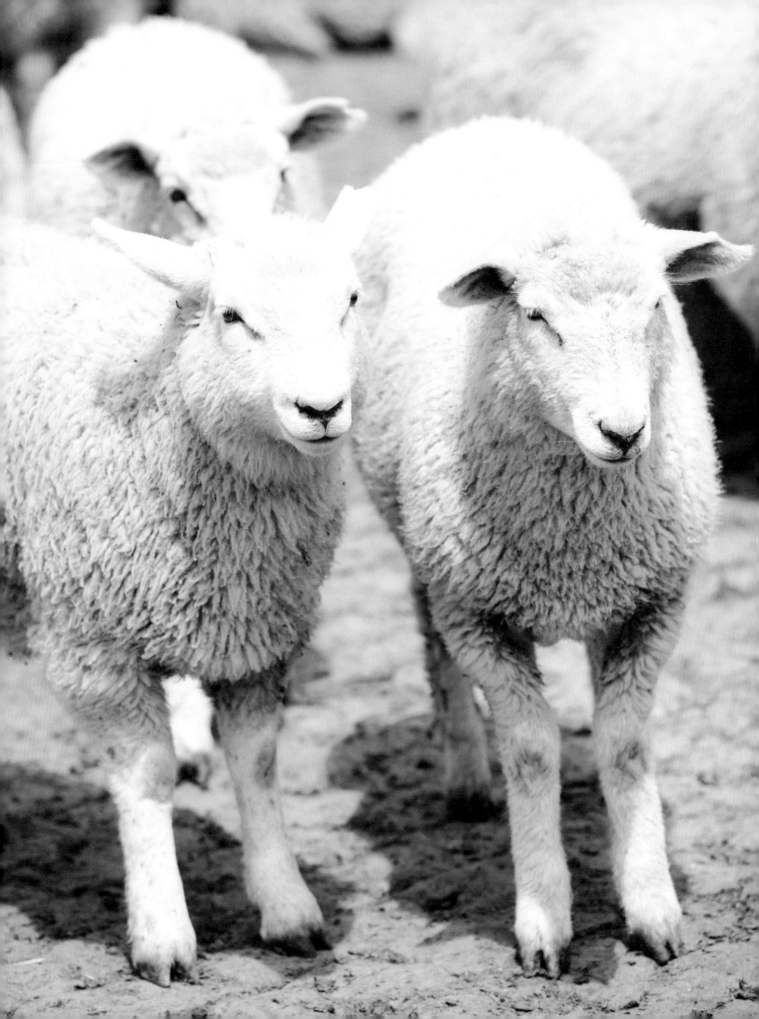

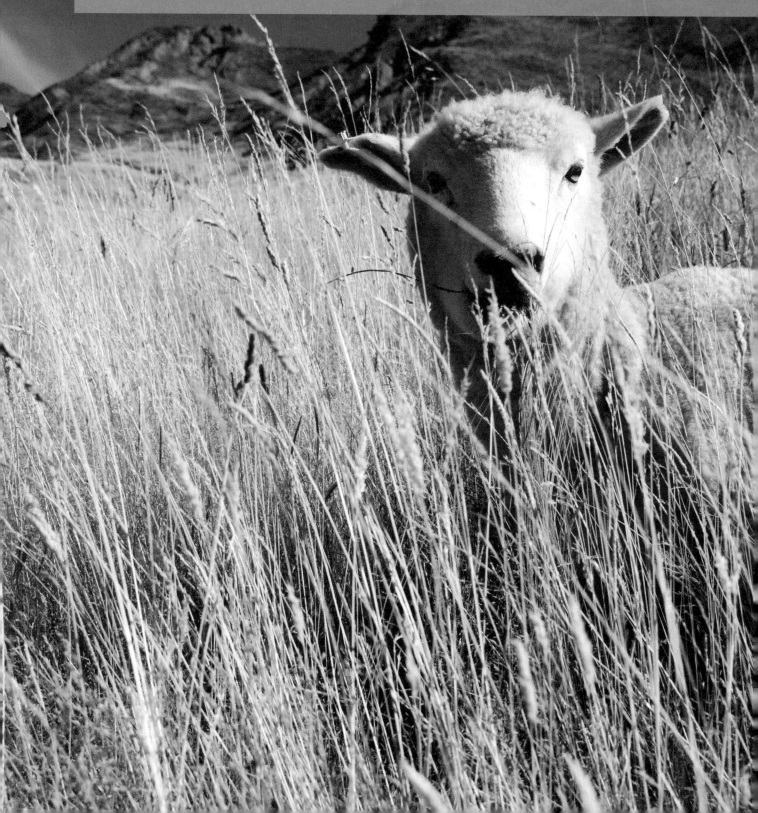

9 Metabolic disorders

Metabolic disorders

Metabolic disorders of sheep are almost invariably caused by poor nutrition. The provision of adequate feed, particularly at crucial stages such as pregnancy and lactation, are the key to prevention of these diseases. The treatment of clinical cases of metabolic disorders is frequently unsatisfactory and is dependent on their early recognition and prompt therapy of affected sheep.

Pregnancy toxaemia

Pregnancy toxaemia (ketosis, twin lamb disease, sleepy sickness, lambing sickness, pregnancy disease) is mainly a condition of multiple-bearing ewes that occurs in late pregnancy. It is characterised by dullness, anorexia, nervous signs, recumbency and eventual death. It arises when the metabolic requirements for glucose by the ewe and the lamb cannot be met. Thus, a falling plane of nutrition or a sudden dietary check during late pregnancy, especially in multiple-bearing ewes, is the most common precipitating factor.

Occurrence and predisposing factors

In the past, widespread outbreaks of pregnancy toxaemia were relatively common and large numbers of ewes were affected and died of this disease. Although pregnancy toxaemia is still a common condition of sheep, it is generally restricted to smaller losses than previously because farmers have a better understanding of the precipitating factors that cause it and also make better provision for winter feeding of ewes. However, outbreaks are still encountered, especially following adverse weather. With the trend to small-block farming in many areas, small properties are often overstocked, causing severe feed restrictions to sheep prior to lambing.

The following factors are commonly associated with pregnancy toxaemia:

- A falling plane of nutrition in the last 2 months of pregnancy. This is the period when 70% of the foetus's birthweight is gained. The effect of nutrition of the ewe on the birthweight of the lamb and its subsequent viability and growth are most important.
- Any sudden restriction of feed during late pregnancy, such as yarding for crutching or shearing or inclement weather such as a snowstorm, may precipitate an outbreak.
- Inadequate shelter during inclement weather or pre-lamb shearing may decrease the feed intake of the ewe but at the same time increase the feed requirement.
- Any disease that restricts the ability of the sheep to feed. Such conditions as footrot, foot abscess, dental abnormalities, gastrointestinal parasitism, pinkeye and hypocalcaemia should be considered.
- In some intensive rotational grazing systems, some ewes are not able to compete for feed and become starved.
- Older ewes are considered to be more at risk than are two-tooth ewes.
- Ewes with twins or triplets are more susceptible than ewes with a single foetus.
- Lack of exercise is often quoted by graziers as a predisposing factor. Lack of exercise may have physiological implications that affect the animal's desire to graze vigorously.

Although the condition has a wide spectrum of features, it is possible to recognise two distinct syndromes that are important in understanding the control of the disease.

1. The under-nutrition syndrome

This is seen in multiple-bearing ewes that have experienced prolonged and progressively more severe under-nourishment during the last 6 weeks of pregnancy. This syndrome is common where available feed from pasture is inadequate or where no supplementary feed has been given.

2. The stress syndrome

This is seen in ewes that have been well nourished but have suddenly been subjected to a complete fast, often as a result of some severe environmental stress. This syndrome is seen during crutching or pre-lamb shearing, particularly during inclement weather.

It has been suggested that the bulk of the uterine contents (twins or triplets) interferes with the capacity of some sheep to ingest adequate feed, and other factors such as age and failing teeth may contribute to this type of case. It is important to realise that although pregnancy toxaemia can occur as a primary clinical condition, it is frequently secondary to one or more predisposing factors. The relative importance of these should be assessed in the control and prevention of the disease.

Pathogenesis

During the last two months of pregnancy the feed requirements of the ewe with twin foetuses rises to nearly twice maintenance level (Table 9.1).

The glucose requirement of the foetus is obligatory and cannot be controlled by the ewe. Once blood glucose from the ewe passes to the lamb, it is utilised as fructose and does not re-enter the ewe's circulation; thus, if the ewe cannot meet the foetal requirements from her diet she must draw on her own body reserves to maintain the foetal demand for glucose. The total foetal demand for glucose is about 8–9 g per kg/foetus/day or about 30–40 g per day for a single foetus. This represents over 35% of the 110 g of glucose available to a 50 kg ewe fed a maintenance diet of roughage.

It must also be remembered that not only is the glucose utilisation *per se* high in the foetus at the terminal stages of pregnancy, but foetal reserves of glycogen are also rapidly increasing in the liver, lung and muscle. This is vital to lamb survival after birth.

The blood glucose of the ewe is derived mainly from propionic acid, one of the three end products of starch and cellulose degradation. Significant glucose also comes from amino acids by gluconeogenesis, either from protein in the diet or from muscle wasting during starvation. In pregnancy toxaemia, the propionic acid and glycogenic precursors derived from the diet and body reserves are unable to maintain glucose requirements. Thus hypoglycaemia is the earliest abnormality detected in pregnancy toxaemia.

Liveweight (on a conceptus-free basis)	Maintenance	Late pregnancy Single-bearing Maintenance x 1.5	Late pregnancy Multiple-bearing Maintenance x 1.9	Lactation Maintenance x 3+
40 kg	0.70	1.1	1.3	2.1
45 kg	0.76	1.1	1.4	2.3
50 kg	0.82	1.2	1.6	2.5
55 kg	0.88	1.3	1.7	2.6
60 kg	0.94	1.4	1.8	2.8
65 kg	1.00	1.5	1.9	3.0
70 kg	1.10	1.6	2.0	3.2

Table 9.1 Daily dry matter requirements (in kilograms, assuming an average of 11.5 MJ ME/kg DM i.e. spring pasture) for various liveweights of sheep.

At the same time, there is an increased requirement for tricarboxylic acids to facilitate the catabolism of fatty acids as an alternative energy source. Where there is a deficiency of glucose precursors, there is a reduction in the intermediate products of the tricarboxylic acid cycle, particularly oxaloacetate which is required if acetyl coenzyme A is to be utilised by the tricarboxylic acid cycle. As a result, acetyl coenzyme A accumulates and is diverted into the production of ketone bodies. The excessive production of ketone bodies and resulting hyperketonaemia produces acidosis and dyspnoea and exacerbates the depression of the central nervous system to the stage where the original hypoglycaemic encephalopathy becomes irreversible. This is followed rapidly by the development of acidosis, dehydration, uraemia, terminal coma and death.

While inadequate propionate and protein intake are the main predisposing factors, deficiencies in other nutritional factors, such as choline and biotin, may contribute to the development of pregnancy toxaemia.

A notable feature of the latter stages of pregnancy toxaemia is the appearance of free fatty acids in the circulation of the ewe. These come as a direct result of lipolysis replacing lipogenesis and only a percentage of the glycerol available from the higher fatty acids (palmitic or oleic) being metabolised.

A consistent finding in pregnancy toxaemia is the hyperactivity of the adrenal gland, possibly as a result of the hypoglycaemia. This is particularly noticeable in the prolonged starvation syndrome. The circulating levels of cortisol are increased and effectively inhibit glucose utilisation by the sheep. Notable evidence of adrenal hyperactivity in the ewe under stress is shown by a developing lymphocytopenia and wool break and shedding of the fleece.

The fatty liver is probably associated with incomplete fat metabolism due to a shortage of oxaloacetic acid and is an important feature of pregnancy toxaemia.

Clinical signs

The typical history in an affected flock is a period of feed restriction followed by the appearance of clinically affected ewes. Early in the syndrome the affected ewe separates herself from the flock and appears depressed. There is a loss of appetite and a disinclination to move, which can often be detected while the flock is being shifted as affected sheep will usually lag behind. If the flock is set stocked, these changes may go unnoticed for a longer period.

As the condition progresses, the affected ewe becomes more depressed, the head may be carried in an unnatural position, the ewe appears blind, may wander aimlessly and show little reaction to the presence of a human or dog. If forced to move, the ewe may stagger and lean awkwardly

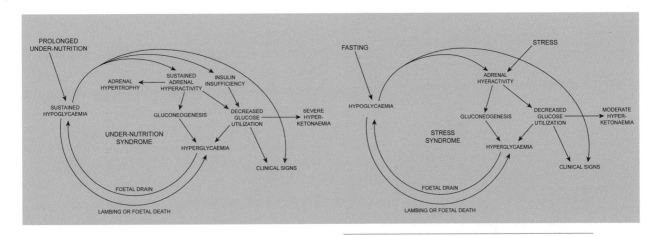

Figure 9.1 Major physiological and biochemical events in the two principal pregnancy toxaemia syndromes (Reid, 1960).

against obstacles and even press its head into fences or gates. A characteristic feature is 'wool pull', where the wool plucks readily. The cardinal signs are mostly normal. In some cases, neuromuscular disturbances occur in the form of fine myoclonic twitching of the ears, periorbital muscles and muzzle with champing of the jaws and the production of a white froth about the mouth.

In the latter stages the ewe will become recumbent, may stargaze and eventually become comatose and die.

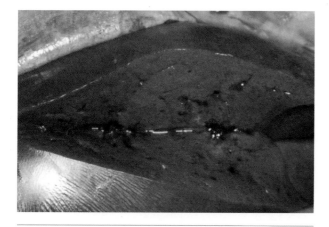

Figure 9.2 A fatty liver from a ewe that died of pregnancy toxaemia.

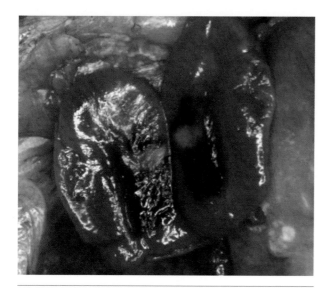

Figure 9.3 Haemorrhage in the adrenal gland of a ewe that died of pregnancy toxaemia.

Occasionally some ewes abort. The onset of parturition during the course of the disease increases the chances of the ewe recovering, although the lambs are often born dead. Foetal death is common when pregnancy toxaemia is prolonged.

Some ewes may be showing concurrent signs of severe lameness, parasitism, pinkeye or some other contributing disease. Once the disease appears, a number of ewes may be affected each day and these normally show a regular progression of clinical signs over a period of 3–7 days. In some instances, particularly following stress, a number of ewes may be affected quite suddenly.

Clinical pathology

Hypoglycaemia is the earliest abnormality detected in pregnancy toxaemia, but as the condition progresses blood glucose levels tend to stabilise and some ewes even become hyperglycaemic. In such cases the prognosis is poor as the foetuses are usually dead.

Hyperketonaemia and ketonuria are characteristic findings in pregnancy toxaemia. The presence of ketone bodies in the urine can be detected using sodium nitroprusside reagents such as Rothera's test, test strips or tablets, and this can be readily performed on the farm. Blood urea nitrogen levels may be increased due to the development of renal failure, and this is associated with a poor prognosis. In more advanced cases there is a ketoacidosis, haemoconcentration, hyperglycaemia and uraemia.

Pathology

At postmortem examination the uterus is usually found to contain two or more developed foetuses, although single-bearing ewes occasionally are affected. The liver is pale, fatty and friable. The adrenal glands are enlarged and may have a darkened cortex due to haemorrhage. In the prolonged starvation syndrome there may be little body fat remaining. The rumen and gut will usually be empty.

Treatment and prognosis

In general, the treatment of pregnancy toxaemia is difficult and the results are variable and often disappointing. Before embarking on the treatment of clinically affected ewes, it is pertinent to consider some guiding principles:
- Because the metabolic events become irreversible in

the latter stages of pregnancy toxaemia, early vigorous treatment is essential for a reliable result. While the ewe is in the mildly depressed, hypoglycaemic, ketotic state, recovery following therapy is common. However, once the nervous signs become severe or the animal is recumbent, renal failure has usually occurred and death is inevitable.
- Maintaining appetite is essential to ensuring a favourable outcome. If, following therapy, the ewe begins to forage then the prognosis is good, but if she remains recumbent and refuses food then the outcome is hopeless. In all cases it is best to leave affected ewes with normal ewes to encourage feeding. Allowing easy access to water is also important.

The following measures may be considered in treatment. Basically they include the provision of carbohydrate, stimulation of gluconeogenesis and the removal of the foetuses.

1. Glucose/dextrose therapy

Intravenous glucose may be given to elevate blood glucose levels initially, but this is often impractical and costly. Following a single loading dose, the renal threshold for glucose is exceeded and surplus glucose is lost in the urine. Approximately 60–100 ml of 40% w/v dextrose may be given intravenously. In addition, it has sometimes been recommended to inject long-acting insulin preparations (40 iu) to prevent hypoglycaemia rebound. This should only be used in the early stages of the disease.

A more popular way of increasing blood glucose levels is oral dosing with glucose precursors such as glycerol or propylene glycol (60–120 ml twice daily).

2. Fluid therapy

Dehydration is a feature of pregnancy toxaemia, and fluid therapy is an important adjunct to treatment. It is usually given orally due to ease of administration and reduced cost. A range of oral rehydration solutions are available and some of these incorporate the glucose precursors mentioned previously. It is also important to ensure that ewes have easy access to water, a point frequently overlooked.

In valuable ewes, intravenous treatment may be given. Solutions administered should include dextrose, bicarbonate or bicarbonate precursors such as lactate and a balanced electrolyte solution.

3. Corticosteroids

Corticosteroids have not given consistent results in the treatment of pregnancy toxaemia, which is not surprising given the high levels of cortisol that are present in affected ewes. Corticosteroids have been used to abort ewes in the very early stages of pregnancy toxaemia but ewes in the latter stages are unresponsive.

4. Caesarean section

Reducing the metabolic drain on the ewe by removing the foetus by caesarean section is a successful procedure for affected ewes that are in the early stages of pregnancy toxaemia.

5. Non-steroidal anti-inflammatory drugs

An overseas study reported increased survival of affected ewes treated daily with 2.5 mg/kg flunixin meglumine, although this has not been assessed under New Zealand conditions. Note that flunixin is not licenced for use in sheep in New Zealand. Care should be taken with dehydrated animals.

6. Other

Other suggested measures for treatment include shearing of ewes to stimulate appetite, and giving calcium borogluconate subcutaneously as decreased calcium levels have been shown to predispose to pregnancy toxaemia. Calcium borogluconate is frequently given to recumbent, pregnant ewes as sometimes the differentiation between pregnancy toxaemia and hypocalcaemia is not clear.

Prevention

The presence of pregnancy toxaemia in a flock is an opportunity to explain to the farmer the effect that under-nutrition may have on the subsequent performance of the flock. It needs to be pointed out that there may be increased lamb deaths at birth and decreased birthweights unless nutrition can be improved significantly and immediately. Further, if the prolonged under-nutrition persists there will be a depression of lactation, impaired mothering ability of the ewes and decreased wool production.

When dealing with an outbreak of pregnancy toxaemia,

it is important to identify those factors that precipitated the problem. This is necessary not only to achieve the best advice for the present season but also to plan for the following year so that there is not a recurrence of the disease.

To avoid pregnancy toxaemia occurring due to progressive starvation, a feeding programme for pregnant ewes should be developed that provides a gradual increase in energy intake to cover the requirements of the developing foetuses without a reduction in body reserves. Weighing and body condition scoring ewes pre-tupping and mid-winter (mid-pregnancy) is a useful way of monitoring their progress.

Ewes carrying multiple foetuses may be detected by ultrasound pregnancy diagnosis and given preferential feeding during late pregnancy. Stocking rates may be reduced by the disposal of surplus stock. However, it is usually too late to gain from this procedure once pregnancy toxaemia has occurred. It needs to be emphasised to the farmer that the early disposal of lambs and dry sheep in the next year is essential to the provision of winter feed stores. It may be necessary to provide supplementary feed either as hay, grain or a crop. In some cases a long-term review of the fertiliser programme is necessary to ensure adequate grass growth. Where controlled winter grazing is practised, it may be necessary to increase the rate of rotation and select out the poorer ewes for preferential treatment.

To avoid pregnancy toxaemia following a sudden fast, unnecessary mustering and holding off feed for long periods should be avoided. Particular care should be exercised when yarding ewes for pre-lamb crutching or shearing.

In conclusion, this important and production limiting condition was aptly explained by one of New Zealand's earlier veterinarians, Alan Leslie: 'When farmers feed sheep judiciously they don't get pregnancy toxaemia; when on the other hand they feed them injudiciously pregnancy toxaemia will occur.'

Hypocalcaemia (milk fever)

Clinical hypocalcaemia (milk fever) in pregnant ewes occurs when there is insufficient intake and absorption of calcium, and insufficient resorption from skeletal reserves to meet foetal demands. Up to 2.8 g of calcium per day is required to meet foetal needs; hypocalcaemia is usually associated with plasma calcium levels below 1.7 mmol/l. It is often complicated by low blood magnesium and low serum phosphorus levels. It occurs mainly in mature ewes during late pregnancy, but occasionally occurs after lambing and has been reported in dry sheep as well.

As in pregnancy toxaemia the losses due to death from hypocalcaemia and overt milk fever are important, but even more important are the production losses that may arise from ewes which have recovered from hypocalcaemia or those which have had subclinical hypocalcaemia. The lambs born from such ewes have a poorer chance of survival, as was shown in one study where 22% of lambs died after having been born from ewes that were hypocalcaemic during late pregnancy. In the normocalcaemic ewes of the same trial, only 3% of lambs died.

Calcium requirements of the pregnant ewe

Two important predisposing factors are necessary before hypocalcaemia occurs. These are the high requirement for calcium by the pregnant ewe and a low dietary intake over a period of weeks or months. Normal circulating serum calcium levels are reported to be 2.0–3.0 mmol/l; in cases of hypocalcaemia, levels as low as 0.80 mmol/l may occur. Dietary calcium levels should be 1.5–2.6 g Ca/kg DM.

Irrespective of calcium intake, ewes do not absorb sufficient dietary calcium to meet their requirements during late pregnancy and for milk secretion in early lactation. Ewes may mobilise up to 20% of their skeletal calcium reserves during this time, with the proportion mobilised depending on the pre-existing degree of mineralisation and on the calcium content of the diet. Replacement of lost skeletal reserves is usually complete by 130 days after parturition on diets providing plentiful calcium (250 mg Ca/kg liveweight/day) and phosphorus (160 mg P/kg liveweight/day). Because the rate of accretion of calcium onto bone decreases with age, the replenishment of the partly depleted skeleton will take longer in older ewes. If skeletal reserves are not replaced adequately, ewes may become susceptible to hypocalcaemia during subsequent pregnancies.

Calcium deficiency can occur in sheep on a variety of diets. Under drought conditions, sheep fed wheat or concentrate diets (<1.0 g Ca/kg DM) containing low calcium and high phosphorus may become calcium-deficient. Further, low phosphorus intake associated with mature or dry summer grass may also limit repletion of skeletal reserves. Under wet conditions and when pasture is growing rapidly, the calcium level may be at its lowest. Hypocalcaemia frequently occurs in sheep grazing lush pasture or in sheep fed diets such as oat crops which have a very low calcium content.

Predisposing factors

In many cases the factors that precipitate hypocalcaemia are similar to those associated with pregnancy toxaemia. Usually sudden changes in feed, either in feed type or the grazing regimen, will cause short-term starvation and lead to clinical hypocalcaemia. Sudden increases in green feed or management procedures such as holding for crutching or shearing are all contributing factors. Extensive droving of sheep and access to sorrel (or other oxalate-containing plants) have also been associated with hypocalcaemia.

Clinical signs and diagnosis

The diagnosis of hypocalcaemia is usually based on a history of a sudden feed check or change, the characteristic clinical signs and a rapid response to treatment. Serum calcium levels may also be assessed to confirm a diagnosis, but this is seldom necessary. Blood samples should be collected from at least 5 different ewes.

Affected ewes are initially ataxic and hyperactive but rapidly become recumbent and comatose. There may be no corneal reflex. They are generally found in sternal recumbency with the head turned into the flank, but seldom go into lateral recumbency like cattle. Tympany usually occurs and regurgitation of rumen contents is often seen. In some cases prolapse of the vagina may also occur. Untreated animals usually go into a deep coma after 24 hours and die.

It should be noted that similar clinical features to hypocalcaemia are seen in ewes suffering from phosphatic fertiliser toxicity, which is also more common in pregnant ewes. This is discussed in further detail later in this chapter.

Treatment

Many sheep with hypocalcaemia also have low blood magnesium and low glucose levels, so treatment with calcium borogluconate, magnesium sulphate and glucose solutions is desirable, although in most cases calcium borogluconate is used on its own.

Ready-made solutions of calcium borogluconate are available at concentrations of 25% and 37.5% w/v, and depending on the concentration 30–100 ml should be given. The higher-concentration solutions should be injected subcutaneously because if given intravenously they may cause cardiac arrest. The response of the ewe following treatment is usually quick and dramatic. It will usually get up within 15–30 minutes, urinate, show muscle tremor and walk away and feed. Sheep which do not respond quickly should be checked for pregnancy toxaemia as this may be a sequel to hypocalcaemia in ewes.

If a number of ewes are treated, it is wise to go around those that have not risen of their own accord and try to gently prod them into movement.

Prevention

The prevention of hypocalcaemia largely depends on avoiding stressful conditions for ewes in late pregnancy or early lactation. Avoid unnecessary mustering and holding for long periods without feed. Do not initiate sudden changes in feed, and introduce sheep to crops gradually over several days. Avoid droving for long periods and do not transport sheep that are heavily pregnant.

Dusting pasture with 5–10 g per head per day of magnesium oxide for the three weeks prior to lambing has been suggested by some practitioners.

Under drought conditions, as seen in parts of Australia, limestone as a calcium supplement should be given to sheep that are grain-fed. Usually 1.5% limestone is recommended (1.5 kg to 100 kg grain).

Hypomagnesaemia (grass tetany)

Hypomagnesaemia (grass tetany) is an occasional cause of sudden death in sheep. It is seen primarily in mature lactating ewes although it has been reported in dry sheep as well.

Magnesium metabolism in the ewe and predisposing factors

The absorption of magnesium from the rumen is dependent on its concentration in the rumen fluid and is affected by other factors such as potassium and ammonia concentrations. If potassium concentrations in herbage

Time of sampling	Magnesium (mmol/l)	Calcium (mmol/l)
When first showing clinical signs	0.43	2.41
18 hours later, during tetany	0.24	2.19
24 hours after treatment	0.97	2.20
Normal	0.7–1.2	2.0–3.0

Table 9.2 Serum magnesium and calcium levels of a ewe showing signs of tetany.

Magnesium (mmol/l)	Calcium (mmol/l)
0.16	2.53
0.26	2.28
0.27	2.44
0.34	2.66
0.41	2.58
0.44	2.79
0.55	2.61
0.56	2.87
0.58	2.21
0.66	2.46
0.71	2.35
0.72	2.37
0.72	2.33
0.74	2.53
0.78	2.38
0.80	2.18
0.80	2.05
0.82	2.68
0.94	2.79
0.99	2.58
mean 0.61	mean 2.47
'normal values' 0.7–1.2	'normal values' 2.0–3.0

Table 9.3 Serum magnesium and calcium levels from a ewe flock in which clinical cases of hypomagnesaemia had occurred (West and Bruère, 1981).

increase (from 10 to 40 g/kg DM) and/or salivary secretions decrease, there is an increase in rumen potassium (from 5 to 40 nmol/l) and a decrease in rumen sodium (from 135 to 80 nmol/l). As a result, active magnesium absorption is decreased by the direct effects of high potassium on the magnesium pump. High ammonium ion concentrations (30 nmol/l) also decrease magnesium absorption, and this effect is additive and independent of the effects of potassium. Simply changing the diet from hay to lush pasture, which may not directly affect mineral uptake, can lead to similar effects because reduced mastication and salivary secretion increases the rumen sodium : potassium (K+/Na+) ratio.

There are virtually no available body reserves of magnesium, so animals are dependent on a continued dietary intake to meet their requirements. This intake is affected by a number of factors. There is good evidence to suggest that prior to clinical hypomagnesaemia occurring, the ewe may already have a low blood magnesium level. The situation is exacerbated as the ewe is unable to quickly mobilise magnesium reserves within her body.

Seventy-five per cent of magnesium reserves are in the skeleton and the other 25% are in muscle and other soft tissues. The demand of the lactating ewe for magnesium is very high. It is twice that of a lactating dairy cow and is at its peak about two weeks into lactation.

The loss of magnesium in milk probably predisposes ewes to hypomagnesaemia, and some researchers have suggested that hypomagnesaemic tetany does not occur unless there is a concomitant hypocalcaemia. This has not been the finding in reported cases in New Zealand.

Finally, it is the failure of the Mg^{2+} ion to reach the central nervous system that produces the severe convulsions associated with the disease. The precipitating factor for clinical hypomagnesaemia is energy imbalance. This may be brought about by either inadequate feed over a period of time or the sudden stress of inclement weather. It may also be induced as a result of other disease such as parasitism, pinkeye or foot lameness (foot abscess and footrot).

Clinical signs

Ewes with hypomagnesaemia are usually found dead in the paddock. Initially, affected sheep may become dull and stop eating. Usually, such ewes if disturbed will develop muscle tremors and severe nervous excitement. They will collapse on one side with the head thrown back and throw convulsions with severe limb paddling. Frothing at the mouth is a common feature, as are nystagmus, rapid heartbeat and rapid respiration. Death usually occurs in 4–6 hours.

Diagnosis

Special mention needs to be made of the diagnosis of hypomagnesaemia, as samples from overt cases for clinical pathology are not easy to obtain. Obtaining a good history of the feeding and management of the flock prior to the suspected occurrence of the disease is very important. Along with this must be a careful assessment of the condition of the ewes and the stage of lactation at which deaths have occurred. Knowledge of previous applications of fertiliser to the farm is also helpful as the outbreak may be associated with the previous heavy use of potassic topdressing. Typically a number of lactating ewes are found dead.

Postmortem examination of dead ewes is seldom helpful, but exclusion of clostridial diseases is important. Gas-filled intestines and some pericardial fluid are seen at autopsy in some cases; these are also seen in deaths from clostridial diseases. A history of flock vaccination will also help to eliminate these diseases as a cause of death. If ewes are found within 12 hours of death, the magnesium levels in the cerebrospinal fluid or vitreous humour can be analysed.

If clinical cases are seen, blood samples collected from them for serum magnesium and serum calcium estimations may be helpful. Also, the response to treatment of such cases may aid diagnosis (Table 9.2).

In general, it is necessary to obtain blood samples from at least 10 other ewes from within the flock. Although these may not be showing overt signs of hypomagnesaemia, some will have very low serum magnesium and the mean of the sample will be lower than normal (Table 9.3).

Treatment

If clinical cases are treated quickly there is a good chance of recovery. The subcutaneous injection of 50–70 ml magnesium sulphate (20%) and calcium borogluconate (25%) is recommended. These can usually be purchased as one solution primarily for use in cattle. In some instances intravenous administration is used in addition to subcutaneous injection. Ewes that respond to treatment may also be identified and drenched with magnesium oxide to boost their magnesium intake.

Magnesium oxide at a rate of 10 g/sheep/day may be administered to the rest of the flock if this is practical. Simply increasing the hay ration may be useful to avert further cases in the remainder of the flock by encouraging salivation and thus increasing the rumen Na+/K+ ratio. If it is considered that access to lush green feed was the cause of the hypomagnesaemia, the flock should be gradually re-introduced to such feed. Again the use of good-quality hay supplement to see ewes through the danger period may be helpful.

Prevention

Recommendations for preventing further cases of hypomagnesaemic tetany should aim at increasing the daily magnesium intake, particularly that of older ewes that might be rearing twins. Magnesium in the form of calcined magnesite or Causmag (magnesium oxide), sprayed onto hay, is an effective preventative measure, but unless sheep are preconditioned to eating hay it may not be eaten. In addition, all procedures such as yarding, trucking and droving should be kept to a minimum to reduce stress and lessen the chances of precipitating an outbreak of the disease.

When introducing ewes to lush feed, this should be done gradually and for a few hours initially. Shelter should be provided during cold, windy weather, either by grazing on undulating country or utilising sheltered paddocks. Attention should also be given to dealing with any concurrent disease. Parasite levels should be monitored and the ewes treated if necessary.

In some instances it may be necessary to seek advice on fertiliser use. Magnesium fertilisers may need to be considered and the use of potassium fertiliser should cease unless shown to be necessary.

In the UK, pasture sodium deficiency has been

associated with the occurrence of hypomagnesaemia tetany in sheep. This was probably caused by soil depletion of sodium following many years of cereal cropping in the country away from coastal winds. The reduced sodium intake induces a rise in potassium concentration in both the alimentary and the circulatory systems, leading to reduced magnesium absorption.

Phosphatic fertiliser toxicity

Aetiology and pathogenesis

Phosphatic fertiliser toxicity is most commonly seen in heavily pregnant or lactating ewes, and therefore it is commonly confused with the metabolic disorders. Sheep grazing pasture that has recently been topdressed with phosphate-based fertilisers such as superphosphate or diammonium phosphate (DAP) are at risk. It has also been reported in ewes that have access to fertiliser bins or sheds. In ewes, the major risk period is during late pregnancy or lactation (late winter and early spring), although there is the potential for toxicity to occur at other times. Toxicity has also been reported in lactating cows, goats close to kidding and deer.

The major toxic principle is believed to be fluorine, which is present at concentrations of 1–3% as a contaminant of the phosphate rock used in fertilisers. The fluoride causes toxic nephrosis of the kidney followed by severe uraemia and death. The role, if any, of phosphorus in the pathogenesis of the disease has not been identified. It has been estimated that 200–300 g of superphosphate would be sufficient to kill most sheep, although this will vary depending on the fluoride concentration in the superphosphate. It is not uncommon for secondary hypocalcaemia or salmonellosis to also be present.

Despite large quantities of phosphatic fertiliser being applied each year in New Zealand, fertiliser toxicity is relatively uncommon. Several predisposing factors are important in the occurrence:
- application of fertiliser in spring with little or no rain falling between application and grazing (it is suggested that at least 25 mm of rain needs to fall before pasture can be considered 'safe')
- grazing pregnant or lactating ewes, which have a high feed demand, on topdressed pasture
- high stocking rates and low pasture covers
- dew at the time of topdressing may allow fertiliser to adhere to the blades of grass, increasing the likelihood of toxicity

Other fertilisers have also been associated with toxicity. Basic slag, a byproduct of steel making that is used to raise the pH of acid soils, has caused deaths predominantly in dairy cattle but also in sheep. It has been suggested that vanadium toxicity may have been involved.

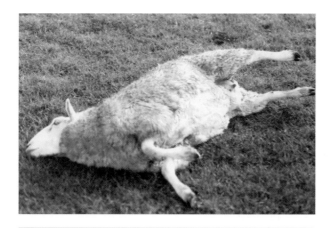

Figure 9.4 A seizuring ewe with hypomagnesaemia (grass tetany).

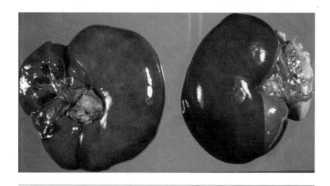

Figure 9.5 Swollen kidneys from a ewe that died of phosphatic fertiliser toxicity.

Clinical signs

Signs usually appear 3–5 days after exposure and include ataxia, muscle tremors, depression, thirst, diarrhoea and death. These signs are similar to those of hypocalcaemia, and because affected ewes may show a temporary improvement following treatment with calcium borogluconate it is important to distinguish between the two conditions. Often ewes are simply found dead, which again may be mistaken for deaths due to other metabolic diseases. The presence of watery diarrhoea may be mistaken for enteric salmonellosis. Mortality rates are typically in the order of 1–5% although on occasion can be as high as 10%.

Pathology and diagnosis

Necropsy findings vary, although a common finding is pale, swollen kidneys. Ewes may have reddened and ulcerated abomasal, and sometimes intestinal, mucosa and watery yellow-brown diarrhoea. In some ewes the liver has been slightly enlarged and pale with an accentuated lobular pattern, although this is not a characteristic finding.

The characteristic histological finding is toxic nephrosis of the kidney. Serum biochemistry of affected ewes almost always shows marked haemoconcentration due to dehydration, and uraemia. In some cases, hypocalcaemia and hyperphosphataemia are present. Diagnosis is based on the history, necropsy findings, histopathology of the kidney, and analysis of rumen or serum fluoride levels. Rumen fluoride concentrations of greater than 200 mg/kg are consistent with fluoride toxicity. Granules of fertiliser may be visible at the base of the pasture on which the ewes have been grazing.

Treatment

There is effectively no treatment for primary fertiliser toxicity. Treatment of clinically ill ewes for hypocalcaemia may result in a temporary improvement, but this will not alleviate the underlying kidney damage.

Prevention

Fertiliser toxicity of grazing livestock is uncommon compared with the amount of fertiliser that is applied annually in New Zealand. Pasture is more likely to be 'safe' when 25 mm of rain has fallen or at least a week after application. The most effective preventative strategy would be to avoid topdressing in spring, or to only topdress part of the farm and graze stock on the other part until the pasture is safe. However, for many farmers this may not be practical. Pregnant or lactating ewes are at greater risk, so keeping them on pasture that has not been topdressed until the rest of the farm is 'safe', or keeping them lightly stocked on long pasture, may reduce the risk.

Lactic acidosis (rumen acidosis, grain overload, rumen impaction)

In New Zealand, lactic acidosis mainly occurs in sheep that are suddenly introduced to grain feeding, or in sheep that are turned onto stubble where they rapidly ingest harvest gleanings.

CASE EXAMPLE

The following outlines a case of fertiliser toxicity. Note that the mortality rate of 12% is higher than would usually be expected.

On this property, DAP fertiliser was applied at 125 kg/ha by aerial topdressing in late August onto paddocks where 770 mixed-age ewes were grazing. No rain fell for five days following the application. The ewes had been set stocked about two weeks beforehand onto very short pasture and were due to start lambing at the time the fertiliser was applied. When the ewes were checked three days after fertiliser application, about 30 were found dead and over the following week a further 56 died, bringing the total number of mortalities to 86.

Serum collected from three affected ewes showed increased blood urea nitrogen (BUN) levels and hypocalcaemia. One ewe had hyperphosphataemia. The consistent postmortem feature from six ewes examined was pale, swollen kidneys. In some of the ewes the liver was slightly enlarged with rounded margins. In one ewe there was severe reddening of the abomasal mucosa and in another there were numerous erosions on the margins of the fundic mucosa. Histologically, the kidneys of all the ewes had a severe toxic nephrosis. In the livers there was varying degrees of cytoplasmic swelling of hepatocytes.

Aetiology and pathogenesis

The aetiology and pathogenesis of lactic acidosis has been studied extensively in cattle; for a review of the subject the reader is referred to *Veterinary Medicine* by Blood and Radostits. In sheep that suddenly become engorged from grain feeding, the grain is not digested properly but instead ferments in the rumen. High levels of lactic acid are produced along with other toxins, and these are absorbed into the circulation and produce a severe acidosis that ultimately ends in an endotoxic shock syndrome.

The smaller the grain, the more quickly the syndrome develops. Some sheep are natural gorgers and consume grain very quickly. It is these that usually become affected first and die.

Clinical signs

The severity of the clinical signs depends largely on the amount of grain eaten. In the first few hours after engorging, the animal will cease eating, become restless and show signs of mild colic. The signs usually become more severe, and depression, a staggering gait and even signs of blindness appear. No rumen movements can be heard and the rumen is distended and doughy. Occasionally there is straining and mild diarrhoea.

Sheep usually become recumbent and refuse to move. As the acidaemia increases, the body temperature falls and mucous membranes become pale and cyanotic. All the signs of acidosis develop with an accelerated pulse, a rapid respiration and severe dehydration. Less acute cases may develop lameness associated with laminitis.

Pathology

The main feature of the autopsy is the distended rumen filled with fermenting, undigested grain, which gives off an acidic smell. In some cases the rumen contents resemble watery porridge. The carcass is dehydrated and congested. The rumen mucosa may be reddened and often the epithelium strips off easily. The rumen pH, if tested, will be 4.0–5.0, depending on the time of death. Few live protozoa are seen in the rumen fluid, but massive numbers of bacteria may be seen in smears of the rumen fluid.

Treatment

In most cases of lactic acidosis the prognosis is rather hopeless, particularly when signs of shock have developed. Treatment depends on the amount of grain ingested and the time since ingestion. If ingestion has been very recent, then some forms of therapy may be helpful. Sheep that have not ingested large quantities may recover if moved onto alternative grazing or if food is withheld for a day to allow ingested grain to be digested. Mildly affected cases can be treated with fluid therapy and dosing with milk of magnesia (15 ml orally), which provides a good antacid that does not convert to a metabolic alkalosis if excess is given. The dose may be repeated every few hours.

In valuable animals, rumen lavage or ruminotomy may be attempted, although unless these are tried early in the course of the disease they are rarely successful. For further information on the aggressive treatment of severe cases of lactic acidosis the reader is referred to *Veterinary Medicine* by Blood and Radostits. Under New Zealand conditions, the treatment of lactic acidosis in sheep is generally an unrewarding exercise, and veterinary effort is better put into advice on the feeding of grain so that the situation does not arise.

The feeding of grain to sheep

There are many circumstances under which grain is fed to sheep, ranging from drought feeding to feedlot systems, winter supplementary feeding and the specialised feeding of pedigree sheep.

Sheep must be trained to eat grain well before the anticipated full use of grain in the diet. It is essential that the grain is either fed in long troughs with access for all the sheep in the flock, or by being dribbled along the ground over a wide area. Wet conditions naturally preclude the latter procedure. In areas prone to drought, some farmers may choose to pre-emptively train their young sheep to eat grain.

To bring sheep up to a maximum quantity of grain in their diet, about 3–4 weeks of training is required. Consideration also has to be given to the type of grain used. Oats are less likely to cause problems than wheat or barley.

For mature sheep, 50 g/head/day is adequate for the initial two days. This can be built up in 50 g increments every second day so that by day 10 sheep may be consuming 200–250 g/head/day. This is then increased to 300 g/head/day for 4–5 days after which time the feed level can either be maintained on a daily basis or fed at twice the rate on alternate days. Access to other feed such as hay or grass requires an adjustment in the amount of grain fed.

Anecdotally in New Zealand, it would seem a small proportion of sheep, perhaps 5%, refuse to eat grain and so careful management of the flock is required to identify these sheep and provide alternatives.

Exposure–starvation syndrome

In New Zealand, large numbers of sheep have died as a result of prolonged exposure to severe cold, snow and wind. Losses are often, but not always, associated with shearing sheep and releasing them into cold, windy weather. Similar losses have been reported in other countries. In July 1992, it is estimated that 1.5 million sheep and 74,000 cattle were lost in New Zealand during a period of inclement weather. Most ewes were some weeks off lambing and were without access to food or water for several days.

The main losses in New Zealand have occurred in the South Island and have often been associated with pre-lamb shearing in the case of ewes, or hogget shearing before inclement weather, particularly snow storms and blizzards. Usually the sheep have been yarded for a longer period than is desirable, and may have been several days without food. When such sheep are released into cold, windy weather, they will walk before the wind seeking shelter. Unless adequate shelter is provided they eventually reach a fence or other obstacle and collapse. Other sheep press in, and frequently whole heaps of sheep are found that have died from the exposure–starvation syndrome.

Critical factors in cold stress

An increase in metabolism due to cold will not normally be elicited unless the environmental temperature to which the sheep is exposed is below the zone of thermoneutrality. This is the range of environmental temperature where the animal does not need to employ thermoregulatory devices to maintain a state of homeothermy.

At the colder end of the thermoneutral zone is the critical temperature. This is the air temperature at which the animal must increase its heat production to maintain body temperature. Before this temperature is reached, vasoconstriction and alteration of the blood supply to the extremities, piloerection and change of body posture are sufficient to control body temperature. The critical temperature will be affected by the level of nutrition and the type and length of the fleece. It will also vary with factors that affect the coldness of the environment such as wind, rain and solar radiation.

A longer fleece not only lowers the critical temperature but also minimises the effect of a fall in temperature below the critical level. Further, increasing the feed of recently shorn sheep lowers the critical temperature from 39°C to 24°C but, in contrast to the effect of fleece length, does not affect the rate of heat loss below the critical temperature.

Once the animal is below its critical temperature, heat production will increase in an attempt by the animal to maintain homeothermy. However, the metabolic rate cannot increase indefinitely and eventually a summit or peak heat production is attained. In the presence of voluntary muscular activity, heat production can increase far beyond the limits of summit metabolism for short periods.

From a practical stand-point, apart from the newborn lamb the pregnant ewe is the most vulnerable to cold stress. A combination of the obligatory demands of the foetus on the blood glucose of ewes, high energy demand for heat production and a reduced energy intake lead to the following crisis responses:
1. The ewe's adipose tissue releases fatty acids and glycerol.
2. Muscle catabolism releases glucogenic amino acids.
3. Liver glucose production is impaired by fatty infiltration.
4. Diversion of metabolites into oxaloacetic acid is limited.

Eventually these crisis mechanisms are unable to meet the challenge, and death is inevitable.

Clinical features

Sheep normally face away from driving rain and wind, and walk for shelter or food. If these cannot be found they either drop from exhaustion or continue walking until they meet an obstacle such as a fence. As a result, in many of the losses recorded in New Zealand recently shorn sheep have been found crowded into the trap of a fence and frequently piled into heaps. Body temperatures are usually subnormal and the sheep are unresponsive to stimuli. The back fat of some sheep is firm and solidified even before the sheep is dead.

Pathology

A characteristic finding in deaths due to cold exposure has been the good preservation of tissues. The gut lining, for example, may remain intact for many hours. In some cases extensive haemorrhages may be found in the proximal two-thirds of the small intestine. Usually the liver is enlarged and pale tan or brown and the adrenal glands are also enlarged and haemorrhagic.

Sometimes subcutaneous oedema of the distal limbs has been reported. Pancreatic changes are commonly found in humans that have died from cold exposure and have been reported in sheep and cattle.

Factors predisposing to cold stress

Although prolonged low temperatures will induce cold stress, in practice the condition is usually brought about by the combined effects of adverse weather (wind, rain and snow) and a lack of food and shelter. In addition, as mentioned above, the pregnant ewe is at a further serious disadvantage.

Other factors affect the onset of the syndrome, including the time interval between the shearing and the inclement weather. In New Zealand, losses occur within 14 days of shearing but in general most losses occur within the first week. There is also a strong association between mortalities and the loss of bodyweight prior to shearing. Sheep that gain weight during this period show increased tolerance to cold exposure; hence, a good plane of nutrition is a help in preventing the syndrome.

Other important influences include the length of wool left after shearing, previous acclimatisation prior to bad weather, the time spent in yards before shearing, and the age and breed of sheep. Shelter from prevailing winds is also essential in preventing losses.

Treatment of cold stress

When confronted with a flock of sheep suffering from cold exposure, the main objective is to save as many as possible. Thus, available manpower and materials must be utilised to the best advantage. If conditions producing exposure are continuing, then priority treatment must be given to sheep that can still walk.

It is usually very difficult or impossible to drive sheep into a strong wind. Two alternatives are available: either move them downwind or truck them to shelter. Fences may have to be moved and sheep lifted manually onto transport. Snow presents further problems, as sheep cannot always be reached. It is worth noting that sheep with sufficient wool will survive under snow for many days even without food.

The rescued sheep must either be taken to sheltered paddocks, if they are able to walk and feed, or moved to sheds and covered yards. Suitable shelter may include tree lines, hedges, implement sheds, hay sheds, forestry blocks, or even warm gullies provided that these are accessible.

The first principle of treatment is to provide warmth, which is a considerable task with hundreds or even thousands of sheep. With such large numbers they are best stacked into sheds close together and covered with hay or old wool (crutchings, etc.) to trap heat of respiration. Sacks may also be used, as may any material, to provide insulation. Another suggestion is to fill the grating area of the wool shed with unaffected sheep. The heat generated from such sheep is quite significant.

Individual sheep may be treated with subcutaneous injections of calcium borogluconate or mixtures containing glucose, magnesium sulphate and calcium borogluconate. Warmed oral fluids may also be used to help raise body temperature and combat dehydration.

Some authors mention the use of hot baths to treat individual or valuable sheep but such are beyond the scope of most operations.

Although the results of treatment are unpredictable, sheep can be helped by the use of the above measures. Often animals that recover will crawl out from the stacked sheep and should be moved to sheltered grazing as soon as possible. Some recovered animals, particularly hoggets, subsequently develop pneumonia.

Prevention of losses from exposure

Most measures taken to prevent losses following shearing during inclement weather are commonsense procedures. These include watching local weather predictions and providing shelter and feed for newly shorn sheep.

Avoiding prolonged and excessive yarding at shearing is essential; in the event of cold weather developing, grazing animals should be kept close to shelter so that they can be moved quickly if necessary.

In New Zealand there is a renewed interest in farm

shelter and farm forestry blocks. These should be planned and utilised sensibly. In areas where losses from exposure are likely to be a risk (e.g. South Island high country), blade shearing and shearing with a snow comb are practised.

REFERENCES

Allcroft Ruth, Burns KN. Hypomagnesaemia in cattle. *New Zealand Veterinary Journal* 16, 109-27, 1968

Andrews AH. Effects of glucose and propylene glycol on pregnancy toxaemia in ewes. *Veterinary Record* 110, 84-5, 1982

Bailey KM. Experiences of cold stress in sheep. *Proceedings of the 23rd Annual Seminar of the Society of Sheep and Beef Cattle Veterinarians, New Zealand Veterinary Association,* 87-98, 1993

Blood DC, Radostitis OM. *Veterinary Medicine,* 9th edition. Baillière Tindall, London, 2000

Bruère AN. Biochemical changes in sheep under stress. *Proceedings of the 5th Annual Seminar of the Sheep Society of the New Zealand Veterinary Association,* Massey University, 32-7, 1975

Clark RG. The effect of cold and rain on adult sheep; pathological considerations. *Proceedings of the 5th Annual Seminar of the Sheep Society of the New Zealand Veterinary Association,* Massey University, 15-21, 1975

Cunningham IJ. Grass staggers and magnesium metabolism. *New Zealand Journal of Science and Technology* 18, 424-8, 1936

Ford EJH, Samad AR, Pursell H. The effect of trenbolone acetate on glucose metabolism in normal and ketotic sheep pregnant with twins. *Journal of Agricultural Science* 92, 323-7, 1979

Gibb J. Grain feeding sheep in drought. *Proceedings of the Society of Sheep and Beef Cattle Veterinarians, New Zealand Veterinary Association,* 91-4, 2014

Grace ND, Healy WB. Effect of ingestion of soil on faecal losses and retention of Mg, Ca, P, K and Na in sheep fed two levels of dried grass. *New Zealand Journal of Agricultural Research* 17, 73-8, 1974

Halliday R, Sykes AR, Slee J, Field AC, Russel AJF. Cold exposure of Southdown and Welsh Mountain sheep 4: Changes in concentrations of free fatty acids, glucose, acetone, protein bound iodine, protein and antibody in blood. *Animal Production* 11, 479-91, 1969

Haughey KG. Cold injury in newborn lambs. *Australian Veterinary Journal* 49, 554, 1973

Hemingway RG, Inglis JSS, Ritchie NS. Factors involved in hypomagnesaemia in sheep. Conference on hypomagnesaemia. *Proceedings of the British Veterinary Association,* Victoria Halls, London WC1, 1960

Herd RP. Fasting in relation to hypocalcaemia and hypomagnesaemia in lactating cows and ewes. *Australian Veterinary Journal* 42, 269-72, 1966b

Herd RP. Supplementary magnesium for the prevention of hypocalcaemia, hypomagnesaemia and grass tetany in sheep. *Australian Veterinary Journal* 42, 369, 1966c

Hughes PL. A cluster of cases of fertiliser toxicity in ewes in the Taihape region. *Proceedings of the 29th Annual Seminar of the Society of Sheep and Beef Cattle Veterinarians, New Zealand Veterinary Association,* 135-9, 1999

Hunt ER. Treatment of pregnancy toxaemia in ewes by induction of parturition. *Australian Veterinary Journal* 52, 338-9, 1976

Joyce JP. Thermoregulation by sheep in cold environments. *Proceedings of the 5th Annual Seminar of the Sheep Society of the New Zealand Veterinary Association,* Massey University, 38-44, 1975

Mavor NH. Clinical impressions in dealing with the post shearing exposure syndrome. *Proceedings of the 5th Annual Seminar of the Sheep Society of the New Zealand Veterinary Association,* Massey University, 47-52, 1975

McDonald IW. Ewe fertility and neonatal lamb mortality. *New Zealand Veterinary Journal* 10, 45-53, 1962

McNaught KJ, Dorofaeff FD, Ludecke TE, Cottier K. Effect of potassium fertiliser, soil magnesium status, and soil type on uptake of magnesium by pasture plants from magnesium fertilisers. *New Zealand Journal of Experimental Agriculture* 1, 329-47, 1973

McNaught KJ, Dorofaeff FD, Karlvosky J. Effect of some magnesium fertilisers on mineral composition of pasture on Horotiu sandy loam. *New Zealand Journal of Experimental Agriculture* 1, 349-63, 1973

O'Hara PJ, Cordes DO. Superphosphate poisoning of sheep: A study of natural outbreaks. *New Zealand Veterinary Journal* 30, 153-5, 1982

O'Hara PJ, McCausland IP, Coup MR. Phosphatic fertiliser poisoning of sheep: Experimental studies. *New Zealand Veterinary Journal* 30, 165-9, 1982

O'Hara PJ, Fraser AJ, James MP. Superphosphate poisoning of sheep: The role of fluoride. *New Zealand Veterinary Journal* 30, 199-201, 1982

Panaretto BA. Some metabolic effects of cold stress on undernourished non-pregnant ewes. *Australian Journal of Agricultural Research* 19, 273-82, 1967

Reid RL. The physiopathology of undernourishment in pregnant sheep with particular reference to pregnancy toxaemia. *Advances in Veterinary Sciences* 12, 161-238, 1968

Sargison ND, Mcrae AI, Scott PR. Hypomagnesaemic tetany in lactating Cheviot gimmers associated with pasture sodium deficiency. *Veterinary Record* 155, 674-6, 2004

Smith GS, Middleton KR. Sodium and potassium content of topdressed pastures in New Zealand in relation to plant and animal nutrition. *New Zealand Journal of Experimental Agriculture* 6, 217-25, 1978

Suttle NF, Field AC. Studies on magnesium in ruminant nutrition 9: Effect of potassium and magnesium intakes on development of hypomagnesaemia in sheep. *British Journal of Nutrition* 23, 81-90, 1969

Sykes AR, Feild AC, Slee J. Cold exposure of Southdown and Welsh Mountain sheep: 3. Changes in plasma, calcium, phosphorus, magnesium, sodium and potassium levels. *Animal Production* 11, 91-9, 1969

West DM, Bruère AN. Hypomagnesaemic tetany in sheep. *New Zealand Veterinary Journal* 29, 85-7, 1981

Zamir S, Rozov A, Gootwine E. Treatment of pregnancy toxaemia in sheep with flunixin meglumine. *Veterinary Record* 165, 265-6, 2009

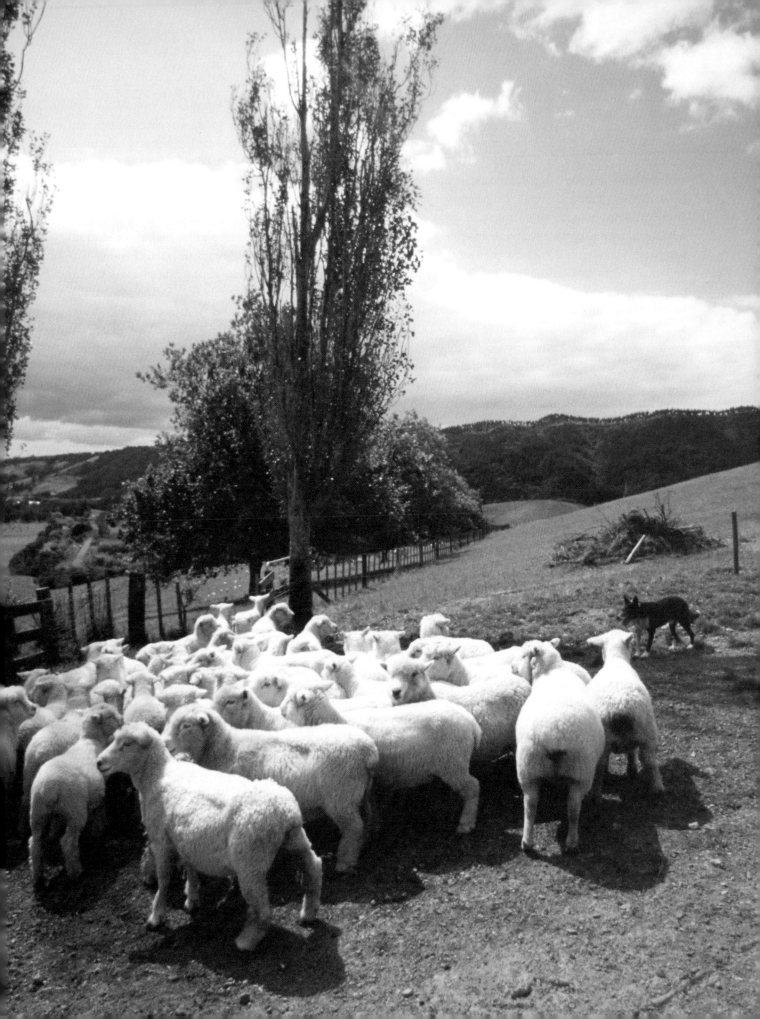

10

Poor thrift in adult ewes

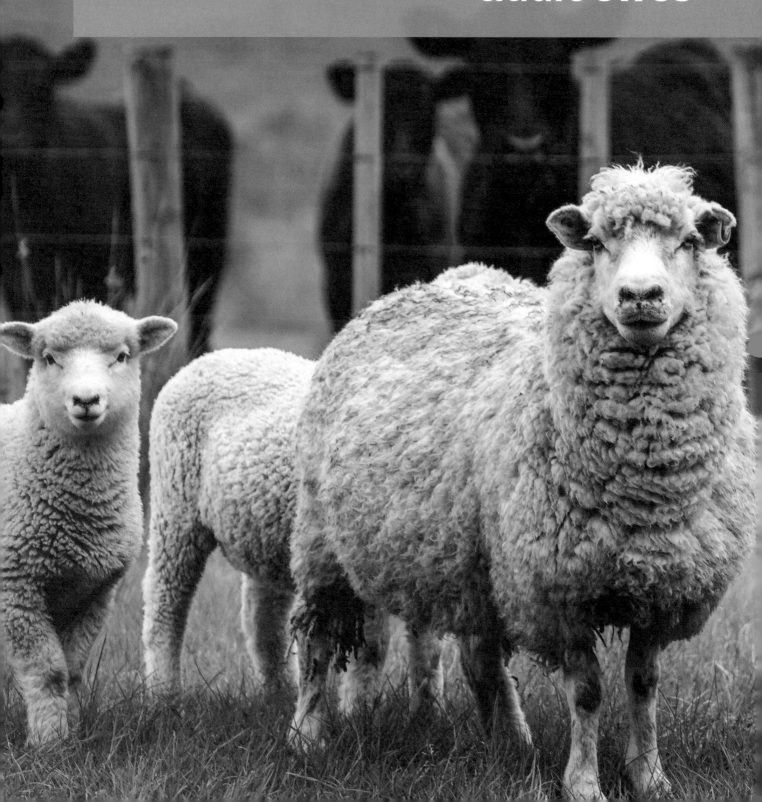

Introduction

The thrift of adult ewes, usually assessed by body condition score (BCS), is an important factor in achieving high levels of production in sheep flocks. The major factor influencing ewe BCS is nutrition, but a range of diseases including dental disorders, Johne's disease, gastrointestinal nematode parasitism, liver fluke and others may also have an impact. While poor BCS can occur throughout the year, poor thrift of ewes appears to be a particular problem during the winter period, presumably due to nutritional restriction and the demands of pregnancy in late winter/spring.

Mortality rates of adult ewes in New Zealand are not well documented, but are likely to range from around 3% per annum up to 16% or greater on some farms. The majority of deaths are likely to occur during the period from lambing through to weaning. Ewe mortalities represent a significant economic loss as well as being a welfare consideration. Preliminary data suggests that ewes in poor BCS at key times of year are more likely to die on-farm than those in better body condition, and so early identification of these at-risk ewes, followed by either preferential feeding or culling, may help reduce losses.

Body condition scoring

Body condition scoring is preferred over weighing as a method of assessing the thrift of adult ewes. This is because in contrast to weighing, BCS is not influenced by frame size, physiological status, wool length or gut fill. In sheep, body condition scoring cannot be done by visual assessment and it is necessary to use a hands-on approach by palpation of the lumbar spine region. Sheep BCS is assessed on a 1 to 5 scale with 1 being very thin and 5 being obese. A BCS diagram can be found in Chapter 6, Figure 6.5.

Body condition score and production

The relationships between BCS and production parameters have been reviewed by Kenyon et al. (2014). In general, poor BCS is associated with reduced production. The relationship for most production parameters is curvilinear, such that for each increase in BCS the relative production response diminishes. For many of these parameters, the most production gains are made from raising BCS from ≤2.0 up to ≥2.5.

Production responses associated with low BCS are listed below. However, it should be noted that for most of these parameters there have been inconsistent results between studies and this might be related to breed, study design, BCS ranges used and feeding levels.

- delayed start to breeding season, although this is a minor effect
- reduced ovulation rates, litter size and lambs born per ewe
- reduced conception rates and/or increased returns to service
- increased embryonic losses
- reduced pregnancy rates
- reduced lamb birthweights
- reduced lamb survival
- reduced lamb growth to weaning and weaning weights
- reduced ewe milk production.

There is no single BCS that could be considered optimal for sheep and it is important to recognise that increasing BCS comes with economic costs. However, it is generally recommended that the BCS of ewes should be maintained in the range 2.5–3.5. It is common for ewes to lose condition during lactation; however, at weaning their BCS should not be below 2.0 and post-weaning they should be managed to ensure that target BCS is met prior to breeding.

Body condition score and welfare

The use of BCS to assess welfare has limitations, but it is a parameter that is sometimes used to assess the welfare of sheep. The Code of Recommendations for the Welfare of Sheep in New Zealand recommends that adult sheep should be BCS 3.0–4.0 at all times and that urgent remedial action is required for any sheep that is BCS 1.0 or below.

Achieving target body condition scores

For optimal production it is important that ewe BCS is adequate during the breeding and lambing periods. However, it takes time for ewes to gain condition and therefore it is recommended that the BCS of all ewes in a flock is assessed at least 6 weeks prior to these critical periods. At the very least, all ewes in the flock should have BCS undertaken at weaning as this allows thin ewes to gain condition prior to breeding, and at pregnancy scanning/in mid-pregnancy as this allows ewes to gain condition prior to lambing. Ideally a further assessment would be undertaken prior to lambing and low-BCS ewes would be offered higher feeding levels in lactation.

Many farmers appear to be resistant to the idea of condition scoring their ewes, and either don't do it, score 'by eye' (which has poor accuracy) or only score a small sample of ewes. However, given that the greatest gains are to be made from increasing the BCS of thin ewes, it is highly recommended to use the hands-on approach to BCS all ewes in the flock with the aim of separating off and preferentially feeding those in poor BCS (BCS <2.5). These thin ewes may also benefit from anthelmintic treatment. Any thin ewes that do not respond to this regimen within 2–3 weeks are likely to have a disease issue and should be humanely euthanased.

Investigation of poor thrift in adult ewes

Firstly a thorough history must be obtained, including:
- time period over which the problem has occurred
- proportion of the flock affected
- whether specific mobs or age groups are more severely affected
- feeding history and stocking rate
- parasite control history (nematodes and trematodes)
- whether the sheep are home-bred or bought in
- history of facial eczema on the property
- previous problems on the property.

A distance examination of the ewes as a mob should be carried out, specifically noting issues such as diarrhoea, lameness, sub-mandibular oedema and other health issues. The thinnest sheep should then be drafted for a more careful clinical examination. In the live sheep, diagnostic samples may be collected if appropriate, e.g. faeces for FEC, serum for liver fluke ELISA and trace-element analysis.

Where very thin (BCS ≤2.0) ewes are present it is highly recommended to euthanase a number of the most severely affected for necropsy examination. Careful consideration should be given to the number of sheep that are necropsied; often a range of issues will be found and it is recommended that a minimum of 3–5 but preferably more ewes are selected.

Many of the causes of poor thrift in adult ewes can be easily identified by gross pathology seen at necropsy. If necessary, the gastrointestinal tract can be collected to perform worm counts. Failure to identify gross pathology, along with a suggestive history, may indicate that under-nutrition was the primary reason for the poor thrift.

Humane euthanasia of adult ewes

Veterinarians have the option of euthanasing ewes using intravenous pentobarbitone, but if the farmer wishes to use the carcasses for pet food or is unable to safely dispose of the carcasses then this is not a good option. The traditional farmer method of on-farm euthanasia of ewes is to cut the throat, including the carotid arteries. However, this method takes at least 2–8 and maybe up to 8–20 seconds to render the sheep insensible and, as such, more-humane practices are preferable. Use of a captive bolt gun to render the sheep insensible, followed by exsanguination, is recommended. Provided that the shot is accurately placed, this is a highly effective method of producing immediate and irreversible concussion. In polled sheep, the recommended shot placement is at the highest point of the head, aiming directly down towards the back of the throat. There are a number of reasonably priced captive bolt guns on the market and a firearms licence is not required to own or operate one. Alternatively a free bullet from, for example, a .22 calibre rifle can be used but it can be more difficult to accurately place the shot and this method also presents additional safety concerns.

Dental abnormalities

The productive life of a sheep is largely determined by its ability to graze. Throughout many sheep-raising countries, dental abnormalities have become an important reason for culling sheep. Premature culling has a major impact on the profitability of a sheep enterprise, and dental abnormalities, whether perceived or real, are important to the sheep industry. Unfortunately a degree of 'quackery' has developed within the industry where lay people pass judgements on sheep's mouths and dental position without knowledge of the special features of ruminant dentition. Therefore it becomes very important for veterinarians who service sheep farms to have a good clinical and scientific knowledge of both normal and abnormal dentition of this species.

It is common for farmers to examine the incisor teeth of their ewes and make culling decisions based on these. However, it is very difficult to examine the molar teeth of live sheep. Abnormalities of the molars often go unnoticed but can have severe effects on production, and any necropsy investigation of ewes in poor thrift should include removal of the cheek muscles and careful examination of the molar teeth.

Historical

In New Zealand the majority of sheep are still farmed on developed hill country. Many of the aged ewes from hill-country farms find their way onto lowland properties where they may be used for one or two more breeding seasons. Historically, the age of 5½ years (5-year-old ewes) is the time when most ewes are either sold for slaughter or culled for selling to lowland properties.

It has been stated by farmers for many years that excessive wear and tooth deterioration has been evident in certain parts of New Zealand since the early stages of the sheep industry. Barnicoat (1957), one of the first scientists to work on the problem in New Zealand, claimed that it had become aggravated during the preceding 30 or 40 years, particularly on the better-class hill country of the North Island. As a result, ewes were often culled one or two years before the 5-year or 6-year stage.

The rejection of otherwise useful breeding ewes on account of failing mouths causes a loss not only to the individual farmer but also to the whole sheep-farming industry. The problem, and it remains an unsolved problem, is complex and involves several 'syndromes'.

The original observations of Barnicoat are worth repeating, for they largely formed the basis for the research that has subsequently followed and serve to emphasise the multifactorial aetiology of the dental problems encountered.

It was commonly stated that unusually good mouths were retained by sheep on properties in the initial stages of grassing after the bush had been cleared by burning. This applied to the North Island, but did not fit the position in the South Island where some different dental problems have been reported. The fact that sheep's mouths were good when grazed on the softer native grasses was confirmed by the exceptionally good dentition of high-country Merino sheep of the South Island.

A number of developments in sheep-farming practices, resulting in greatly increased carrying capacities, have most likely contributed to the dental problems now encountered. These include:

- application of artificial manures, especially phosphates and lime
- introduction of European grasses and clovers, which largely replaced the low-yielding, fine, native grasses
- close subdivision
- close grazing and rotational grazing
- differences in chemical composition of pastures
- easily available feed, resulting in less dental exercise
- replacement of Merinos and other fine-woolled breeds by Romneys, and later the use of Border Leicester cross sheep
- heavier stocking rates leading to increased soil ingestion.

The cost of dental problems

The main economic effects of premature tooth deterioration can be summarised as follows:

- The overhead cost of maintaining the flock is increased. Ewes are sold one or two years earlier and may have given only two or three profitable lambing seasons. In addition, more ewe lambs must be retained as replacements so that each year fewer lambs are available for sale.
- Sheep with failing mouths may produce less wool and fewer lambs.
- Ewes culled at an early age may possess otherwise

desirable characteristics and are removed from the flock before they have attained their highest fertility. Hence, any selection for genetic gain is seriously affected.
- In premature culling, farmers may be forced to buy inferior replacement stock or retain animals for breeding that would normally be culled.
- Ewes with poor mouths may not be accepted by buyers as true-to-age, even if age marked. Ewes with failing mouths command lower prices than ewes with a 'sound' mouth and this point has frequently been voiced by farmers.

Dentition of the sheep

To understand the clinical aspects of dental abnormalities and be able to professionally advise farmers on their problems, it is important to have a full understanding of normal dentition. Veterinarians who become involved in sheep practice and deal with dental problems need to carefully inspect the mouths of many sheep of all ages to become fully conversant with the variations that are encountered. No amount of book description can adequately describe the complex nature of this problem.

Sheep have 32 permanent teeth distributed according to the dental formula:

| Upper | Incisor | 0 | Premolar | 3 | Molar | 3 |
| Lower | | 4 | | 3 | | 3 |

Strictly speaking, the fourth incisor tooth is a canine but as it functions as, and morphologically resembles, an incisor, it can be considered as an incisor for purposes of discussion.

In the lamb there are 20 temporary teeth, there being no temporary molars. The eruption times vary considerably, particularly in the permanent teeth, but Table 10.1 gives the average eruption periods.

Temporary or milk teeth

The temporary incisor teeth of the lamb begin development during the fifth week of foetal growth. Each tooth develops from a tooth bud that forms beneath the surface in the area of the primitive mouth that will develop into the jaws. A tooth bud consists of the enamel organ derived from the oral ectoderm which produces enamel; the dental papilla, derived from mesenchyme which produces pulp and dentine; and finally the dental sac, which forms the cementum and the periodontal membrane.

Calcification of the tooth is first seen at about 17 weeks, and at 21 weeks the first deciduous incisor enters the oral cavity. By birth the deciduous teeth have reached a relatively advanced stage of development and by 4 weeks of age the entire set of temporary teeth is functional.

The eruption of the incisor teeth occurs in two distinct phases, pre-functional and functional. The pre-functional eruption, which is the movement of the tooth from the jaw tissues towards the occlusal plane, takes place before the birth of the lamb. The functional eruption is the gradual exposure of the crown (after the occlusal plane is reached) by the separation of the epithelial attachment from the enamel and by recession of the gingiva. This process occurs to a small degree throughout the life of the sheep (permanent incisors as well) and partly compensates for the wear of the teeth. However, the former belief that the incisors moved upwards to compensate for wear has now

Teeth	Temporary	Permanent
I1	At birth or 1 week	1–1½ years
I2	1–2 weeks	1½–2 years
I3	2–3 weeks	2½–3 years
I4 (canine)	3–4 weeks	3½–4 years
P1)		
P2)	2–6 weeks	1½–2 years
P3)		
M1		3 months (lower) / 5 months (upper)
M2		9–12 months
M3		1½–2 years

Table 10.1 Eruption times of sheep's teeth.

been shown to be incorrect. The apparent eruption of the crown of the tooth is actually due to gum recession.

The teeth are considered to be fully functional when they have met their respective antagonists, which in the case of the incisor teeth is the dental pad.

The permanent incisors

The permanent incisor tooth tapers from a spade-shaped crown to the root apex with no intervening neck (the deciduous teeth are smaller and have a discernible constricted neck). Approximately a third to a half of the fully erupted incisor is visible above the gum margin as the 'clinical crown'. The unworn incisor may be up to 33 mm long and just under half shows above the gum as the clinical crown. It is postulated that the length of time a tooth lasts under conditions causing wear is dependent on the amount of tooth substance present. Permanent incisor teeth vary considerably in the amount of tooth substance in sheep of identical ages.

The eruption times of the permanent incisor teeth vary by as much as 8 months and care must be exercised when ageing sheep using teeth eruption time. The fourth incisor has the most variable eruption pattern and may be totally absent or displaced in up to 5% of sheep.

Before eruption, the two central permanent incisors develop in the jaw with their lingual (tongue) sides facing. As they erupt they rotate 90° into their final position. Although some degree of rotation may be seen during the development of the other incisor teeth, for the most part they develop in much the same plane that they eventually assume after eruption. The rotation of the central incisor has some clinical importance, since the process may not be complete as the tooth first erupts through the jaw. Since the eruption time is highly variable, it is possible that two-tooth rams or ewes are culled on this basis and adequate time should be allowed to give teeth a chance to attain a normal position.

The development and anatomy of the permanent incisors

The incisor tooth consists of a hard, mineralised enamel cap over mineralised but slightly less hard dentine, and a sensitive core, the pulp cavity. Before eruption the permanent incisor is almost completely formed within the jaw. For the central incisors, this process begins in lambs at

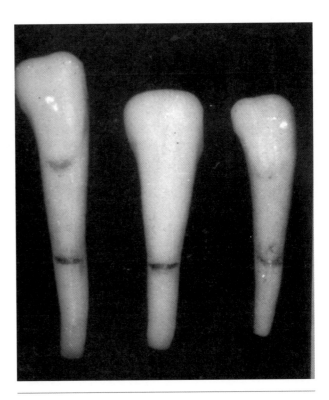

Figure 10.1 Dissected central permanent incisor teeth of sheep of same age and breed showing marked variation in tooth substance (from Barnicoat CR, 1957).

approximately 5 months of age and continues throughout the first 12–18 months. The sequence of events is: firstly, the ameloblasts differentiate; secondly, these ameloblasts induce the differentiation of odontoblasts from the dental papilla; thirdly, the odontoblasts produce dentine; and fourthly, the dentine induces the ameloblasts to produce enamel. This is a progressive process that begins at the tip of the incisor and moves towards the root as the tooth develops and matures. Once the genetically determined length of enamel has been laid down in the developing tooth, the ameloblasts cease to produce enamel substance. They still have, however, the important function of initiating the production of dentine necessary for the root. Root formation continues after eruption has started and in the molar teeth for as long as root elongation continues. Although the root of the tooth can in some cases elongate by perhaps 1–2 mm due to the deposition of cementum, with this exception the teeth of sheep are basically formed before or very soon after eruption and cannot grow after that time.

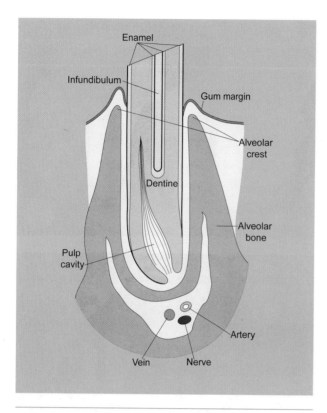

Figure 10.2 Diagrammatic cross-section of an incisor tooth.

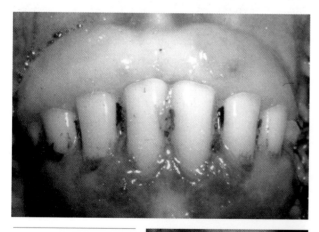
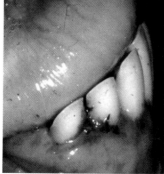

Figure 10.3 Anterior and lateral aspects of a good full mouth of permanent incisor teeth. Note the position of the teeth relative to the dental pad.

The incisor is held in place in its bony socket by the periodontal ligament, which in ruminants is very large. In fact, it is approximately 10 times the width of the comparable structure in humans. The wide periodontal ligament (membrane) allows relatively extensive movement of the incisor teeth (up to 2–3 mm), which is necessary as they occlude with the soft cartilaginous maxillary pad. It is important that this point is recognised during the clinical inspection of teeth in sheep.

Another important feature of the incisor teeth in sheep is that the alveolar bone in which they are socketed is constantly undergoing remodelling. A prominent radiographic feature of periodontal disease in sheep is the severe loss of alveolar bone that takes place.

The fully developed incisor tooth has a bevelled tip (occlusal surface) and is abraded to a flat surface biting against the hard dental pad, which develops corresponding shallow depressions. As the tooth wears, the pulp canal becomes closed with a hard plug of secondary dentine deposited by special cells of the pulp. This plug of dentine is usually stained darker than the surrounding true dentine and is often mistaken for decay. As the sheep's teeth wear further with age, tooth substance disappears and the teeth appear separated or 'gapped'. Eventually the teeth can become very small, mere spikes or pebbles with little biting ability. Finally the remnant falls out and the sheep becomes either 'broken mouthed' (one or more incisors missing) or a 'gummy' with all the incisors missing.

Permanent molars

The length of most cheek teeth and their snug fit within the alveolar bone means that these teeth are lost less often than incisors even when their ligamentous support has been destroyed. The periodontal membrane of the cheek teeth is designed to hold the tooth in place against the downward and lateral forces of cudding.

The molars are frequently black due to grass staining and this should not be taken as an abnormality. Less than a third of the molar tooth is visible as the clinical crown.

Occlusion

In animals with normal dentition the incisors meet the upper dental pad within 5 mm of its anterior edge, the position depending on the relative lengths of the mandible and the maxilla, the angles of the anterior incisors within their sockets and the length of the clinical crown. All three change with age. In the UK it is reported that the incisors drift forward on the upper dental pad with age. Our own observations in New Zealand flocks in which tooth wear is occurring is that the incisors appear to become more upright as the sheep age.

Franklin (1950) studied the effects of feeding grain to young sheep after weaning for periods of 5–8 months. The resultant calcium deficiency and imbalance in the calcium : phosphorus ratio resulted in a number of dental defects in later life, including:
- retarded eruption of permanent incisors
- overcrowding of the teeth in the mandible
- forward angulation (proclination) of the incisors so that they failed to register with the dental pad in severe cases
- defective enamel formation.

Recent research suggests that proclination, and resulting malposition of incisors, most often results from periodontal disease and is neither a highly heritable trait nor a prime cause of broken mouth as suggested in the past. The importance placed on subtle differences in the 'bite' of rams by breeders and other sheep farmers is misplaced unless prognathia and brachygnathia is severe.

Clinical examination

Sheep do not lend themselves to protracted dental examination except for the incisor teeth. These can be readily examined by retracting the lips without occluding the nostrils. Examination of the lingual aspect of the incisors and lower dental pad is possible by further retraction of the lips until the mouth opens.

Clinical examination of the cheek teeth can be performed with the use of a gag and torch, but is difficult. Palpation of the ventral and lateral aspects of the mandible through the cheek will detect gaps left by missing teeth or the presence of impacted grass around the molar teeth. More-detailed examination may require slaughter of a sample of sheep. To assist with record keeping, the list of terms (following page) used when describing sheep's teeth and jaws is given.

Excessively worn incisors

Excessive wear of incisor teeth is common in New Zealand

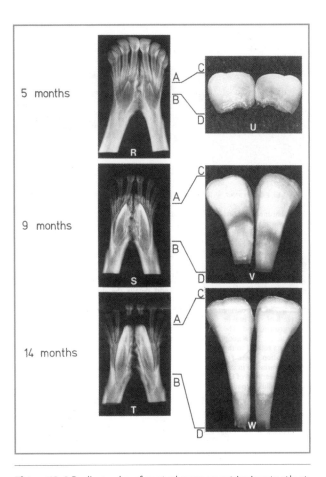

Figure 10.4 Radiographs of central permanent incisor teeth at different stages before eruption and the same teeth dissected at postmortem (from Suckling GW, 1979).

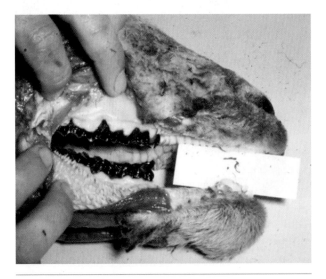

Figure 10.5 Permanent molar teeth exposed to show grass stain and irregular gum-tooth margin.

Terms used in clinical descriptions of sheep's teeth	
Brachygnathia	Lower jaw short relative to the upper jaw (undershot).
Broken mouth	The partial or complete loss of permanent incisor teeth.
Calculus	Calcified deposit on the tooth surface.
Dentigerous cyst (Odontogenic cyst)	Localised swelling of the bone (caused by a cyst containing an unerupted or partially erupted incisor).
Enamel defects	Hypoplasia — alterations in the surface of the enamel with a decrease in enamel thickness occurring as shallow pits, grooves or larger areas of missing enamel. Usually stained brown. Opacity — alteration in enamel translucency. Either white, or yellow, circumscribed or diffuse.
Excessively worn incisors	Labial incisor wall level with or below the lower dental pad.
Gum recession	Apical movement of the gum margin.
Gummy	All incisors absent or worn to smooth pebbles.
Long incisor	Incisor crown over 16 mm in height with a wear facet or a subjective assessment made by an experienced observer.
Loose incisor	Abnormal movement (e.g. greater than 3 mm) on the exertion of firm digital pressure.
Maleruption	Abnormality in the tooth eruption process, e.g. outside the normal age range.
Malposition	Deviation of a tooth from the vertical axis or rotation of tooth on long axis or eruption outside the arcade.
Pocket	Abnormal deepening of the gingival sulcus.
Periodontal or parodontal	Pertaining to tissues that support the tooth.
Proclination	Forward angulation of the incisors.
Prognathia	Lower jaw long relative to the upper jaw (overshot).
Retroclination	Backward angulation of the incisors.

sheep flocks, and in some districts sheep mouths are worn down to gum level by the age of 3½ years. This rapid wear of the permanent incisors is also reflected in the temporary incisors of younger sheep. On some farms the incisors of ewe replacements may be worn down to gum level by 12 months of age.

In some areas of New Zealand, tooth wear problems are endemic and it is rare to find a flock of sheep with 'normal' teeth. As with earlier investigations (Barnicoat, 1947), more-recent findings also point to the variation in wear seen between individual sheep of the same age and breed within a given flock. This variation has been measured carefully by some researchers and as an example the following quote from Barnicoat (1957) is pertinent:

1. During four years of use, central incisors of the better, unworn mouths lost, on average, 0.2 g of tooth substance and those on the poorest mouths 0.7 g, equivalent to average yearly losses of about 0.05 g and 0.17 g respectively per tooth.
2. Since the roots of incisors from 'gummy' teeth weighed about 0.3 g on average, the weight of useful crown remaining at five years varied from about 0 to 0.5 g.

3. The weight of an incisor at the initial two-tooth stage varied from about 0.8 to 1.3 g, a range of 0.5 g, which is of the same order of weight difference between the best and poorest teeth from 5-year-old ewes.

These variations in initial size of incisors may be an important factor in determining the duration of tooth substance. However, in practice the problem is not as simple as this and other factors contribute to this complex problem.

Aetiology

Since the problem of excessive incisor wear was first described, many contributing aetiologies have been suggested. These have included heredity, nutrition, erosion by pasture juices, the use of fertilisers and lime, mechanical factors, oral conformation, environmental factors, endocrine factors, premature eruption, soil abrasion, plant abrasion and soil solubilisation. Despite this considerable body of work, the precise aetiology of incisor tooth wear has not been found. However, a number of factors have been established and appear to be of considerable significance.

1. Soil ingestion

Abrasion due to soil ingestion has been generally accepted as the main cause of incisor deterioration in sheep. It has been proposed that the abrasive action of soil at the time of prehension results in excessive wear. It was shown from a study of farms in the Wairarapa district that the rate of wear on each farm was correlated with the amount of soil ingested, particularly over the winter period. Approximately 70% of wear was observed between July and October when the soil content of faeces was over 40%. Ways of avoiding soil ingestion such as rotational grazing or the provision of crops have been promoted.

It was found that peak soil intakes were reduced by up to 75% and tooth wear reduced by over 50% when supplementary feed was supplied for about 8–10 weeks over the winter period when pasture growth was low and animal appetite high.

The Wairarapa studies also showed that within a relatively close geographical area farms could be found that were classified as high-wear, medium-wear and low-wear. A more detailed study of those individual farms

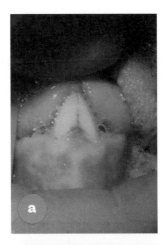

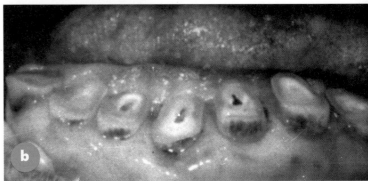

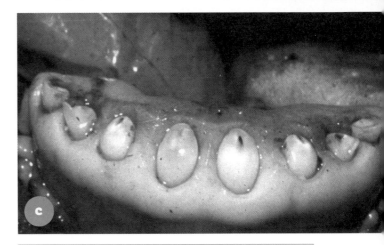

Figure 10.6 Tooth wear. **(a)** Mouth of a 14-month-old ewe showing severe wear of temporary incisor teeth and non-rotation of the permanent and central incisors. **(b)** Excessive wear of permanent incisors of a 4-year-old ewe. **(c)** Excessive wear of permanent incisors. Note pebble-like appearance of teeth.

suggested that soil type, earthworm activity, stocking rate and pasture improvement may all have affected the tooth-wear problems.

The Wairarapa work was a considerable advance in the understanding of the tooth-wear problem. From subsequent work it has been shown that the yellow-brown loams, yellow-brown pumice soils, yellow-brown earths, red and brown loams and brown granular clays are associated with low rates of soil ingestion and generally lower wear rates. Yellow-grey earths, recent soils from silty alluvium, podzolised yellow-brown earths and podzoles in general were associated with high levels of soil ingestion.

In Otago and Southland tooth wear has been found to be highest on yellow-grey earths with a low phosphorus retention.

However, the clinical picture of wear is not always typical of wear caused simply by abrasion. This was recognised by Barnicoat in 1957, who closely monitored the progress of wear in sheep grazing on improved pastures. The teeth were not observed to simply shorten from the top but to dissolve and 'wear' from the sides as well as the tip so that the incisors were eventually reduced to 'pebbles'.

2. Defective tooth development

Developmental defects of the teeth of sheep have been reported experimentally with nutritional deficiencies and excesses, parasitism and trauma. Observations by the authors on a sheep farm severely affected by drought in the autumn of 1983 indicated that defective tooth formation also occurs in the field and can contribute to rapid wear. On this farm many hoggets erupted central permanent incisors with enamel defects. Severely affected teeth crumbled away rapidly and were soft and chalky when drilled.

In addition, enamel hypoplasia associated with rapid tooth wear has been observed by the authors on a number of farms and more details are given later in this discussion. However, excessive wear also occurs in apparently normal teeth and differences in tooth composition do not account for the total problem.

Poor nutrition, be it due to a defective diet *per se* or induced as a result of parasitism, has appeared clinically and experimentally to play an important role in dental problems of sheep.

Teeth contain approximately 90% calcium phosphate, the main ingredient of apatite,[1] with many other minerals and micro-elements including magnesium, sodium, tin, fluorine, zinc, barium, iron, aluminium, chromium, cobalt, antimony, magnesium, gold, chlorine, bromium and copper. With the exception of fluorine, calcium and phosphorus, little is known of the role of other elements in tooth mineralisation. Protein, energy and vitamins are also important in tooth structure and formation.

Calcium and phosphorus are clearly important in tooth formation. Australian work demonstrated that lambs fed diets low in calcium and high in phosphorus, such as cereals and grains, had dental development problems even though their diet was corrected later in life. These problems were prevented by the addition of calcium supplements. Sheep fed an improper ratio of Ca : P developed abnormalities including delayed eruption, undershot mandibles, overcrowding of incisors and abnormal wear of molars.

The ratio of calcium to phosphorus may have significance in the development of teeth. The available calcium and phosphorus in pastures varies widely. Strangely, studies have shown that the sheep showing the greatest degree of tooth wear were often found grazing pastures with a high level of calcium and phosphorus. Paradoxically, the application of lime to some farms in Northland appeared to improve tooth wear problems.

The role of parasites may also be important, since interference with the absorption of minerals, in particular calcium and phosphorus, may result from parasite infestation.

The role of fluorine in tooth development is also poorly understood in relation to the major dental problems of sheep in New Zealand. Fluorine increases structural stability of the tooth apatite by replacing the $-OH$ group of the carbonate hydroxyapatite. Adequate amounts of dietary fluorine lead to more durable teeth; however, excessive fluorine intake causes problems in developing teeth or excessive wear along with pitting, enamel hypoplasia, discolouration, delayed eruption, recession of alveolar bone and gingiva, maleruption and misshapen teeth.

Mineral analysis of sheep's teeth from many parts of New Zealand has shown a wide variation in fluorine levels (28–320 ppm). Teeth with low fluorine levels showed no faster wear than those with 'normal' levels and there was no

---

1 A series of minerals of the general formula $3Ca_3(PO_4)_2, CaF_2$.

evidence of fluorosis in teeth with higher levels of fluorine. Defects reported on a number of farms in the Wairarapa in 1977–1978 (see below) were quite similar to those seen in fluorosis, but fluorine levels of bone of affected animals varied widely.

Other minerals, including copper and molybdenum, have been investigated as contributing to developmental defects of teeth but as yet no conclusive associations have been demonstrated.

3. Chemical attack

From observations of wear of incisor teeth in sheep on improved pasture, Barnicoat (1957) postulated that pasture juices may contain substances capable of dissolving teeth. However, he was unable to substantiate this hypothesis. More recently, Mitchum and Bruère (1984) proposed that acids in soil may dissolve teeth as it is recognised that citric acid from citrus fruit can have this affect. This solubilisation hypothesis has yet to be fully tested *in vivo*, but in conjunction with physical abrasion could account for the excessive rates of tooth wear observed in many New Zealand flocks.

An *in vitro* study on demineralisation and incisor wear demonstrated that sheep dentine demineralises in buffered sodium lactate solution at pH levels within the range of, or above, those reported for herbage and soil, in the presence of Ca^{2-} and PO_4^{3+} ions. It was concluded by Otago Dental School workers (Bloxham and Purton, 1991) that this sensitivity to chemical erosion might be a contributing factor to incisor tooth wear.

The solubilisation hypothesis suggests that two things must take place before solubilisation of the incisors occurs. Firstly, soil must contain high concentrations of substances capable of dissolving apatite. Concentrations of these substances are dependent on microbial mass and production, which in turn is dependent on food supply and other environmental factors. Sheep manure serves as a good source of microbial food and is present in soil in quantities directly related to stocking rate. Secondly, the incisors must contact the solubilising substances present in soil. Thus excessive loss of incisor substance is related to soil ingestion but is also dependent on soil content.

4. Genetic influence

It has been demonstrated that there is a significant inherited component to the rate at which teeth wear, and heritability estimates of 0.46 ± 0.13 have been suggested. Experimental studies have supported farmer and veterinary opinion that incisors of Border Leicester sheep and their crosses wear faster than Romney sheep, which in turn wear faster than Merino types.

The mechanisms for breed or sire differences in rate of wear are not known, but may depend on inherited grazing behaviour rather than differences in composition of the incisor teeth. Such differences in composition have not been demonstrated to date.

A study on the abrasion of incisor teeth from high-wear and low-wear farms conducted at Wallaceville Animal Research Centre by Erasmusen (1985) demonstrated only small differences in resistance to abrasion for the teeth of either type of farm. They also showed that dentine resists abrasion as effectively as enamel, but also pointed out that dentine has a much higher protein content than enamel and may be more susceptible to chemical erosion and possibly wear.

5. Workload

Heavier ewes and those rearing more lambs are reported to suffer more tooth wear, probably as a result of greater use of incisors to ingest grass. Because short grass is more difficult to ingest and more 'bites' are required, constantly grazing short grass is probably a major causative factor. Thus stocking rate may be modified to improve longevity of ewes in a flock.

6. Early eruption of incisors

Although premature eruption of permanent incisor teeth has been reported under occasional and extreme conditions of husbandry and feeding as described in the 'dental abnormality syndrome' in the Wairarapa in 1977–1978, there is little evidence to suggest that the eruption times of the incisor teeth have any significant relationship to wear.

Mineralisation of the central permanent incisors takes place from 5–7 months of age and maturation is complete between 10 and 12 months (300–365 days). While it has been shown that those sheep receiving better nutrition in the first year of life have earlier erupting teeth than those receiving poorer nutrition, the median age for tooth eruption in all breeds is beyond the stage when maturation of the teeth is completed. The estimated median age of eruption of the central permanent incisors for Romneys, Perendales, Suffolks and Southdowns have been given as 475, 465, 460 and 430 days, respectively.

Control

The aetiology and pathogenesis of this widespread syndrome is obviously complex and has defied clarification. In an effort to assist individual farmers to reduce the effects of the problem, advice has been directed towards achieving a high standard of animal health and growth and improved and alternative feed sources. The aim of these procedures has been to preserve both the deciduous and permanent teeth from excessive wear and provide a continuing range of nutrients for skeletal growth and tooth development, particularly in replacements from weaning until first mating. Measures such as careful parasite control, the application of appropriate trace elements plus the use of alternative feedstuffs can considerably improve the development and subsequent wear of permanent incisor teeth. The following steps are suggested.

1. Ensure that the permanent teeth of replacement sheep are well formed. These develop during the hogget stage, and attention to nutrition (including micro-nutrients) and parasite control is essential for this group. Every effort should be made to retain as much of the temporary incisor teeth as possible, as these might be important for the normal eruption of the permanent teeth.
2. Avoid overgrazing, especially at times when soil ingestion can be high, such as during winter and during summer and autumn droughts. Supplementary feeding such as crops or hay from covered racks can reduce tooth wear.
3. It is thought that shifting sheep daily or every second day during the winter onto clean pasture (not contaminated with soil) will reduce tooth wear compared with sheep that are set stocked.
4. Changes in the cattle : sheep ratio may be important to give better control of grazing and also more effective parasite control in sheep. Total sheep grazing in the absence of cattle has proved a difficult farming system to maintain for prolonged periods in New Zealand.
5. Genetic selection has yet to be proven to be feasible, but changing from the Border Leicester breed and its crosses may reduce the problem.

Enamel defects

Developmental defects of enamel result from some disturbance to the activity of ameloblasts during tooth development. These defects include enamel hypoplasia seen as pitting of the enamel, and enamel opacities in which there is a change in the translucency of the enamel.

Defective enamel formation in sheep has been associated with feeding grain diets high in phosphorus and low in calcium, parasitism, under-nutrition resulting from drought conditions, and excessive fluorine ingestion.

During the investigation of dental abnormalities in sheep in the Wairarapa district, mottling and pitting of the enamel of permanent teeth was found to be common, affecting in some instances up to 90% of an age group on a farm. The defects were most readily seen in recently erupted incisors and in many instances the abnormality became lost with time as the tooth became worn beyond the level of the pitting.

Within an age group such as two-tooths, the lines of pitting were often observed in the same place in recently erupted central incisors and in some sheep two distinct lines were present. This suggested a periodic insult altering ameloblast activity during the time of incisor tooth mineralisation, which begins in lambs between 5 and 8 months of age and continues until shortly before eruption.

Similar defects have been observed when recently weaned lambs were fed grain diets low in calcium and high in phosphorus. In addition, the dramatic effect of parasitism on calcium and phosphorus nutrition has been reported. Subsequent work demonstrated that enamel defects could be reproduced by infecting lambs 8–9 months of age with relatively high worm burdens of *Trichostrongylus* spp and *Ostertagia* spp. In addition, the problems of enamel hypoplasia have disappeared on farms once appropriate parasite control programmes have been followed.

In situations where enamel defects could arise from fluorine toxicity, such as farms in close proximity to aluminium smelters, the fluorine levels in bone ash can be estimated to confirm the diagnosis.

Defects of the enamel associated with fluorosis have been reported in some industrialised countries. The defects produced are usually much more severe than just enamel hypoplasia, and include other severe dental abnormalities such as delayed eruption of permanent teeth, brown discolouration of teeth, chipping and severe dental pain. In addition there are usually severe skeletal changes as well, characterised by marked lameness and fracture of a variety of bones. Fluorosis has been reported mainly in cattle.

Periodontal disease (parodontal disease, broken mouth)

Periodontal disease is one of the most common chronic diseases of humans and a common dental disease of sheep in Australia, New Zealand and Britain.

Earlier reports of periodontal disease in sheep described a condition affecting mainly the molars, characterised by inflammation and ulceration of the gingivae, food impaction and tooth loss. Other reports have described a periodontal disease that affected the incisors with an acute periodontitis, tooth loosening and frequent tooth loss.

It has been suggested that two forms of periodontal disease affect sheep: an acute form associated with an acute necrotising, ulcerative gingivitis which may affect both incisor and molar teeth; and a more chronic form affecting mainly the incisor teeth and resulting in eventual tooth loss. Whether these two conditions are manifestations of the one disease remains to be established. It has been noted that in sheep developing broken mouth, the severity of clinical gingivitis fluctuates with time and eventual tooth loss may be preceded by 2–3 years of chronic gingivitis interspersed with acute episodes of severe gingivitis.

Clinical findings

Periodontal disease is an inflammatory disease of the tooth supports, which includes the periodontal ligament, connective tissue, alveolar bone and gingiva around the tooth. The characteristic finding is long incisors that protrude in front of the dental pad, become loose and are sometimes lost. Pockets form around the base of the tooth and a variable amount of gingivitis is present.

The molars can also be affected, and when this happens the sheep may experience severe dental pain which may result in reduced grazing and weight loss. For example, in a necropsy survey of ill-thrifty ewes on a large commercial farm, chronic periodontal disease of the molar and premolar teeth was considered to be the major cause of ill thrift in 13 out of 120 ill-thrifty ewes slaughtered. In most

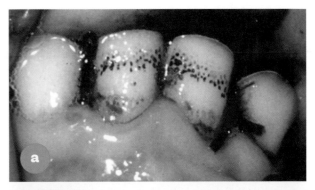
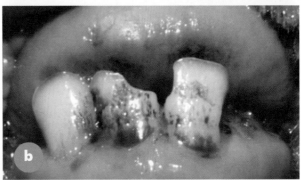
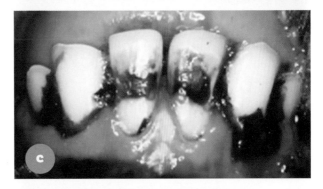
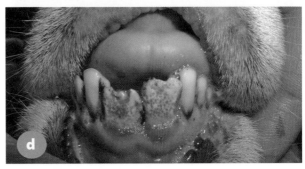

Figure 10.7 Enamel hypoplasia.
(a) Severe enamel hypoplasia with staining of tooth substance. **(b)** Severe enamel hypoplasia. Note fragile nature of central incisors. **(c)** Severe enamel defect. **(d)** Severe enamel defect as a result of excessive fluorine in the diet during tooth development. (Photograph courtesy RG Clark)

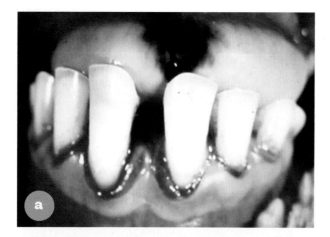

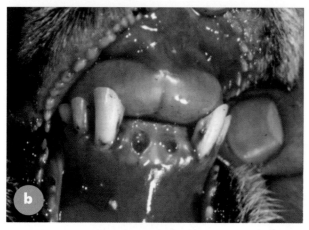

Figure 10.8 (a) Acute periodontal disease showing gingivitis. **(b)** Loss of loosened central incisors as a result of periodontal disease.

of these ewes, the tooth was loose with pocketing of the gum margins containing impacted plant material.

Aetiology and pathogenesis

The primary factors that initiate periodontal disease remain controversial and are poorly defined, but the pathogenesis of periodontal disease, like the human condition, appears to be associated with the progression of bacterial plaque-induced gingivitis which damages the attachment of the periodontal ligament to the tooth, leading to incisor loosening and eventually loss. This suggests a microbial aetiology originating in the mouth. However, this does not explain the geographical distribution of periodontal disease and its endemic prevalence on affected farms. Attempts to incriminate specific bacteria or to treat sheep with antibiotics for over 3 months (tetracyclines, metronidazole) have not been successful in confirming a primary bacterial aetiology.

The fact that periodontal disease occurs as a chronic problem on some farms and not others has led to the suggestion of nutritional factors that could result in degeneration of the supporting structures of the tooth, including the periodontal ligament and alveolar bone. A range of nutritional possibilities has been investigated, including calcium and phosphorus imbalances, low selenium, low vitamin D, high molybdenum and high vitamin A, and all have been largely discounted.

Most investigators who have studied periodontal disease in sheep agree that unknown farm factors and plaque-associated bacterial infection play a part in the development of the disease, although their inter-relationship is not understood.

A consistent finding is that periodontal disease affecting incisor teeth is generally not observed in flocks that suffer from excessive tooth wear. This suggests that short incisor teeth are less susceptible to periodontal disease, possibly because there is less mechanical force exerted on the supporting structures of the incisors. In addition, if the incisors are excessively long then, when the molar teeth are apposed, the incisors would be forced to move forward of the dental pad to allow the upper and lower molar teeth to meet when chewing takes place. This has led to the suggestion that trimming of the incisors would prevent the development of periodontal disease, but to date this benefit has not been demonstrated.

Control

As explained previously, the specific cause or causes remain unknown, but despite this there are suggestions for prevention, or even amelioration of early cases. These have included:

1. The shifting of ewes from lush improved pasture to unimproved land such as native tussock or rough hill grazing.
2. Not feeding root crops to ewes as this can exacerbate the loosening and precipitate the loss of incisors.
3. Grazing sheep at higher stock density, which may prevent periodontal disease. Presumably this would increase the rate of tooth wear.
4. Various methods of shortening the incisors have been suggested and used on farms. These range from the 'Caldow technique' in which an electric grinder running at approximately 11,000 rpm cuts the incisors level with the lower dental pad, to a milder technique in which 2–4 mm of the top of the incisors is removed, sometimes using an electric grinder at 5500 rpm, although the faster 11,000 rpm has also been used for this purpose. In Australia, tooth grinding has been used and it has been suggested that it should be carried out on ewes at 3–4 years of age to improve the bite of the animal and prevent broken mouth.

Tooth grinding has raised concerns for two reasons: animal welfare and efficacy.

1. **Animal welfare:** The potential for severe dental pain during and after the procedure and the potential exposure of the pulp cavity to infection has been studied in Australia. It was concluded that it was not a serious animal welfare problem, but the technique has been banned in Britain and is discouraged in New Zealand.
2. **Efficacy:** There is a lack of information on the effects of tooth grinding on flock productivity. In controlled studies in New Zealand and Australia there has been no significant improvement in bodyweight, fleece production and lambing percentage following tooth grinding. However, there is a cosmetic difference that may influence the market price of aged ewes and this is probably the main reason for the use of the technique.

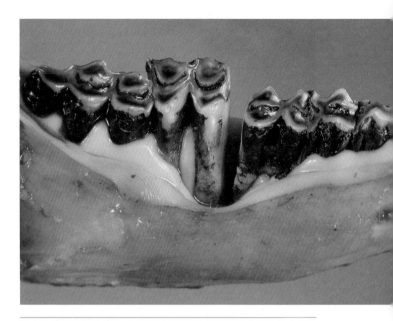

Figure 10.9 Gum recession and pocket resulting from periodontal disease of molar teeth.

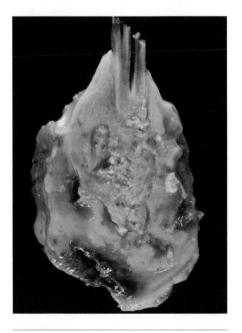

Figure 10.10 Molar tooth root abscess and osteomyelitis of the lower jaw resulting from periodontal disease. (Photographs courtesy KG Thompson)

Dentigerous cysts (odontogenic cysts)

Dentigerous cysts, although uncommon, have been observed most frequently in flocks with excessive wear of incisors, especially temporary incisors. They are also believed to be associated with feeding on root crops and have been reported mainly from the southern South Island of New Zealand. The jaw in the incisor region is swollen, and one or more teeth may be missing and the rest malpositioned. When radiographed, the 'missing' tooth is found to be unerupted and contained in the cyst structure. While an infective aetiology has been proposed, it is possible that these are an extreme form of malpositioning and maleruption.

Dental caries

Dental caries are rare in sheep, but they have been reported. The condition is usually associated with concentrate or root crop feeding and the condition resembles that seen in humans. Deep holes develop in the enamel, usually at the base of the tooth, which may snap off leaving a ragged stump at gum level.

Defects in conformation of the jaw

No problems encountered by sheep breeders raises more controversy than those arising over jaw definition. It would be reasonable to suggest that many immature sale animals have been rejected by lay inspectors on the grounds that the animal was 'undershot' or 'overshot'. In many instances, no consideration has been given for the variation that may be seen in 'normal' mouths (with respect to incisor teeth).

Incisor teeth projecting forward of their normal position are described as overshot, while those meeting the dental pad behind this position are undershot. The terms prognathia and brachygnathia are synonymous.

Undershot (brachygnathia)

The severe undershot condition is inherited and, contrary to the belief of most people that the mandible is the only bone affected, it has been shown that sheep with this defect have longer skulls (maxilla and premaxilla) as well as shorter mandibles than normal sheep. It has been suggested that the inheritance is under the control of several pairs of genes, both dominant and recessive acting in different ways in the development of the skull and the mandible. For practical purposes, if the tips of the incisor teeth are either 2 mm or less forward of the dental pad or 5 mm behind the front edge of the dental pad, the 'defect' is unlikely to be hereditary.

Seriously undershot jaws (Figure 10.12) are obvious from birth but may go undetected in a flock until after weaning, when the poor growth of the affected lamb or hogget usually makes it obvious. Perhaps surprisingly, some affected sheep appear to suffer no ill effects and grow at the same rate as their peers.

Overshot (prognathia)

This situation is less common than undershot jaw. It is also believed to be hereditary and associated with the development of the bones of the skull. In addition, both foetal and post-natal malnutrition may contribute to the fault.

Concentrated diets deficient in calcium may contribute to the defect, as seen in sheep fed grain alone. Hoggets

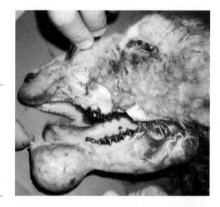

Figure 10.11 Dissected lower jaw of a 2-year-old ewe showing severe dentigerous cysts.

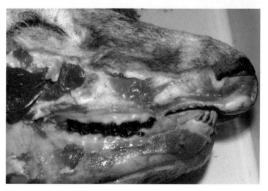

Figure 10.12 Severely undershot jaw of a ewe hogget.

grazing lush clover and ewes grazing sparse native pastures have been associated with the development of overshot jaws (see Figure 10.13).

Slightly overshot jaws tend to last (or wear) well, but the teeth may become jagged with wear and form spikes. This is associated with uneven attrition against the dental pad during eating and cudding. As the wear advances, the central incisors tend to wear rapidly and form a V-shape to the mouth.

Dental abnormality syndrome

A syndrome involving severe and extreme dental abnormalities has been described on individual sheep farms and occasionally on several farms within a geographical area. In most instances the severe dental changes are seen follow extraordinarily severe environmental conditions involving flooding, drought and severe food shortages.

The features of the syndrome have included excessive wear of deciduous incisor teeth, early eruption, maleruption and malpositioning of permanent incisor teeth, associated with osteopathy of the mandibular bone and the frequent formation of dentigerous cysts. Periodontitis of incisor teeth may be present in some cases, and excessive incisor wear and premature tooth-loss have been recorded in sheep as young as three years old. In some instances severe enamel hypoplasia characterised by pitting of the permanent incisors was also noted.

On some properties where the syndrome has been recorded dental defects of cattle have also been seen.

Johne's disease

Johne's disease is a bacterial disease of all domesticated grazing ruminant species. In sheep and cattle it results in chronic, untreatable wasting and death of a small proportion of adult animals. It is a difficult disease to control because the causative organism has a long environmental viability and a long incubation period. Further, apparently healthy sheep may still shed the organism and the currently available diagnostic tests have poor sensitivity, particularly in the subclinical stages of the disease.

History of Johne's disease in New Zealand

The earliest report of Johne's disease in sheep was in

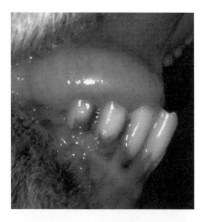

Figure 10.13 Lateral view of a sheep's jaw showing overshooting of the permanent incisors.

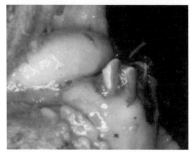

Figure 10.14 Lateral view of a severely overshot jaw.

Bosnia in 1908. It was first diagnosed in New Zealand in 1912 in a cow that had been recently imported. The first locally acquired case of bovine Johne's disease was diagnosed in Taranaki in 1928, but it was not until 1952 that ovine Johne's disease was confirmed on a sheep property in South Canterbury. The owner had observed the chronic wasting disease in his ewes over the previous 11 years. Ewes that were bred on the property were affected as two-tooths and onwards, the condition being noticed as progressive wasting until death occurred.

By 1961, nine years after the disease was first reported, it had been diagnosed in 30 more sheep flocks along the foothills and in coastal areas of South Canterbury. By 1970, 150 farms were recognised as having the disease, 70 in South Canterbury, 67 in mid-Canterbury, 10 near Gore, one near Oamaru, one at Westport and one at Hokitika. Many farmers had recognised progressive emaciation in their ewes for a number of years before Johne's disease had been diagnosed.

Johne's disease of sheep was reported first in the North Island in 1972 in Hawke's Bay, and by 1979 the disease had been diagnosed on 284 sheep farms. This information was used to predict the numbers of farms likely to be infected in 5-yearly intervals. The predictions were justified, and by 1986 a further review reported 759 affected farms, an even higher figure than expected. A study published in 2014 estimated the flock-level prevalence in New Zealand as 76%, although the average annual incidence of clinical disease is likely to be less than 1%. Until September 2001, Johne's disease was a notifiable disease in New Zealand but it has since been removed from the notifiable disease register.

Eradication of ovine Johne's disease is very challenging and is unlikely to be achievable in New Zealand, so the aim of control measures is to minimise exposure and therefore the incidence of clinical disease.

Aetiology and epidemiology

Johne's disease is caused by *Mycobacterium avium* subsp. *paratuberculosis* (*M. paratuberculosis*). There appears to be a strain that is adapted to sheep and a strain that is adapted to cattle, and thus it is possible to have one animal species on a property affected with Johne's disease while the other species remains unaffected. However, there is occasionally cross-species infection. Goats and deer may be affected with either strain. *Mycobacterium paratuberculosis* can survive in the environment for some months, and it has also been isolated from wildlife such as rabbits and stoats. The relative importance of wildlife infection in the epidemiology of the disease in livestock is unclear.

Mycobacterium paratuberculosis has also been isolated from some humans with Crohn's disease, but the association between the organism and this disease is unclear. The presence of *M. paratuberculosis* in a percentage of Crohn's disease patients may be that it is either associated with the pathogenesis of the disease or that Crohn's disease patients are more likely to be colonised by this organism. This unanswered question raises the issue of meat, milk and water contamination by *M. paratuberculosis* and public health. Internationally there is an awareness of this food safety issue and some countries have adopted a precautionary approach.

Transmission of the organism is predominantly by the faecal–oral route, either from contaminated teats during suckling or ingestion of contaminated soil, pasture or water. Infection *in utero* has also been reported in sheep and deer and the organism has been isolated from the milk of infected cows. It has been isolated from the semen of rams and bulls. Young animals appear more susceptible to infection than adult animals, and it is thought that infection generally occurs at a young age. However, because the disease has a long incubation period, clinical signs are not seen until later in life.

It is important to recognise that while a large proportion of young animals may be exposed to the organism, many clear the infection while a proportion go on to become subclinical carriers. These apparently healthy animals probably maintain the infection within a flock because they shed small numbers of *M. paratuberculosis* in the faeces. Some subclinical carriers eventually develop the full clinical disease.

In New Zealand, the annual incidence of clinical Johne's disease within most flocks appears to be low, with 0–2% of adult ewes per year showing clinical signs and either dying or being destroyed. In a few flocks this figure may be up to 4–5%. Merino sheep are reported be more susceptible than Romney-type sheep. This contrasts with other countries such as Australia and Norway, where in the past up to 10–20% of adult ewes have reportedly become clinically affected per year. In Iceland, the mean mortality rate was 8–9% annually and approached 40% in some flocks. Under completely different climatic and husbandry conditions, an annual mortality rate of 4% was seen in Cyprus. On individual properties, the overt incidence of clinical disease may vary from year to year.

Factors that possibly influence the flock mortality rates include:
- differences in virulence between strains of *M. paratuberculosis*
- differences in host susceptibility
- climatic factors
- husbandry factors
- nutritional stress
- concomitant disease such as gastrointestinal parasitism.

The relative importance of these factors is unknown and constitutes a gap in our understanding of the epidemiology of ovine Johne's disease. The high mortality rate recorded in Iceland was possibly due to a number of factors, including a susceptible population of sheep, housing animals indoors during winter, intimate contact between sheep from different farms and a wet, cold climate. It is also believed that close contact of sheep and their progeny at lambing has a major influence on the spread of the disease.

Pathogenesis

Following exposure, the organism is taken up by macrophages in the epithelial dome overlying Peyer's patches in the small intestine. Over time, small granulomatous lesions develop in the ileal Peyer's patches and extend to the adjacent lamina propria and villi, becoming locally extensive and finally generalised. Thus, a chronic granulomatous enteritis develops. There is also involvement of the lymph nodes and lymphatics draining the intestine.

Clinical features

Due to intestinal malabsorption, sheep in the clinical stages of the disease become progressively emaciated and, if they are not destroyed, eventually die. Clinically affected ewes may have sub-mandibular oedema and occasionally diarrhoea, although the latter is not a feature of the disease in sheep, in contrast to cattle. The clinical signs usually develop progressively over 2–4 weeks, with the ewes becoming more emaciated and lifeless. Until the terminal stages the appetite is generally maintained.

Clinical signs are usually seen in adult animals, with many affected ewes being over two years of age. The majority of clinical cases are seen during the winter, and this is probably because the stressors of pregnancy, colder weather and decreased nutrition precipitate clinical disease.

It should be recognised that a number of other diseases will also cause chronic ill thrift in adult ewes, particularly when nutrition is marginal. It is probable that within an infected flock, only a proportion of unthrifty ewes can be attributed to Johne's disease. For example, in one large commercial flock of 14,000 ewes, up to 10% showed progressive wasting each year and had to be destroyed. The farmer considered that this problem was due predominantly to Johne's disease, yet on slaughter of 120 ill-thrifty ewes only 18 out of 120 (15%) were found to have clinical Johne's disease.

It is unclear what production effects, if any, subclinical Johne's disease may have, but they appear to be minor. Thus the main financial loss is the constant wastage of ewes with clinical disease.

Pathology and diagnosis

The diagnosis of Johne's disease can be difficult because many animals that are 'infected' are subclinical carriers. For clinical cases, diagnosis is best based on recognition of the clinical features and postmortem examination. Lesions are usually confined to the terminal ileum, caecum, colon and associated lymph nodes. Characteristic postmortem findings include:

- thickening of the ileal mucosa, which in some cases can take on a corrugated appearance
- thickening of the intestinal lymphatics on the serosal surface of the ileum and caecum; these vessels appear more pronounced than normal and have pinpoint yellow/white nodules throughout their length
- enlargement of the mesenteric lymph nodes, which are diffusely pale and occasionally necrotic and mineralised.

The diagnosis can be confirmed by histopathological examination of the ileum and/or mesenteric lymph node. A smear of the ileal mucosa, stained with Ziehl-Neelson stain, may reveal red acid-fast organisms.

Faecal smears can be examined for the presence of acid-fast organisms following Ziehl-Neelson staining, but this test lacks sensitivity during the early stages of the disease due to low levels of shedding and intermittent shedding. Faecal culture is possible but is difficult because the organism is fastidious and slow-growing. Pooled faecal culture can be used as a flock screening test.

A number of serological tests including ELISA and agar gel immunodiffusion (AGID) have been developed. For detecting clinical disease these tests have a reasonably high sensitivity, but they have poor sensitivity for detecting subclinical stages of the disease. Other tests such as polymerase chain reaction (PCR) may be useful in sheep. This method has high specificity and results can be obtained rapidly, but its potential for diagnosis of Johne's disease is yet to be fully realised.

Worthington's (2004) recommendations for the diagnosis of this disease provide a sound but complex basis to follow: 'Diagnosis of infected flocks is easier than the diagnosis in an individual animal. When the objective is to identify non-infected flocks and maintain them free from the disease an appropriate combination of cell-mediated immune (CMI) tests, culture or PCR, absorbed ELISA and histological examination in culled animals should be confirmed by re-testing and the use of highly specific methods. If the purchase of non-infected animals is important, they should be acquired from flocks identified as free from infection.'

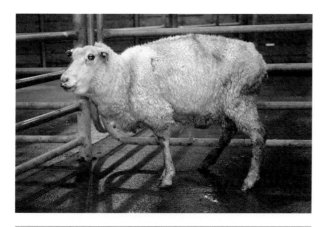

Figure 10.15 Sheep affected with Johne's disease. Note the emaciation, bottle jaw and diarrhoea.

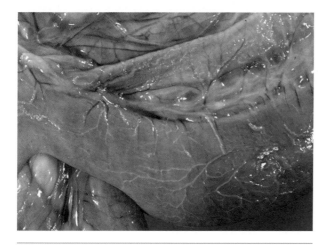

Figure 10.16 Enlargement of the lymphatics over the ileum and caecum of a ewe with Johne's disease. (Photographs courtesy KG Thompson)

Production losses from Johne's disease

There is a lack of information on the size of the production losses caused by this disease. It is currently believed that Johne's disease does not cause large economic losses to the New Zealand cattle and sheep industries, relative to the value of these industries. However, there are reports of the disease causing production losses in deer herds, where significant numbers of deaths of 8- to 15-month-old animals have been caused by Johne's disease. In contrast, clinical Johne's disease in sheep and cattle is rare in animals less than 2 years of age.

It should also be emphasised that on individual sheep farms where Johne's disease is endemic, the constant loss of a small number of fading pregnant ewes each year can become a depressing annoyance to the flock owner.

Control

As stated previously, the control of Johne's disease is not straightforward. The reasons for this must be emphasised:
- Johne's disease has a long incubation period.
- Most infected animals are subclinical cases.
- Infection spreads before it is detected.
- Diagnostic tests have variable sensitivity.
- Prevalence is always underestimated.
- Losses are minor until infection is well established and the benefits of control may be difficult to explain to some farmers.
- The organism has a long environmental viability.

Therefore, control programmes may reduce the levels of infection to some extent but will not result in eradication of the disease. Because of the high prevalence of infection in New Zealand, and the relatively low incidence of clinical disease within each flock, the emphasis is on controlling the disease rather than trying to eradicate it. Control measures that have been advocated include identifying and eliminating infected animals, hygiene and husbandry measures, grazing management and vaccination.

Identifying and eliminating infected animals

Under all circumstances, suspected cases of Johne's disease should be removed from the flock before lambing commences because this is likely to be a time when the spread of the disease is at a peak. Ewes suspected of having Johne's disease should be separated out from the flock and if they do not respond to anthelmintic treatment and better feeding, they should be destroyed. It may not be practical to rear replacements on a heavily infected property.

Most importing countries require certification of freedom from Johne's disease for sheep importations.

Hygiene and husbandry

Attention to areas where faecal contamination is heavy may be useful in reducing the levels of exposure to the organism. This may include placing water troughs in higher positions, fencing areas of dams that are contaminated and muddy, and avoiding lambing in wet, dirty paddocks.

Ensuring good animal health through effective parasite control, control of other diseases such as facial eczema and providing adequate nutrition may help in reducing the levels of clinical disease.

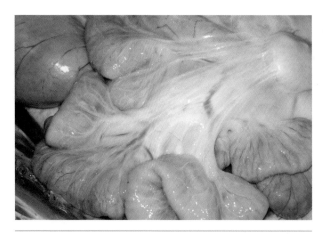

Figure 10.17 Terminal ileum with marked lymphadenitis. Note enlarged mesenteric lymph node.

Grazing management

The reduction of pasture contamination by *M. paratuberculosis* and hence the exposure of young, susceptible animals to the causative organism has been well studied in Australia. The suggested recommendations from this work may be hard to adopt in their entirety in New Zealand, but they are a guide to grazing management that could be helpful in controlling Johne's disease. They are:

- Produce low-contamination pastures by removing infected adult sheep for as long as possible, preferably over summer. Leave pastures ungrazed, or grazed by adult cattle or unaffected sheep.
- Use a narrow joining period so that lambs are born in a tight period and weaning is not delayed. Remove clinically affected (low condition score) ewes before lambing and again at marking. Move the lambing flock onto low-contamination pasture before lambing and use a low stocking rate.
- Wean lambs as early as possible, which can be when the youngest are 7 weeks old, provided that pastures are highly nutritious. If low-contamination pastures are scarce it is more important to use them for weaning rather than lambing.
- Leave weaned lambs in the low-challenge environment for as long as possible. These paddocks will remain low risk because the weaner sheep are expected to shed very few *M. paratuberculosis* in their first year of life.

Other steps that can be taken to reduce transmission rates include avoidance of very high stocking rates, and use of rotational grazing with sufficient time between rotations to allow die-off of *M. paratuberculosis*. Spells of one month during summer are beneficial to reduce viable counts of *M. paratuberculosis* in the environment and should reduce the impact of ovine Johne's disease.

Vaccination

In New Zealand a *M. paratuberculosis* vaccine is available. It is an inactivated vaccine of the organism adjuvanted with mineral oil in a multiple emulsion (Gudair®; Zoetis New Zealand Ltd). Because clinical Johne's disease is a disease of adult sheep, only replacement ewes should be vaccinated. In most New Zealand flocks vaccination is done at weaning or soon after, when replacement ewe lambs have been selected. However, vaccination of older sheep may in some cases be warranted. Only a single dose of vaccine is required.

All vaccinated sheep must be earmarked (permanently identified). After vaccination, a firm swelling usually develops at the injection site (subcutaneously behind the ear) and may become bigger than 5 cm in diameter. Also, when some infected animals are injected the vaccine may cause a secondary immune response with an even more intense reaction; thus, vaccination requires particular care. The vaccination site lesions can persist for long periods of time and the local lymph nodes may also contain lesions, some of which contain oil droplets from the vaccine adjuvant and acid-fast organisms that could be confused with tuberculosis lesions. Because vaccinated animals are permanently identified, the meatworks must be notified before they are sent for slaughter.

Human safety is important in the use of this vaccine, as accidental self-injection can result in severe tissue damage and a painful injury. However, in spite of the caution required in using Johne's vaccine and the fact that it does not prevent infection *per se*, in most cases it does prevent clinical disease. In one flock of 3000 Romney sheep surveyed by Massey University veterinarians, there was an incidence of approximately 100 cases of Johne's disease per year. Following six years of vaccine use in the ewe lambs, clinical cases of the disease had disappeared from the flock. Australian studies have shown that vaccination reduces the shedding of *M. paratuberculosis* in the faeces by up to 90% and a reduction of flock mortalities also by 90%.

As stated, in New Zealand the within-flock incidence of clinical Johne's disease appears to be low, of the order of < 1% per annum. In some flocks it may be higher. Therefore, before embarking on a vaccination programme in a flock, very careful consideration should be given to the possible benefits. Modelling studies have suggested that a clinical incidence needs to be ≥2% before vaccination is cost-effective, but some farmers with lower clinical incidence may choose to vaccinate due to the distress caused by seeing clinically affected sheep.

Small-intestinal carcinoma

Small-intestinal carcinoma is a relatively common cancer of adult sheep in New Zealand. Abattoir surveys of ewes in New Zealand in the late 1960s found 1.25% of British-bred ewes and 0.24% of fine-wool ewes affected. The condition has also been reported in Australia and the UK. The cause is unknown.

Clinical features

The characteristic clinical signs are chronic wasting progressing to emaciation and death in adult ewes. These signs are easily confused with other conditions causing ill thrift in this age group.

Diagnosis and pathology

A diagnosis of small-intestinal carcinoma is made on postmortem examination. The lesion may affect any part of the jejunum and ileum, and the gross appearance of these lesions is variable. They generally appear as a dense white ring of fibrous tissue encircling the intestine, with thickening of the mucosal and muscle layers at the primary site causing constriction of the intestinal lumen. Large sections of the intestine may be involved. The tumours metastasise to the local lymph nodes and liver, but can also implant on the serosal surfaces of other abdominal viscera. Histological examination of affected tissue reveals heavy infiltration of the mucosa and submucosa with fibrous tissue, and disruption of the glandular structure'.

Gastrointestinal nematode parasitism

While adult ewes are generally considered relatively immune to nematode parasitism, high faecal egg counts and high worm counts are a common finding in thin ewes. Necropsy studies and worm counts of thin ewes performed at Massey University have frequently found high worm counts with a large range of genera present. It is unclear whether the nematode parasites are a cause or

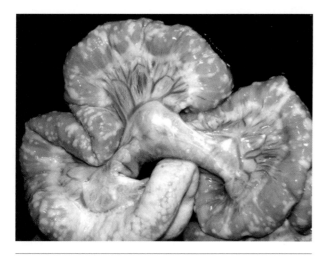

Figure 10.18 Small-intestine carcinoma.

a consequence of the poor thrift, but nevertheless in the management of thin ewes it is recommended to treat them with an effective anthelmintic along with increasing their nutrition. While the correlation between FEC and adult worm burden is not as strong in adult sheep as it is in lambs, FEC can still be a useful tool in the investigation of poor thrift in ewes provided that the results are interpreted with caution and in light of the history and clinical findings. See also Chapter 8.

Liver fluke; chronic fascioliasis

Adult liver fluke (*Fasciola hepatica*) live in the bile ducts of adult sheep and can cause poor thrift (see Chapter 8). Clinical signs are usually seen during the autumn and winter, and affected sheep have loss of BCS, anorexia, anaemia and sometimes submandibular oedema. At necropsy there is varying degrees of hepatic fibrosis and bile-duct thickening along with compensatory hepatic hypertrophy. Liver fluke may be found within the bile ducts. As this is a treatable condition, it is important to rule it in or out during any investigation of poor thrift in adult ewes.

Facial eczema

Facial eczema often results in damage to the liver with subsequent fibrosis (see Chapter 18). Some degree of liver regeneration may occur, but in severe cases the amount of remaining functional liver tissue is much reduced. While the production effects of chronic liver damage due to facial eczema have not been quantified, it is likely that, particularly during times of nutritional or physiological stress, affected sheep are likely to lose BCS. For example, 120 thin ewes were necropsied on a large commercial property with a severe poor-thrift issue in their adult ewes. Chronic liver damage due to facial eczema was considered to be the primary reason for poor thrift in 30% (36/120) of the ewes.

Lung abscesses

Enzootic pneumonia is common in New Zealand lambs, particularly in the warmer northern regions (see Chapter 6). In most cases the lesions largely resolve by adulthood, but on occasion abscesses are found in the lungs of thin ewes and are considered to be the primary reason for poor

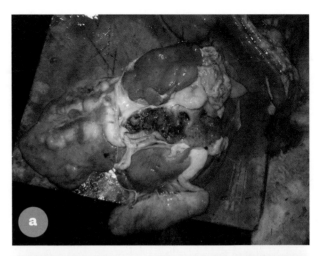

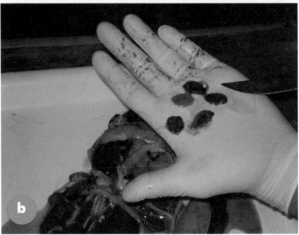

Figure 10.19 (a) A deformed liver due to chronic fascioliasis. **(b)** Adult liver fluke from the bile ducts.

thrift. On rare occasions these abscesses may rupture, resulting in death.

Lameness

Any condition that affects the ability of a ewe to graze will result in loss of BCS, particularly if nutritional levels are at maintenance levels or below, such as during winter rotational grazing. Lameness can be due to a variety of reasons, but is most usually due to lesions in the foot (see Chapter 11). On occasion, severely overgrown hooves have been noted to cause lameness sufficient to result in poor thrift.

REFERENCES

INTRODUCTION

Gibson TJ, Ridler AL, Lamb CR, Williams A, Giles S, Gregory NG. Preliminary evaluation of the effectiveness of captive-bolt guns as a killing method without exsanguination for horned and unhorned sheep. *Animal Welfare* 21 (S2), 35-42, 2012

Johnson CB, Mellor DJ, Hemsworth PH, Fisher AD. A scientific comment on the welfare of domesticated ruminants slaughtered without stunning. *New Zealand Veterinary Journal* 63, 58-65, 2015

Kenyon PR, Maloney SK, Blache D. Review of sheep body condition score in relation to production characteristics. *New Zealand Journal of Agricultural Research* 57, 38-64, 2014

Ridler AL, Griffiths KJ. Improving the welfare of ewes. *Achieving sustainable production of sheep*, edited by Greyling J. Burleigh Dodds Science Publishing, Cambridge UK, 2017

DENTAL ABNORMALITIES

Armstrong MC. Paradontal disease of sheep in South Canterbury. *New Zealand Journal of Agriculture* 100, 429-31, 1960

Baker JR, Britt DP. Dental calculus and periodontal disease in sheep. *Veterinary Record* 115, 411-12, 1984

Barnicoat CR. Some results of surveys of the problem of wear in sheep teeth. *Proceedings of 10th Annual Meeting of Sheep Farmers*, Massey College, 98-101, 1947

Barnicoat CR. Wear in sheep's teeth. *New Zealand Journal of Science and Technology* 38, 583-632, 1957

Barnicoat CR. Wear in sheep's teeth. *New Zealand Journal of Agricultural Research* 2, 1025-40, 1959

Barnicoat CR. Mechanism of hard tissue destruction. *American Association for the Advancement of Sciences Publication* 75, 155-70, 1963

Benzie D, Cresswell E. Studies of the dentition of sheep. IV. Radiological studies from investigations into the shedding of permanent incisor teeth by hill sheep. *Research in Veterinary Science* 3, 416-28, 1962

Bircham JS, Crouchley G, Aitken MW. Effects of superphosphate, lime and stocking rate on pasture and animal production on the Wairarapa plains. *New Zealand Journal of Experimental Agriculture* 9, 69-72, 1981

Bloxham GP, Purton DG. Demineralisation and incisor wear: An in vitro study. *New Zealand Journal of Agricultural Research* 34, 277-9, 1991

Bruère AN, West DM, Orr MB, O'Callaghan MW. A syndrome of dental abnormalities of sheep: 1. Clinical aspects on a commercial sheep farm in the Wairarapa. *New Zealand Veterinary Journal* 27, 152-8, 1979

Cocquyt G, Driessen B, Simoens P. Variability in the eruption of the permanent incisor teeth of sheep. *Veterinary Record* 157, 619-23, 2005

Coop IE, Clark VR. The influence of method of rearing as hoggets on the lifetime productivity of sheep. *New Zealand Journal of Science and Technology* 35A, 214-28, 1955

Cutress TW. Histopathology of periodontal disease in sheep. *Journal of Periodontal Research* 47, 643-50, 1976

Cutress TW, Healy WB. Wear of sheep's teeth. II. Effects of pasture juices on dentine. *New Zealand Journal of Agricultural Research* 8, 753-62, 1965

Cutress TW, Suckling GW, Healy WB, Mattingley J, Aitken WM. Periodontal disease in sheep. II. The composition of sera from sheep with periodontosis. *Journal of Periodontal Research* 43, 668-76, 1972

Duckworth J, Hill R, Benzie D, Dalgarno AC, Robinson JF. Studies of the dentition of sheep. 1. Clinical observations from investigations into the shedding of permanent incisor teeth by hill sheep. *Research in Veterinary Science* 3, 1-17, 1962

Erasmuson AF. Abrasion of ovine teeth from high-wear and low-wear farms. *New Zealand Journal of Agricultural Research* 28, 225-31, 1985

Franklin MC. Diet and dental development in the sheep. Bulletin No. 252, *Australian Commonwealth Scientific and Research Organisation*, Melbourne, Australia, 1950

Frisken KW, Laws AJ, Tagg JR, Orr MB. Environmental influences on the progression of clinical and microbiological parameters of sheep periodontal disease. *Research in Veterinary Science* 46, 147-52, 1989

Gardner DG, Orr MB. Dentigerous cysts (ovine odontogenic cysts) in sheep. *New Zealand Veterinary Journal* 38, 148-50, 1990

Gunn GR. The effects of calcium and phosphorus supplementation on the performance of Scottish Blackface hill ewes, with particular reference to the premature loss of permanent incisor teeth. *Journal of Agricultural Science, Cambridge* 72, 371-8, 1969

Gunn RG. A note on the effect of broken mouth on the performance of Scottish Blackface hill ewes. *Animal Production* 12, 517-20, 1970

Hart KE, Mackinnon MM. Enzootic paradontal disease of adult teeth in the Bulls-Santoft area. *New Zealand Veterinary Journal* 6, 118-23, 1958

Hatt SD. The development of the deciduous incisor in the sheep. *Research in Veterinary Science* 8, 143-50, 1967

Healy WB, Ludwig TG. Wear of sheep's teeth. 1. The role of ingested soil. *New Zealand Journal of Agricultural Research* 8, 737-52, 1965

Healy WB, Cutress TW, Michie C. Wear of sheep's teeth. IV. Reduction of soil ingestion and tooth wear by supplementary feeding. *New Zealand Journal of Agricultural Research* 10, 201-9, 1967

Hindson JC. Trimming sheep teeth. *Veterinary Record* 118, 706, 1986

Krook L, Maylin GA. Industrial fluoride pollution. Chronic fluoride poisoning in Cornwall Island cattle. Supplement B, *Cornell Veterinarian* 69, 1979

Ludwig TG, Healy WB, Cutress TW. Wear of sheep's teeth. III. Seasonal variation in wear and ingested soil. *New Zealand Journal of Agricultural Research* 9, 157-64, 1965

McGregor BA. Incisor development, wear and loss in sheep and their impact on ewe production, longevity and economics: A review. *Small Ruminant Research* 95, 79-87, 2011

Mackinnon MM. A pathological study of an enzootic paradontal disease of mature sheep. *New Zealand Veterinary Journal* 7, 18-26, 1959

McRoberts MR, Hill R, Dalgarno AC. The effects of diets deficient in phosphorus, phosphorus and vitamin D or calcium on the skeleton and teeth of growing sheep. 1. The mineral status of the skeleton and clinical appearance of the teeth. *Journal of Agricultural Science, Cambridge* 65, 1-14, 1965

Meyer HH, Aitken WM, Smeaton JE. Inheritance of wear rate in the teeth of sheep. *Proceedings of the New Zealand Society of Animal Production* 43, 189-91, 1983

Michum GD. Tooth deterioration in sheep. *Masterate Thesis*, Massey University, Palmerston North, New Zealand, 1985

Michum GD, Bruère AN. Solubilization of sheep's teeth: A new look at a widespread New Zealand problem. *Proceedings of the 14th Annual Seminar of the Society of Sheep and Beef Cattle Veterinarians, New Zealand Veterinary Association*, 44-56, 1984

Millar KR, Allsop TF, Kane DW, Webster MC. Failure of copper or vitamin D supplements to affect the dental condition of young sheep on two Wairarapa farms. *New Zealand Veterinary Journal* 33, 41-6, 1985

Northey RD, Hawley JG, Suckling GW. The tooth to pad relationship in sheep — some mechanical considerations. *New Zealand Journal of Agricultural Research* 18, 133-8, 1975

Orr MB. Periodontal disease in sheep in New Zealand. *Proceedings of the 14th Annual Seminar of the Society of Sheep and Beef Cattle Veterinarians, New Zealand Veterinary Association*, 33-8, 1984

Orr MB. A study of the effect of large worm burdens in lambs on their incisor dentition as adults. *New Zealand Veterinary Journal* 37, 38, 1989

Orr MB, Chalmers M. A field study of the association between periodontal disease and body condition in sheep. *New Zealand Veterinary Journal* 36, 171-2, 1988

Orr MB, Gardner DG. Prevalence of dentigerous cysts (ovine odontogenic cysts) in ewes in the South Island of New Zealand. *New Zealand Veterinary Journal* 44, 198, 1996

Orr MB, O'Callaghan MW, West DM, Bruère AN. A syndrome of dental abnormalities of sheep. II. The pathology and radiology. *New Zealand Veterinary Journal* 27, 276-8, 1979

Orr MB, Mason P, Crosbie SF. The effect of gastro-intestinal parasitism on the temporary dentition of lambs. *New Zealand Veterinary Journal* 33, 48-52, 1985

Orr MB, Christiasen KM, Kissling RC. A survey of excessively worn incisors and periodontal disease in sheep in Dunedin City Silver Peaks, Bruce, and Clutha counties. *New Zealand Veterinary Journal* 34, 111-15, 1986

Orr MB, Laws AJ, Frisken KW. Sheep incisors and cutters and grinders. *New Zealand Veterinary Journal* 35, 14-15, 1987

Porter WL. Premature tooth loss in sheep. *FRCVS Thesis*, Massey University, Palmerston North, New Zealand, 1972

Purser AF, Wiener G, West DM. Causes of variation in dental characters of Scottish Blackface sheep in a hill flock, and relations to ewe performance. *Journal of Agricultural Science, Cambridge* 99, 287-94, 1982

Ridler AL, West DM. Examination of teeth in sheep health management. *Small Ruminant Research* 92, 92-5, 2010.

Salisbury RM, Armstrong MC, Gray KG. Ulcero-memranous gingivitis in sheep. *New Zealand Veterinary Journal* 1, 51-2, 1953

Spence J, Aitchison G. Clinical aspects of dental disease in sheep. *In Practice* 8, 128-35, 1986

Spence JA, Aitchison GU, Sykes AR, Atkinson PJ. Broken mouth (premature incisor loss) in sheep. The pathogenesis of periodontal disease. *Journal of Comparative Pathology* 90, 275-92, 1980

Spence JA, Aitchison GU, Fraser J. Development of periodontal disease in a single flock of sheep: Clinical signs, morphology of subgingival plaque and influence of antimicrobial agents. *Research in Veterinary Science* 45, 324-31, 1988

Suckling GW. Mineralization of the enamel of ovine permanent central incisor teeth using microhardness and histological techniques. *Calcified Tissue International* 28, 121-9, 1979

Suckling GW. Defects of enamel in sheep resulting from trauma during tooth development. *Journal of Dental Research* 59, 1541-8, 1980

Suckling GW, Elliott DC, Thurley DC. The production of developmental defects of enamel in the incisor teeth of penned sheep resulting from induced parasitism. *Archives of Oral Biology* 28, 393-9, 1983

Surveillance

(1982) 2: 31	Broken incisors in hoggets — caries?
(1982) 3:25	Ovine incisor faults change after management changes
(1982) 4: 22	Paradontal disease
(1982) 4: 24	Paradontal disease in dairy cattle
(1983) 1: 8	Sheep study shows teeth problems cause early culling
(1983) 1: 19	Sheep incisor wear and acute periodontitis.
(1987) 2: 14-15	Sheep incisor grinder

Sykes AR, Field AL, Gunn RC. Effects of age and state of incisor dentition on body composition and lamb production on sheep grazing hill pastures. *Journal of Agricultural Science, Cambridge* 83, 135-43, 1974

Sykes AR, Coop RL, Angus KW. The influence of chronic *Ostertagia circumcincta* infection on the skeleton of growing sheep. *Journal of Comparative Pathology* 87, 521-9, 1977

Sykes AR, Coop RL, Angus KW. Chronic infection with *Trichostrongylus vitrinus* in sheep. Some effects on food utilisation, skeletal growth and certain serum constituents. *Research in Veterinary Science* 26, 372-7, 1979

Thurley DC. The normal anatomy, histology and development of sheep's teeth. *Proceedings of the Sheep and Beef Cattle Society of the New Zealand Veterinary Association* 15, 3-14, 1984

Thurley DC. The pathogenesis of excessive wear in the deciduous teeth of sheep. *New Zealand Veterinary Journal* 32, 25-9, 1984

Thurley DC. The pathogenesis of excessive wear in the permanent teeth of sheep. *New Zealand Veterinary Journal* 33, 24-6, 1985a

Thurley DC. Erosion of the non-occlusal surfaces of sheep's deciduous teeth. *New Zealand Veterinary Journal* 33, 157-8, 1985b

West DM, Spence JA. Diseases of the oral cavity. *Diseases of Sheep*, 3rd edition, pp 125-31, edited by Martin WB, Aitkin ID. Blackwell Science, 2000

West DM, Thompson KG, Holloway PM. Ill-thrift in ewes — a necropsy survey. *Proceedings of the 31st Annual Seminar of Society of Sheep and Beef Cattle Veterinarians, New Zealand Veterinary Association*, 189-93, 2001

West DM. Dental disease of sheep. *New Zealand Veterinary Journal* 50, 102-4, 2002

JOHNE'S DISEASE

Armstrong MC. Johne's disease of sheep in the South Island of New Zealand. *New Zealand Veterinary Journal* 4, 56-9, 1956

Armstrong MC. Johne's disease of sheep in South Canterbury. *New Zealand Journal Agriculture* 103, 2637, 1961

Britton A. Gudair™ — a new killed ovine Johne's disease vaccine. *Proceedings from the 31st Annual Seminar of the Society of Sheep and Beef Cattle Veterinarians, New Zealand Veterinary Association*, 41-9, 2001

Bruère AN. Ovine Johne's disease. The dilemma for the veterinarian and the stud breeder. *Proceedings of the 16th Annual Seminar of the Society of Sheep and Beef Cattle Veterinarians, New Zealand Veterinary Association*, 191-8, 1986

Collett MG, West DM. A comparison of the injection site and draining lymph node pathology induced by an attenuated live and a killed Johne's disease vaccine in sheep. *Proceedings of the 5th International Sheep Veterinary Congress*, Stellenbosch, South Africa, 2001

Corpa JM, Perez V, Sanchez MA, Garcia Marin JF. Control of paratuberculosis (Johne's disease) in goats by vaccination of adult animals. *Veterinary Record* 146, 195-6, 2000

Davidson RM. Ovine Johne's disease in New Zealand. *New Zealand Veterinary Journal* 18, 28-31, 1970

Davis GB. A sheep mortality survey in Hawke's Bay. *New Zealand Veterinary Journal* 22, 39-42, 1974

de Lisle GW. Johne's disease in New Zealand: The past, present and a glimpse into the future. *New Zealand Veterinary Journal* (Suppl.) 50, 53-6, 2002

de Lisle GW. Johne's disease — a New Zealand perspective. *Proceedings of the 35th Annual Seminar of the Society of Sheep and Beef Cattle Veterinarians, New Zealand Veterinary Association*, 1114, 2005

de Lisle GW, Cannon MC, Yates GF, Collins DM. Use of polymerase chain reaction to subtype *Mycobacterium avium* subspecies *paratuberculosis*, an increasingly important pathogen from farmed deer in New Zealand. *New Zealand Veterinary Journal* 54, 195-7, 2006

Eppleston J, Whittington RJ. Isolation of *Mycobacterium avium* subsp. *paratuberculosis* from the semen of rams with clinical Johne's disease. *Australian Veterinary Journal* 79, 776-7, 2001

Gautam M, Ridler A, Wilson PR, Heuer C. A review of paratuberculosis control in New Zealand pastoral livestock. *New Zealand Veterinary Journal*, in press

Gilmour NJL. The pathogenesis and control of Johne's disease. *Veterinary Record* 99, 433-4, 1976

Gumbrell RC. The history and current status of ovine Johne's disease in New Zealand. *Proceedings from the 16th Annual Seminar of the Sheep and Beef Cattle Society of the New Zealand Veterinary Association*, 173-84, 1986

Gwozdz JM, Thompson KG, Murray A, West DM, Manktelow BW. Use of the polymerase chain reaction assay for the detection of *Mycobacterium avium* subspecies *paratuberculosis* in blood and liver biopsies from experimentally infected sheep. *Australian Veterinary Journal* 78, 622-4, 2000

MacDiarmid SC. Prospects for the control of ovine Johne's disease. *Proceedings from the 16th Annual Seminar of the Society of Sheep and Beef Cattle Veterinarians, New Zealand Veterinary Association*, 206-9, 1986

Mackintosh CG, de Lisle GW, Collins DM, Griffin JFT. Mycobacterial diseases of deer. *New Zealand Veterinary Journal* 52, 163-74, 2004

Morris CA, Hickey SM, Henderson HV. The effect of Johne's disease on production traits in Romney, Merino and Merino x Romney-cross ewes. *New Zealand Veterinary Journal* 54, 204-9, 2006

Surveillance

(1978) 3: 21	Johne's disease of sheep
(1976) 3: 22	How good is the geldiffusion test for Johne's disease in sheep?
(1982) 9 (4): 12-13	Serological diagnosis of Johne's disease in sheep
(1983) 10 (4): 2-3	Colloquium on Johne's disease
(1988) 15 (2): 5-6	Vaccination against Johne's disease in sheep
(1990) 17 (4): 24	Sheep and cattle with Johne's

disease are infected with different strains of *Mycobacterium paratuberculosis* (1994) 21(1): 14–15 An update on Johne's disease in New Zealand

Thompson KG, West DM, Anderson PVA, Burnham DL. Subclinical Johne's disease in sheep. *Proceedings of the New Zealand Society of Animal Production* 62, 284–7, 2002

van Kooten HCJ, Mackintosh CG, Koets AP. Intra-uterine transmission of paratuberculosis (Johne's disease) in farmed red deer. *New Zealand Veterinary Journal* 54, 16–20, 2006

Verdugo C, Jones G, Johnson WO, Wilson PR, Stringer L, Heuer C. Estimation of flock/herd-level true *Mycobacterium avium* subspecies *paratuberculosis* prevalence on sheep, beef cattle and deer farms in New Zealand using a novel Bayesian model. *Preventive Veterinary Medicine* 117, 447–455, 2014

Wakelin R. Efficacy of vaccination of lambs with a Johne's disease vaccine at 3 to 4 months of age. *Proceedings of the 25th Annual Seminar of the Society of Sheep and Beef Cattle Veterinarians, New Zealand Veterinary Association*, 201–5, 1995

Walker A. Vaccination programmes for control of OJD: Cost-benefit consideration. *Proceedings of the 35th Annual Seminar of the Society of Sheep and Beef Cattle Veterinarians, New Zealand Veterinary Association*, 115–9, 2005

West DM. Johne's disease in New Zealand: History from first cases to current situation. *Proceedings of the 4th International Congress for Sheep Veterinarians*, Armidale, NSW, Australia, 151–5, 1997

West DM, Thompson KG, Holloway PM. Ill-thrift in ewes — a necropsy survey. *Proceedings of the 31st Annual Seminar of the Society of Sheep and Beef Cattle Veterinarians, New Zealand Veterinary Association*, 189–93, 2001

Whittington R. Johne's disease — an Australian perspective. *Proceedings of the 35th Annual Seminar of the Society of Sheep and Beef Cattle Veterinarians, New Zealand Veterinary Association*, 91–110, 2005

Whittington RJ, Sergeant ESG. Progress towards understanding the spread, detection and control of *Mycobacterium avium* subsp. *paratuberculosis* in animal populations. *Australian Veterinary Journal* 79, 267–78, 2001

Williamson GT, Salisbury RM. Johne's disease in sheep. *New Zealand Veterinary Journal* 1, 15–17, 1952

Windsor PA, Eppleston J. Lesions in sheep following administration of a vaccine of a Freud's complete adjuvant nature used in the control of ovine paratuberculosis. *New Zealand Veterinary Journal* 54, 237–41, 2006

Windsor PA. Paratuberculosis in sheep and goats. *Veterinary Microbiology* 181, 161–9, 2015

SMALL-INTESTINAL CARCINOMA

Ross AD. Small intestinal carcinoma in sheep. *Australian Veterinary Journal* 56, 25–8, 1980

Simpson BH. The geographic distribution of carcinomas in the small intestine of New Zealand sheep. *New Zealand Veterinary Journal* 20, 24–8, 1972

Simpson BH. An epidemiological study of carcinoma of the small intestine in New Zealand sheep. *New Zealand Veterinary Journal* 20, 91–7, 1972

Webster WM. Neoplasia in food animals with special reference to the high incidence in sheep. *New Zealand Veterinary Journal* 14, 203–14, 1966

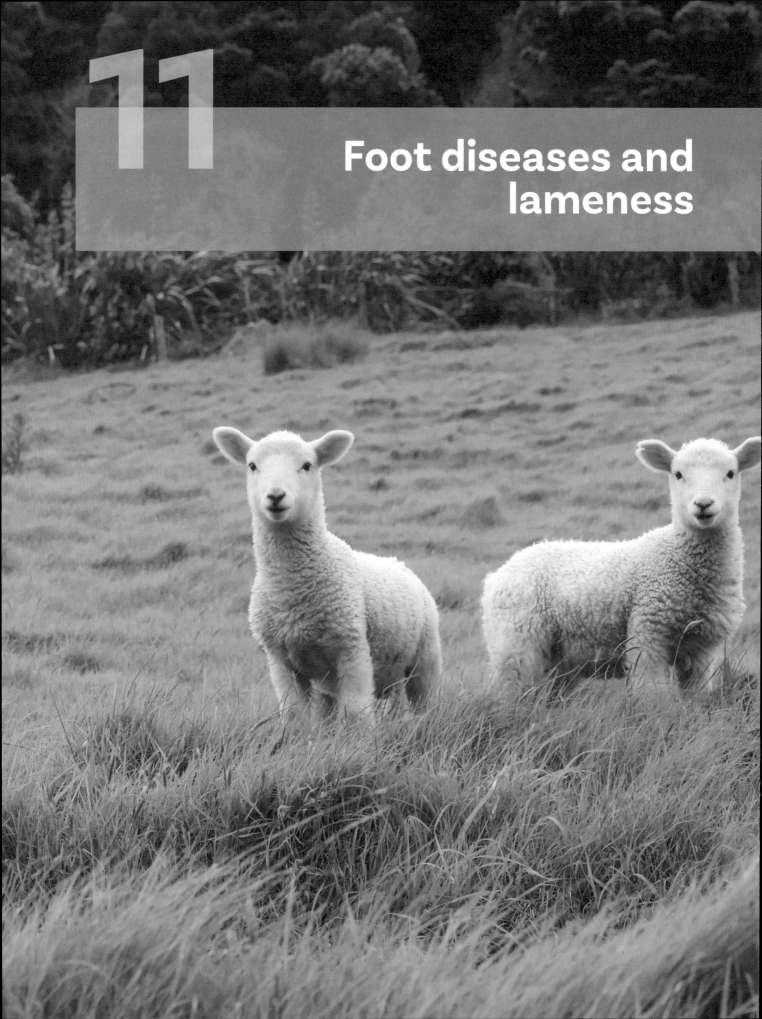

11

Foot diseases and lameness

Lameness in sheep is a significant issue, particularly among fine-wool breeds. Lameness is painful for sheep and frequently results in production losses. Furthermore, increasing scrutiny of lame sheep being transported to slaughter has re-emphasised the importance of controlling ovine lameness. The vast majority of ovine lameness occurs in the foot and the majority of cases are caused by ovine interdigital dermatitis (OID, sometimes also known as 'scald') and footrot. Less frequently, a range of other conditions including foot abscess, toe abscess and toe granuloma are seen.

It is important to note that development of OID and particularly footrot are likely due to complex interactions between the pathogen, the host and the environment. Limited research on OID and footrot has been undertaken in New Zealand and much of the information presented here is from research carried out in Australia and the UK. Differences in climatic conditions and host susceptibility means that care should be exercised when extrapolating these data to New Zealand conditions.

It is thought that healthy intact interdigital skin is difficult for bacteria to invade, and therefore predisposing factors exert a profound influence on the occurrence, persistence and, in some cases, transmission of foot diseases. Water maceration following continued contact with wet pastures and mechanical trauma are considered to be the most important.

Ovine interdigital dermatitis (OID) and footrot

Aetiology

In the past it was thought that OID and footrot were two different disease conditions, that OID was caused primarily by *Fusobacterium necrophorum* and that OID was required before footrot, caused by *Dichelobacter nodosus*, could develop. However, recent research suggests that OID and footrot may be presentations of the same disease, and that both are likely primarily due to *D. nodosus*. *Dichelobacter nodosus* is commonly isolated from the feet of healthy sheep in the UK and the same would probably be found in New Zealand. Development of disease is likely due to a complex interaction of pathogen factors, host factors and environmental conditions. Predisposing factors are important for disease development; most commonly these are water maceration or mechanical damage of the interdigital skin.

Dichelobacter nodosus is found predominantly in the feet of ruminants and has very limited environmental survival. It destroys the epidermal matrices of the hoof, leading to separation of the horn tissue, which is the characteristic lesion of footrot. The role of *F. necrophorum* is debated. It was thought to be the main causative agent for OID and an integral contributor to the pathogenesis of footrot by facilitating infection by *D. nodosus*. However, recent research suggests it may be an opportunistic secondary pathogen. *Dichelobacter nodosus*, by virtue of its proteolytic activity, is the only organism able to invade the epidermal matrix. It has been shown that *D. nodosus* varies in its keratinolytic protease activity and that this is directly related to the extent of invasion of the hoof matrices. Strains of low protease activity induce only mild lesions of footrot; the horn separation, if it occurs at all, being restricted to the axial part of the heel and the posterior half of the sole. Strains with high protease activity, however, produce much more severe lesions that may extend to complete separation of the horn of the sole and wall of the hoof. It is suggested that the former condition be designated benign (non-progressive) footrot

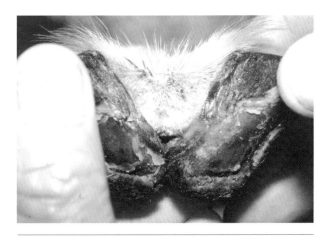

Figure 11.1 Normal interdigital space.

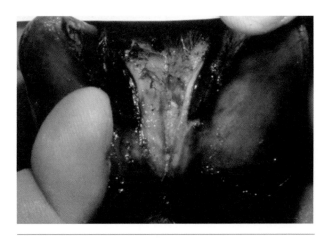

Figure 11.2 Ovine interdigital dermatitis.

and the latter virulent (progressive) footrot. In Australia, a condition midway between these two forms of footrot has been called intermediate footrot.

Other organisms including *Trueparella pyogenes*, *Treponema species* and *spirochaetes* may possibly contribute to the disease process, although their role is not well understood.

For the remainder of this chapter, OID and footrot will be discussed as two separate entities.

Ovine interdigital dermatitis ('scald')

Note: 'Scald' is a non-specific term that has been used to describe any interdigital dermatitis. It has been suggested that this term should no longer be used, but unfortunately it is well entrenched in farmer and veterinary vocabulary.

Epidemiology

Ovine interdigital dermatitis is common wherever underfoot conditions are persistently wet and heavy stocking is practised. All ages are susceptible and up to 90% of a mob may be affected, many in all four feet. The disease may persist for months, particularly in sheep on wet, legume-dominated pastures.

Ram hoggets in their first winter (approximately 8 months of age) appear to be particularly susceptible to OID because of their behaviour and sexual activity. Young rams often congregate in groups and indulge in riding and sexual activity. As a result of these forays the pasture is trampled and becomes muddy and heavily contaminated with faeces. In addition, there is the increased risk of physical damage to the interdigital skin when rams are mounting or being mounted.

Clinical findings

The predominant clinical sign of OID is lameness affecting a number of sheep, at a time when underfoot conditions are moist or muddy. When the affected sheep are examined closely, a range of lesions affecting the interdigital area is evident. In mild cases the interdigital skin is red and swollen and often covered by a moist film of whitish necrotic material. In more severely affected cases the foot is 'carried' and the interdigital skin is necrotic and eroded, thus exposing the sensitive subcutaneous tissues. Suppuration and swelling of these deeper tissues may be present. The characteristic odour and under-running of the wall or sole associated with footrot is absent.

Diagnosis
A diagnosis of OID can usually be made from the careful examination of as many affected feet as is practical under the circumstances. Examination may be facilitated by first washing the feet using a soft brush and water.

Treatment and control
Ovine interdigital dermatitis, especially in its mild form, recovers spontaneously if the flock can be moved to dry pastures. However, during periods of high rainfall this is often not possible and foot bathing at regular intervals is advisable. This can be undertaken as regularly as once a week, although foot bathing at 2- and 4-week intervals can markedly reduce the prevalence of OID. Zinc sulphate as a 10% solution is the most commonly used foot bathing agent and has largely replaced 5% formalin. A combination of zinc sulphate and the penetrating agent sodium lauryl sulphate is a more expensive alternative. For individual cases, topical antimicrobials such as oxytetracycline spray can be used. Prompt treatment of affected sheep is recommended to reduce the likelihood of footrot development.

Because lesions of OID are relatively superficial, the sheep are often treated by walking them slowly through a footbath at least 6 metres long rather than keeping them standing in a suitably constructed pen. A contact period of at least 1–2 minutes is recommended. Following treatment they should preferably stand in a dry area such as the grating of a woolshed, to allow the disinfecting agent to dry on the feet. Treatment such as that described may also be important in reducing the risk of foot abscess or footrot.

Severe cases of OID in which the interdigital skin is eroded and infection has entered the deeper tissues should be treated as potential cases of foot abscess (see later). It may be appropriate to house these sheep for up to a week to allow the feet to dry. In addition, selected use of antibiotics such as penicillin may limit the infection and prevent it spreading to the distal interphalangeal joint.

Footrot
Virulent footrot is a specific non-suppurative disease of the feet of sheep, goats, cattle, deer and probably other

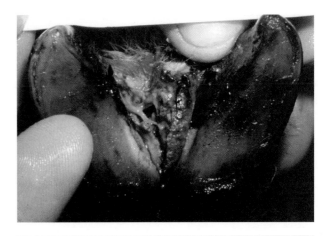

Figure 11.3 Ovine interdigital dermatitis with necrosis.

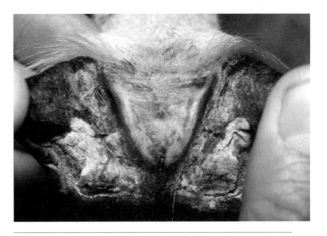

Figure 11.4 Footrot largely confined to the interdigital area.

ruminants, characterised by a progressive necrosis of the intermediate layers of the epidermis resulting in separation of the horn from the soft tissues of the foot and by varying degrees of lameness. Although worldwide in distribution, the incidence varies considerably, being highest under wet conditions conducive to the development of OID.

Footrot is an important disease problem in the New Zealand, Australian and UK sheep industries. In Australia it is considered a major production-limiting disease, particularly in Merino sheep. This has led to the introduction of footrot-free areas and eradication schemes to rid flocks of at least the virulent strains of the disease.

Prevalence, production losses and cost of treatment
It is difficult to accurately measure both the incidence and the economic impact of footrot in New Zealand. Surveys conducted in New Zealand between 1979 and 1982 estimated that between 4% and 8% of sheep were affected with footrot. It is likely that footrot is relatively uncommon in the coarse-woolled breeds, but a survey of footrot prevalence in New Zealand Merino sheep from 304 farms, reported by Hickford et al. (2005), stated that 78% of respondents claimed to have had footrot in the previous five years. The footrot prevalence during two preceding years was estimated to be 7.7% for ewes, 5.6% for hoggets, 4.5% for wethers and 5.5% for rams, giving an overall weighted average of 6.4% for Merino sheep in New Zealand.

From the same survey, it was shown that production losses in wool weight and quality were also significant. The average loss of greasy fleece weight was estimated to be 0.3 kg for ewes, leading to a 5% reduction in wool value. Also, an estimated decline in lambing percentage for sheep affected by footrot of 8.25% was reported as well as additional annual deaths of sheep. The cost of treatment and control included chemicals used for foot bathing, vaccines, antibiotics and labour, plus the losses of production that can be a significant farm expenditure.

As well as these aspects of the disease, its overall effect on the husbandry and welfare of sheep is of major consequence. Affected sheep are difficult to drove, grazing is impeded and it may induce pregnancy toxaemia in pregnant ewes. At the same time, when lambing is imminent or long periods of wet weather occur, effective treatment and control of footrot is virtually impossible.

Footrot also affects the international movement of sheep. Live sheep exported from New Zealand to Australia and other countries must be certified by a veterinarian as free from footrot. In Australia, footrot is classified as either 'benign' or 'virulent', with virulent footrot being a notifiable disease.

Aetiology
As described above, *D. nodosus* is the only organism that induces footrot lesions in suitably predisposed feet and is therefore regarded as the essential transmitting agent of footrot.

Dichelobacter nodosus organisms live only in diseased feet and probably survive for no longer than 7–14 days in faeces, soil and pasture. Indeed, some experiments have shown that viable organisms can only persist in muddy soil for a maximum of 4 days.

There are many strains of *D. nodosus* with a wide spectrum of virulence ranging from benign to virulent. It is believed that these strains do not mutate readily. Different strains with different virulence can be found on the same property, the same sheep and even within the same feet of sheep. Virulent strains are more easily eradicated from a sheep flock because infected sheep are identified more readily and eradication programmes are aimed at virulent footrot rather than against all strains of *D. nodosus*. Frequently, benign strains may persist in a flock following a successful footrot eradication programme. However, the expression of virulence on a property is probably dependent on the environmental conditions and the relative susceptibility of the sheep, as well as the virulence of the *D. nodosus* strains involved. Thus, under the right conditions it is likely that 'benign' footrot can cause lameness in a small proportion of the flock.

Epidemiology
Predisposing factors
Predisposing factors exert a profound influence on the occurrence, persistence and transmission of footrot. Effective eradication requires an appreciation of how environmental factors affect the occurrence of new cases, the spread to unaffected sheep and the cessation of spread.

Footrot spreads under restricted environmental conditions requiring moisture and warmer temperatures. Australian studies demonstrated that transmission of footrot required at least 3 months of rainfall averaging 50 mm per month in the cooler part of the year and falls of at least 125 mm per month in summer. In those studies, transmission of footrot occurred when the mean ambient temperature rose above 10°C, so in cooler climates transmission of footrot may be restricted during winter time. However, these transmission parameters may not necessarily be the same in wetter, more temperate climates such as New Zealand or the UK. Footrot is more prevalent when there is a dense sward of clover-dominant pasture to maintain moisture.

Under Australian conditions, spread is seasonal with outbreaks occurring in the late autumn (April/May), particularly when rain has fallen, but more commonly in late spring (October/November). Outbreaks can also occur in the summer on irrigated pasture. Transmission does not occur after pasture dries and, although during droughts the prevalence of the disease is substantially reduced, the disease does not disappear. Thus in Australia, the period of transmission of footrot may be restricted to as short as 3–4 weeks, although 6–12 weeks is more usual.

In New Zealand, conditions are suitable for the transmission of footrot during most of the year and this factor has a major influence on the success of eradication schemes in New Zealand compared with Australia. Furthermore, the stocking rates and stocking densities of New Zealand properties are generally higher than those in many parts of Australia. High stocking densities facilitate transmission of the organism and may result in larger outbreaks of disease. Sheep and goats straying between properties may also be more common in New Zealand.

Host susceptibility

All ages of sheep are susceptible to footrot. Young lambs will often develop superficial 'OID' lesions in all four feet, but are easily cured using footbath treatment.

All breeds are susceptible, but British breeds are more tolerant than Merino sheep. There is a range of susceptibilities between sheep of the same breed. Susceptibility to footrot is a heritable characteristic with an estimated heritability of between 0.15 and 0.30. This indicates that selection for footrot tolerance is feasible and some farmers have made substantial progress by selecting tolerant sheep in the face of natural challenge.

Alternative hosts

Cattle, goats and deer are suitable alternative hosts for *D. nodosus*. Cattle strains of *D. nodosus* are usually benign for sheep and are therefore not important as a reservoir of virulent footrot, which is the important target of eradication schemes. However, some *D. nodosus* isolates from goats are virulent for sheep, and on properties where footrot eradication is being attempted goats would have to be included in the control programme.

Clinical findings

The characteristic lesion is a progressive necrosis of the intermediate layers of the epidermis leading to detachment of the horn. Although the appearance of affected feet varies somewhat, in outbreaks the disease takes a well-defined course. The earliest sign is swelling and moistening of the skin of the interdigital cleft; it can be difficult to clinically differentiate between early footrot and OID. A break occurs at the skin–horn junction and from there the infection spreads under the horn tissue, working down the axial wall, under the sole and eventually up the abaxial wall so that the hoof is finally attached only at the coronet. When extensive under-running has occurred lameness is severe, the animal may carry the leg and, if more than one foot is affected, may walk on its knees or remain recumbent. Usually both claws are affected. There is a characteristic black foul-smelling discharge which is always small in amount.

The detached horn can be lifted up and pared off in large pieces. Loss of condition soon follows, and flystrike is a common complication.

Diagnosis

In most cases, diagnosis can be made on clinical evidence of extensive separation of the horn tissue of the sole and wall of the hoof and the characteristic odour associated with *D. nodosus* infection. In some instances it is necessary to demonstrate by bacteriological examination the presence of *D. nodosus* organisms. This can be done by making a smear of material from deep within the lesion and staining with Gram stain. *Dichelobacter nodosus* is visible as large Gram-negative rods that often have pronounced swollen ends. Experimentally at Lincoln University a polymerase chain reaction (PCR) technique has also been used.

Laboratory tests are available to assess the virulence

of the strain of *D. nodosus*. These are expensive and time-consuming and are seldom justified in New Zealand. However, on the farm it is preferable to make a clinical assessment of the flock situation. A representative sample of the flock should be examined and if there is extensive under-running of the hoofs of many of the sheep, then virulent footrot is present.

A number of scoring systems for assessing the severity of footrot lesions have been described. The following is adapted from an Australian scoring system (modified after Egerton, 1989).

0 = Normal.
1 = Slight to moderate inflammation of the interdigital skin with erosion of the epithelium. This may be due to ovine interdigital dermatitis, benign footrot or early virulent footrot.
2 = Necrotising inflammation of the interdigital skin, involving part or all of the soft horn of the axial wall of the digit.
3 (a, b, c) = Any lesion of the claw which results in under-running of the soft horn of the heels or sole but not extending to the abaxial edge of the sole of the hoof.
4 = Under-running of the hard horn of the claw (under-running extends to the abaxial edge of the sole of the hoof).

The virulence classification of the disease should be based on the prevalence of sheep with score 4 lesions relative to the number of sheep affected with footrot (lesion score 2, 3 or 4). If 20 sheep with lesions of score 2 or greater are examined and 5 or more have score 4 lesions, then the strain of affecting organism is classified as virulent.

Treatment
Treatment should be initiated promptly, as affected sheep are a likely major source of infection to other sheep. Prompt treatment also leads to a more rapid recovery for the affected sheep.

Injected antibiotics
Sheep affected with footrot can be treated with parenteral antibiotics; in many cases a single high dose will result in a cure. Antibiotics that have been used include penicillin (75,000 units/kg), streptomycin (75 mg/kg), erythromycin (12 mg/kg), long-acting oxytetracycline (20 mg/kg), lincomycin (5 mg/kg)–spectinomycin (10 mg/kg) and tilmicosin (5 mg/kg). There have been reports of sheep deaths, probably due to salmonellosis, following the use of lincomycin–spectinomycin. Topical treatment of the interdigital skin using oxytetracycline spray, or similar, can also be used.

Footrot cure rates vary but are usually in the order of 80–100%. It is important that the sheep remain in a dry environment for at least 24 hours after treatment. Studies in the UK have highlighted that early parental antibiotic treatment of individual sheep with moderate to severe footrot results in much faster recovery compared with 'traditional' topical treatment. It may also lead to a reduction in subsequent cases of footrot within the flock, presumably due to reduced exposure of the flock to *D. nodosus*. Disadvantages of using antibiotics to treat footrot include cost, meat residues and resistance issues, so on a flock basis antibiotics should only be used in a rational way as an adjunct to a targeted management/control plan. Sheep that fail to respond to antibiotic treatment should be culled.

Topical treatments
The traditional approach to treatment was to pare affected feet and then apply an antibacterial chemical. More recently there has been debate about the role of foot trimming, and UK authors have demonstrated that it may delay recovery time. If foot trimming of sheep is undertaken it should be done with care to minimise damage to healthy tissue. It should also be noted that foot trimming has no role in the prevention of footrot.

Topical antibacterial chemicals are very useful for the treatment of OID and prevention of footrot and are usually applied in foot baths. Formalin (5%) and zinc sulphate (10%) solutions are those most commonly used, although the former is falling out of favour due to health concerns. Sodium lauryl sulphate may be added to zinc sulphate as a penetrating agent. While foot bathing sounds like a relatively straightforward procedure and allows a large number of sheep to be treated in a relatively short time period, in reality it is a complex procedure which is sometimes done very poorly. The following points are relevant to foot bathing:

- Foot bathing is not an appropriate treatment for

moderate to severe cases of footrot. These are better treated with parenteral antibiotics (see above).
- It is not practical to foot-bathe sheep during tupping or lambing time.
- It is difficult to ensure adequate contact time with the chemical. Depending on the chemical used and the severity of the condition, a contact time of 1–30 minutes is required.
- It is important that the correct concentration of chemical is used and that replenishment occurs as necessary.
- Foot bathing sheep once a week, or even once a fortnight, will greatly reduce the spread of footrot.
- Excessive formalin foot bathing, that is more than twice a week, in concentrations greatly exceeding 10% can cause foot damage.
- The sheep should be released to a dry environment, preferably on a wooden grating such as in a shearing shed, for at least 1 hour to allow the chemical to dry onto the feet.
- Zinc sulphate is less effective if formalin has been used within the previous two months.
- During the dry summer months, an 80–100% cure rate can be expected, but in wet conditions it may be much lower.
- Persistent cases should be culled.

Vaccination

A multi-strain *D. nodosus* vaccine is available in New Zealand (Footvax®; MSD Animal Health). It is recommended that a sensitiser dose be given and then boosted just before the expected footrot disease risk period. The booster should be at least 6 weeks after but within 12 months of the sensitiser. This will have two effects. Within a few weeks of completion of the schedule, most unaffected sheep will be protected against footrot. Sheep already affected will heal more quickly and the severity of the disease in those remaining affected will, for the most part, be reduced. The overall effect of vaccination is to reduce the prevalence and severity of the disease in a flock. However, the length of protection afforded is relatively short, up to 4 months, which highlights the importance of strategic timing of the booster dose. Vaccination on its own will not eradicate the disease and is costly if it is to be maintained on an annual whole-flock basis, but is a useful aid to footrot control in some flocks. Since the vaccine contains an oil adjuvant, some degree of local tissue reaction should be anticipated at the site of vaccination.

The use of Footvax is not recommended within 4 weeks of tupping or lambing, or in young lambs less than 4 weeks of age. It should not be used in conjunction with injectable moxidectin formulations. Accidental self-injection can lead to severe tissue damage. If self-injection occurs, medical attention should be sought immediately.

Overseas research with specific monovalent footrot vaccines has shown promise in reducing the incidence of footrot in treated flocks. One flock so vaccinated remained footrot-free for a year. Whether such therapy will become commercially possible still requires further work.

Breeding for tolerance

As mentioned previously, the heritability of footrot tolerance has been estimated at 0.15–0.30. In New Zealand, several flocks such as the Broomfield Corriedale and the Patterson Merino have a high level of genetic tolerance to footrot. These have been developed by culling or not breeding from sheep that show footrot. However, these breeding systems require sheep to be exposed to the disease to allow the expression of susceptibility or tolerance.

A genetic marker associated with tolerance has been identified at Lincoln University (Hickford, 2001). They have found that genes known as the major histocompatibility complex (MHC) are important in controlling the immune response to footrot. Within the MHC, alleles have been identified that are associated with footrot tolerance and susceptibility. Therefore, genetic variation within the MHC can be used as a 'genetic marker' of relative footrot susceptibility and this can be used in a breeding programme to select more-tolerant sheep. It is important to realise that other genes probably also affect an individual's response to the disease.

Oral zinc sulphate dosing

While there have been some overseas reports of oral zinc sulphate treatment curing footrot, trials in New Zealand, Australia, USA and Spain have given no response.

Control

Many New Zealand flocks have endemic footrot. However, the significance of this infection varies and many British-breed-based flocks in drier areas of the country are not troubled to any great extent. On such farms, limited treatment may be undertaken to check the occasional outbreak of OID and sheep with chronic lameness may be culled.

For farmers who wish to undertake some degree of footrot control, options range from the strategic use of foot bathing and/or vaccination through to an intensive control programme or even eradication. If strategic control (foot bathing and/or vaccination) is used, seasonal variation in the severity of disease should be expected so that in some years outbreaks will still occur. Precisely what therapeutic or prophylactic procedures are appropriate will have to be established with due consideration of the costs of footrot to the farmer, whether eradication is feasible, what facilities or resources are available and whether the owner wishes to accept a degree of footrot in the flock.

It should be noted that in the control of footrot it is preferable to recognise danger periods (warmth and moisture) and institute control measures early, rather than wait until an outbreak occurs.

Intensive control programme

This is the best control option for high-risk properties to get rid of most of the footrot on the property. To be successful, an intensive control programme requires considerable ongoing commitment from the farmer and farm staff. It also requires adequate facilities. Staff must have skills in diagnostic foot paring to recognise lesions of footrot. Diagnostic foot paring differs from therapeutic foot paring in that the primary objective is to make a diagnosis of a clean foot. To do this, excess lateral wall, heel and toe horn is removed, and the abaxial grooves and heels are inspected for lifting and infection.

The basic principles of the intensive control programme are to separate the sheep into either the 'clean mob' (all four feet normal) or the 'treatment mob' (one or more feet not normal). The objective is to keep the clean mob clean and, through the use of paring and foot bathing, with or without antibiotic use, turn the treatment mob into a cured mob. It is essential that the mobs are kept separate. Sheep that do not respond to treatment should be culled. For more detailed information on designing an intensive control programme, see 'A guide to the management of footrot in sheep' by Mulvaney (2013). This booklet is available from Merino New Zealand.

Control during an outbreak

There are a number of factors to consider when undertaking footrot control. The initial task is to reach a satisfactory diagnosis and assessment of the severity of the problem. The following checklist should be considered:

- It is important to determine what precipitated the outbreak.
- How interested and skilled is the flock owner in footrot control/eradication?
- What facilities are available for inspecting the feet of sheep and for foot bathing?
- What methods of control are available?
- The value and productivity of the flock.
- Is the flock open, closed or does it have a ram-only entry scheme?
- Are goats present on the farm?
- Stage of the 'sheep year'. For instance, it may not be appropriate to attempt control in heavily pregnant sheep or to interfere with sheep during tupping. Likewise, the initiation of footrot control during lactation can also be extremely difficult. Under these conditions careful individual treatment may be necessary as a holding operation until conditions are more suitable for a full control programme to be started.

If the flock is not affected during tupping or close to lambing, the clinical effects of footrot, and to some extent, transmission to unaffected sheep, can be controlled by treating flocks in foot baths. For many years farmers have applied such treatments using 5% formalin or 10% zinc sulphate by walking sheep through a 6-metre-long footbath once a week. Using portable footbaths, up to 10,000 sheep have been treated weekly. Less frequent treatments at once a fortnight also reduces the spread of infection appreciably, as the incubation period for under-running infections to develop is 10–14 days.

In addition to foot bathing, the use of vaccine has to be considered. In Australia and the drier parts of New Zealand (e.g. Central Otago), many farmers may prefer to eradicate rather than simply control footrot.

Eradication

Eradication of footrot, especially virulent footrot, has been successfully achieved in many districts in Australia and on a limited number of farms in New Zealand; mainly in the South Island. It should be noted that differences in climatic conditions and host susceptibility mean that eradication on New Zealand farms is unlikely to be as straightforward as in many areas of Australian. Eradication should not be embarked on lightly, as it requires a full commitment of resources if it is to be successful. Also, neighbouring sheep with footrot that stray onto the property, the presence of feral goats on the farm or the introduction of sheep such as breeding rams may all compromise the eradication programme.

The following methods have been employed:

1. Complete disposal

This is the simplest approach but it is costly to replace a complete flock. There must also be a source of footrot-free sheep from which restocking can take place. Restocking should not occur until at least 14–21 days after de-stocking to ensure that there are no viable *D. nodosus* organisms in the environment.

2. Identification and disposal of infected sheep

This is based on the accurate identification of infected sheep. This has to be done manually by diagnostic paring. The feet of each sheep are examined while the sheep is restrained in a suitable cradle and the horn pared using secateurs. As soon as footrot lesions are found, the sheep is classified as infected and separated accordingly. If no footrot is found after all feet have been trimmed, the sheep is classified as free. Re-inspection is required. This procedure should not be undertaken during a transmission period as sheep incubating infection will be missed.

3. Identification and treatment of infected sheep

This approach requires the use of foot bathing following careful foot paring. In addition, parenteral chemotherapy and vaccination might be used.

The following strategy has been used in Australia for the eradication of footrot. If we assume that footrot occurs in August during a transmission period, then intensive control cannot be undertaken during this time because it would interfere with lambing. Thus the control phase would occur from August until weaning (around January). The eradication phase would be undertaken during January and February with follow-up surveillance.

1. The diagnosis and acceptance phase

The acceptance phase requires the individual owner to believe the diagnosis and to accept that action is required if footrot is to be eradicated.

2. The control phase

The objective during the control phase is to reduce the prevalence of footrot to a level below 5%. This low prevalence will usually allow the culling of affected sheep.

The measures taken to reduce the prevalence will vary depending on the time of year and the likelihood of spread of footrot. If the outbreak occurs during a major spread period, then vaccination plus weekly foot bathing is needed until the period of spread passes or until vaccination takes effect. In some instances the use of systemic antibiotics, either to all sheep or to all lame sheep, is used to reduce the prevalence.

3. The eradication phase

The eradication phase requires a careful diagnostic paring of the feet of every sheep and disposal of affected sheep. The responsibility of inspection should rest with one person, often the veterinarian. The 'clean' sheep should be foot-bathed and put into a paddock that has not been stocked for 7 days. Between 4 and 6 weeks later, the whole inspection procedure is repeated. If no footrot is found then footrot is probably eradicated and the flock can progress to the surveillance phase.

4. The surveillance phase

The surveillance phase requires continued vigilance, as especially in large flocks there will probably be breakdowns. Surveillance should continue for at least 12 months, or until the flock has passed through a period of transmission.

The following costs associated with eradication need to be considered:
- formalin or $ZnSO_4$
- footrot vaccine

- antibiotic
- mustering time and yard time
- inspection time (1000 sheep/day)
- depreciation of equipment
- loss of sale of 2%.

The development of control or eradication plans for owners requires the skill of the veterinarian to instil confidence that the plan can be carried through. It is essential also to be realistic about the pitfalls that may occur along the way and to ensure that these are explained to the owners.

In Australia, footrot eradication is a major means of entry for veterinarians who wish to contribute to the sheep industry. This does not necessarily apply in New Zealand, where the transmission period of footrot is so extended. However, in areas such as Central Otago, veterinarians have successfully applied these schemes in their client's flocks.

Foot abscess and toe abscess

Suppurative conditions of the foot can be separated into two distinct entities with different pathogenesis. The first, and by far the most common and important, is foot abscess (infective bulbar necrosis, heel abscess); and the second, lamellar suppuration (toe abscess).

The two organisms most consistently isolated from cases of foot abscess are *F. necrophorum* and *Trueparella (Arcanobacterium) pyogenes*, and the condition can be defined as an infection of the distal interphalangeal joint by these two bacteria. *Trueparella pyogenes* produces a specific growth factor that increases the invasiveness of *F. necrophorum*, which in turn secretes an exotoxin that protects *T. pyogenes* and itself from phagocytosis. Most commonly, foot abscess develops as a complication of OID by extension of the necrotic process into the subcutis and thence into the distal interphalangeal joint. In early cases of foot abscess the process is necrotic rather than suppurative due to the predominance of *F. necrophorum* but, with time, *T. pyogenes* is cultured more consistently and suppuration is evident. The possibility of other micro-organisms playing an essential or supporting role cannot be dismissed.

Toe abscess (lamellar suppuration) arises from a mixed infection in which *F. necrophorum* predominates, but prior infection with OID is not involved in its pathogenesis. In most cases it is presumed that the organisms gain entry through minute fissures in the horn tissue, especially at the sole wall junction (white line).

Foot abscess

Pathogenesis

Foot abscess of sheep is an acute, often purulent infection usually involving one digit of the foot.

It is generally accepted that most cases of foot abscess arise as a sequel to OID. Both conditions often occur simultaneously in a flock and in several instances OID has been seen to precede foot abscess. In addition, the

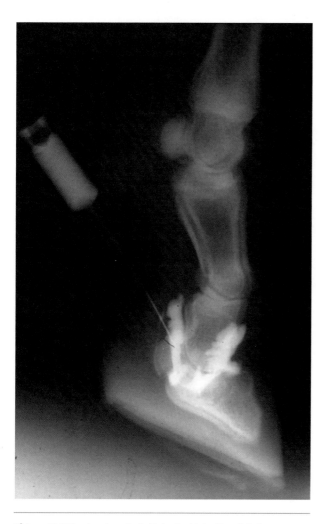

Figure 11.5 Contrast material injected into the distal interphalangeal joint showing the extent of the dorsal and volar pouches.

bacterial flora of the two conditions is similar.

A clearer understanding of the pathogenesis of foot abscess has come from studies on the anatomy of the digit and in particular the distal interphalangeal joint. This joint is most vulnerable to infection or trauma on the axial or interdigital aspect where the joint capsule protrudes above the coronary border as the dorsal and volar pouches. At these two sites the joint capsule is protected only by the interdigital skin layer and a small amount of subcutaneous tissue. Therefore, it is understandable that outbreaks of OID in which the interdigital skin becomes necrotic and eroded may result in cases of foot abscess. Indeed, any severe interdigital skin damage arising from such things as injury or excessive use of formalin foot baths increases the susceptibility of the foot to infection and to the development of foot abscess.

Occasionally, sporadic cases of foot abscess arise because bacteria gain entry to the distal interphalangeal joint from sources other than OID. A common source is from infections in the lamellar region of the foot (toe abscess). In many instances unintentional damage may be inflicted on the foot by the owner attempting to drain toe abscess lesions, and the trauma produced may be sufficient to allow infection to gain entry to the distal interphalangeal joint.

Incidence and economic importance

The incidence of foot abscess is low and seldom rises above 2%. Much of the importance of foot abscess undoubtedly arises because of the severe nature of the lesion and because ewes close to lambing and rams are more frequently affected. Production losses may therefore arise if sheep breeding programmes are disrupted by rams developing foot abscess close to the period of mating or if ewes develop pregnancy toxaemia as a consequence of the severe lameness associated with foot abscess.

Surveys conducted in New Zealand have shown that about three-quarters of farms experience cases of foot abscess, but the overall incidence is only 0.15%. Only 3% of respondents reported an incidence greater than 1%. However, on occasions, particularly following periods of heavy rain, severe outbreaks of foot abscess affecting up to a third of a flock may occur. Similar outbreaks have been reported in Australia.

Predisposing factors

Predisposing factors exert a profound effect on the prevalence of foot abscess and of prime importance are wet and muddy underfoot conditions. It is only under such circumstances that outbreaks of foot abscess have been reported, usually in association with OID.

Interdigital skin damage

It is apparent that some prior interdigital skin damage is necessary to facilitate the deeper bacterial invasion of the subcutaneous tissues and ultimately the distal interphalangeal joint. Experimentally, such tissue damage has been reproduced by applying liquid nitrogen to a small area of the interdigital skin for between 2 and 3 minutes. Following this treatment the sheep were housed in moist, dirty underfoot conditions and foot abscess was consistently reproduced. While this may appear a rather extreme means of creating tissue damage, the lesions produced are similar to the severe interdigital necrosis and erosion that has been observed in naturally occurring cases of OID.

A number of causes of interdigital tissue damage have been suggested as predisposing to foot abscess. These include walking on sharp stones, stubble and thistles. It has also been suggested that friction between the digits may play an important role. A common finding during outbreaks of foot lameness and foot abscess is the accumulation of mud and straw into a plug, which becomes hard when wedged between the claws and predisposes sheep to foot abscess. When the plug is removed, the underlying interdigital skin is seen to be inflamed, eroded and necrotic.

Outbreaks of foot abscess have also been reported following the excessive use of formalin foot baths. The suggested pathogenesis was that primary damage to the interdigital skin resulted from the misuse of formalin and that this permitted the bacterial invasion of the deeper tissues and the distal interphalangeal joint of the foot.

Animal behaviour

The attack rate of foot abscess is higher for rams than for ewes and a possible explanation for this has been advanced. The behaviour of rams, especially young rams, is different from that of ewes; rams often congregate in groups and

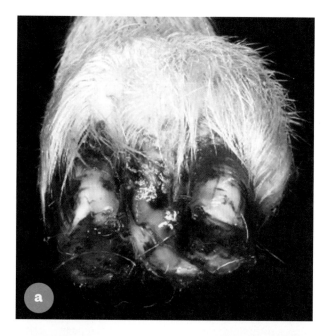

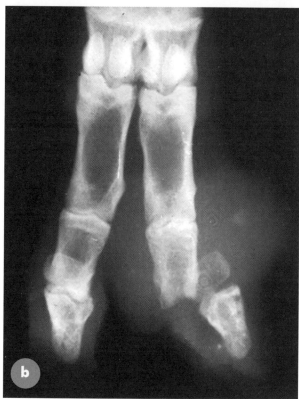

Figure 11.6 Foot abscess.
(a) Affecting lateral digit. **(b)** Radiograph: note dislocation of third phalanx.

indulge in riding and sexual activity. As a result of these forays the pasture is trampled and becomes muddy and heavily contaminated with faeces.

Clinical findings

The disease causes an acute lameness, usually restricted to one foot. On examination, usually one claw is found to be hot and swollen, particularly in the interdigital space, and this swelling displaces the affected digit abaxially. Sinus tracts discharging bloody, necrotic material and pus are usually present in the interdigital area and extend into the distal interphalangeal joint. Later the sinuses may extend to break out at one or more points above the coronet. In older lesions the discharge becomes more purulent. In up to half the cases there is exaggerated movement of the affected digit, indicating that the necrotising joint infection has ruptured the axial collateral ligaments and the interdigital ligament. In these cases it is likely that there will be displacement of the digit during locomotion and permanent deformity. Once the infection is established in the distal interphalangeal joint, healing is slow and takes approximately 2 months. Even after this period of time there may be residual lameness, deformity and a degenerative arthropathy. Despite this, most sheep perform satisfactorily.

Diagnosis

This can usually be made on the clinical findings. It differs from footrot in that:

- The lesions extend beyond the limits of the epidermal skin or matrix of the hoof.
- The disease is almost invariably restricted to one digit of one foot.
- There is no characteristic odour as is associated with *D. nodosus*.
- The prevalence rarely exceeds 15%.

Radiology is particularly useful to confirm distal interphalangeal joint involvement and also provides information on the likely outcome and degree of deformity. In very early cases there may be difficulty in distinguishing between severe cases of OID and foot abscess; that is, in deciding if the distal interphalangeal joint is infected. In addition to looking carefully for swelling above the abaxial coronet, radiology of the foot is valuable.

Treatment

In most cases attempting to drain the abscess or using antibiotic therapy is of limited value and does not appear to markedly accelerate healing, which is not surprising given that the infection is centred on the distal interphalangeal joint. Purulent joint infections erode articular cartilage very quickly, resulting in permanent joint damage. In addition, the joint is contained within the hoof and is almost impossible to drain without creating further damage to joint structures such as ligaments. To significantly alter the outcome of infection, therapy would have to be early enough to either prevent the infection becoming established in the joint or prevent damage to the axial collateral ligaments with the possibility of subsequent rupture. Bandaging the foot to prevent splaying of the digits should reduce the chances of the axial collateral ligaments rupturing, by reducing pressure on the ligaments. Bandaging also reduces the risk of further bacterial contamination of the lesion from the environment.

Although sheep do not respond rapidly to therapy, the prognosis for functional recovery is good in most cases. The healing process is protracted, but after a period of about 2 months most sheep can walk normally; however, the discomfort and pain experienced during this period should be considered. Other options are to amputate the digit or cull the animal. Digit amputation is relatively straightforward but the cost, nursing during the healing phase and likely return to normal function (especially for rams) should be borne in mind.

Control

The sporadic occurrence of foot abscesses and the ubiquitous nature of the causative bacteria make prevention of the disease difficult. Control has been based on minimising the factors that predispose to outbreaks of the condition.

Outbreaks of foot abscess occur during wet environmental conditions that are conducive to injuring the interdigital skin. Such things as maintaining rams and ewes in late pregnancy on wet country, or yarding sheep in wet muddy yards, should be avoided. Where practical, temporary yards should be erected on a drier part of the farm. Care should be taken if sheep, especially late pregnant ewes or rams, are grazed on crops during the wet winter months as the muddy conditions may be ideal for the development of OID and foot abscess.

If, under such circumstances, severe OID occurs in a flock, consideration should be given to instituting treatment before foot abscess develops. This may include careful foot bathing of sheep in 10% zinc sulphate or 5% formalin solution and providing dry underfoot conditions. Providing dry conditions may be impossible in many situations, but it may be appropriate to house the sheep for up to a week to allow the feet to dry. In addition, selected use of antibiotics such as penicillin may limit the infection and prevent joint involvement.

Attempts to immunise animals against infection by *F. necrophorum* have been disappointing. Although commercial *F. necrophorum* vaccines have been made and marketed, there is little published record of their efficacy and farmers are unsure of, or have been dissatisfied with, the protection given. Experimental use of these vaccines results in detectable levels of circulating serum antibodies, but the protection afforded against infection is meagre. However, an effective *F. necrophorum* vaccine would have wide application in the livestock industries and there remains considerable interest in developing a product such as this.

Toe abscess (lamellar suppuration)

Confusion has arisen between differentiating the condition of toe abscess and that of foot abscess. Toe abscess, like foot abscess, is an acute suppurative condition commonly affecting only one digit. Unlike foot abscess it arises sporadically in any flock and not as a complication of OID. The condition occurs mainly at the toe of the forefeet, and the opportunist infection probably gains entry to the sensitive laminae region through minute fissures in the horn in the area of the white line, especially in misshapen or overgrown hooves. Occasional cases may also arise following injudicious paring of the feet.

In the majority of cases, the earliest sign of infection is an acute lameness which is so painful that the sheep refuses to bear any weight on the foot. Examination may fail to reveal any obvious lesion, but generally one claw is found to be hot and pressure applied to the wall causes the sheep to flinch. Careful paring away of the horn at the toe reveals the presence of imprisoned pus. If the original site of injury on the plantar surface becomes sealed by mud, faeces or exudate, infection can track upwards and produce a sinus above the coronet. *Fusobacterium necrophorum* and *Trueparella pyogenes* can often be cultured from the pus along with other organisms found in the environment.

In contrast with foot abscess, toe abscess responds rapidly to drainage of the lesion.

Toe granulomas

Toe granulomas are sometimes seen on the sole or toe of the hoof. They can be 2–3 cm in size and are usually caused by over-zealous hoof trimming. Treatment is by careful paring of the hoof to expose the granuloma, removal of the granuloma with a scalpel and then application of a pressure bandage for 3–5 days. Severely affected sheep may need to be culled.

Interdigital fibromas

Interdigital fibromas are occasionally seen as fibrous growths in the interdigital space of the hoof. They are mainly seen in older and heavy rams and may cause lameness during tupping.

Foot and mouth disease

This virus infection affects all cloven-hoofed animals and characteristically produces vesicles on the coronet and in the interdigital space. Following rupture, the vesicles may be invaded by *F. necrophorum*. Separation of the hooves starts first at the coronet, and the high morbidity and other systemic effects differentiate it from foot abscess. Foot and mouth disease does not occur in Australia or New Zealand and both countries maintain strict quarantine procedures to exclude it. More information is included in Chapter 21.

Contagious pustular dermatitis (scabby mouth)

This proliferative dermatitis is caused by the scabby mouth virus (Chapter 18). It mainly affects lambs. Scabs tend to build up and coalesce about the lips and coronet and sometimes in the interdigital space. Secondary infection of these lesions with *F. necrophorum* and *Dermatophilus congolensis* frequently occurs. Spontaneous recovery is common. The age group affected, the characteristic sites and proliferative nature of the lesion and the high morbidity differentiate it from other foot conditions. Prevention is either by vaccination or removal of the predisposing factors such as thistles which causes initial skin damage (see Chapter 18).

Dermatophilus congolensis infection

Infection of the coronet region with *Dermatophilus congolensis* is seen occasionally during outbreaks of dermatophilosis. The infection appears in the form of multiple raised scabs between the coronet and the knee or hock. Characteristic filaments and coccoid forms of *D. congolensis* may be seen in stained smears made from the underside of the scab material. *Dermatophilus congolensis* is a frequent secondary invader of skin lesions such as contagious pustular dermatitis and may be further complicated by *F. necrophorum* infection. Moisture is important in the spread of the condition (see Chapter 18).

Erysipelothrix arthritis

Erysipelothrix arthritis is a fibrinous polyarthritis caused by the soil-borne pathogen *E. rhusiopathiae*.

Epidemiology

The organism persists for long periods in the soil and gains entry to the body in the following circumstances.

1. Contamination of fresh wounds at lambing and docking. The lambs then develop a polyarthritis characterised by prolonged lameness and stunted growth. This form of the disease is less important in New Zealand than in Britain because the ewes lamb outdoors and docking and castration are usually performed in temporary pens on 'clean' pasture.
2. Post-dipping lameness, once a not infrequent occurrence following the plunge-dipping of sheep, is no longer a problem since changed methods of controlling lice and fly have been introduced (see Chapter 19). Plunge-dips have fallen into disuse, and shower-dipping is also less commonly used. The temporary, but acute, lameness occurring following plunge-dipping was caused by the rapid proliferation of *E. rhusiopathiae* in stale dip solutions which had had either insufficient bacteriostat added or had become exhausted. The organism was able to multiply

very rapidly in very short time in such dip solutions and reach dangerous levels of contamination within 24 hours.

Where shower-dips are still used, constant replenishment of bacteriostat should be used during showering and sumps should be emptied at the end of each day's dipping and replenished with fresh dip for following use.

Clinical findings

Severe lameness develops 2–4 days after exposure and may affect up to 90% of sheep, although 25% is more usual. Despite the severe lameness, often in all four legs, the lesions are almost imperceptible. There may be minor swelling of the joints and pain on manipulation. At necropsy very little joint change is evident although there may be excessive turbid synovial fluid present. Suppuration is not a feature.

Culturing the organism from the joints is often difficult and, if available, detection of antibodies in the joint fluid may be more rewarding.

Treatment

Many of the milder cases recover spontaneously in about 7–10 days and for this reason treatment is not always undertaken. However, the condition can become chronic unless treated in the early stages, particularly in lambs. The organism is sensitive to penicillin and this is often administered as a single dose. The decision to administer antibiotics will depend on the particular circumstances of the case.

Control

Control of *Erysipelothrix* arthritis is based on prevention of wound contamination by:
1. Hygiene at lambing and docking time. All instruments used should be cleaned and disinfected and these procedures should be carried out in clean surroundings.
2. Preventing the multiplication of *Erysipelothrix* organisms in sheep dips by:
    (a) only using fresh dip
    (b) correct use of bacteriostats.

Suppurative arthritis

Whereas *Erysipelothrix* arthritis is a serous or fibrinous arthritis, there are a number of other bacteria that can result in a suppurative arthritis if they gain access to the joints of sheep. The most common is likely to be *Streptococcus dysgalactiae* but may also include *F. necrophorum*, *A. pyogenes*, *Staphylococcus* spp and *Escherichia coli*. The severe and often permanent joint damage that results from these infections means that many of the affected lambs die or are destroyed.

Clinical findings

1. The predisposing factors, such as unhygienic lambing or docking conditions are similar to those for *Erysipelothrix* arthritis and thus a number of lambs can be affected at once.
2. There is gross swelling of the joints, particularly the carpus, metacarpus and hock.
3. In many cases more than one joint is affected, as well as other organs such as the liver and lung.
4. Characteristically, grey/green pus accumulates in the joints and tendon sheaths and may discharge to the exterior.
5. Because of the permanent joint damage, the course is chronic, resulting in severe muscle wasting and emaciation.

Treatment

If identified early, daily treatment with penicillin for a minimum of 5 days can be undertaken. However, because of the permanent and painful joint damage, many cases are not worth treating and affected lambs should be destroyed on humane grounds. It is wise to resist the temptation to leave the farmer with a supply of antibiotics to repeatedly inject these suffering lambs.

Prevention

Emphasise the importance of hygiene during lambing, castration and tailing.

Laminitis in sheep (nutritional, aseptic)

Laminitis is rarely reported in sheep in New Zealand and when it is encountered, it is usually associated with excessive concentrate or grain feeding. Most cases recover spontaneously if the diet and exercise are restricted, although severe cases can result in marked separation of the horn of the feet.

Shelly hoof

This condition appears as a hole or gap on the outer wall of the claw that becomes packed with mud. It generally does not affect the sheep, but it is an important condition because it needs to be differentiated from footrot.

REFERENCES

Abbott KA. The epidemiology of intermediate footrot. *PhD Thesis*, University of Sydney, Australia, 2000

Abbott KA, Lewis CJ. Current approaches to the management of ovine footrot. *The Veterinary Journal* 169, 28-41, 2005

Allworth B. Footrot — control and eradication. *Proceedings of the Post-Graduate Committee in Veterinary Science*, University of Sydney. No 141 — Sheep medicine, 443-9, 1990

Allworth MB. Exploring the footrot maze. *Proceedings of the 2nd Pan Pacific Veterinary Conference (Sheep)*, 159-62, 1996

Beveridge WIB. Footrot in sheep: A transmissible disease due to infection with *Fusiformis nodosus* (n.spp). *Bulletin of the Council for Scientific and Industrial Research*, Melbourne, Australia, 140, 1941

Casey RH, Martin PAJ. Effect of foot paring of sheep affected with footrot on response to zinc sulphate/sodium lauryl sulphate foot bathing treatment. *Australian Veterinary Journal* 65, 258-9, 1988

Clifton R, Green L. Pathogenesis of ovine footrot disease: A complex picture. *Veterinary Record* 179, 225-7, 2016

Dhungyel OP, Lehmann DR, Whittington RJ. Pilot trails in Australia on eradication of footrot by flock specific vacccination. *Veterinary Microbiology* 132, 364-71, 2008

Egerton JR. Control and eradication of footrot at the farm level — the role of the veterinarian. *Proceedings of the 19th Annual Seminar of the Society of Sheep and Beef Cattle Veterinarians, New Zealand Veterinary Association* (2nd International Congress for Sheep Veterinarians), 215-22, 1989

Egerton JR, Burrell DH. Prophylactic and therapeutic vaccination against ovine footrot. *Australian Veterinary Journal* 44, 275-83, 1970

Egerton JR, Ghimire SC, Dhungyel OP, et al. Eradication of virulent footrot from sheep and goats in any endemic area of Nepal and an evaluation of specific vaccination. *Veterinary Record* 151, 290-5, 2002

Egerton JR, Parsonson IM, Graham NPH. Parenteral chemotherapy of ovine footrot. *Australian Veterinary Journal* 44, 275-83, 1968

Frosth S, Koenig U, Nyman AK, Pringle M, Aspan A. Characterisation of *Dichelobacter nodosus* and detection of *Fusobacterium necrophorum* and *Treponema* spp. in sheep with different clinical manifestations of footrot. *Veterinary Microbiology* 179, 82-90, 2015

Graham NPH, Egerton JR. Pathogenesis of ovine footrot: The role of some environmental factors. *Australian Veterinary Journal* 44, 235-40, 1968

Green LE, Wassink GJ, Grogono-Thomas R, Moore LJ, Medley GF. Looking after the individual to reduce disease in the flock: A binomial mixed effects model investigating the impact of individual sheep management of footrot and interdigital dermatitis in a prospective longitudinal study on one farm. *Preventive Veterinary Medicine* 78, 172-8, 2007

Green LE, George TRN. Assessment of current knowledge of footrot in sheep with particular reference to *Dichelobacter nodosus* and implications for elimination and control strategies for sheep in Great Britain. *Veterinary Journal* 175, 173-80, 2008

Gurung RB, Dhungyel OP, Tschering P, Egerton JR. The use of autogenous *Dichelobacter nodosus* vaccine to eliminate clinical signs of virulent footrot in a flock of sheep in Bhutan. *Veterinary Journal* 172, 356-63, 2006

Hickford JGH. A new approach to footrot control. *Proceedings of the 31st Annual Seminar of the Society of Sheep and Beef Cattle Veterinarians, New Zealand Veterinary Association*, 75-80, 2001

Hickford JGH, Davies S, Zhou H, Gudex BW. A survey of the control and financial impact of footrot in the New Zealand Merino industry. *Proceedings of the New Zealand Society of Animal Production* 65, 117-22, 2005

Hooper RS, Jones TW. Corono-pedal abscessation following the excessive use of formalin as a treatment for footrot in sheep. *Veterinary Record* 90, 697-9, 1972

Jopp AJ, Jackson R, Mulvaney CJ. A survey on the prevalence, treatment and control of footrot in Central Otago. *New Zealand Veterinary Jounal* 32, 172-3, 1984

Kaler J, Daniels SLS, Wright JL, Green LE. Randomized clinical trial of long acting oxytetracycline, foot trimming, and flunixin meglumine on time to recovery in sheep with footrot. *Journal of Veterinary Internal Medicine* 24, 420-5, 2010

Maboni G, Frosth S, Aspan A, Totemeyer S. Ovine footrot: new insights into bacterial colonisation. *Veterinary Record* 179, 228, 2016

Mulvaney C. A guide to the mangement of footrot in sheep. Merino New Zealand, 2013

Parsonson IM, Egerton JR, Roberts DS. Ovine interdigital dermatitis. *Journal of Comparative Pathology* 77, 309-13, 1967

Paterson R, Paterson H. The selection and breeding of Merino sheep for footrot resistance. *Proceedings of the New Zealand Society of Animal Production* 51, 283-6, 1991

Roberts DS, Egerton JR. The aetiology and pathogenesis of ovine footrot. II. The pathogenic association of *Fusiformis nodosus* and *F. necrophorus*. *Journal of Comparative Pathology* 79, 217-26, 1969

Roberts DS, Graham NPH, Egerton JR, Parsonson IM. Infective bulbar necrosis (heel abscess) of sheep, a mixed infection with *Fusiformis necrophorus* and *Corynebacterium pyogenes*. *Journal of Comparative Pathology* 78, 1-7, 1968

Robertson DRH. Comparison of tilmicosin and lincomycin/spectinomycin combination for treatment of footrot in merino sheep. *Proceedings of the Society of Sheep and Beef Cattle Veterinarians, New Zealand Veterinary Association*, 5-14, 2014

Skerman TM, Moorhouse SR. Broomfield Corriedales: A strain of sheep selectively bred for resistance to footrot. *New Zealand Veterinary Journal* 35, 101-6, 1987

Vizard AL. The rational use of antibiotics in an eradication programme for virulent footrot. *Proceedings of the 2nd Pan Pacific Veterinary Conference (Sheep)*, 163-70, 1996

West DM. Anatomical considerations of the distal interphalangeal joint of sheep. *New Zealand Veterinary Journal* 31, 58-60, 1983

West DM. Observations on an outbreak of foot abscess in sheep. *New Zealand Veterinary Journal* 31, 71-4, 1983

West DM. A study of naturally occurring cases of ovine foot abscess in New Zealand. *New Zealand Veterinary Journal* 31, 152-6, 1983

Winter AC. Lameness in sheep. *Small Ruminat Research* 76, 149-53, 2008

Witcomb LA, Green LE, Kaler J, Ul-Hassan A, Calvo-Bado LA, Medley GF, Grogono-Thomas R, Wellington EMH. A longitudinal study of the role of *Dichelobacter nodosus* and *Fusobacterium necrophorum* load in initiation and severity of footrot in sheep. *Preventive Veterinary Medicine* 115, 48-55, 2014

Witcomb LA, Green LE, Calvo-Bado LA, Russell CL, Smith EM, Grogono-Thomas R, Wellington EMH. First study of pathogen load and localisation of ovine footrot using fluorescence in situ hybridisation (FISH). *Veterinary Microbiology* 176, 321-7, 2015

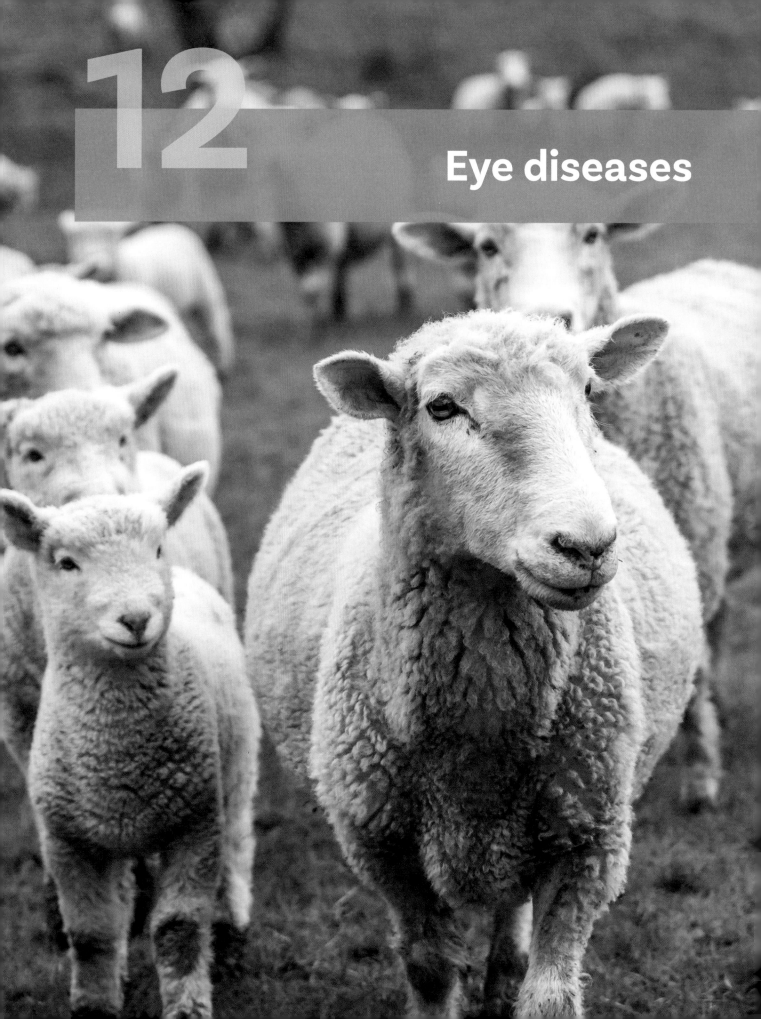

12

Eye diseases

Pinkeye

Pinkeye (ovine infectious keratoconjunctivitis, OIKC, contagious ophthalmia) is a worldwide common condition affecting sheep and goats. It is characterised by a severe conjunctivitis and keratitis that causes temporary blindness. As a problem it becomes particularly significant when it affects pregnant ewes, making feeding difficult and often leading to the occurrence of pregnancy toxaemia.

Aetiology

In New Zealand *Chlamydophila* spp have been associated with most outbreaks of the disease. In 2001 *Mycoplasma conjunctivae* was identified as a cause of pinkeye by the then National Centre for Disease Investigation. It appears to cause a more severe disease compared with that caused by *Chlamydophila* spp. A serological survey for *M. conjunctivae* infection in sheep and goats, conducted in 2003, reported a prevalence of antibodies to *M. conjunctivae* of 71% in 45 flocks tested in seven different provinces, suggesting it to be a more common causative agent of pinkeye than previously thought. Both *Chlamydophila* and *Mycoplasma* are considered the primary causative agents either alone or in combination. In Australia *Rickettsia conjunctivae* and *Mycoplasma* spp are believed to be the main causative agents, while in Britain *M. conjunctivae* is considered a main causative agent with *Branhamella ovis*, *Escherichia coli* and *Staphylococcus aureus* playing a secondary part in increasing the ocular reaction. It is possible that there may be different aetiological agents producing similar clinical findings in different countries.

Epidemiology

The disease is found wherever sheep are kept. Most *Chlamydophila* outbreaks in New Zealand, although temporarily distressing to the sheep, are mild and most commonly occur annually in adult sheep during the summer and autumn; more severe attacks may appear suddenly after several years of low incidence or freedom from the disease. Some of the latter more severe cases may be attributed to *M. conjunctivae*. Whatever the aetiological agent, the disease may occur at any time of the year and in sheep of any age (Figure 12.1).

Chlamydophila spp is spread indirectly by dust, pollen in grass and flies that have been contaminated by the lachrymal secretions of infected sheep. Sheep may also be infected directly from the eye secretions of other infected animals. It is believed that the handling of the face and head of sheep when drenching may also be an important means of spread. It is frequently seen in pregnant ewes in the South Island when they are being fed hay. Generally the disease is more common in dry, warm weather when large numbers of flies and dusty farm conditions predominate.

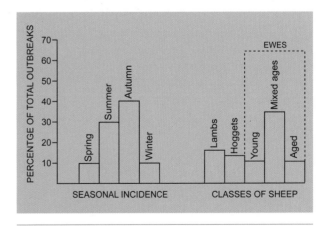

Figure 12.1 Seasonal incidence and classes of sheep affected in *Chlamydophila* pinkeye outbreaks.

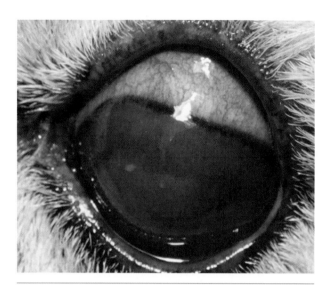

Figure 12.2 A mild pinkeye lesion with conjunctivitis and injection of the scleral blood vessels.

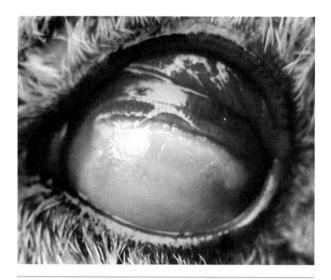

Figure 12.3 Severe pinkeye with possible permanent damage to the cornea.

Outbreaks may be severe in some flocks with the morbidity rate as high as 50% but usually it is 10–15%.

After clinical recovery the eyes of most sheep continue to harbour the *Chlamydophila* organisms for periods of up to a year, and such carrier animals are a source of reinfection in subsequent years. More than 50% of recovered animals remain resistant for periods up to a year. *Mycoplasma conjunctivae* may persist in the eye or nares of recovered sheep for up to 3 months.

Clinical findings

Pinkeye starts as a simple conjunctivitis with photophobia and lacrimation. A wet face extending ventrally from the medial canthus of the eye is usually the first sign of the disease. This is followed about 24 hours later by keratitis with cloudiness of the cornea and some increase in vascularity. The next stage is a severe pannus formation with vascularisation from the periphery of the eye. The cornea then appears pink. This finally turns yellow due to the presence of desquamating cells and other debris, and finally corneal ulcers may develop. In extreme cases the anterior chamber of the eye may rupture. In most cases recovery commences in 3–4 days and is complete in 10–14 days, although in some animals the cloudiness of the cornea may persist for several weeks or even permanently. In many cases both eyes are affected and spread through the flock is rapid. Pinkeye caused by *M. conjunctivae* may be more severe, with outbreaks persisting for some weeks or even months. Resolution of infection may be protracted and in some sheep the disease may recur after apparent recovery.

Diagnosis

The diagnosis of pinkeye is straightforward because of the specific lesions and the epidemiology. In particular the corneal vascularisation is a characteristic feature and in conjunctival smears, epithelial cells display the intracytoplasmic inclusions that are associated with the *Chlamydophila* agent. However, identification of whether the condition is caused by *Chlamydophila* or *M. conjunctivae* requires laboratory investigation.

The condition needs to be differentiated from grass seed (barley grass in particular) contamination of the eye and, in young lambs, entropion (see later).

Treatment

Because of the relatively quick and spontaneous recovery that occurs with *Chlamydophila* pinkeye it is often questionable whether treatment and isolation of mildly infected sheep is warranted. Such matters as the time of the year and the nature of the environment are important. For example, dry ewes during a hot dry summer are probably best left to recover spontaneously, rather than yarding under dusty conditions that may exacerbate the spread of the disease. However, pregnant animals may be at risk of pregnancy toxaemia and treatment may therefore be desirable.

Although most cases recover spontaneously, early treatment does aid recovery and reduce the number of animals that develop an ulcerative keratitis; however, treated sheep are more likely to relapse and become re-infected than untreated sheep.

Treatment is a tedious process and should be done with care. If an outbreak is severe and occurs during the grass seed season, care must be taken to inspect eyes for penetrating grass awns. The common treatment used in pinkeye is topical treatment with oxytetracycline, which can be administered as a puffer or a spray at a 10% concentration. In moderate to severe cases, parenteral administration of long-acting oxytetracycline is warranted. For treatment of refractory cases caused by *M. conjunctivae*, overseas some researchers have recommended the off-label use of tilmicosin at the cattle dose rate of 10 mg/kg. It is important to ensure that this dose rate is not exceeded and that an appropriate meat withholding period is adhered to. Animals weighing less than 15 kg should not be treated with this drug.

Note that, particularly in the case of *M. conjuntivae* pinkeye, relapses after treatment may occur.

Entropion (inverted eyelids)

Entropion of newborn lambs is a defect of eyelid formation in which the eyelids become inverted causing a severe irritation to the cornea and, if it is not corrected, may lead to permanent blindness. It occurs in all breeds of sheep, but is seen commonly in Corriedales, halfbreds, Merinos, Border Leicesters and Romneys.

Aetiology

It is believed that entropion is an inherited condition of sheep, possibly inherited as a dominant trait, but the exact nature of the inheritance is uncertain.

Clinical findings

The inverted eyelashes and facial hairs cause irritation of the sensitive conjunctivae, resulting in a severe conjunctivitis and keratitis (not unlike pinkeye in appearance). Ulcers may form on the cornea. Lacrimation is usually severe and the eye may be cloudy and filled with pus following bacterial infection.

Entropion may affect one or both eyes, and unless treated some lambs may have permanently damaged eyes. In some cases spontaneous recovery apparently occurs. Affected lambs are more susceptible to mismothering, starvation and death.

The diagnosis of the condition is not difficult and is based on the ocular examination of affected lambs. However, it is important not to confuse the condition with pinkeye and institute topical treatment without correcting the underlying condition.

Treatment

Mildly affected cases may be treated by manually everting the eyelids. Sometimes this exercise needs to be repeated, but many cases will respond to this simple attention. If the inversion recurs after manual eversion, careful injection of 0.5 ml of procaine penicillin subcutaneously into the area below the lower eyelid is often effective.

Under some circumstances large numbers of lambs will be severely affected. These can be effectively treated by inserting a Michel clip into the lower eyelid — this should be removed after 7 days. Alternatively a simple surgical operation involving the removal of an elliptical strip of skin from above and below the eyelids can be performed with a pair of sharp surgical scissors and a pair of rat-toothed forceps. The skin may be sutured, but when numbers of lambs are involved this is a tedious process and if left the purse-string effect of the resulting scar tissue is sufficient to keep the lid everted. Lambs treated in this way should be permanently marked and not used for breeding.

Prevention

The ewe and the ram, if they can be identified, should be culled from the breeding flock, particularly if the incidence of entropion is high.

Inherited cataract

Blindness due to a form of inherited cataract has been reported on one occasion in New Zealand Romney sheep. The condition is not widespread; should it occur, because it is thought to be caused by an autosomal dominant gene the culling of affected animals will quickly resolve the problem within a flock.

Microphthalmia

Three blind lambs with abnormally small eyes were born in a Texel flock in the Manawatu region of New Zealand in 1999. In the same flock seven more were born the next year. Macroscopically, the optic globes were about one half normal size and the optic nerves at the chiasma were approximately half the normal diameter. It was concluded that these lambs were affected with congenital microphthalmia. It is estimated that 5–10% of Texel or Texel-cross sheep in New Zealand are microphthalmia carriers of the recessive gene causing the disorder. Microphthalmia was first recognised in European Texels and has now been reported in flocks in a number of countries including Australia, New Zealand and South America.

Control of the condition has been limited to the culling of rams and ewes known to have produced affected progeny. Fortunately, Texel rams in New Zealand are mainly used as terminal sires over other breeds, so the disorder is unlikely to show in crossbred lambs. There is a predictive DNA test now available that identifies carriers of the gene defect (Zoetis NZ). This diagnostic test may be useful for pedigree Texel breeders to both help eliminate the disorder and ensure that buyers of their rams are not purchasing carrier sheep. The interpretation of the i-Scan test gives the probability that an animal is a carrier of the microphthalmia gene and the risk involved if used for breeding.

REFERENCES

PINKEYE

Cooper BS. Transmission of a *Chlamydia*-like agent isolated from contagious conjunctive-keratitis of sheep. *New Zealand Veterinary Journal* 22, 181-4, 1974

Cooper BS. Contagious conjunctive-keratitis of sheep (CCK) in New Zealand. *New Zealand Veterinary Journal* 15, 79-84, 1967

Egiwu GO, Faull WB, Bradbury JM, Clarkson MJ. Ovine infectious keratoconjunctivitis: A microbiological study of clinically unaffected and affected sheep's eyes with special reference to *Mycoplasma conjunctivae*, *Veterinary Record* 125, 253-6, 1989

Hosie BD. Ocular diseases. *Diseases of sheep*, 3rd edition, pp 301-5, edited by Martin WB and Aitken ID. Blackwell Science, 2000

Motha MXJ. A serological survey for *Mycoplasma conjunctivae* infection in sheep and goats. *Surveillance* 30, 9-10, 2003

Spadbrow PB, Marley J. Ovine kerato-conjunctivitis, possible T strain mycoplasmas in the conjunctival sac. *Australian Veterinary Journal* 47, 116-18, 1971

Thornton R. Ovine infectious keratoconjunctivitis (atypical pinkeye; OIKC). *Proceedings of the 33rd Annual Seminar of the Society of Sheep and Beef Cattle Veterinarians, New Zealand Veterinary Association*, 105-9, 2003

ENTROPION

Taylor M, Catchpole J. Incidence of entropion in lambs from two ewe flocks put to the same ram. *Veterinary Record* 188, 361, 1986

INHERITED CATARACT

Brooks HV, Jolly RD, West DM, Bruère AN. An inherited cataract in New Zealand Romney sheep. *New Zealand Veterinary Journal* 30, 113-14, 1982

MICROPHTHALMIA

Roe WD, West DM, Walshe MT, Jolly RD. Microphthalmia in Texel lambs. *New Zealand Veterinary Journal* 51, 194-5, 2003

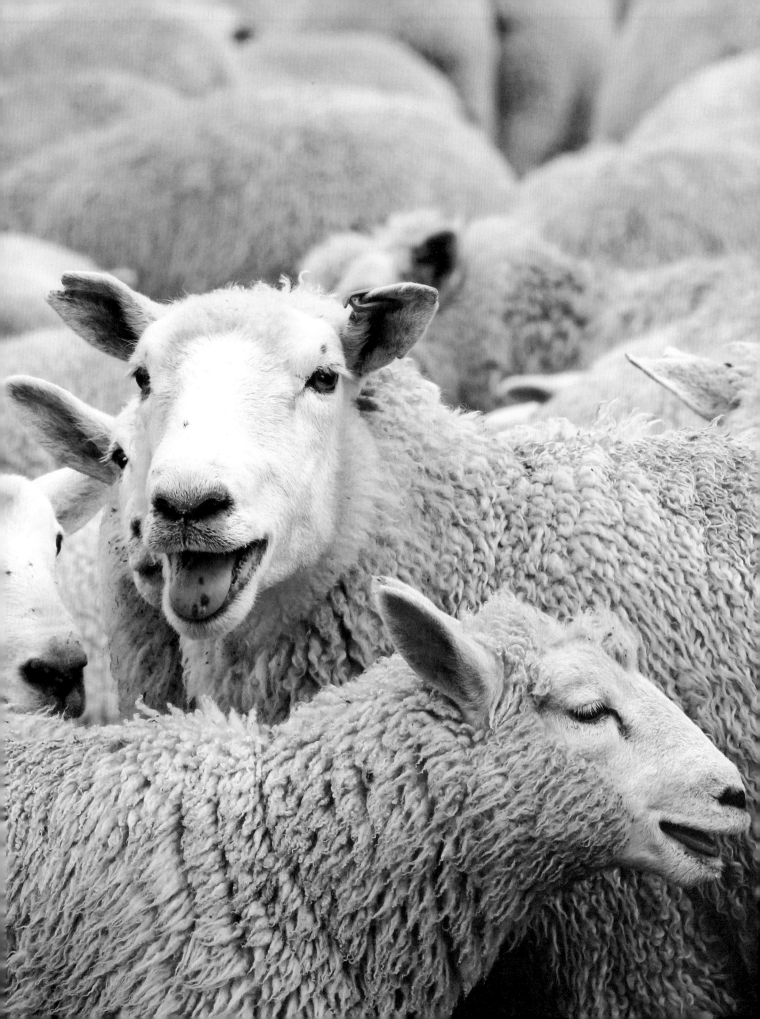

13 Caseous lymphadenitis

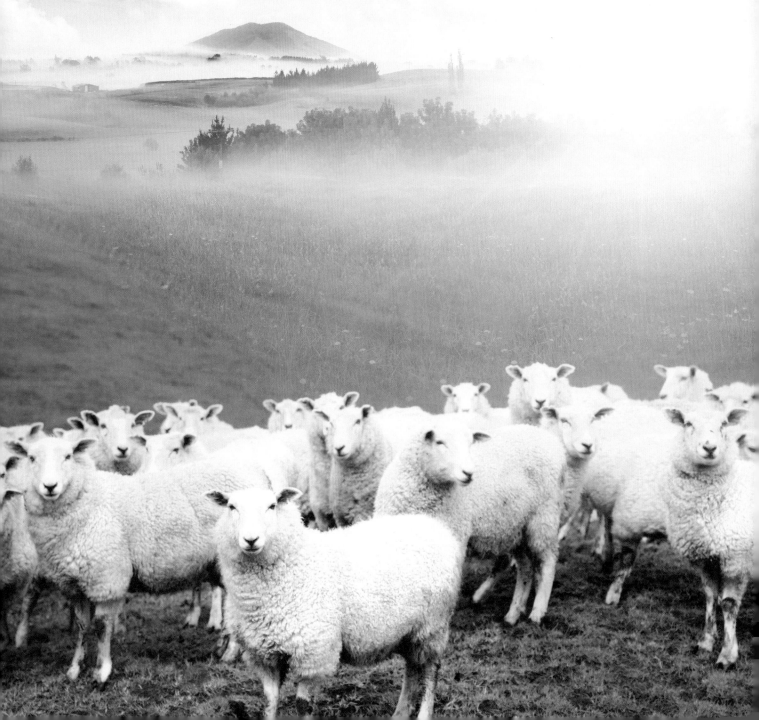

Caseous lymphadenitis (CLA, cheesy gland, lympho) is a common bacterial disease of sheep and goats in New Zealand and other sheep-raising countries. It was first reported in the UK relatively recently, in 1991. It is a chronic disease that causes formation of abscesses in lymph nodes. It is a problem of concern to some farmers, particularly Merino farmers, and it causes considerable economic loss to the sheep industry primarily due to reduced wool production, carcass inspection costs and trimming of affected carcasses.

Aetiology

Caseous lymphadenitis is caused by *Corynebacterium pseudotuberculosis*, a very short Gram-positive rod appearing as a coccus or coccobacillus. The organism is able to remain viable in the environment for many weeks. Experimentally it has been recovered from purulent material placed in shaded areas of a shearing shed for up to 20 weeks and from fomites such as straw, hay and wood for up to 8 weeks. It is able to survive for at least 24 hours in prepared commercial sheep dips and has been shown to grow in sheep faeces. It has also been isolated from faecal material in sheep camps and from the faeces of both infected and non-infected sheep.

The pathogenic properties of *C. pseudotuberculosis*, which include clumping, cytotoxicity and induction of caseation, are largely attributable to bacterial lipid which occurs as a floccular layer external to the cell wall. The lipid of *C. pseudotuberculosis* is highly pyogenic and is associated with abscess formation. In addition, the organism also produces an exotoxin which is thought to enhance bacterial dissemination by increasing vascular permeability.

Transmission

The majority of disease spread is thought to occur at shearing. This may be due to the accidental rupture of affected lymph nodes during shearing contaminating the environment, and infection then entering other sheep via skin wounds. Merino sheep with large neck wrinkles are particularly prone to these accidental shearing cuts. Infection may enter any skin wound from such material, or from ground heavily contaminated with the organism, e.g. sheep camps, yards, woolsheds, etc. The organism is also able to penetrate freshly shorn unbroken skin. Another route of transmission may be by aerosol spread when sheep with lung abscesses cough and discharge the organism onto fresh shearing cuts of other sheep. Keeping sheep penned together under cover for an hour or more after shearing is associated with an increased risk of infection. In addition, dipping up to 2 weeks after shearing may facilitate spread via contaminated dip wash. It is theoretically possible that infection could be transmitted between flocks via contaminated shearing equipment, clothing or mobile handling equipment.

Pathogenesis

In most cases in sheep, progressive caseous lymphadenitis follows the infection of a superficial wound with spread of the organism to the superficial or regional lymph node. These suppurate, and their lymphatogenous and haematogenous extension may produce abscesses in internal organs. The progression of the disease is slow and may reach the bloodstream only in older animals. In younger animals the disease tends to be confined to the superficial lymph nodes of which the prescapular, popliteal and prefemoral are the most frequently affected. In rams, the superficial inguinal lymph nodes may become infected, producing a palpable abscess near the genitalia and rendering the ram unsound. In the UK, however, the most common site for abscesses is in the lymph nodes of the head (parotid, retropharyngeal and submandibular) and this may be due to intensive husbandry practices with transmission via such things as contaminated feeding troughs.

The initial lesion in lymphoid tissue progresses through stages of necrosis and capsule reformation. This gives the lesion its characteristic lamellations, which become particularly prominent when calcareous granules are deposited in successive layers at the margin of the expanding lesion (the onion appearance).

Spread from the lymph nodes may produce lesions in the lungs. These are more common with advancing age.

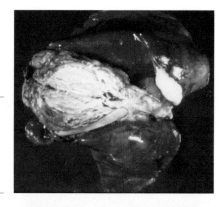

Figure 13.1 Caseous lymphadenitis affecting the lungs.

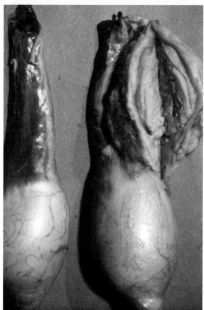

Figure 13.2 Caseous lymphadenitis affecting the scrotal lymph node.

Similar lesions are found in young lambs on occasions when the disease has disseminated very quickly. Although dissemination to other viscera is uncommon, metastases are occasionally seen in the renal cortex as discrete abscesses or a descending pyelonephritis. Other viscera, chiefly the liver and spleen, may contain solitary abscesses.

Occasionally in lambs and older sheep organisms are disseminated to other organs such as the central nervous system or joints.

Progress of the infection at primary or secondary sites involves phagocytosis, intracellular multiplication of *C. pseudotuberculosis*, and death of host cells. Liberated bacteria are engulfed by remaining or infiltrating phagocytes, which again go through the process of degeneration and death while the organism continues to multiply and divide. This cycle of phagocytosis, multiplication of organism and cellular degeneration provides the basis of the chronic lesions observed in caseous lymphadenitis of sheep.

The size of lesions varies and probably depends on several factors including the initial number of organisms, the rate of multiplication and accessibility of a lesion to host cells. Size might also reflect the quantity of cytotoxic lipid accumulated during development.

Clinical features

If the disease affects the superficial lymph nodes there may be palpable enlargement of these glands. Affected nodes may rupture, or be accidentally 'lanced' by shearing, causing a discharging wound and leading to heavy contamination of the environment. At slaughter, these lesions must be removed from the carcass and in severe cases the entire carcass may be condemned. However, in most cases the sheep remain healthy.

When internal lesions occur, lungs and thoracic nodes are the most commonly involved sites. Sheep with severe lung lesions may have focal or generalised pneumonia, or pleurisy. Coughing may result. Sheep with extensive internal infections may occasionally show signs of ill thrift and emaciation.

Australian research in Merino sheep has suggested that in the first year of infection wool production may be decreased by 4–7%, although in subsequent years there is no significant effect on wool production.

Diagnosis

Overt and discharging lesions may be seen in advanced cases of caseous lymphadenitis but many cases are not diagnosed until necropsy or during the meat inspection process. Where necessary, the organism may be cultured from purulent material.

A number of serological tests have been developed and used for research purposes and overseas. These include bacterial agglutination tests, haemolysis inhibition test, an ELISA test, and an agar gel immunoprecipitation test.

Prevalence

Although the national system of reporting on this disease is now very accurate, the overall prevalence appears to have altered little from earlier reports, particularly in respect to breed and location.

The New Zealand sheep meat industry has a nationwide distribution of slaughtering and processing plants with a well-trained inspection service under close veterinary supervision. It also keeps excellent computer-based disease and defects records. In addition the industry relies largely on the slaughtering and processing of prime lamb carcasses for export; thus, a very large proportion, nearly 50%, of the total sheep population is slaughtered and inspected annually. These inspection data provide a comparatively accurate picture of the national and regional prevalence of slaughtered and culled sheep. Similar information is also available for slaughtered goats.

Data reviewed from these more recent New Zealand records largely reconfirm previous information, which may be summarised as follows:

1. The prevalence of caseous lymphadenitis is higher in the South Island than the North Island. This can be accounted for by the greater number of fine-woolled breeds (Merino, halfbred and Corriedale) grazed in the South Island.
2. Merinos are more commonly affected than Corriedales or halfbreds, which in turn have a higher prevalence than Romneys and crossbreds. The finer skin and neck wrinkles of Merinos makes them very susceptible to skin damage at shearing.
3. The prevalence is higher in older sheep. This is simply a reflection of greater exposure to shearing and skin damage.
4. There is a large variation between farms, presumably the result of breed differences and farm practices.

In Australia the sheep industry is dominated by fine-wool production rather than the more dual-purpose nature of the New Zealand industry. Hence the predominant breed is the Merino and a high percentage of animals are slaughtered as adults, and have been shorn many times. Such features account for the comparatively high prevalence of caseous lymphadenitis found in Australian stock at slaughter.

Human infection

A very small number of cases of human infection with *C. pseudotuberculosis* have been documented. Most have been recorded in shepherds and meatworkers. Infection in humans is usually manifested as abscessation of either the axillary or superficial inguinal node consistent with entry via the corresponding limb and results from working in unhygienic conditions.

Prevention and control

Prior to the availability of an effective vaccine against *C. pseudotuberculosis* infection, great emphasis was given to hygienic methods of control. Such methods, if properly applied, were effective in reducing the disease on individual properties but the overall incidence of the disease was not reduced.

Vaccination

A caseous lymphadenitis vaccine is available in New Zealand, combined with clostridial vaccines (Glanvac 6®; Zoetis New Zealand). Vaccination does not provide complete protection but does provide significant protection to immunised sheep by reducing the incidence of lesions and also reducing the number of abscesses found in infected sheep that have been immunised. Lambs should be vaccinated twice before being shorn, the first vaccination given at docking/marking and the second at weaning (at least 4–6 weeks apart). Subsequently, adult sheep should receive an annual booster at least 2 weeks prior to shearing.

Hygiene

It would be unwise to ignore hygienic methods of control in any programme designed to control caseous lymphadenitis on a property where it is a problem. There are three main areas to consider:

1. Prevention of unnecessary wounds

Every effort should be made to reduce the wounding of sheep to a minimum by encouraging clean, smooth shearing. Selection of 'plain bodied' sheep in preference to wrinkly strains may reduce wounding at shearing. Other factors such as rough dogs, badly constructed yards and so on are all sources of wounding in yarded sheep. Blade shearing also reduces the incidence of skin damage significantly.

2. Prevention of wound infection

To prevent wound infection, sheep should be moved from the shearing shed or yards to clean paddocks as quickly as possible. Further, the construction of the shearing shed and yards is important. For example, shearing sheds with two-tier holding pens are not to be recommended as this may result in sheep that have just been shorn being held in the lower tier to become fouled by those above. The construction of sheds should also allow the shearing board to be cleaned and dried easily. Shears and combs and cutters should be treated with disinfectant. Attention should also be drawn to the importance of good personal hygiene of the shearers.

The order of shearing is also important. In general, shear younger sheep first. Any sheep with obviously discharging abscesses should be separated and shorn last. Other measures to minimise post-shearing contamination include:

- Do not overcrowd sheep in counting-out pens.
- Release sheep as soon as possible after shearing.
- Avoid dust at all cost. Either use concrete yards or dampen down dusty yards with water before use.
- Do not draft sheep until wounds have healed.
- Do not attempt to dip sheep until all wounds have healed (two weeks).

3. Reduction of the source of wound contamination

A number of areas should be considered in a control programme:

- Separate and dispose of sheep with open abscesses.
- Regularly inspect flocks for developing or discharging abscesses.
- Pay attention to areas where sheep may congregate, e.g. yards, water troughs, unfenced plantations and old sheep camp areas.

REFERENCES

Augustine JL, Renshaw HW. Survival of *Corynebacterium pseudotuberculosis* in axenic purulent exudates on common barnyard fomites. *American Journal of Veterinary Research* 47, 713-15, 1986

Baird GJ, Fontaine MC. *Corynebacterium pseudotuberculosis* and its role in ovine caseous lymphadenitis. *Journal of Comparative Pathology* 137, 179-210, 2007

Batey RG. Pathogenesis of caseous lymphadenitis in sheep and goats. *Australian Veterinary Journal* 63, 269-72, 1986

Brown CC, Olander HJ. Caseous lymphadenitis in Goats and Sheep: A review. *Veterinary Bulletin* 57, 1-12, 1987

Eggleton DG, Middleton HD, Doidge CV, Minty DW. Immunisation against ovine caseous lymphadenitis: Comparison of *Corynebacterium pseudotuberculosis* vaccines with and without bacterial cells. *Australian Veterinary Journal* 68, 317-19, 1991

Ensor CR. Caseous lymphadenitis in sheep. *New Zealand Journal of Agriculture* 108, 34-5, 1964

Hughes JG, Barton J. A survey of the incidence of lympho in the high country. *Tussock Grasslands and Mountain Lands Institute* 17, 57-71, 1969

Nuttall WO. Caseous lymphadenitis in sheep and goats in New Zealand. *Surveillance* (MAFQual) 15, 10-12, 1988

Paton MW. New concepts in the epidemiology and control of caseous lymphadenitis. *23rd Proceedings of the Sheep and Beef Cattle Society of the New Zealand Veterinary Association*, 25-37, 1993

Paton MW, Mercy AR, Wilkinson FC, Gardner JJ, Sutherland SS, Ellis TM. The effects of caseous lymphadenitis on wool production and bodyweight in young sheep. *Australian Veterinary Journal* 65, 117-19, 1988

Paton MW, Rose IR, Hart RA, Sutherland SS, Mercy AR, Ellis TM, Dhaliwal JA. New infection with *Corynebacterium pseudotuberculosis* reduces wool production. *Australian Veterinary Journal* 71, 47-9, 1994

Paton MW, Sutherland SS, Rose IR, Hart RA, Mercy AR, Ellis TM. The spread of *Corynebacterium pseudotuberculosis* infection to unvaccinated and vaccinated sheep. *Australian Veterinary Journal* 72, 266-9, 1995

Paton M, Rose I, Hart R, Sutherland S, Mercy A, Ellis T. Post-shearing management affects the seroincidence of *Corynebacterium pseudotuberculosis* infection in sheep flocks. *Preventative Veterinary Medicine* 26, 275-84, 1996

Sheik-Omar AR, Shah M. Caseous lymphadenitis in sheep imported from Australia for slaughter in Malaysia. *Australian Veterinary Journal* 61, 410-16, 1984

Surveillance

(1979) 4: 8-9	CLA on the increase
(1981) 4: 17-18	Sheep prevalence of *C. ovis* at meatworks
(1982) 2: 4-5	Caseous lymphadenitis vaccine trials get underway
(1988) 15: 10-12	Caseous lymphadenitis in sheep and goats in New Zealand

Williamson LH. Caseous lymphadenitis in small ruminants. *Veterinary Clinics of North America Food Animal Practice* 17, 359-71, 2001

14 Diseases of the mammary gland

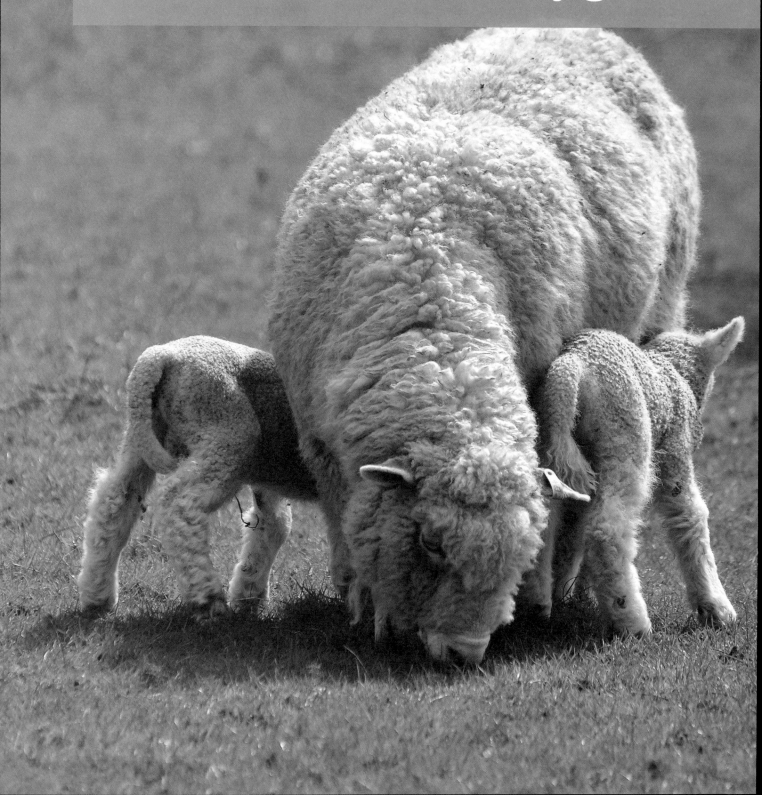

Limited New Zealand survey data has shown that between 2% and 6% of breeding ewes have defective udders at weaning. Australian surveys have reported a higher culling of ewes with udder defects (6–14%). Unfortunately there are few substantial reports on ovine mammary disease in New Zealand, although anecdotal information suggests that some farmers have experienced significant losses of both ewes and lambs as a result of udder defects. It is common practice for New Zealand sheep farmers to palpate the udders of ewes, usually after weaning, to identify those with udder defects for culling. However, there has been limited research on how udder defects such as lumps, teat size and symmetry affect lamb survival or growth, or how these defects change over time. Hence it is difficult to provide firm guidelines on the appropriateness or otherwise of culling ewes with various udder defects.

Mastitis

Mastitis is the most important ovine mammary disease; but in relation to some more-important diseases, mastitis is probably of minor importance to the New Zealand sheep industry. It is probably of greatest concern to sheep milking flocks. For example, in a 1999 case, 50 of 400 ewes in a milking flock developed gangrenous mastitis caused by *Staphylococcus aureus*. In countries where sheep are maintained under intensive conditions, particularly for milk production, mastitis is considered to be a serious health problem of sheep. Because of the extensive grazing of sheep, in New Zealand and Australia mastitis is essentially a wastage disease causing death and stunting of suckling lambs and wastage through culling of affected ewes.

Aetiology

The organisms associated with mastitis in ewes are numerous. However, in New Zealand and Australia the main aetiological agents are considered to be *Mannheimia (Pasteurella) haemolytica* and *Staphylococcus aureus* with *Streptococcus* spp, *Micrococcus* spp, *Escherichia coli* and *Trueperella pyogenes* as common isolates from infected udders. On rare occasions *Pseudomonas aeruginosa*, *Corynebacterium pseudotuberculosis* and *Clostridium perfringens* have been incriminated. In Australia, subclinical mastitis has primarily been associated with coagulase-negative staphylococci.

Overseas a variety of organisms including *Histophilus somni*, *Pasteurella multocida*, *Streptococcus* spp, *Klebsiella pneumoniae* and *Mycoplasma* spp have also been identified as aetiological agents of mastitis in ewes.

Predisposing factors and pathogenesis of mastitis in sheep

In New Zealand, most reported cases of clinical mastitis in sheep are associated with *Staph. aureus*, so that in this text the pathogenesis and predisposing factors are particularly related to this organism.

As with mastitis in cattle, infection is considered to be via the teat canal, except for *Mycoplasma* spp which appear to localise in the udder following a septicaemia.

In mastitis caused by *Staph. aureus* a potent toxin is produced causing a severe gangrene of the udder. Other organisms generally produce a suppurative reaction in the ducts and acini of the mammary gland, progressing from acute to chronic inflammation with involution of the acini and mammary gland fibrosis.

In flocks where a regular incidence of mastitis due to *Staph. aureus* occurs, a carrier state exists not only in ewes with chronic mastitis but also in ewes that are clinically normal. Pathogenic staphylococci have been isolated from over 30% of clinically normal udders in some flocks with a mastitis problem. Even in flocks with a low prevalence of clinical mastitis, staphylococci may be isolated from up to 8% of udders. Staphylococcal mastitis (gangrenous mastitis or 'black' mastitis) may develop from organisms in the milk cistern once the host–parasite relationship is disturbed. Other factors such as the quantity of milk produced, serum antitoxin titres, stage of lactation and the 'state' of the host all have an influence on the development of mastitis.

Environmental factors, especially cold stress, play an important role in the development of mastitis in ewes. Cold possibly predisposes to mastitis by reducing blood flow to the mammary gland and causing tissue devitalisation. A further contributing factor may be the increased plasma cortisol secretion stimulated by cold stress, which may reduce phagocytosis and impair antibody response. The association of bare, muddy paddocks with mastitis also suggests the involvement of cold and nutritional stress plus soil contamination of the teats.

In New Zealand, clover-dominant pasture and improved pasture have been associated with a higher incidence of mastitis. The reason for this is unknown but it is suggested it may be related to higher milk production or even the oestrogenic effect of clover. Experimentally, ewes with a low milk production were less susceptible to mastitis than high-yielding ewes when challenged with pathogenic bacteria.

Other factors that may predispose to mastitis in ewes include udder damage and even over-stocking of the udder caused by the loss of the suckling lamb. Scabby mouth may damage the teat end and allow entry of bacteria. In machine-milked dairy ewes, mastitis has been associated with high machine vacuum and poor hygiene. Overseas, mastitis has been linked to intensive husbandry systems and high litter sizes.

Clinical features

The severity of the clinical signs of mastitis appears to be closely related to the stage of lactation. The more acute forms of mastitis, particularly staphylococcal mastitis, occur during early lactation while the more chronic forms such as those caused by *T. pyogenes* are often seen after weaning.

In acute forms of the disease in ewes the first feature noted by the farmer may be a starving or dead lamb. Usually the disease is well advanced before it is noticed in the ewe. Gangrenous or black mastitis due to *Staph. aureus* will usually produce severe lameness in affected sheep. The ewe may be lying down a lot and cease eating.

Within hours the udder will be hot and swollen and an elevated rectal temperature (40–42°C) may be recorded. The skin of the mammary gland becomes reddened at first and then turns dark purplish and finally black in colour, as the udder finally becomes gangrenous. As the udder changes colour the skin often peels and becomes moist to touch (moist gangrene). The udder secretions are usually a small amount of blood-tinged watery fluid, which finally dries up.

Ewes with gangrenous mastitis may die within a few days. In some the udder may slough out or shrivel, but the affected ewe usually remains thin and unthrifty for some time.

Other forms of mastitis are less severe. The udder may be hot and swollen and the milk may be coagulated or even contain blood. Such cases if not treated will usually result in permanent udder induration on the affected side. Post-weaning mastitis caused by *T. pyogenes* may not be detected until shearing, when the affected side of the udder will be a discharging abscess of greenish-grey pus.

Treatment

The treatment of ovine mastitis is often unsatisfactory because of the stage at which it is detected and, as stated above, most cases in New Zealand and Australia are due to staphylococcal infections that are inherently difficult to treat successfully.

The usual recommendations include the use of appropriate antibiotics given both parenterally and into the teat canal after first milking out the udder. Treatment must be instigated within a few hours of the appearance of clinical signs. Ewes severely affected with gangrenous mastitis should be euthanased.

Control

Various recommendations have been made in an effort to reduce the incidence of mastitis in problem flocks. The provision of shelter in lambing and early lactation paddocks may be very important during inclement weather. In flocks where scabby mouth has been known to occur, vaccination may be warranted.

It has been suggested that 'over-stocking' of the udder may be reduced by grazing recently weaned ewes on a lower plane of nutrition and hence reducing the predisposition to mastitis. In dairy sheep, 'dry sheep' treatment has been recommended but some trial information suggests that it does not give the same result as 'dry cow' treatment in dairy cattle.

The udders of ewes should be routinely inspected by the farmer and sheep that have recovered from mastitis or have an affected udder should be culled. However, the culling of affected ewes appears to have little effect on the overall incidence of mastitis. Unfortunately, as with a number of diseases of grazing animals, mastitis in ewes is one that causes a slow persistent wastage but is extremely difficult to control effectively.

Hard udder

A syndrome of 'hard udder' has been reported occasionally by shepherds and farmers. There is only one report in the New Zealand literature. The condition seems to appear on some farms in a given lambing season and may result in a number of ewes that are unable to suckle their lambs.

At a casual inspection the udder of affected ewes appears to be full of milk and causes the ewe no pain. On palpation the udder is literally as hard as board with a very sharp antero-dorsal border similar to a case of udder oedema in a heifer. No milk can be expressed from the teats. Either or both sides may be affected.

At autopsy the essential gross feature is the presence of numerous irregularly shaped fibrous tags firmly adherent to the teat sinus. The teat sinuses are usually blood-filled. Histologically, granulation tissue is present in the teat sinus and duct.

No causative agent has been diagnosed. It is postulated that the cause of the condition may be trauma that has occurred months previously. On incision the mammae are found to be full of colostrum. After weeks the affected mammary glands gradually become soft again and appear normal. Affected ewes should be culled.

Agalactia

Agalactia in ewes, a syndrome of variable description, has been reported in New Zealand. In some reports the udder is hard and swollen, while in others no change from normal was seen. No cause for this condition has been found.

Contagious agalactia, a disease of sheep and goats, is caused by *Mycoplasma agalactiae*. It is found in small ruminants worldwide, but has not been reported in New Zealand although extensive surveillance has been carried out (see Chapter 21).

REFERENCES

Barber S. Clinical mastitis of sheep — causes, prevention and treatment. *Proceedings of the Society of Sheep and Beef Cattle* Veterinarians, *New Zealand Veterinary Association*, 27-9, 2016

Barber S. Sub-clinical mastitis of sheep — causes and prevention. *Proceedings of the Society of Sheep and Beef Cattle* Veterinarians, *New Zealand Veterinary Association*, 55-7, 2016

Clark RG. Field observations on ovine mastitis. *2nd Proceedings of the Sheep Society of the New Zealand Veterinary Association*, 47-54, 1972

Clark RG. Ovine mammary diseases. A Review. *10th Proceedings of the Sheep and Beef Cattle Society of the New Zealand Veterinary Association*, 16-29, 1980

Davis GB. A sheep mortality survey in Hawkes Bay. *New Zealand Veterinary Journal* 22, 39-42, 1974

Ekdahl, M. Characteristics of some organisms causing ovine mastitis. *2nd Proceedings of the Sheep Society of the New Zealand Veterinary Association*, 41-6, 1972

Hayman RH, Turner HN, Turton E. Observations on survival and growth to weaning of lambs from ewes with defective udders. *Australian Journal of Agricultural Research* 6, 446-56, 1955

Jackson R, King C. *Mycoplasma mycoides* subspecies *mycoides* (large colony) infection in goats. *Surveillance* 29, 8-12, 2002

Kittelberger R, O'Keefe JS, Meynell R, Sewell M, Rosati S, Lambert M, Dufour P, Pepin M. Comparison of four diagnostic tests for the identification of serum antibodies in small ruminants infected with *Mycoplasma agalactiae*. *New Zealand Veterinary Journal* 54, 10-15, 2006

Menzies PI, Ramanoon SZ. Mastitis of sheep and goats. *Veterinary Clinics of North America Food Animal Practice* 17, 333-58, 2001

Moule GR. Observations on mortality amongst lambs in Queensland. *Australian Veterinary Journal* 30, 153-71, 1954

Quinlivan TD. Survey observations on ovine mastitis in New Zealand stud Romney flocks 1. The incidence of ovine mastitis. *New Zealand Veterinary Journal* 16, 149-53, 1968a

Quinlivan TD. Survey observations on ovine mastitis in New Zealand stud Romney flocks 2. The bacteriology of ovine mastitis. *New Zealand Veterinary Journal* 16, 153-60, 1968b

Quinlivan TD. Ovine mastitis. *2nd Proceedings of the Sheep Society of the New Zealand Veterinary Association*, 32-40, 1972

Skyrme HP. Hard udders in ewes. *New Zealand Veterinary Journal* 18, 96, 1970

Surveillance

(1979) 3: 19	Mastitis in sheep
(1979) 5: 21	Dairy ewes
(1983) 2: 11	The normal bacterial flora of the milk of suckled and machine milked ewes
(1999) 26(1): 15	Mastitis in East Friesian ewes

Wallace LR. Observations of lambing behaviour in ewes. *Proceedings of the 9th Seminar of the New Zealand Society of Animal Production* 85-95, 1949

Watson DL, Franklin NA, Davies HI, Kettlewell P, Frost AJ. Survey of intramammary infections in ewes on the New England Tableland of New South Wales. *Australian Veterinary Journal* 67, 6-8, 1990

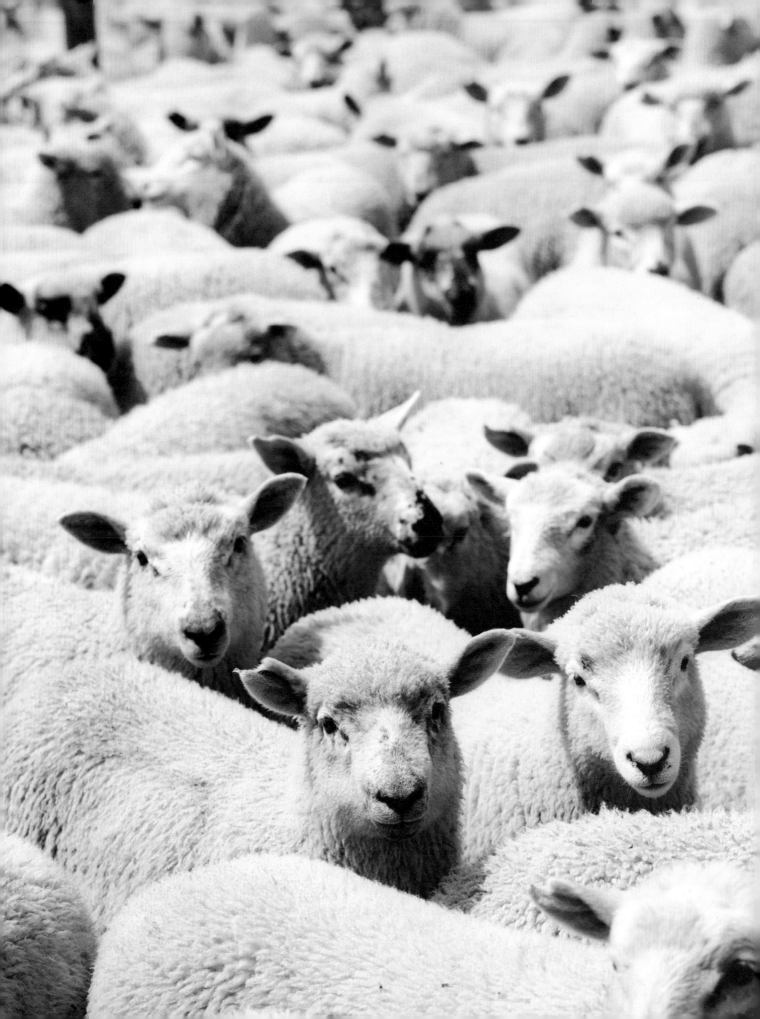

15

Clostridial diseases

The clostridial diseases of enterotoxaemia, tetanus, blackleg, malignant oedema and black disease are endemic in sheep flocks throughout New Zealand. They are of major importance to farm animals and, except for tetanus, are characterised by severe disease of brief duration and death. The clostridial organisms are ubiquitous in nature, rendering their eradication impossible. Although the widespread use of multi-component vaccines has markedly reduced losses from these diseases, they are still prevalent and losses from enterotoxaemia and tetanus are still common. Those losses that are reported in *Surveillance* have occurred almost invariably when preventative vaccination has not been carried out or vaccination programmes have lapsed.

A number of clostridial diseases such as botulism, braxy, lamb dysentery and struck have not been diagnosed in sheep in New Zealand but are present in other parts of the world. Botulism has been found in New Zealand waterfowl.

Enterotoxaemia (pulpy kidney)

In the early 1900s, New Zealand sheep farmers on better developed farms were troubled by a fatal disease of lambs between 3 and 4 weeks of age. The first full description of this disease in New Zealand is recorded in the Annual Report of the New Zealand Department of Agriculture in 1907.

The pattern is still similar, although enterotoxaemia

Organism	Disease in sheep	Disease in cattle
C. perfringens type A strain	Gas gangrene, enterotoxaemia, haemorrhagic enteritis	Gas gangrene, sudden death, enterotoxaemia
C. perfringens type B strain	Lamb dysentery,* enterotoxaemia	Enterotoxaemia in calves
C. perfringens type C strain	Struck,* enterotoxaemia	Enterotoxaemia
C. perfringens type D strain	Enterotoxaemia (pulpy kidney)	Enterotoxaemia
C. chauvoei	Blackleg, post-parturient gangrene	Blackleg
C. novyi	Black disease, infectious necrotic hepatitis, big head	Black disease
C. septicum	Malignant oedema, braxy,* navel infection	Malignant oedema
C. tetani	Tetanus	Tetanus
C. sordellii	Sudden death syndrome, gas gangrene	Sudden death syndrome, gas gangrene
C. haemolyticum		Red water disease

* Not reported in sheep in New Zealand.

Table 15.1 Clostridial diseases of sheep and cattle.

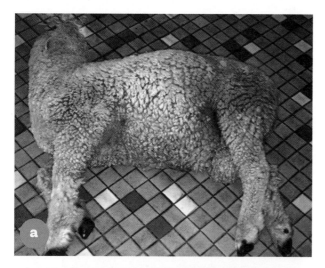

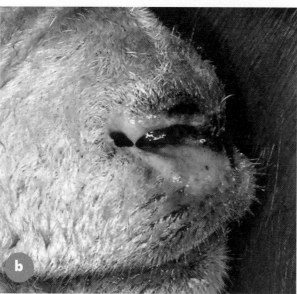

Figure 15.1 Ram hogget dead from pulpy kidney. Note that **(a)** the head is arched backwards and **(b)** froth is present at the nostrils.

has been reported in sheep of all ages. Its main occurrence is in the best-grown lambs between 3 and 10 weeks of age, although due to the widespread practice of vaccinating ewes prior to lambing many cases are now seen in weaned lambs following waning of passive maternal antibodies. It is more prevalent on well-developed farms with high-quality pastures. In North Island east coast districts, outbreaks have occurred in lambs during the early summer and may have been associated with a heavy infestation of tapeworms (*Moniezia* spp). Outbreaks are sometimes associated with feed changes, particularly in weaned lambs grazed on kale, turnips or lucerne and, rarely, in older sheep on wheat or barley stubble.

Enterotoxaemia is still an important disease of sheep in spite of the control methods used. In fact, the widespread use of vaccination indicates its importance; if vaccination were relaxed, one would anticipate a return to the epidemics that were prevalent prior to the 1950s when vaccination became a popular procedure.

Aetiology and pathogenesis

Enterotoxaemia is an acute, fatal toxaemia of sheep caused by the proliferation of the normal gut inhabitant *Clostridium perfringens* type D and the liberation of lethal toxins.

Clostridium perfringens type D is normally present in the intestines. The organism is acquired by ingestion early in life. It multiplies slowly, but is continuously passed in the faeces so that bacterial numbers and toxin levels never build up greatly. However, sudden changes in the diet, particularly to an increasing plane of nutrition, results in fermentable carbohydrate flowing on to the small intestine and providing a substrate in which the organisms may readily proliferate. It is also possible that bowel stasis, which may be caused by insufficient roughage in the diet, or possibly the presence of heavy tapeworm burdens, may contribute to this build-up of toxin in the gut.

The non-toxic prototoxin produced by the bacteria is converted into epsilon toxin by the action of proteolytic enzymes, including trypsin. Epsilon toxin produced by *C. perfringens* type D may reach high concentrations in the intestine where it causes increased vascular permeability, thereby promoting its own absorption. The epsilon toxin produces a profuse mucoid diarrhoea but, more importantly, when it is absorbed it has a strong affinity for brain tissue where it binds to receptor sites on vascular endothelial cells and disrupts the blood–brain barrier, causing brain oedema and haemorrhage. This vascular endothelial damage also occurs in other tissues, especially the lungs and myocardium. Most of the clinical and pathological findings are explainable in terms of this widespread vascular damage. These include the accumulation of protein-rich effusions in the pericardial sac, in the brain and lungs and the rapid postmortem autolysis of the kidney; hence the name pulpy kidney.

The acute pain and anxiety associated with severe brain oedema results in the increased release of catecholamines, which induce the mobilisation of hepatic glycogen to produce hyperglycaemia and glycosuria.

Clinical features

Most sheep or lambs with enterotoxaemia are found dead, usually with some signs of an agonal struggle. The disease develops very rapidly and it is unusual to see clinical signs. These are mainly characterised by a short period of anorexia, dullness, terminal convulsions and frothing at the mouth. Older sheep may survive a little longer than lambs, but usually for only a few hours. Some lambs may show nervous signs associated with focal symmetrical encephalomalacia (Chapter 17).

Pathology

Dead animals are usually found in lateral recumbency with the head arched backwards. Froth, with blood, may be present at the mouth or nostrils. In older sheep the carcass may be slightly bloated, the wool pulls away from the skin easily and decomposition is rapid. Lambs are usually large and well grown for their age (large, single lambs).

The necropsy findings usually present certain characteristics, although in a few cases the findings may be atypical. Usually the following features are found:
- The intestines are gas-filled and decomposing rapidly. In milk-fed lambs the gut contents are soft and 'mayonnaise-like'.
- As early as an hour after death there is diffuse leakage of blood in the kidney cortex, which becomes soft and pulpy. The kidney substance may become virtually liquid and when washed only the more fibrous kidney pelvis remains intact. These changes may not be present in an animal necropsied soon after death.

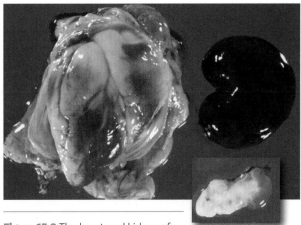

Figure 15.2 The heart and kidney of a lamb that died of pulpy kidney. There was excess fluid containing a fibrin clot in the pericardial fluid (inset).

- Almost invariably there is excessive, often clotted, pericardial fluid. Petechial haemorrhages may be present on the epicardium and endocardium.
- The lungs are oedematous and congested.
- Glycosuria is characteristic but with time this may disappear due to bacterial proliferation in the urine.
- Focal symmetrical haemorrhage and/or necrosis may be present in the brain, particularly the internal capsule, midbrain and cerebellar peduncles.

Diagnosis

The diagnosis of enterotoxaemia is usually based on a history of sudden death in animals fed a high-risk diet. The lack of protective immunisation for the flock is also important in reaching a diagnosis. Usually these points, coupled with a necropsy examination, are sufficient to provide a diagnosis.

Histological examination of the brain and kidney may support a diagnosis. Evidence of acute vascular damage can be seen in the form of perivascular proteinaceous effusions or microhaemorrhages, especially in the forebrain and midbrain. Focal areas of acute haemorrhage and necrosis, usually bilaterally symmetrical, may accompany these vascular lesions. Oedema of the cerebral grey matter, similar to acute polioencephalomalacia, may also be present and in such cases droplets of extravasated protein can often be found histologically in pericapillary spaces. The best areas for examination are the basal ganglia in the cerebellar white matter near the fourth ventricle.

Prevention

The prevention of enterotoxaemia is almost completely reliant on vaccination of susceptible sheep (see later). Before vaccination was available, prevention was based on grazing control, which involved reducing the intake of high-quality feed. Such a procedure was a useful aid in controlling a sudden outbreak of enterotoxaemia, but in young sheep it interrupted growth and was not compatible with prime-lamb production.

Dealing with an outbreak

Outbreaks of enterotoxaemia are still common and may arise under the following circumstances:
- lambs being 'finished' for sale or slaughter
- ewes being 'flushed' at tupping time
- hogget deaths, particularly ram hoggets on autumn feed.

In deciding on what action to take, it is important to consider the number of animals involved and whether a check in feeding will greatly affect their condition. It is also important to inquire whether the ewes have been vaccinated previously, especially in the case of lamb deaths.

In an outbreak the immediate use of purified toxoid of *C. perfringens* containing an alum adjuvant is recommended. If the animals have been vaccinated previously, the response to revaccination is very rapid. Even in cases where prior vaccination has not occurred, the use of the vaccine is recommended because many animals will be naturally sensitised, as has been shown from field trials. Under these circumstances, significant protection can be achieved within 48 hours of vaccination. The yarding of animals for vaccination and restricting feed are usually sufficient to hold the progress of the epidemic until the vaccine is effective.

Tetanus

Aetiology

Tetanus is a fatal paralysing disease caused by a neurotoxin released by *Clostridium tetani*, which proliferates in damaged tissue.

Epidemiology

Clostridium tetani is found in every country in the world and its spores are commonly found in soil and faeces. All animals and humans are susceptible. The disease occurs when the spores gain entry into deep wounds with sufficient devitalised tissue to provide the anaerobic conditions necessary for its multiplication and the elaboration of its specific neurotoxin.

Docking wounds in lambs, particularly following the use of rubber rings, are an ideal site for the proliferation of *C. tetani*. The neurotoxin reaches the central nervous system via the peripheral nerve trunks and produces increasing stimuli to muscles, maintaining them in a state of contraction. Death occurs by asphyxiation due to paralysis of the respiratory muscles.

Clinical features

The incubation period may be from 1 to 3 weeks. The main feature of tetanus is the severe spasm of voluntary muscles, producing a general rigidity. Any stimulus promotes the rigidity. As the disease progresses, lambs become permanently fixed in lateral recumbency and in an extended

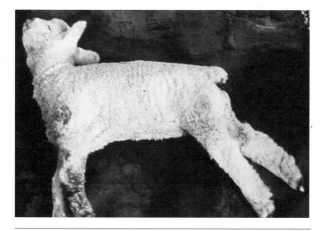

Figure 15.3 A lamb affected by tetanus 8 days after tailing.

'saw horse' position. The facial muscles are contracted at the margin of the mouth and produce a 'grinning' appearance. The disease is very painful and affected animals should be quickly destroyed on humane grounds.

Diagnosis
The diagnosis is readily made from the clinical features described above. A precise confirmation may be made by fluorescent staining of tissue taken from the wound, but in most cases this is unnecessary.

Control
During an outbreak of tetanus it is wise to ascertain when the first cases were seen and if, for example, the disease is the result of docking wound contamination, when that occurred. From this information it is possible to give a reasonable prognosis on numbers of animals likely to be further affected, bearing in mind that the incubation period is 1–3 weeks. The remaining healthy lambs may be given tetanus antitoxin which will give them immediate protection lasting for about 3 weeks.

Prevention
When tetanus occurs, it is most important to discuss the cause of the condition and the common association of tailing with rubber rings or searing irons. The veterinarian must then emphasise the preventative measures that must be taken against this disease, which include:
- modifying the tailing method
- vaccinating ewes to provide passive protection for the lamb via the colostrum (see later)
- routinely using tetanus antitoxin at docking time.

Blackleg

Aetiology
Blackleg is caused by *Clostridium chauvoei*, a common intestinal inhabitant. It is spore-forming and can survive in soil for many years.

Epidemiology
Blackleg of sheep is a myonecrosis, accompanied by toxaemia and gas formation resulting from infection by *C. chauvoei*. As well as sheep, it is reported in a variety of species including cattle, pigs, fish and whales. Humans and equidae are resistant. In New Zealand, blackleg is more commonly associated with cattle than sheep. In sheep, rather than causing sporadic deaths as in cattle, it usually causes severe losses involving numbers of animals and associated with some predisposing factor. Such factors include tailing lambs in dirty yards, wintering hoggets on root crops and injecting sheep with contaminated needles. It may also occasionally occur as a sequel to abortion or lambing assistance.

In cattle, the organism is presumed to gain access to the body in the alimentary tract and lies dormant in muscle until activated by anaerobic conditions. In sheep, the majority of outbreaks appear to be associated with wounds inflicted by shearing, docking and other forms of farm surgery. The incubation period is short, usually 1–3 days.

In the past there has been some difficulty in differentiating between disease due to *C. chauvoei* and to *C. septicum*. While *C. septicum* is commonly isolated from lesions of blackleg, it rapidly invades carcasses and often swamps the growth of *C. chauvoei*. The fresher the material and the more careful the bacteriological examination, the fewer cases of *C. septicum* as the pathogen are identified.

Clinical features
The appearance of lesions is related to the site of the trauma. After injuries at parturition, the vaginal mucosa may be eroded and the perineal and adjacent tissues swollen, dark red and gassy. Blood-stained droplets will usually ooze from the skin. In lambs with blackleg following docking it is noticeable that wether lambs in particular may be affected, particularly if open castration has been practised. In an epidemic, all stages of disease may be present and lambs may be walking but lame, recumbent, or in the final stages of toxaemia. The skin is a dark red/blue/black colour and affected tissues are swollen and crepitous. The cardinal signs are elevated and death usually follows within 24 hours.

Pathology
In dead animals, the typical blackleg lesions can be seen extending from the initial wound. The carcasses appear bloated and have a bloody nasal discharge. As with other clostridial diseases, sheep dying from blackleg putrefy rapidly. It should be remembered that *C. septicum* is a

common postmortem invader, so that a lesion caused by *C. chauvoei* often becomes invaded by *C. septicum* after death. Since the latter is far easier to grow and to isolate, the underlying *C. chauvoei* has often been overlooked. *Clostridium chauvoei* and *C. septicum* infections can be distinguished by the use of the specific fluorescent staining.

Histopathology of the lesions of blackleg is a most useful aid to confirming a diagnosis. Therefore, formalin-fixed sections taken from the edge of the lesions are an important laboratory submission.

Treatment
The use of broad-spectrum antibiotics has been recommended for the treatment of blackleg. However, these are often ineffective and the occasional animal that may recover usually loses skin and muscle from the affected region by sloughing. In practice affected animals should be euthanased to avoid suffering.

Prevention

Vaccination

Vaccination is an important preventative strategy (see later).

Hygienic measures

Often outbreaks of blackleg are associated with careless farm practices. *Clostridium chauvoei* multiplies in carcasses, so the disposal of dead sheep is important in reducing contamination on the farm. It is important to emphasise this point, as carcasses and tails from docking left rotting under trees are an ideal site for the concentration of blackleg spores.

Other procedures that may cause blackleg include the use of dirty dip solutions, or dipping sheep too soon after shearing, before shearing wounds have closed. Lambs may be affected following tailing and castration, particularly when these procedures are conducted in dirty surroundings or the lambs have been kept in such surroundings either before or after tailing. Similarly, vaccinating sheep in dusty yards with unhygienic instruments has been associated with cases of blackleg. Hence in all instances it is necessary to give advice on hygienic measures that should be followed to reduce losses from blackleg.

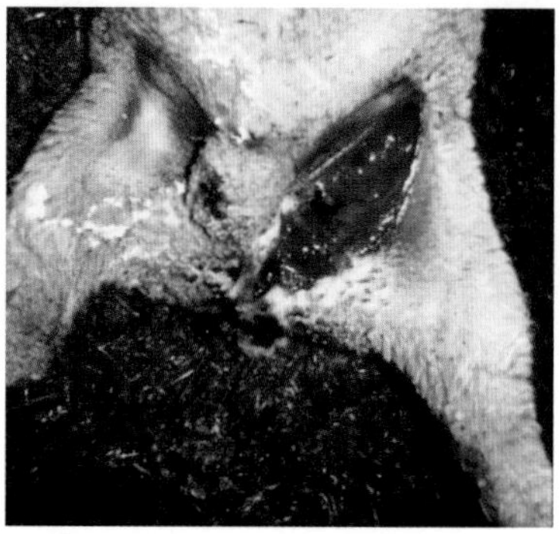

Malignant oedema

Aetiology
The significance of *Clostridium septicum* as a wound contaminant is not always clear because of its ability to invade dead sheep carcasses. Attaching pathological significance to its presence depends on establishing that characteristic lesions are present. *Clostridium septicum* may swamp initial infections such as *C. chauvoei*. In addition, the role of *C. novyi* type B as a cause of wound and navel infection is uncertain.

Clinical features
In New Zealand it is generally considered that *C. septicum* is the cause of many cases of navel illness in lambs and is frequently associated with many conditions described as blackleg.

In uncomplicated cases, the smell is similar to that found in *C. chauvoei* infections.

Pathology
At autopsy a gelatinous serosanguinous exudate is seen both interstitially and subcutaneously around the wound or navel. In the latter there is also an intense hyperaemia of the peritoneal blood vessels but little or no gas is present.

Diagnosis
Confirmation of malignant oedema is dependent on the demonstration of the causal organism in characteristically affected tissue, using fluorescent antibody technique. Culture of the organisms from affected tissue or an intact

Figure 15.4 A lamb affected by blackleg two days after castration.

rib is, by itself, of limited value and must be considered along with the other clinical and autopsy features.

Prevention
Vaccines are used (see later). To prevent navel infection in lambs the ewes should receive a booster dose 2–6 weeks before lambing so that the lamb is protected passively via the ewe's colostrum.

Hygiene
Those points stressed for blackleg also apply to malignant oedema.

Braxy (bradshot)
The exception to *Clostridium septicum* as a wound invader occurs in the disease braxy, a common condition of wintering hoggets in Scotland. This disease follows an invasion through the abomasal mucosa, the original lesion presumably being caused by the ingestion of frozen food. Despite similar predisposing factors in parts of New Zealand, particularly in Southland, it has not been reported in sheep but has been diagnosed in goats.

Clinical features
Death from braxy is sudden and at autopsy typical ulcerations, congestion and haemorrhage are seen in the abomasum and small intestine. As for blackleg, fixed tissues are a useful aid for diagnosis. Before vaccination became available, losses of up to 50% of a flock were recorded in Scotland.

Prevention
Prevention is by vaccination.

Black disease (infectious necrotic hepatitis)

Aetiology
Black disease is mainly a disease of sheep, but in some countries it has been reported in cattle also. It is caused by *Clostridium novyi* associated with liver damage. *Clostridium novyi* is the third member of the group that causes what is recognised in New Zealand as 'blood poisoning'. In Australia, it is often associated with 'crowpeck' infections and 'swelled head' in Merino rams as a result of infection of fighting wounds. In New Zealand the organism has been isolated from navel infections of calves and lambs and is suspected as a cause of some wound infections. However, *C. novyi* is recognised mainly for its role in black disease of sheep.

Epidemiology
In New Zealand, black disease is mainly associated with liver fluke infections. *Clostridium novyi* is part of the normal flora of many soils and sheep intestines but some organisms pass through the intestinal wall and become lodged as spores in the liver. As many as 60% of the livers of healthy sheep from an area known to be affected with black disease will contain *C. novyi* spores, while in non-affected areas up to 30% of livers may contain spores. Damage by immature migrating flukes is the most important precipitating cause of black disease, but there are a number of cases reported where no specific precipitating lesions were seen. Black disease has also been seen in animals grazed or fed under intensive systems.

Clinical features
All ages may be affected, but it is usually seen in adult sheep during the summer/autumn period when the young liver flukes are migrating. The incidence is usually low but deaths may occur for up to 6 weeks after sheep leave an endemic fluke area.

The course of the disease is rapid with, at most, only a few hours between the first appearance of signs and death. Affected animals are dull, but attempt to remain with the flock. When approached they will attempt to rise, even though the effort is beyond them. Death, unlike that resulting from enterotoxaemia, occurs quietly.

Pathology and diagnosis
In endemic fluke areas, deaths in adult sheep in the summer/autumn period and the presence of characteristic necropsy findings usually allow a diagnosis to be made.

In the fresh cadaver, the combination of peritoneal and pericardial effusions coupled with circular areas of liver necrosis is virtually pathognomonic. Smears from the periphery of the necrotic foci show exceptionally large Gram-positive rods, often with subterminal spores.

In addition to the above lesions there may be subcutaneous and intermuscular oedema and marked subcutaneous injection of blood vessels, hence the name black disease.

For laboratory confirmation of diagnosis, samples of necrotic foci — fixed and fresh, together with air-dried films from their margins — should be sent to the laboratory as soon as possible for histological examination and fluorescent antibody tests. As with blackleg, bacterial invasion of the carcass may prevent the confirmation of *C. novyi*.

Prevention
Prevention is by vaccination (see later).

Lamb dysentery

Aetiology
Lamb dysentery is caused by *Clostridium perfringens* type B, an organism that is present in New Zealand but has not been associated with lamb dysentery in this country. The disease can be a serious problem in Britain where it usually occurs in lambs under 1 week of age, but lambs up to 3 weeks old can be affected occasionally. The condition is associated with the use of permanent lambing paddocks or rearing facilities; once the disease appears in a given year, it tends to increase as the lambing season progresses. The more voracious and robust lambs suffer most, thus putting the progeny of high-milk-yielding ewes at the greatest risk. In an outbreak, lambs of one particular breed may be severely affected, while those of another breed may be almost totally unaffected. The mortality rate may approximate 100%. Foals and calves may also be affected.

Clinical features
Most cases occur in the first week of life, many lambs being affected by the second or third day. A lamb that has been suckling vigorously ceases to suck, bleats continuously and shows acute abdominal pain. The diarrhoea may be blood-stained and eventually becomes tarry. Prostration and death may occur within a few hours. The occasional, less-acute case may linger for 2–3 weeks.

Pathology
At necropsy characteristic ulcerations are seen on the reddened and inflamed mucosa of the small intestine. The mesenteric lymph nodes are enlarged and the liver is large and friable. Smears made from intestinal scrapings show numerous Gram-positive rods.

A supporting diagnosis is dependent on demonstrating the beta and epsilon toxin ELISA from the gut contents or peritoneal fluid.

Prevention
Previously, shepherds gave newborn lambs a lamb dysentery antitoxin. However, it is now common practice to immunise ewes prior to lambing so that the lamb receives passive colostral protection from its dam (see later).

Struck

Struck is a disease of adult sheep due to *Clostridium perfringens* type C. It is reported in Britain and in certain areas of the USA. *C. perfringens* type C is present in New Zealand but it has not yet been identified as a cause of sudden deaths as in overseas countries.

Botulism

Botulism of sheep caused by *Clostridium botulinum* is not recorded in New Zealand, although the organism does exist here. In Australia, botulism has been reported occasionally in dry or drought periods when feed is short and sheep resort to feeding on carrion such as rabbit carcasses and on rotting vegetation.

In New Zealand, botulism has caused large-scale mortalities among waterfowl and has also been diagnosed in dogs and trout.

The spores of *C. botulism* occur in the soil, where they can survive for long periods. If the ground is warm and moist, the spores will germinate and multiply in decomposing animal and plant material. As the bacteria multiply, a highly potent toxin is produced which persists. Water contaminated with rotting vegetation can also contain sufficient toxin to cause the death of sheep.

The toxin is absorbed from the small intestine. It adheres to certain nerve endings and blocks the transmission of nerve impulses.

Clinical features
The rate at which signs develop depends on the amount of toxin ingested, so that where this has been large, signs can appear within a few hours and death follows within 18 hours. In such cases the flaccid paralysis may not be obvious and even though the gait is uncoordinated and spastic, the animal may be able to walk until near death.

In sheep, grazing and the mastication of food become very difficult. Excessive salivation and nervous twitching and jaw champing are common. Generally, affected sheep lie down quietly as the flaccid paralysis develops and soon die as a result of respiratory failure.

Prevention
In Australia a vaccine is available. Two doses are given, 1 year apart and this gives animals a lifelong protection against the disease.

Clostridium sordellii
Clostridium sordellii has been implicated as a cause of sudden death of sheep and cattle in New Zealand and overseas. Overseas, in some cases it has been isolated as the sole pathogen and in others *C. perfringens* types A or D have also been isolated from the same animals. However, in many cases a pathological lesion has not been associated as a site of multiplication and there is still some debate over the contribution of *C. sordellii* in causing death.

Clostridium sordellii is an ubiquitous anaerobe producing several toxins, of which the most important are a lethal toxin and a haemorrhagic toxin.

Clinical features
A variety of clinical syndromes have been associated with *C. sordellii* infection. The most common of these is sudden death of sheep (and cattle) of all age groups. It has also been associated with acute infection of the wall of the abomasum, a blackleg-like condition and, in one case, haemorrhagic enteritis. In ewes, the majority of reported deaths have occurred around lambing time, often associated with feed changes.

Pathology
The characteristic finding is rapid autolysis of the carcass, as is seen with most clostridial diseases. Overseas, abomasitis has been reported from sheep of all age groups with congestion, oedema and haemorrhage of the abomasal mucosa. In some cases abomasal ulceration has been reported, and in a few cases perforation of an abomasal ulcer has resulted in peritonitis. Lambs of 4–12 weeks of age have been described as having a displaced abomasum lying across the abdomen immediately distal to the xiphisternum. Various other features such as excessive abdominal and pericardial fluid, petechial haemorrhages on the epicardium and caecum, and congested intestines have also been reported in some cases.

Diagnosis
Acute death of sheep in a flock with rapid carcass autolysis and where other disease processes are not identified may be suggestive. At postmortem examination, every effort should be made to identify a primary lesion such as abomasitis. Culture of the organism from the liver, muscle and/or abomasum may be attempted. Large chunks of tissue should be collected, and transported to the laboratory in airtight bags as soon after collection as possible.

Prevention
Clostridium sordellii is a component of some clostridial vaccines. Hence if this disease is of concern, vaccination procedures as outlined below may be used in its prevention. However, it is still not clear whether *C. sordellii* is an important pathogen causing sporadic losses due to sudden death, or if it is simply a postmortem invader or incidental finding. Other specific prevention strategies are not defined, although ensuring good hygiene during husbandry procedures (docking, vaccinating, etc.) and avoiding sudden changes of feed are sensible precautions.

Vaccination against clostridial diseases
Almost all prime-lamb producers, stud sheep farmers and significant numbers of hill-country farmers routinely vaccinate their sheep against clostridial diseases. Vaccination is not costly and is usually very effective if carried out correctly.

The main clostridial diseases in New Zealand are enterotoxaemia, tetanus, blackleg, malignant oedema and black disease, and thus the majority of clostridial vaccines available are '5-in-1', containing toxoids of *C. perfringens* type D, *C. tetani*, *C. chauvoei*, *C. novyi* type B and *C. septicum*. The 5-in-1 vaccines are available with a number of additions such as selenium, anthelmintics or in association with *Corynebacterium pseudotuberculosis* vaccine (Glanvac 6®; Chapter 13) or leptospirosis vaccine (Ultravac 7-in-1®; Chapter 20). For lambs whose dams were not vaccinated, a further option is a vaccine containing tetanus antitoxin and *C. perfringens* type D toxoid which is primarily intended to protect against tetanus at docking.

In addition to the five clostridial toxoids listed above, there are also clostridial vaccines containing *C. sordellii* and sometimes other *Clostridia* not thought to cause disease in New Zealand. These may be used under circumstances where protection against additional bacteria is required. In this respect, veterinary advice is recommended to ensure that the appropriate product is used for the animals concerned.

To confer a good immunity, two vaccinations should be given. The first is referred to as the sensitiser and should be followed at least 4 weeks later by a second or booster dose. If the two doses are as close as 4 weeks, their effect is very much reduced. Sheep sensitised 18 months previously show an immediate and strong response to booster vaccination. Experimentally the best results have been achieved by giving three doses, but this is generally unnecessary.

Time of vaccination

The most common vaccination procedure followed in New Zealand is to actively immunise the ewe flock at an early age with a multiple component vaccine. This is generally the recommended option and is preferred over vaccination of the lambs at docking time. The procedure is as follows:

- Vaccinate all replacement ewe lambs (and ram lambs if a ram breeding flock) as soon after weaning as possible. This is the sensitiser dose. Depending on the perceived risk, non-replacement lambs can be vaccinated as well if they are to stay on the property for a while.
- A booster dose should be given 4–6 weeks later.
- As the ewe lambs enter the breeding flock as two-tooths at approximately 18 months of age, they can be booster-dosed with the mixed-age ewes during the winter period prior to lambing. It is preferable to dose the flock 2–6 weeks prior to lambing to give the best colostral titre of antitoxin. This ensures passive protection to the suckling lambs, which lasts up to 16 weeks in the lambs.
- In flocks where no sheep have been previously vaccinated, all sheep should be given their sensitiser dose either just prior to or 4–6 weeks after tupping is completed. These sheep are then given their booster dose 2–6 weeks prior to lambing.
- In subsequent years all previously vaccinated sheep are given a booster dose prior to lambing.
- In the face of any outbreak of enterotoxaemia sheep may be vaccinated immediately.

In flocks where the ewes are not vaccinated, lambs may be vaccinated at docking time with a *C. perfringens* type D toxoid and a tetanus anti-toxin. Note that for full protection against enterotoxaemia a multiple clostridial vaccine must be given at weaning time to boost the immunity to *C. perfringens* type D.

The general procedure for vaccination of sheep

Preparation

Vaccination should be carried out in fine weather, in clean yards free from dust. It is a good idea to damp the yards down with water from either sprinklers or hoses before commencing. Prepare a suitable work area such as a table to accommodate the vaccination equipment and materials. Have at least 10 needles available in a tray of methylated spirits. Needles should be changed frequently (every 12–24 animals) to reduce the risk of infection. Use short needles. Recommended sizes are 13 mm x 16–18 gauge. Before use, steel vaccination guns may be sterilised by boiling in water for 10 minutes but do not attempt to re-sterilise plastic disposable equipment. Many farmers use plastic vaccination guns and these should be cleaned in warm water after use.

Vaccination

First ensure that the vaccination gun is functioning properly and delivering the correct dose. The vaccine must be injected only under the skin, high in the side of the neck. After parting the wool, lift a fold of loose skin and insert the needle at a slight angle into the 'tent' of the skin so formed, taking care to avoid injection into the muscle tissue.

REFERENCES

Bruère SN. Case studies: Two outbreaks of blackleg in sheep. *Proceedings of the Annual Seminar of the Sheep and Beef Cattle Veterinarians, New Zealand Veterinary Association* 12, 336-8, 1982

Bruère SN. Blacks disease in sheep. *Society of the Sheep and Beef Cattle Veterinarians, New Zealand Veterinary Association – Newsletter* 26, 8-9, 2004

Cooper BS. Transfer from the ewe to lamb of clostridial antibodies. *New Zealand Veterinary Journal* 15, 1-7, 1966

Cooper BS. Clostridial diseases of sheep: Control by vaccination. *Proceedings of the 6th Annual Seminar of the Sheep and Beef Cattle Veterinarians, New Zealand Veterinary Association,* 47-51, 1976

Cooper BS, Jull DJ. Local reactions in sheep to clostridial vaccines. *New Zealand Veterinary Journal* 14, 171-5, 1966

Deprez P. Clostridium perfringens infections – a diagnostic challenge. *Veterinary Record* 177, 388-9, 2015

Gill JM. Clostridial deaths and failure to vaccinate. *Society of the Sheep and Beef Cattle Veterinarians, New Zealand Veterinary Association – Newsletter* 30, 16, 2006

Lewis CJ. Aspects of clostridial disease in sheep. *In Practice,* 494-9, 1998

Lewis CJ, Naylor RD. Sudden death in sheep associated with *Clostridium sordellii. Veterinary Record* 142, 417-21, 1998

Moffat JR. Prelamb ewe vaccination – comparing apples with apples. *Proceedings of the Society of Sheep and Beef Cattle Veterinarians, New Zealand Veterinary Association* 34, 181-9, 2004

O'Connell K. *Clostridium sordellii* vaccination in sheep. *Proceedings of the 32nd Annual Seminar of the Sheep and Beef Cattle Veterinarians, New Zealand Veterinary Association,* 177-88, 2002

Popoff MR. Bacteriological examination in enterotoxaemia of sheep and lambs. *Veterinary Record* 114, 324, 1984

Richards SM, Hunt BW. *Clostridium sordellii* in lambs. *Veterinary Record* 111, 22, 1982

Slaughter RE. Clostridial diseases in lambs and young sheep. *Proceedings of the 6th Annual Seminar of the Sheep and Beef Cattle Veterinarians, New Zealand Veterinary Association,* 27-32, 1976

Smith LDS, Safford JW, Hawkins WW. *Clostridium sordellii* infection in sheep. *Cornell Veterinarian* 52, 62-8, 1962

Stevenson BJ. The diagnosis of clostridial diseases in lambs. *Proceedings of the 6th Annual Seminar of the Sheep and Beef Cattle Veterinarians, New Zealand Veterinary Association,* 44-6, 1976

Surveillance

(1975) 2(3): 15-17	Diagnosis of clostridial diseases.
(1979) 6(4): 27	'Braxy?'
(1980) 7(1): 26	Enterotoxaemia in lambs
(1992) 19(2): 26-7	Botulism in New Zealand
(2005) 32(2): 28-32	*Clostridium sordellii* in a Suffolk ram
(2005) 32(4): 14-19	*Clostridium septicum* deaths in ewe hoggets

Thompson KG. Gross pathology review – the alimentary tract. *Proceedings of the Sheep and Beef Cattle Veterinarians of the New Zealand Veterinary Association* 34, 191-206, 2004

Vatn S, Tranulis MA, Hofshagen M. Sacina-like bacteria, *Clostridium fallax* and *Clostridium sordellii* in lambs with abomasal bloat, haemorrhage and ulcers. *Journal of Comparative Pathology* 122, 193-200, 2000

Wallace GV. Homologous passive protection of lambs against various clostridial diseases. *New Zealand Veterinary Journal* 11, 39-40, 1963

Wallace GV. Homologous passive protection of lambs against various clostridial diseases. *New Zealand Veterinary Journal* 12, 61-2, 1964

Wallace GV. Results from the use of fluorescent in labelled *Clostridium oedematiens* serum. *New Zealand Veterinary Journal* 14, 24-25, 1966

16

Other causes of sudden death including salmonellosis, *Histophilus somni*, septicaemia, redgut, enteric listeriosis and anthrax

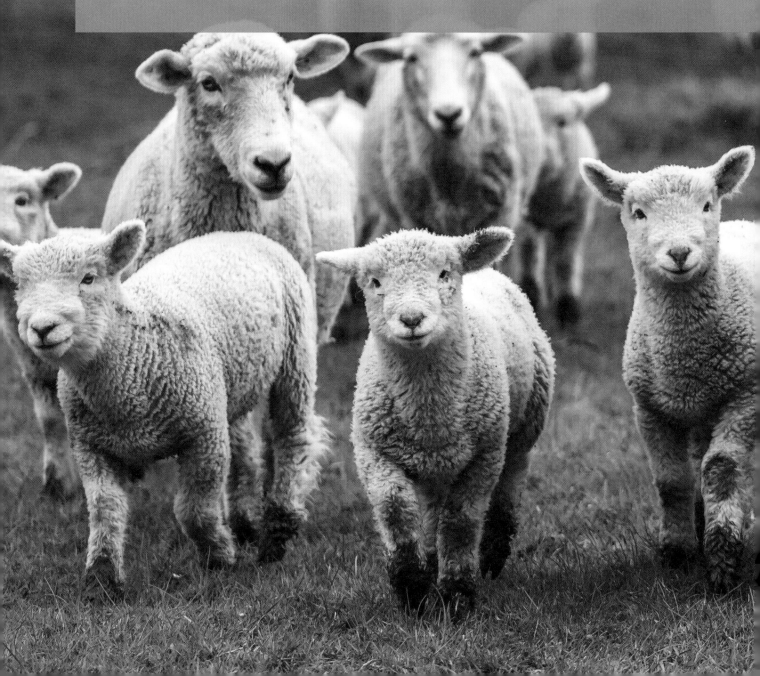

Salmonellosis

The enteric form of salmonellosis of sheep is a bacterial disease characterised by outbreaks of profuse diarrhoea and death. Most outbreaks follow situations that cause stress to sheep, such as transportation, crowding and temporary food deprivation. The disease occurs sporadically in adult ewes but is uncommon in young sheep. In New Zealand, the enteric form of salmonellosis should be distinguished from *S.* Brandenburg abortions (see Chapter 4).

Aetiology

Salmonella bacteria have a wide ecological distribution and perhaps the widest host range of any zoonotic agent. In sheep, the enteric form of salmonellosis is caused by *Salmonella* Hindmarsh, *Salmonella typhimurium* and *Salmonella bovis-morbificans*, with other *Salmonella* serotypes occasionally isolated. On rare occasions, *S.* Brandenburg has caused enteritis in non-pregnant sheep. Originally, *S. bovis-morbificans* and *S.* Hindmarsh species were not differentiated and were reported as *S. bovis-morbificans*. Most of the cases that were identified as *S. bovis-morbificans* prior to the early 1980s were probably *S.* Hindmarsh.

Epidemiology

Geographical distribution

In New Zealand sheep, salmonellosis was first reported in 1949 and during the 1950s the disease was largely confined to the Hawke's Bay, Manawatu and Wairarapa districts. *Salmonella typhimurium* isolates outnumbered *S. bovis-morbificans* by 239 to 4. However, since that time, salmonellosis has become widespread throughout most sheep districts and *S.* Hindmarsh has become the most common serotype isolated.

Seasonal pattern

Since it was first reported in New Zealand, salmonellosis of sheep has been recognised as having a seasonal pattern of occurrence, with most cases ocurring between December and June. It is possible that most cases occur during these months because at these times adult sheep are generally being rotationally grazed or break-grazed and are often yarded relatively frequently for husbandry interventions.

Predisposing factors

It is generally accepted that salmonellosis of sheep is a disease in which carrier animals occur commonly but clinical disease only occurs as a result of some stress factor. The following factors have been cited as predisposing factors:
- sudden changes in nutrition from good feed to poor feed
- holding sheep in yards over long periods (24 hours)
- transhipment over long distances either by droving or by vehicles
- holding sheep at very heavy stocking densities.

These management procedures can lead to rapid transfer of infection from one sheep to another via pasture, particularly around drinking areas. The introduction and confinement of sheep into environments containing viable *Salmonella* organisms can result in the rapid appearance of these bacteria in faeces, even though no clinical signs have been seen. However, anecdotally cases have also occurred in sheep in good condition on apparently good nutrition and without recent predisposing management factors.

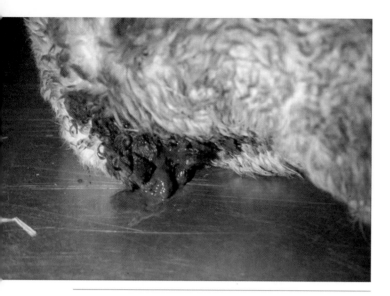

Figure 16.1 Salmonellosis. Note the khaki scour contrasting with the dark dags.

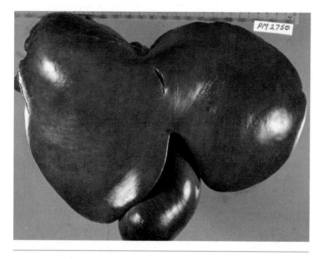

Figure 16.2 Swollen liver from a ewe with salmonellosis. The gall bladder is large because the ewe has not been eating.

Morbidity/mortality

Field data reported by the New Zealand Animal Health Division laboratories indicate that approximately 1–2 farms in every 100 will have an outbreak of salmonellosis, although it has been suggested that the true figure may be higher as in many cases veterinary investigation is not sought. Since 2008 there appears to have been an increase in the number of diagnosed cases of enteric salmonellosis, primarily due to *S*. Hindmarsh, particularly in Otago and Southland.

On affected properties the mean mortality rate recorded has been usually about 1% although on rare occasions the mortality rate may exceed 5%. Losses may occur suddenly and appear only over a few days, while in some instances the disease may cause periodic losses over several weeks unless action is taken to prevent them occurring.

Pathogenesis

During an outbreak of salmonellosis, there is a rapid transfer of infection from infected to non-infected animals. However, there is evidence to suggest that under stress the resistance of the carrier or infected animal is reduced, leading to a rapid multiplication of the bacteria in the rumen and possibly the intestine. This is followed by bacterial invasion and the systemic spread of the disease. Some animals survive this stage of the disease but localisation of the organism occurs in the mesenteric lymph nodes, liver, spleen and particularly the gall bladder. These animals become chronic carriers of the disease and discharge organisms intermittently into the faeces and occasionally into milk.

There is evidence that the normal contents of the alimentary tract have a bacteriostatic or bactericidal effect on *Salmonella* organisms. It is suggested that the volatile fatty acids, particularly butyric acid, may be inhibitory to *Salmonella* spp and that levels of these are reduced during temporary starvation, thus enabling a rapid increase in, and systemic invasion by, *Salmonella* organisms.

Clinical findings

In the majority of salmonellosis epidemics, some sheep are usually found dead and concurrently several ill or dying sheep may be found, usually near to a water source. Sheep with clinical salmonellosis are acutely ill. They have an elevated temperature, are dull, disinclined to move and have a severe and profuse diarrhoea. The faeces are fluid, putrid-smelling, khaki-coloured and usually adhere to the wool of the crutch and hind limbs. They contain large amounts of mucus and occasionally flecks of blood. In per-acute cases, death may occur before the diarrhoea has developed. Less severely affected sheep may die after a sickness lasting from 12 to 24 hours. During the terminal stages of the disease sheep become severely dehydrated; although some sheep may recover, the convalescent period is usually protracted.

In some countries abortion occurs in sheep due to salmonellae, but with the exception of *S*. Brandenburg this is not a usual occurrence in New Zealand.

Pathology and diagnosis

The necropsy findings can be very helpful in the diagnosis of salmonellosis and it is important to visit the farm and perform as many necropsies as necessary to complete a diagnosis. Visiting the farm also enables the veterinarian to undertake a good examination of the environment and assess the factors that may have caused the outbreak. The necropsy features to look for include:
- an enlarged fatty liver with a distended gall bladder
- enlarged oedematous or haemorrhagic mesenteric lymph nodes
- inflammation of the abomasum and intestines
- moderate to severe congestion of the lungs, liver and kidneys
- petechial haemorrhages on serosal surfaces
- typical khaki-coloured diarrhoea with mucus and occasionally flecks of blood.

In advanced cases the carcass will be dehydrated and may show mild signs of jaundice.

A diagnosis of salmonellosis may be confirmed by culture of the organism from the intestinal contents and/or mesenteric lymph node and by histopathological examination of fixed sections of abomasum, intestine and mesenteric lymph node. If the carcass is decomposing, the isolation of *Salmonella* spp is very difficult and the only samples that may be of use are bile or a lymph node. It is probably better to wait for a freshly dead sheep from which to collect samples.

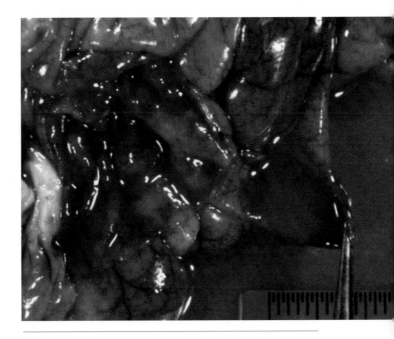

Figure 16.3 Enteritis due to salmonellosis.

Treatment

Public health aspects

Infected animals are a potential source of human salmonellosis, and personal hygiene should be stressed to the farmer concerned. Diseased or recently recovered sheep should not be sent to slaughter.

Clinically affected sheep

Treatment of individual sheep may be attempted, but the prognosis for recovery should be guarded. Treatment is usually based on providing fluid therapy, gut protectives and antibiotics given by both the oral and parenteral routes.

Dealing with an outbreak

It is difficult to predict the disease course of salmonellosis and therefore control of the disease is likely to vary from farm to farm depending on the circumstances. The amount of feed available, whether the flock has been vaccinated previously and the ease and practicality of yarding to administer the vaccine are all factors that need to be considered.

It is usually recommended that the flock be spread out to reduce cross-infection. If practical, the farmer should increase the level of nutrition but in some cases this may be difficult because the disease often occurs during times of feed shortages. Certainly, the sheep should be moved from the paddock where the deaths have occurred and be provided with a good source of water. Clinically affected animals should be isolated to reduce contamination and treated if appropriate. Stress factors should be avoided and any mustering and yarding undertaken with caution. Yards can be effectively decontaminated by spraying with 5% formalin or other effective disinfectant.

Vaccination during an outbreak has proved to be useful in reducing losses, and most veterinarians now recommend that course depending on the particular circumstances on the farm. The combination of vaccination and spreading the ewes out is usually an effective means of curtailing an outbreak within 7–10 days, after which time the farmer can revert to the original management.

Prevention

Increasing awareness of the threat from salmonellosis to animal and human health, and recognition of the implications to New Zealand's meat marketing industry, have emphasised the need for effective measures for controlling this disease. While farmers have learnt to avoid or modify some of the management procedures that precipitate outbreaks, control by management alone is not compatible with modern farming practices, which often require high stock densities. Therefore the use of vaccine is widely recommended. A vaccine containing inactivated strains of *S.* Hindmarsh, *S. typhimurium*, *S. bovismorbificans* and *S.* Brandenburg is available (Salvexin + B®; MSD Animal Health Ltd).

The mechanism by which the vaccine protects individual sheep is unknown, but it appears that the number of organisms shed is considerably reduced following vaccination. This may therefore affect the course of the disease by reducing the challenge to other sheep. Perhaps this is why vaccination of part of a flock appears to alter the occurrence of the disease in the flock as a whole.

Because salmonellosis is primarily a disease of adult ewes, ewes are vaccinated instead of lambs. Used prophylactically it is recommended that ewes be first vaccinated twice at an interval of at least 4 weeks, the first dose being given to the ewes when they are weaned from their lambs and the second dose 4–6 weeks later or at the first sign of an outbreak. In the following years it is probable that a booster injection will be sufficient. Note that the timing of vaccination differs to that recommended if the primary objective is prevention of *S.* Brandenburg abortion (see Chapter 4).

While the above vaccination programme is clearly desirable, its use in the field is often restricted to situations of high risk or for valuable sheep. Because of cost, an alternative programme that is used more widely involves the vaccination each year of introduced or replacement (usually two-tooth) ewes with a single inoculation in January. Should there be a breakdown and appearance of salmonellosis under some extreme conditions, revaccination of all sheep will soon prevent further mortalities. Anectodally, this regimen has proved satisfactory in the field in most cases but on some farms a more comprehensive programme is required. It is not clear what length of protection is afforded by vaccination and because of the sporadic nature of the disease, both in relation to the season and to the husbandry of particular flocks, it is difficult to assess the precise effect of vaccination. Veterinarians need to learn to reach a decision on vaccine use with the help of local knowledge and experience.

Histophilus somni septicaemia

A disease associated with Gram-negative pleomorphic organisms causing pyaemia and joint infection in lambs was first reported in New Zealand in 1962. Following that report there was no further literature about this disease in New Zealand until 1991, but since then there have been reports of these organisms causing sudden death, septicaemia and meningitis in lambs. It has been suggested that the condition is becoming more common but the reasons for this are unclear. It may be that the condition was previously under-reported or mistaken for other causes of sudden death such as enterotoxaemia or pneumonia.

Aetiology and pathogenesis

In the past, Gram-negative pleomorphic bacteria causing disease in sheep and cattle have been called *Histophilus ovis*, *Haemophilus somnus* and *Haemophilus agni*, but it is now suggested that they are all the same organism and have been given the name *Histophilus somni*. They are important causes of epididymitis in young rams (see Chapter 2), but have also been associated with septicaemia resulting in sudden death, meningoencephalitis, arthritis and pneumonia of both male and female lambs. The organisms can be isolated from the reproductive tracts of healthy immature rams and ewes but the pathogenesis of the septicaemia is unclear.

Epidemiology

The disease most commonly affects young growing sheep during the post-weaning period, with affected lambs often well managed and on a good plane of nutrition. Cryptorchid ('short-scrotum') lambs, entire ram lambs and ewe lambs may all be affected. Mortality rates vary but may be as high as 10% in some cases. Dribbling losses may occur, with 2–3 lambs dying each week over a period of several weeks or months.

Clinical findings

Often, affected sheep will simply be found dead and they are usually in good body condition. Generalised septicaemia will result in dullness, depression and death while localisation in the meninges and brain will result in neurological signs including depression, ataxia, head tremors and nystagmus.

Pathology

A range of lesions may be found at necropsy depending on where the organisms have localised. Green-grey purulent material may be present beneath the dura mater of the brain, and throughout the joints. There may be petechial haemorrhages on the serosal surfaces of body organs, serous effusion into body cavities and multiple abscessation throughout the kidneys, lungs, liver and heart.

Various lesions have been reported following histopathological examination of cases, including a fibrinosuppurative meningitis, and microabscesses or thrombi in the brain, kidneys, liver, lungs and heart.

Diagnosis

Septicaemia associated with Gram-negative pleomorphic organisms should always be considered when lambs are found dead in the post-weaning period. The condition

> **CASE STUDY**
>
> Over a period of 5 weeks between mid-February and late March, 20 of a group of 900 Romney-cross cryptorchid ram and ewe lambs were found dead. The lambs were being finished for slaughter on Pasja (forage brassica) and pasture. They had been vaccinated against clostridial diseases and were on a regular worm-drenching programme. Two lambs found while still alive showed signs of ataxia, fine head tremors and recumbency. These two lambs and a further two that were found freshly dead were necropsied. All four had thick green purulent material in the meninges from which *Histophilus somni* was isolated. They also had excess quantities of fluid in the pericardium. A number of lesions were detected on histopathology including a severe fibrinopurulent meningoencephalitis, foci of suppuration in the liver and lungs, and fibrinous thrombi in the kidneys. Fifteen semen samples were collected at random from healthy ram and cryptorchid lambs in the group, and *Histophilus somni* was isolated from 11 of the semen samples. The relationship between the genital infection and the septicaemia is unclear.

can easily be mistaken for enterotoxaemia, particularly in unvaccinated lambs, and therefore examination of the brain at necropsy is recommended. Necropsy and histological examination in association with ruling out other causes of death will support a diagnosis. The diagnosis is confirmed by bacteriological culture of the organisms, although they can be difficult to grow, particularly in the face of contamination. The most recently dead animals should be selected and samples for bacteriology should be collected as cleanly as possible and transported in transport media.

Treatment
Treatment is likely to be unrewarding because by the time affected lambs are identified they are likely to have irreversible damage to the brain, joints or kidneys.

Control and prevention
Because the precipitating factors are not known, firm recommendations for the control and prevention of this disease cannot be made. It is thought that the reproductive tract of young sheep may become invaded by Gram-negative pleomorphic organisms from the environment, particularly in areas where sheep congregate, such as sheep camps and around gateways and in sheep yards. Therefore, keeping lambs away from dirty, contaminated areas and minimising yarding times may reduce the level of exposure to the organism.

Redgut
Redgut is a disease of sheep, usually weaned lambs, grazing high-quality lucerne or clover pastures. The condition is characterised by sudden death and at necropsy an intense reddening of the intestines. In most cases there is a clockwise torsion of the intestinal mass (when viewed from the ventral aspect). It may also affect young cattle on occasion.

Aetiology and pathogenesis
It is suggested that the death of sheep with redgut is due to circulatory shock arising from arrested mesenteric blood flow caused by mechanical torsion and dilation of the intestinal mass. Grazing lucerne and other lush pastures appears to predispose sheep to this condition.

In comparison with lambs on grass pasture, lucerne-fed lambs have smaller rumens and increased large intestinal fermentation, plus increased size and malposition of the large intestines. These features of lambs grazing lucerne possibly account for instability and hyperactivity of the intestinal mass and lead to the torsions often seen with redgut.

Pathology
The sheep are usually found dead. In suspected cases of redgut, the sheep should be necropsied on their backs so that any clockwise intestinal displacement can be seen more readily. (Torsions are not always easy to detect at necropsy. The mesenteric root should be checked before the gut is disturbed.) The rumen is relatively small and empty. The intestines are reddened from an area beginning about 1 metre from the pylorus and extending to the terminal colon. Histological examination confirms that the reddening is due to congestion and haemorrhage and not inflammation.

Diagnosis
The association of sudden death of young weaned lambs grazing high-quality lucerne or clover pastures should alert the veterinarian to the possibility of redgut. It is important to differentiate redgut from enterotoxaemia, but the vaccination history and necropsy findings make differentiation possible.

Control
Redgut can be controlled by grazing lucerne and other high-quality pasture intermittently. This allows the rumen to maintain a size large enough to prevent the predisposing changes in gut position. A regimen of 5 days lucerne grazing and 2 days grass grazing appears to be a practical control method.

Enteric listeriosis
In sheep, *Listeria* spp are usually associated with neurological disease (see Chapter 17) and occasionally as a cause of abortion. However, they can also cause a gastroenteritis resulting in death. The disease is usually associated with feeding poor-quality baleage or silage, although the condition has also been reported in ewes

grazing pasture. High stocking density may also be an important precipitating factor. The majority of diagnosed cases have occurred during winter.

Diarrhoea and depression may precede death, or sheep may simply be found dead. At necropsy there may be severe patchy reddening of the abomasum and caecum. Histology reveals a suppurative or ulcerative abomasitis, enteritis, colitis and typhlitis, and Gram-positive rods may be present within the lesions. *Listeria* can be isolated from intestinal contents. This condition could be confused with other causes of sudden death in ewes such as salmonellosis or possibly clostridial diseases or fertiliser toxicity. Therefore the history of the flock, necropsy, histopathology and bacteriological culture are important in making a diagnosis.

Anthrax

Anthrax has been eradicated from New Zealand, but it should be considered during any investigation of sudden death. *Bacillus anthracis* may cause anthrax in a number of species, including sheep, goats, cattle, humans and other animals. It has not been reported in sheep in New Zealand but it has been reported in cattle, with the last recorded case occurring in 1954.

Epidemiology

Anthrax spores may survive in soil for many years. Sheep usually become infected from grazing spore-infected pasture or soil. Penetrating wounds such as those produced by grass seed awns may also produce anthrax.

On entering the body the spores germinate and multiply. The toxins they produce cause severe damage to blood vessels, leading to death. Prior to death there is a massive number of anthrax bacilli circulating in the blood and in other body tissues. When this blood and secretions are exposed to air, the bacilli form spores that contaminate the soil, frequently for years.

Clinical findings

Affected sheep are usually found dead. The carcass is usually severely distended and blood is frequently discharging from the mouth, nose and anus.

Diagnosis

Postmortem examination of sheep that have died or are suspected of having died of anthrax is most undesirable. Once opened, the body fluids and blood release large numbers of bacilli which sporulate and produce a long-term reservoir for the re-infection of other animals. In addition, anthrax can be transmitted to humans, although most human infections occur as a result of the handling of pelts from infected sheep.

The diagnosis is usually made from a blood smear taken from a superficial skin vein such as on the ear. Microscopic examination of such smears for the presence of the bacteria, following staining with polychrome methylene blue, enables a diagnosis to be made.

Prevention

Prevention is by vaccination, but this is only necessary in endemic areas.

REFERENCES

SALMONELLOSIS

Allworth MB, West DM, Bruère AN. Salmonellosis in ram hoggets following prophylactic zinc dosing. *New Zealand Veterinary Journal* 33, 171, 1985

Beckett FW. The use of salmonella vaccine in outbreaks of salmonellosis in sheep. *New Zealand Veterinary Journal* 15, 66-9, 1967

Belton D. Salmonellosis in New Zealand livestock. *Surveillance* 20, 13-4, 1993

Bruère AN. Animal health problems associated with autumn-winter grazing. *Proceedings of the Society of Sheep and Beef Cattle Veterinarians, New Zealand Veterinary Association* 11, 88-93, 1981

Clark G. *Salmonella* isolates in New Zealand sheep. *Surveillance* 26, 6-7, 1999

Clark RG, Swanney S, Hogan MC, Marchant RM, Fenwick SG. *Salmonella* Brandenburg in non-pregnant 8-month-old sheep. *New Zealand Veterinary Journal* 47, 210, 1999

Clark RG, Robinson RA, Alley MR, Nicol CM, Hathaway SC, Marchant RM. Salmonella in animals in New Zealand: The past to the future. *New Zealand Veterinary Journal* 50 (Suppl.), 57-60, 2002

Josland SW. Observations on the aetiology of the bovine and ovine salmonellosis in New Zealand. *New Zealand Veterinary Journal* 1, 131, 1953

Kane DW. The prevalence of *Salmonella* infection in sheep at slaughter. *New Zealand Veterinary Journal* 27, 110-13, 1979

Kelly K. *Salmonella* Hindmarsh more 'stuff' down south. *Proceedings of the Society of Sheep and Beef Cattle Veterinarians of the NZVA and Cervetec* 309, 61-6, 2015

Midwinter A. *Salmonella typhimurium* phage types in New Zealand. *Surveillance* 25, 5-6, 1998

Robinson RA. *Salmonella* excretion by sheep following yarding. *New Zealand Veterinary Journal* 15, 24-5, 1967

Robinson RA. *Salmonella* infection: Diagnosis and control. *New Zealand Veterinary Journal* 18, 259-77, 1970

Robinson RA, Royal WA. Field epizootiology of *Salmonella* infection in sheep. *New Zealand Journal of Agriculture* 14, 442-56, 1971

Robinson RA, Shortridge EH, MacDiarmid HJ. The effects of monthly formalin treatments on the survival of salmonellae in earthen sheep yard debris. *New Zealand Veterinary Journal* 18, 214-16, 1970

Salisbury RM. *Salmonella* infections in animals and birds in New Zealand. *New Zealand Veterinary Journal* 6, 76-86, 1958

Surveillance

(1979) 3: 21	Salmonellosis of sheep (Otago-Southland)
(1980) 3: 20	Salmonellosis of rams
(1980) 4: 4-5	Salmonellosis data
(2000) 27(3): 18	*Salmonella typimurium* and *Salmonella* Hindmarsh
(2006) 33(2): 30	*Salmonella* Hindmarsh

West DM. Salmonellosis of sheep. *Proceedings of the Society of Sheep and Beef Cattle Veterinarians, New Zealand Veterinary Association* 18, 90-9, 1988

HISTOPHILUS SOMNI SEPTICAEMIA

Agen O, Ahrens P, Kuhnert P, Christensen H, Mutters R. Proposal of *Histophilus somni*; gen.nov., Sp. nov. for the three species incertae sedis '*Haemophilus somnus*', '*Haemophilus agni*' and '*Histophilus ovis*'. *International Journal of systemic and Evolutionary Microbiology* 53, 1449-56, 2003

Gill J. *Haemophilus agni* (*Histophilus ovis*) as a cause of mortality in lambs. *Surveillance* 19 (2), 13, 1992

Kater JC, Marshall SC, Hartley WJ. A specific suppurative synovitis and pyaemia in lambs. *New Zealand Veterinary Journal* 10, 143-4, 1962

Kearney KP, Orr MB. An outbreak of *Haemophilus agni-Histophilus ovis* septicaemia in lambs. *New Zealand Veterinary Journal* 41, 149-50, 1993

Philbey AW, Glastonbury JRW. Thromboembolic meningoencephalitis in sheep due to *Histophilus ovis*. *Proceedings of the Australian Sheep Veterinary Society, Pan Pacific Conference*, 125-7, 1991

Surveillance

(1993) 20 (2): 3	Review of diagnostic cases
(1998) 25 (2): 15	Review of diagnostic cases
(2006): 33 (1): 11	Review of diagnostic cases

REDGUT

Barrel GK, Gumbrell RC, Reid TC. Artificial induction of redgut in sheep. *Research in Veterinary Science* 46, 318-21, 1984

Gumbrell RC. Redgut in sheep. *Proceedings of the 4th Annual Seminar of the Society of Sheep and Beef Cattle Veterinarians, New Zealand Veterinary Association*, 37-42, 1974

Gumbrell RC, Jagusch KT. 'Redgut syndrome' in lambs grazing lucerne. *New Zealand Veterinary Journal* 21, 178-9, 1973

Gumbrell RC. Redgut in sheep: A disease with a twist. *New Zealand Veterinary Journal* 45, 217-21, 1997

Surveillance (1983) 1: 21-2: Redgut in sheep

ENTERIC LISTERIOSIS

Clark RG, Gill JM, Swanney S. *Listeria monocytogenes* gastroenteritis in sheep. *New Zealand Veterinary Journal* 52, 46-7, 2004

Oswald AWR. Sudden death in Merino ewes in late gestation. *Proceedings of the 32nd Annual Seminar of the Society of Sheep and Beef Cattle Veterinarians, New Zealand Veterinary Association*, 227-34, 2002

Surveillance

(1998) 25 (3): 11	Review of diagnostic cases
(2004) 31 (3): 21-5	Ewes with enteric listeriosis
(2007) 34 (4): 13-16	Enteric listeriosis

ANTHRAX

Davidson RM. Control and eradication of animal diseases in New Zealand. *New Zealand Veterinary Journal* 50 (Suppl.), 6-12, 2002

Surveillance (1993) 20 (1)L 21-2 Anthrax — still history after all these years.

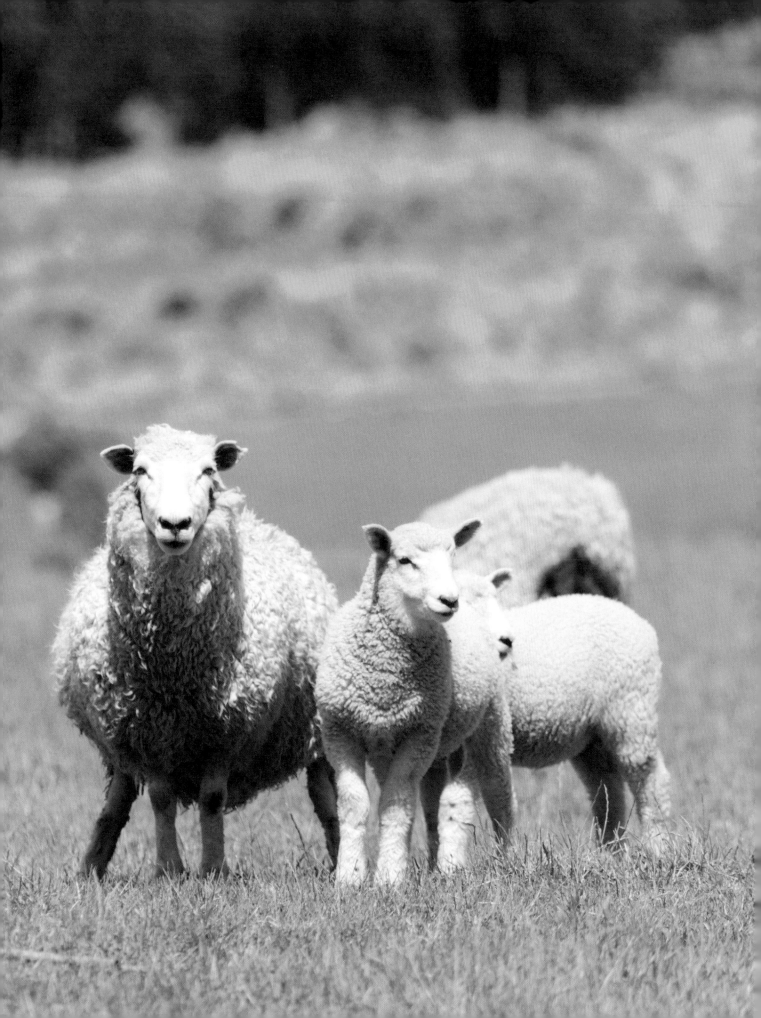

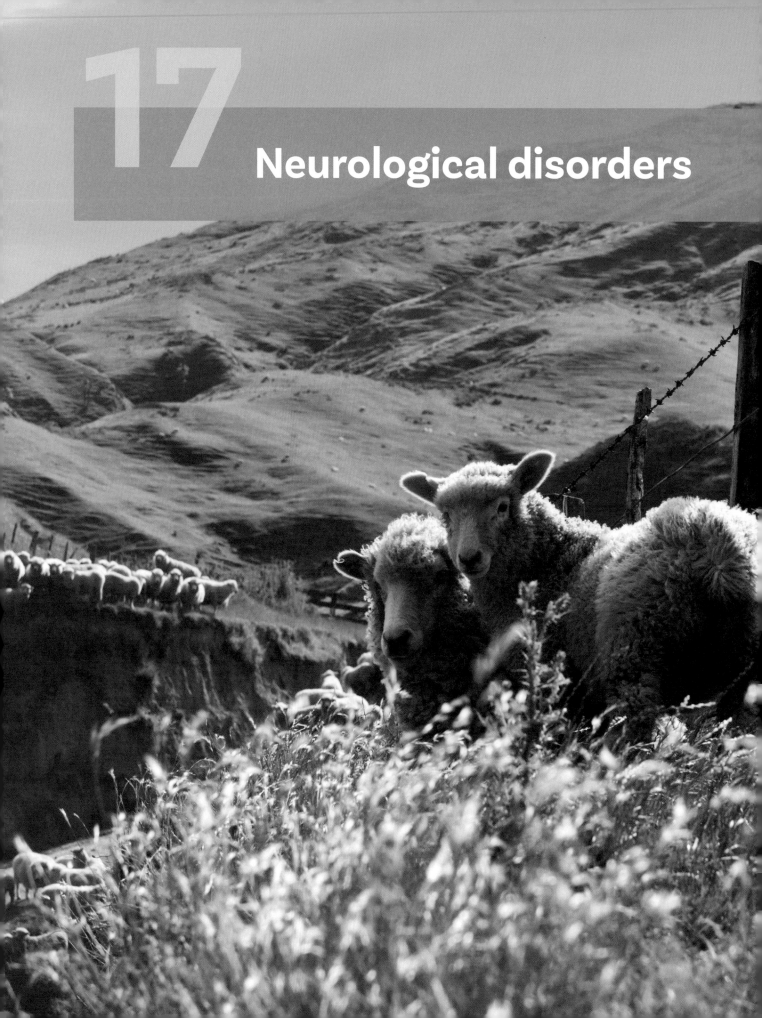

17 Neurological disorders

Sheep may be affected by a variety of neurological disorders, and determining the cause of these frequently poses a challenge to the veterinarian. In many of these conditions, only a single sheep may be affected and treatment is of limited value. However, when a number of sheep in a flock are affected, reaching a diagnosis quickly is important so that prophylactic measures may be applied.

Sheep are not always easy to examine neurologically, as they are less accustomed to human contact than companion animals. Nevertheless it is possible to establish the locality of a lesion and reach an accurate diagnosis of the disease from a careful consideration of the history and clinical findings.

Clinical investigation

The history of the case should be investigated carefully, noting all the usual features including age, sex, breed of affected sheep and any recent changes in management and grazing. It is also important to assess the number of affected animals and the rapidity of progression of clinical signs. In New Zealand, the examination of the environment is very important as so many diseases of sheep with neurological manifestations are related to environmental factors, e.g. ryegrass staggers, Phalaris staggers and pregnancy toxaemia.

Initially the affected animals should be observed when they are undisturbed in the paddock. This will allow a comparative assessment to be made of the condition of the flock and the relationship of affected to normal sheep.

Head carriage and movements

The carriage of the head is most important. The 'hyper-alert' sheep with a high head carriage may have defective vision (pregnancy toxaemia). A tilted head (head rotated) may indicate a lesion of the upper medulla or an ear infection. Lateral deviation of the head may be the result of unilateral blindness, while vertical changes of head position may occur in generalised brain swelling, cerebral or cerebellar cortical lesions, malacias or meningitis.

Head tremors, which are commonly seen in many neurological disorders of sheep, indicate lesions or defects in the cerebellum or diencephalon. Fine head tremors are often seen in the newborn lamb and may indicate gross intracranial malformations.

Compulsive circling may indicate a brain-stem or cerebellar lesion on the side to which the animal turns (e.g. listeriosis), or a cerebral lesion which is usually on the opposite side. Other abnormal features may include knuckling at the fetlocks, ataxia, posterior paralysis, swayback, trotting gait and kangaroo gait.

Close physical examination

The response to approach may be important. In many neurological disorders, sheep are oblivious to human presence (e.g. polioencephalomalacia, listeriosis) while in others their reaction is one of apprehension (e.g. ryegrass staggers). Other features of the head may be noted. The bulging of the cheek caused by cud retention, lingual paralysis or a drooping ear or eyelid may all be indicative of facial paralysis (e.g. listeriosis).

Nystagmus is associated with lesions in the brain stem, the vestibular apparatus or cerebellum; unequal pupil size is suggestive of damage to the hypothalamus or the cervical portion of the autonomic nervous system. The absence of the photomotor reflex may be due to lesions in the eye, optic or oculomotor nerve, while the absence of the eye preservation reflex may suggest lesions of the facial or trigeminal nerves. Obstacle avoidance is the best test for blindness.

The cutaneous and pedal reflexes are probably the most useful means of testing local spinal reflex arcs in sheep and in the detection of spinal abscesses and fractured vertebrae, for example.

In many cases it is necessary to conduct a postmortem examination to confirm a particular diagnosis.

Postmortem examination

During necropsy for a suspected neurological disease, the general postmortem examination should not be neglected. However, careful removal of the brain and spinal cord is essential. It is generally better to euthanase an animal showing advanced clinical signs than to rely on the necropsy of an animal that may have been dead for hours or even a day or more.

Samples of nervous tissue should be placed in a container of adequate size so that 10–20 times the volume of the tissue can be added as 10% formalin. The material should be despatched to the diagnostic laboratory, ideally after several days to allow fixation of the tissue to proceed. As part of New Zealand's surveillance programme for scrapie, veterinarians are encouraged to submit the brain and anterior spinal cord of adult sheep showing progressive neurological signs (see Chapter 21). Financial incentives are available to the veterinarian and the flock owner.

Specific neurological disorders of sheep

The main disorders discussed are listed in Table 17.1.

Plant and chemical poisonings

Sheep may be affected by a number of plant and chemical poisonings that produce severe derangement of the nervous system.[1]

Ryegrass staggers

Ryegrass staggers is a neurological disorder of sheep as well as of cattle, horses, deer and alpacas. It is common in Australia and New Zealand and is reported from several

---

[1] For a fuller description of these see *Veterinary Clinical Toxicology*, Publication No. 249, VetLearn Foundation, Massey University, Palmerston North, New Zealand.

Chemical and plant poisonings+	Ryegrass staggers, lead poisoning, organophosphorus poisoning, Phalaris staggers, tutu poisoning, hepatic encephalopathy
Microbiological diseases	Brain and spinal abscesses, listeriosis, focal symmetrical encephalomalacia, polioencephalomalacia (caused by bacterial toxins), *Histophilus somni* meningoencephalitis
Congenital disorders of lambs	
— Inherited	Ceroid lipofuscinosis, daft lamb disease, neuraxonal dystrophy, cerebellar abiotrophy, encephalopathy, ovine segmental axonopathy, ovine spongiform leucoencephalopathy, familial episodic ataxia
— Other	Microencephaly, cerebellar defects, spina bifida, arthrogryposis toxoplasmosis, enzootic ataxia, hairy shaker/border disease, agenesis of the corpus callosum and hippocampus
Functional disorders	Hypocalcaemia, hypomagnesaemia, pregnancy toxaemia, tetanus, kangaroo gait, axonal degeneration
Microbiological diseases exotic to New Zealand	Louping ill, scrapie, maedi-visna, rabies, Aujesky's disease*
Parasitic diseases	Coenurosis

+ Refer to Parton, Bruère and Chambers (2006) for full descriptions.
* Recorded in pigs in New Zealand.

Table 17.1 Main neurological disorders of sheep seen in New Zealand.

other countries. Ryegrass staggers occurs in sheep grazing pastures dominant in perennial ryegrass (*Lolium perenne*) with outbreaks occurring mainly in summer and autumn under close grazing conditions.

Farmers have repeatedly emphasised the seriousness of ryegrass staggers. Although the direct mortality rate from ryegrass staggers is low, the high morbidity rate may lead to losses through misadventure such as drowning or being caught in ditches or fences, or from attacks by natural predators such as gulls. Losses from such sources may vary from 2% to 10% in serious ryegrass staggers seasons. Further, sheep in affected flocks have reduced growth rates and may have difficulty in mating. Movement of animals is difficult and procedures such as rotational grazing and drenching of lambs may have to be abandoned until the signs have subsided. Under such circumstances, serious occurrences of parasitism (e.g. haemonchosis) have frequently resulted. Farmers may be forced to use additional supplementary feed and labour to reduce the effects of a severe outbreak.

Aetiology

The *Lolium*-endophytic fungus *Neotyphodium* (*Acremonium*) *lolii* is found within the leaf, sheath, stem and seed of many cultivars of perennial ryegrass (*Lolium perenne*). *Neotyphodium lolii* produces toxins, with the major toxin in the aetiology of ryegrass staggers being lolitrem B. This is a neurotoxic complex indole with structural similarity to many other tremorgens such as aflatrem, the penitrems, paspalanines, janthitrems and paxilline. A further effect of this toxin is to have stimulatory and inhibitory effects on the smooth muscle of the gut and peripheral vasculature.

Endophyte spread is seed-borne rather than from plant to plant. The endophyte does not survive storage in the seed for 15 months at room temperature. Endophyte is found most commonly in ryegrass in the summer and autumn, and its highest concentration is in the leaf sheath of the outer or oldest leaves.

The Argentine stem weevil and ryegrass staggers

Another aspect of the presence of the *Lolium* endophyte is that infected ryegrass is resistant to attacks by the Argentine stem weevil (*Listronotus bonariensis*). This is because the endophyte also produces a substance called peramine which reduces the adult-stage feeding of Argentine stem weevil and consequently reduces egg laying and larvae development. Therefore, in terms of grass production, endophyte-infected ryegrass has production advantages over endophyte-free ryegrass.

Cultivars of ryegrass have been developed that are infected with *N. lolii* but produce low levels of lolitrem B while still producing high levels of peramine. In most cases, such ryegrasses should not cause ryegrass staggers while still protecting against Argentine stem weevil.

Clinical signs

The morbidity rates vary considerably between flocks and seasons. There is also a wide range of susceptibility to the disease between animals, which has a heritable component. The heritability of ryegrass staggers is estimated to be up to 0.17.

Sheep develop signs within 7–14 days of being placed on toxic pastures. On casual examination, animals at rest show few obvious clinical signs. However, when disturbed and made to walk or run, the clinical signs immediately become apparent. As forced movement continues, the signs increase in severity until a maximum response is reached which indicates the extent and severity of the disease present in the flock. The mildest clinical signs are a slight trembling of the head and fasciculation of the skin muscles of the neck, shoulder and flank regions. As the neuromuscular disorder progresses there is head nodding and jerky limb movements. Interference with postural reflexes follows, seen as swaying while standing and staggering during movement.

As the condition worsens, a stiff-legged, stilted gait may develop with short prancing steps, usually resulting in collapse to the ground. Sheep roll in lateral recumbency with head extended, back arched and legs held rigidly in a tetanic spasm of several minutes duration. This is followed by sudden muscular relaxation and apparent recovery. The animal then slowly regains its feet and walks away, often still showing tremors but with very little locomotory incoordination.

Pathological and functional changes

No consistent or specific pathological changes have been found in organs or tissues in sheep affected with ryegrass staggers, including the central nervous system. These negative findings, together with the apparent rapid recovery of animals, suggests a very temporary derangement. The incapacity is probably in the transmission of nerve impulses between the brain and functional groups of skeletal muscles whose coordinated activities maintain precise balance and smooth movement during locomotion.

Treatment

Treatment involves supplying the animals with safe feedstuffs, if available, and ensuring they do not suffer from misadventure. Any handling of affected stock should be done quietly and carefully. Various tonics and mycotoxin binders are marketed for the treatment of ryegrass staggers but robust scientific evidence of their efficacy in sheep is lacking.

Control

It is difficult to give general advice on the control of ryegrass staggers when farm conditions show marked variation, both individually and between districts. In some areas, regular summer drought conditions cause little clover growth, wilting and death of ryegrass and the accumulation of litter. Such conditions are common in eastern parts of both the North and the South Island. Also, in most areas the signs of ryegrass staggers have developed and spread through a flock before rotational systems can be applied, and once ryegrass staggers has developed the movement of stock on a daily basis is an impossible procedure.

Control measures can be costly and may not be easily acceptable to many farmers. The following options are available:
- Avoid hard grazing of ryegrass pastures during risk periods.
- Re-sow pastures with cultivars that resist Argentine stem weevil attack but do not contain high levels of lolitrem B.
- Grow rape or other fodder for late summer grazing (cost- and equipment-intensive).
- Develop lucerne; only suitable in certain soil types (difficult to establish in many North Island areas because of clay-based soils).
- Allow reversion of pastures to a low-producing weed state (not acceptable in modern farming).
- Feed silage (labour-intensive and reduces stores of winter feed).
- Breed sheep tolerant to ryegrass staggers (slow, may interfere with other breeding objectives).

Phalaris poisoning

Phalaris spp, namely P. tuberosa (also known as P. aquatica) and P. arundinacea (reed canary grass), have become established in New Zealand and Australia. Both are widespread and have been known to cause toxicity in sheep and cattle. In New Zealand Phalaris poisoning is not commonly reported, which is in contrast to Australia where various species of Phalaris are used extensively for cattle and sheep pasture.

Toxicity

Both plants contain indole alkaloids, which act as inhibitors of monoamine oxidase and interfere with serotonin and catecholamine action, metabolism and detoxification.

The alkaloids vary in toxicity and their concentration in the grass is affected by environmental conditions. Phalaris spp when subjected to dull cloudy weather for some time are likely to be toxic to sheep. If the light intensity is high, Phalaris spp are unlikely to be dangerous unless soil nitrate levels are also high (as a result of several years of clover growth). The danger of toxicity increases when day temperatures are 20°C or above, particularly when light intensities are low, i.e. the autumn period is a favourable time for Phalaris poisoning to occur.

Clinical signs

Peracute, acute and chronic syndromes have all been described, but in New Zealand they all tend to merge into an acute toxicity with sudden deaths in some sheep, while other sheep show persistent nervous signs for several days before death (Phalaris staggers).

In New Zealand the acute syndrome is most likely to occur when Phalaris spp are growing rapidly and when pastures are lightly stocked and young shoots of Phalaris spp are partially shaded by dead litter from a previous season's growth. The more chronic syndrome is said to occur when sheep have prolonged repeated exposure to grass showing new growth.

1. Acute syndrome

This is usually seen within 12 and 72 hours of hungry animals going onto toxic pasture. Animals will suddenly collapse, especially when excited or moved. They will show arrhythmic tachycardia and ventricular fibrillation, and death may occur at this stage. Some animals will lie on their sides, and show convulsive spasms, dorsoflexion of the head and neck, jaw champing with ropy saliva, rigid extension of the limbs and severe tachycardia. Some less severely affected sheep may be hyperexcitable and ataxic, with nodding of the head, twitching ears and tail, chewing and salivation. All these signs are easily triggered by excitement, and sheep that try to run will inevitably fall down.

2. Chronic syndrome

This is characterised by similar neurological signs to those described above, but they persist when the animals are moved from the Phalaris grass because of lesions in the central nervous system. Many of these sheep have persistent uncontrollable head nodding, limb weakness and arrhythmic tachycardia. These clinical signs may last in sheep for months. The morbidity rate is high in most outbreaks and there may be up to 50% mortality on occasions.

Pathology

Sheep dying from the acute syndrome may simply show signs of an acute congestive heart failure (congestion of the abdominal viscera and petechial haemorrhages of the epicardium). There may also be blood-stained nasal discharges.

In the more chronic cases (i.e. those which have shown Phalaris staggers), there is usually a greenish pigmentation of various tissues, mainly the brain and kidneys. The central neurons of the spinal cord and the neurons of the dorsal root ganglia also carry the pigment. In the kidney the pigment is confined to the medulla.

The extensive accumulation of pigment in cell mitochondria probably interferes with their function, leading to secondary demyelination, which is seen in the spinal cords of sheep with Phalaris staggers.

Diagnosis

Confirmed diagnosis may be made from formalin-fixed brain tissue for histopathology.

Treatment

There is no known treatment for Phalaris staggers.

Control

If Phalaris spp are to be grazed, then sheep should be introduced to the pasture over a period of several days and then set stocked with high stocking rates during periods of lush growth. The risk of toxicity is increased by grazing autumn-saved Phalaris pasture, spelling and rotational grazing.

Hungry sheep should never be turned onto Phalaris pasture. Hay made from the pasture is much less toxic than the original pasture, because the alkaloids break down as the plants dry.

Tutu poisoning

Tutu is the classical poison plant of New Zealand, and in our earlier history significant numbers of cattle and sheep were lost from tutu poisoning. Except horses, most species are affected and there are reports of losses in cattle, sheep, pigs, elephants and a dog.

Toxicity

All New Zealand species of *Coriaria* contain the toxin tutin. Younger shoots contain more toxins than the older plant shoots, and leaves contain more tutin than do the stems of all species. The seeds, both green and ripe, contain tutin and are toxic.

The fate of absorbed tutu in the body is not clearly understood, although it is believed that it becomes localised in the brain and spinal cord in a detoxified state.

Clinical signs

The clinical signs are sudden in onset and are usually seen within 24–48 hours of ingestion of the plant. The signs seen are picrotoxin-like in effect and are hence mainly referable to the central nervous system.

Respiration rate is increased and so is the heart rate, with a significant rise in blood pressure. Muscle twitching soon becomes evident and severe. Extreme excitement including blind charging and eleptiform convulsions are seen. Sheep become bloated and regurgitate ingesta. Terminal convulsions and death are the final outcome of most cases of tutu poisoning in livestock.

Pathology
The main feature of the postmortem is the presence of undigested tutu leaves in the rumen. These are a valuable aid to a confirmed diagnosis.

Treatment
Treatment is largely symptomatic; the intravenous use of barbiturates proved useful in the treatment of two circus elephants, but reported cases of successful treatment are rare.

Prevention
It is wise to ensure that adequate feed is available if tutu is present in paddocks. Animals that are hungry should not be allowed access to tutu. Most cases of poisoning have been associated with droving and hungry livestock denied access to normal fodder.

Lead poisoning
While lead poisoning has been reported commonly in cattle and dogs in New Zealand, its occurrence in sheep is quite rare. From overseas experience most cases of lead poisoning in sheep have been associated with grazing smelter-contaminated pasture. The clinical signs displayed are mainly of a subacute nature and are as follows:
- course is over 3–4 days
- anorexia, dehydration and dullness
- incoordination, circling, apparent blindness and salivation
- muscle tremors and hyperaesthesia
- abdominal pain, belly kicking, rumen atony and constipation
- sheep frequently die near water.

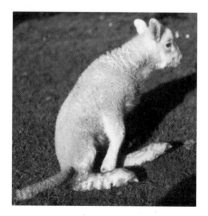

Figure 17.1 Lamb with hind-limb paralysis due to a spinal abscess.

Organophosphorus poisoning
In spite of the extensive exposure of sheep to organophosphorus compounds, notably sheep dips, there are relatively few reports of organophosphorus poisoning in this species. When it does occur, the main clinical signs seen are referable to the nicotinic effects of the poison. These include fasciculation of muscles (shivering and tremors), muscle weakness and paralysis. Occasionally in sheep, torticollis is reported.

Hepatic encephalopathy
Hepatic encephalopathy with widespread spongy vacuolation of the brain has been reported in sheep and cattle in New Zealand that have been affected with facial eczema. A variety of nervous signs have been reported, with most cases ending in recumbency and death.

Microbiological diseases

Spinal abscesses
Spinal abscesses may occur in all ages of sheep but are seen most commonly in lambs following lambing or docking. The clinical signs vary depending on the site and the degree of interference with nerve transmission. The lesions are commonly found in the thoraco-lumbar region, which usually results in posterior paralysis with the lamb seen attempting to drag itself by the forelimbs.

The common bacteria isolated from lesions of spinal abscess include *Fusobacterium necrophorum*, *Staphylococcus aureus* and occasionally *Trueparella (Arcanobacter) pyogenes*. In many cases, additional abscess sites may be found in the liver and lungs, indicating that a bacteraemia has occurred.

Prevention of spinal abscesses involves attention to hygiene at lambing time to minimise navel infections and at docking time to reduce infection of surgical sites. Occasionally, infection at the site of tail docking may ascend along the spinal cord producing posterior paralysis.

Bacterial meningitis and brain abscesses
With the exception of listeriosis, there is no specific bacterial meningitis in sheep and most cases arise as complications of pre-existing disease states. Organisms may reach the brain in three ways: directly as result of

trauma, by local extension from lesions in adjacent tissue, or via the haematogenous route. The last is most common, and bacterial meningitis usually occurs in association with generalised infections with *Escherichia coli*, *Pasteurella* species, *Staphylococcus aureus*, *Trueperella pyogenes*, or *Streptococcus* species.

A more specific form of brain abscess is that of parapituitary abscesses that occur in rams as a consequence of infection of fighting wounds of the head. Septic emboli from the poll area are carried by venous drainage to the vascular rete surrounding the pituitary, where they establish abscesses that spread to ventral parts of the brain.

A variety of nervous signs are seen with brain abscesses depending on the site of the lesion, the speed at which it develops and the degree of disruption to nervous tissue. Abscesses of the brain may result in circling, deviation or rotation of the head, drooping of an ear or eye, retention of cud and inequality in pupil size. However, adult sheep can sometimes tolerate quite extensive brain abscesses and continue to graze with seemingly little discomfort or disability. This is in contrast to cases of listeriosis which usually progress quickly over a period of 3 or 4 days.

It is difficult to reach a diagnosis of brain abscess with certainty in the live animal, although a history of fighting in rams combined with the sudden onset of a generalised or localised neurological dysfunction that continues over a week or more is suggestive of bacterial meningitis. Examination of cerebrospinal fluid for cell type and the presence of bacteria may be useful, but in most instances the diagnosis is made following necropsy. Unless carried out very early, treatment with antibiotics is unrewarding and does little to repair any neurological defect.

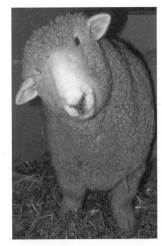

Figure 17.2 Characteristic head tilt in a ram with a brain abscess.

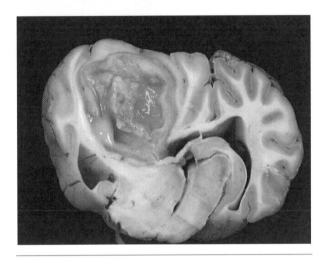

Figure 17.3 Brain abscess.

Listeriosis

Listeriosis occurs in sheep throughout the world and was first described in New Zealand in 1931. It is a common and important condition that may occur in four different forms: meningoencephalitis, abortion, enteritis (Chapter 16) and, in lambs, septicaemia. The meningoencephalitic form has been reported most commonly in New Zealand. The disease is caused by *Listeria monocytogenes*.

Epidemiology

Sheep, cattle, buffalo, goats, horses, pigs, dogs, cats,

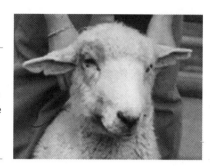

Figure 17.4 Unilateral facial paralysis of a sheep with listeriosis. Note the drooping right ear and upper lip.

rabbits and humans are susceptible to infection. Most human cases arise from sources other than sheep. Women have been known to abort as a result of *L. monocytogenes* infection.

Listeria last for long periods in soil, and the decaying vegetation on the soil surface may provide a suitable environment for multiplication. The alimentary tract is also a haven for the organism and carriers may contaminate the environment.

In New Zealand, meningoencephalitis usually occurs sporadically in older sheep in the period from late summer to winter (February to July). However, overseas it has been suggested that the incidence could be greater in lambs, 2-year-old and aged sheep associated with shedding of teeth and periodontitis. Outbreaks may sometimes occur, and these are usually associated with the feeding of silage or baleage. In one recorded case, 80 of 600 1-year-old Merino sheep died following silage feeding.

The organism does not multiply in well-made silage which has a low pH (4–4.5) but in poor silage contaminated with soil or on the edge of the pit or stack the pH may be above 5.5, allowing the organism to survive and multiply. A possible source of contamination of feed was suggested by the isolation of *L. monocytogenes* from 19.7% of faecal samples collected from seagulls scavenging near sewage works.

Pathogenesis

In sheep the infection is presumed to reach the brain stem via peripheral nerves, especially the trigeminal. It has been suggested that lesions to the mouth of sheep, including shedding of deciduous teeth, may allow infection of branches of the trigeminal nerve and eventually localisation of infection in the brain stem.

Clinical findings

The clinical signs of listeriosis are usually those of severe depression combined with unidirectional circling and unilateral facial paralysis. A careful examination of such cases will often allow a presumptive diagnosis to be made.

In the early stages the sheep is depressed, separated from the flock and progressively develops the signs of circling and facial paralysis. The lips, ear, eyelids and nostrils are paralysed on the affected side and the sheep usually circles in a direction away from the affected side. These signs progress over 1 or 2 days and the sheep becomes comatosed, recumbent and dies. Sometimes it is not until this stage has been reached that the veterinarian is consulted, but even in these cases it is often possible to identify the characteristics of facial paralysis and tendency to fall to one side only, when held in the standing position. Occasionally head pressing against solid objects will be seen.

Diagnosis

A presumptive diagnosis may be made on a consideration of the history and clinical findings, but not all cases display the 'classical' signs and in many cases the sheep is found dead. In live sheep, examination of the cerebrospinal fluid may support a diagnosis of listeriosis. However, confirmation of the diagnosis is usually made postmortem. The macroscopic changes are mild but microabscesses in the region of the mid-brain are characteristic. Bacterial culture is difficult and not always rewarding.

Treatment and control

Although *L. monocytogenes* is susceptible to penicillin and tetracycline, treatment is seldom successful because of the brain damage that has already been caused.

Control of listeriosis has proved to be difficult because of the sporadic nature of the disease. Where silage feeding of sheep is undertaken, farmers should be aware of the need to produce high-quality silage that is stored and used in a manner which prevents spoilage. At present, no vaccine is licensed for use in either Australia or New Zealand.

Focal symmetrical encephalomalacia (FSE)

Focal symmetrical encephalomalacia of lambs is a neurological manifestation of enterotoxaemia. It is caused by the toxins liberated by *Clostridium perfringens* type D which has a strong affinity for vascular endothelium, especially the brain where it disrupts the blood–brain barrier causing oedema and sometimes haemorrhage. From earlier reports in New Zealand by Gill (1927 and 1933) and the later investigation by Hartley (1956), it would appear that mild epidemics of FSE have followed this pattern. Gill claimed three distinct syndromes which he thought were inter-related. Of the 10% of affected lambs he saw alive, 70% showed hyperacute convulsive signs (enterotoxaemia), 20% showed head retraction, and 10% he classified as subacute, lethargic-type disease (focal symmetrical encephalomalacia). These latter lambs rarely showed convulsions typical of enterotoxaemia. Some lived for several days, but recovery was rare.

In the cases cited by Hartley (1956), similar percentages of lambs as described by Gill showed the same features. The pathological picture in both reports was also similar.

Clinical features

Affected lambs may show a wide variety of neurological signs. Some lambs are just found prostrate and are unable to stand even when assisted. Paddling movements with the legs and opisthotonus are seen in some cases. Lambs able to walk may show incoordination, are usually dull and lethargic and may show head pressing. Most lambs are apparently blind and have drooped ears. Aimless wandering in circles is not uncommonly seen. It is claimed that occasionally lambs that are given care may recover but in most cases death is imminent.

Pathology

Some lambs with FSE have postmortem changes identical to those described for enterotoxaemia, i.e. congested and oedematous lungs, serofibrinous fluid in the pericardial sac and pulpy kidneys, but others do not. Careful examination of the brain stem may reveal large bilaterally symmetrical foci of haemorrhage and this can be confirmed by histological examination. In some lambs, distinct focal bilaterally symmetrical haemorrhagic lesions are found in the region of the internal capsule adjacent to the basal ganglia, lateral to and beneath the posterior corpora quadrigemina, and also in the cerebellar peduncles. Diffuse slightly haemorrhagic areas may also be seen in the mid-thalamic region.

Treatment and control

Treatment is unlikely to be rewarding. Control is as for enterotoxaemia (Chapter 15).

Polioencephalomalacia

Polioencephalomalacia is an acute central nervous disease of sheep and other ruminants. It is also a common and important disease of goats. It is considered to be an induced thiamine deficiency, probably caused by the microbiological production of thiaminase and thiamine analogues in the rumen. Experimentally and in the field it has been linked to sulphur intoxication, usually following the feeding of a concentrated feed that contains high levels of sulphur. Several other conditions, including lead poisoning and water intoxication, may present in a similar way to polioencephlomalacia.

Epidemiology

All ages of sheep are susceptible to polioencephalomalacia but the incidence is highest in lambs 2–12 months of age; especially in lambs on feedlots, where it has been estimated to account for up to 20% of all deaths. The condition is usually associated with a feed change to less roughage, which is thought to favour the multiplication of thiaminase-producing bacteria in the rumen.

A milder form of the disease which has been associated with temporary blindness appears to be related to periods when young sheep have been confined to woolsheds or yards and may have been without feed for several days. Such occurrences are rare nowadays.

In New Zealand losses from polioencephalomalacia have been experienced at all times of the year and under various systems of farm management. The morbidity in most outbreaks has rarely been greater than 5% but affected sheep, unless treated, usually die. The duration of outbreaks may extend over a period of a few days to several weeks. In ewes there is an apparent seasonal incidence (March to July) associated with pregnancy.

In New Zealand, polioencephalomalacia outbreaks have often been associated with the feeding of grain or improved pasture, or feed changes as one example from a *Surveillance* report demonstrates. This case involved a group of 1-year-old ewes that had been fed on swedes, then shorn and put onto long pasture. Over the next few days, about 30 developed signs of polioencephalomalacia and this was confirmed on necropsy.

Pathogenesis

Thiamine is an essential component of several enzymes involved in carbohydrate metabolism, and a state of deficiency results in increased blood concentration of pyruvate, a reduction in the lactate to pyruvate ratio and a depression of erythrocyte transketolase. It is suggested that the high and specific requirement of the cerebral cortex for oxidative metabolism of glucose could explain the acute cerebral oedema and laminar necrosis that characterise polioencephalomalacia. It may also explain why cobalt deficiency has been incriminated as a possible contributing cause of polioencephalomalacia.

Clinical features

Two forms of polioencephalomalacia in sheep have been recognised clinically: a severe form and a mild form, although the latter seems to be rarely reported in New Zealand in recent years. In the severe form, affected sheep may be found prostrate, lying on their sides; they usually show nystagmus, absence of the eye preservation reflex and opisthotonus, together with intermittent convulsions.

Less severely affected sheep may stand with assistance, but when left alone either attempt to circle and fall over or adopt a 'dog-sitting', 'star-gazing' posture. Still less severely affected animals may be dejected and blind, and often wander aimlessly showing a 'star-gazing' appearance. Some animals circle continuously, and many severely affected animals display hyperexcitability when handled.

Neurological signs may last from 24 hours to about a week. In prolonged cases the brain damage is irreversible and animals are usually destroyed on humane grounds.

In the mild form of polioencephalomalacia (first described in New Zealand as amaurosis), blindness usually appears suddenly in sheep that have been yarded for a period. Some animals may show dejection and head pressing. However, affected sheep, once they become adapted to their disability, may graze normally and the majority will make a complete clinical recovery after 4 to 6 weeks.

Diagnosis

The acute nervous signs of polioencephalomalacia resemble those of focal symmetrical encephalomalacia (enterotoxaemia) or hypomagnesaemia and can be confused with listeriosis or brain abscesses. The clinical signs of these last two conditions, however, do not have the characteristic symmetrical nature of polioencephalomalacia. The history of cases may be helpful, since hypomagnesaemia is usually seen in lactating ewes and rarely are animals seen displaying clinical signs.

Support for a clinical diagnosis of polioencephalomalacia can come from biochemical tests such as the blood level of thiamine (normal between 75 and 185 nmol/l; below 50 nmol/l is indicative of deficiency). In addition, raised levels of blood pyruvate and lactate, together with reduced transketolase activity, may help establish a diagnosis. However, most cases of polioencephalomalacia are acute and thiamine therapy is instituted before the results of biochemical tests are available. Response to this therapy may assist the diagnosis.

Pathology

In almost all cases of severe polioencephalomalacia, distinct macroscopic lesions are visible on critical examination of either fresh or preserved brains. Characteristically the lesions involve the cerebral cortex and are usually roughly bilaterally symmetrical, but occasionally unilateral, areas of yellow discoloured friable cortical grey matter. The lesions usually extend from frontal to occipital poles and there is often a distinct line of demarcation of the affected tissue from the underlying white matter. Additional cranial lesions such as distinct small haemorrhages are often seen also. The affected areas of the brain fluoresce under a Wood's lamp, which has been attributed to the accumulation of ceroid lipofuscin in macrophages.

Treatment

If sheep are treated early in the course of the disease before much irreversible necrosis has occurred, complete recovery may occur with treatment with thiamine (10 mg/kg) given intravenously and then followed by twice-daily intramuscular injections for up to 3 days. Within 1 or 2 hours of treatment, one expects a reduction of the acute neurological signs and the sheep is quieter. Within 24 hours complete recovery may occur, although sight may take longer to return on occasions.

In valuable animals the use of hypertonic solutions to reduce cerebral oedema in the early stage may be of benefit.

Control

It is reasonable to examine the diet and perhaps suggest a change to include more roughage, especially if deaths occur at specific times such as following mustering for shearing. In contact sheep might be injected with thiamine or perhaps given oral supplementation, but the prevalence seldom justifies such intervention unless the sheep are on a feedlot.

Tetanus

See under clostridial diseases (Chapter 15).

Histophilus somni meningoencephalitis

See under other causes of sudden death (Chapter 16).

Congenital abnormalities

Congenital defects of the nervous system are common in lambs, and veterinarians are sometimes presented with a number of defective lambs from one flock or farm. The owner usually wishes to know whether more such cases will occur in that season or in future years and what can be done to prevent a recurrence of the problem. The more common defects seen in New Zealand are listed in Table 17.1. Many of these have resulted from foetal viral infections such as hairy shaker/border disease and the Akabane disease (not recorded in New Zealand). Other defects are inherited conditions or of unknown aetiology.

Ovine ceroid-lipofuscinosis

Ovine ceroid-lipofuscinosis is an inherited disease originally reported from an inbred flock of South Hampshire sheep in New Zealand. It has now been reported in Borderdale sheep in the South Island. It is characterised pathologically by microencephaly, and the intracellular accumulation of autofluorescent lipopigments in neurons and other cells. It has features in common with a heterogeneous group of storage diseases of children known as Batten's disease. The mode of inheritance is autosomal recessive.

Affected lambs appear normal at birth, but between 9 and 12 months of age they tend to separate themselves from the flock, become blind and develop nervous signs of spontaneous episodes of head nodding, champing of jaws and twitching of ears, eyelids, lips and muzzle. The frequency and severity of these episodes increases with age, and affected sheep lose weight and have difficulty feeding. The wool of the lower jaw is often constantly wet with water from periods of sham drinking. Few survive beyond 2 years of age.

Daft lamb disease (cerebellar cortical atrophy)

'Daft' lamb disease is uncommon, but has been reported in Britain, Canada, Australia and New Zealand. It has occurred in a variety of breeds and is considered to be an inherited disease with an autosomal recessive mode of transmission. The disease has been reported in Corriedale, Drysdale and Border Leicester sheep in New Zealand.

The clinical signs are evident at birth or soon after, and are variable. Some lambs are found recumbent while others adopt an extreme dorsoflexion of the neck so that the head is pointing upwards. The abnormal head movements and head carriage cause difficulties in feeding and moving such that the majority of lambs have to be destroyed.

Tear scald is often present on the cheeks and lambs are prone to conjunctivitis, and when bottle-fed may also develop middle ear infections.

Neuraxonal dystrophy

Neuraxonal dystrophy is a familial degenerative disease characterised by progressive hind-leg ataxia in lambs after weaning. It has been reported in Suffolk sheep in California and in Romney, Coopworth, Perendale and Merino sheep in New Zealand. It is thought to be inherited as an autosomal recessive trait, but this has not been confirmed.

The condition usually affects a small number of lambs each year, although in an occurrence in Southland in 1990, 60/1000 lambs were affected and died. At 6–8 months of age these lambs develop ataxia of the hind legs, which becomes progressive until they become recumbent and either die or are destroyed. The signs are similar to those of delayed swayback (see later). No gross abnormalities are present at necropsy and the microscopic lesions that have been described consist of axonal spheroids in the proprioceptive pathways of the spinal cord, medulla and mid-brain.

Cerebellar abiotrophy

A disease characterised by fine head tremors and hind-limb weakness which develops at several weeks of age was diagnosed in Wiltshire sheep in New Zealand in 2002. The disease was not present at birth and the clinical signs differed from daft lamb disease. The history suggested it had an autosomal mode of inheritance, as cases presented following sire/daughter matings.

Encephalopathy of Poll Dorset sheep

On one farm in New Zealand, polled Dorset lambs have been born that grew well for the first few months of life. They then became dull and progressively lost weight in spite of various treatments. The affected lambs all had the same sire. Histology of the brain showed status spongiosis in the grey matter of the anterior basal nuclei of the thalamus.

Ovine segmental axonopathy of Merino sheep

Sporadic cases of a neurological disease in which affected sheep show mild hind-limb ataxia, some proprioceptive deficits and slow progression to recumbency have been reported in a Merino flock in New Zealand. Signs were first seen from around 12 months of age. It compares to ovine segmental axonopathy described in Australian Merino flocks. Histopathologically, the main lesions are reported as Wallerian degeneration and axonopathy extending from the mid-brain to the lumbar spinal cord and more distally. The cause is unknown.

Ovine spongiform leucoencephalopathy

A presumed inherited neurological disease of New Zealand Romneys was recorded on at least six farms in Otago between 1967 and 1987 (Manktelow et al., 1997). It affected 2–3% of lambs at 2–3 months of age and was characterised by a rapidly developing and progressive posterior paresis and flaccid paralysis. The condition was presumed to be inherited.

Familial episodic ataxia

An inherited neurological disorder in newborn lambs affecting two flocks in New Zealand has been described. The severity of clinical signs varied in affected lambs but the condition was most notable when they were forced to move or otherwise put under stress. Signs included asymmetric gait, hypometria of forelimbs and hypermetria of hind-limbs and sometimes nystagmus. After walking with an assymetric gait many would fall to one side, but if undisturbed would recover within minutes. As lambs aged, the clinical signs progressively reduced until they became normal.

Swayback (enzootic ataxia)

Swayback is a well-described disorder characterised by ataxia of the hind-limbs of lambs. The condition is uncommon in New Zealand. It is associated with low copper status of the ewe during pregnancy. Lambs may be affected at birth (congenital) or develop ataxia at any time up to 5 months of age (delayed swayback). The diagnosis can be confirmed by histological examination of the brain and spinal cord along with estimation of copper levels in the liver and blood of affected lambs and ewes.

Swayback can be effectively prevented by the prophylactic supplementation of copper to ewes from mid-gestation onwards. How this supplement is provided will depend on the particular circumstances on the farm, but the common methods are topdressing the pasture with copper compounds, injecting the ewes with one of the commercially available copper preparations, or dosing each ewe with cupric oxide capsules (see Chapter 7).

Congenital toxoplasmosis

Neuropathological examination of aborted lambs or newborn lambs that are weak may provide specific or supportive evidence of toxoplasmosis (see Chapter 4).

Hairy shaker disease, border disease

Hairy shaker disease has been reported from most of the major sheep-rearing countries of the world and is caused by a placentae-crossing pestivirus closely related to the viruses of bovine viral diarrhoea/mucosal disease, and hog cholera/swine fever.

The lambs are affected by a congenital tremor and show a variety of signs ranging from fine tremors of the head which are only discernable on close inspection, to violent rhythmic contractions of the hind legs, body and head. These tremors become worse with stimulation but if the lambs survive, tend to regress with age (see Chapter 4).

Functional disorders

Metabolic diseases

Sheep affected by metabolic conditions of pregnancy toxaemia, hypocalcaemia and hypomagnesaemia have nervous signs that are not associated with specific structural alterations in nervous tissue (these three conditions are discussed in Chapter 9).

Kangaroo gait

A locomotor disorder of lactating ewes called 'kangaroo gait' was first described in New Zealand in 1978. It has also been reported in sheep in the United Kingdom. Affected sheep show gait defects including difficulty in placing the forelimbs with knuckling of the fetlocks, abnormal cranial positioning of the hind-limbs with shortened strides, and a characteristic bounding gait when forced to move rapidly. The condition has been reported only in ewes in lactation and up to 1 month post-weaning. Most affected ewes recover when their lambs are weaned.

The cause of the condition is unknown, but several pathological studies have found morphological evidence suggesting a polyneuropathy with preferentially severe involvement of the radial nerves. However, this has not been found in all cases. Spongy changes in neuropil, dorsal root ganglionopathy and neuronal degeneration in the hippocampus and cervical cord have also been variably recorded. There does not appear to be any hereditary basis, as it usually affects a small number of unrelated ewes in individual flocks. The disease is usually seen in inadequately fed ewes suckling twins.

Exotic diseases presenting with nervous signs

For descriptions of these diseases (scrapie, maedi-visna, louping ill), see Chapter 21.

Parasitic diseases

Coenurosis (gid, sturdy)

Coenurosis is caused by *Coenurus cerebralis*, the intermediate stage of the cestode *Taenia multiceps*. In some countries of the world (e.g. Britain) it remains a problem in sheep. It apparently does not occur in Australia and its survival in New Zealand is doubtful as a consequence of the programme to eradicate hydatids.

Early New Zealand reports were from Canterbury where it was diagnosed first by Gilruth in 1902. As late as 1962, occasional cases were still being reported from that province between Cheviot and Timaru and from North Otago.

Clinical features

Occasionally lambs become infected with large numbers of infectious tapeworm embryos, which produce severe nervous depression, aimless wandering, blindness and convulsions. Such lambs may die quite suddenly in a few days and unless the brain is very carefully examined at postmortem the lesions will not be diagnosed.

In the majority of cases of coenurosis the signs develop slowly as the cyst develops, causing pressure on the surrounding brain tissue. Initially the sheep may be dull, lethargic and anorexic. Later signs will depend on the location of the cyst. Features seen include the head held high or to one side. Vision may be impaired and animals may become blind in one or both eyes. Some animals may circle; some become excited, stumble, rear and lunge uncontrollably.

In classical cases the frontal bones of the skull may soften due to the pressure of the cyst. Untreated cases will eventually become comatose and die but the course of the disease may be over some weeks.

Treatment and control

In countries where the disease is endemic, treatment of the cyst surgically is often undertaken with apparently about 70–80% of cases recovering.

The prevention of the disease is the same as for hydatids, namely not feeding dogs raw offal and regular bi-monthly treatment of dogs with an anthelmintic, e.g. Praziquantel (Droncit, May & Baker N.Z. Ltd).

REFERENCES

Barlow RM. Neurological disorders of sheep. The clinical and pathological investigation. *Proceedings of the 15th Annual Seminar of the Society of Sheep and Beef Cattle Veterinarians, New Zealand Veterinary Association*, 71-8, 1985a

Barlow RM. Border (hairy shaker) disease in sheep. The pathology and pathogenesis of bovine virus diarrhoea mucosal disease. *Proceedings of the 15th Annual Seminar of the Society of Sheep and Beef Cattle Veterinarians, New Zealand Veterinary Association*, 99-104, 1985b

Barlow RM. Differential diagnosis of nervous diseases of sheep. *In Practice* 9, 76-81, 1987

Gemmell MA. Coenurosis in New Zealand. *New Zealand Veterinary Journal* 7, 30, 1959

Gitter M, Stebbings RS, Morris JA, Hannam D, Harris C. Relationship between ovine listeriosis and silage feeding. *Veterinary Record* 118, 207-8, 1986

Gooneratne SR, Olkowski AA, Christensen DA. Sulphur-induced polioencephalomalacia in sheep: Some biological changes. *Canadian Journal of Veterinary Research* 53, 462-7, 1989

Gould DH. Polioencephlomalacia. *Journal of Animal Science* 76, 309-14, 1998

Hartley WJ. A focal symmetrical encephalomalacia of lambs. *New Zealand Veterinary Journal* 4, 129-35, 1956

Hartley WJ, Kater JC. Polio-encephalomalacia of sheep. *New Zealand Veterinary Journal* 7, 75-80, 1959

Hartley WJ, Kater JC. Observations on diseases of the central nervous system of sheep in New Zealand. *New Zealand Veterinary Journal* 10, 128-42, 1962

Hartley WJ, Kater JC, Andrews ED. An outbreak of Polioencephalomalacia in cobalt-deficient sheep. *New Zealand Veterinary Journal* 10, 118-20, 1962

Hartley WJ, Rofe JC. Neurological diseases in sheep in New Zealand. *New Zealand Veterinary Journal* 50 (Suppl.), 91-2, 2002

Haughey KG, Hartley WJ, Della-Porta AJ, Murray MD. Akabane disease of sheep. *Australian Veterinary Journal* 65, 136-40, 1988

Jolly RD, Blair HT, Johnstone AC. Genetic disorders of sheep in New Zealand: A review and perspective. *New Zealand Veterinary Journal* 52, 52-64, 2004

Jolly RD, Janmaat A, West DM, Morrison I. Ovine ceroid-lipofuscinosis: A model of Batten's disease. *Neuropathology and Applied Neurobiology* 6, 195-209, 1980

Jolly RD, Johnstone AC, Williams SD, Zhang K, Jordan TW. Segmental axonopathy of Merino sheep in New Zealand. *New Zealand Veterinary Journal* 54, 210-17, 2006

Low JC, Scott PR, Howie F, Lewis M, FitzSimons J, Spence JA. Sulphur-induced polioencephalomalacia in lambs. *Veterinary Record* 138, 327-9, 1996

Manktelow BW, Hartley WJ, Gill JM. A presumed inherited spongiform leucoencephalomyelopathy of Romney lambs in New Zealand. *New Zealand Veterinary Journal* 45, 199-201, 1997

Mavor NH. Outbreaks of Listeriosis in sheep. *Proceedings of the 15th Annual Seminar of the Society of Sheep and Beef Cattle Veterinarians, New Zealand Veterinary Association*, 88-91, 1985

Mayhew IG, Jolly RD, Burnham D, Ridler AL, Poff GJ, Blair HT. Familial episodic ataxia in lambs. *New Zealand Veterinary Journal* 61, 107-10, 2013

Moffat SA. Kangaroo gait in ewes. *Proceedings of the 8th Annual Seminar of the Society of Sheep and Beef Cattle Veterinarians, New Zealand Veterinary Association*, 22-3, 1978

Morris CA, McKay AD. Moving towards low-chemical farming with sheep and cattle: The potential of a breeding approach. *New Zealand Society of Animal Production* 62, 81-5, 2002

Morris CA, Wheeler TT, Henderson HV, Towers NR, Phua SH. Animal physiology and genetic aspects of ryegrass staggers in grazing sheep. *New Zealand Veterinary Journal* 65, 171-5, 2017

Mullins J, Hartley WJ, Salisbury RM. An outbreak of blindness (amaurosis) in sheep. *New Zealand Veterinary Journal* 6, 52-3, 1958

Orr M. Central nervous system diseases of sheep — laboratory findings. *Proceedings of the 15th Annual Seminar of the Society of Sheep and Beef Cattle Veterinarians, New Zealand Veterinary Association*, 79-82, 1985

O'Toole D, Wells GAH, Green RB, Hawkins SAC. Radial and tibial nerve pathology of two lactating ewes with 'kangaroo gait'. *Journal of Comparative Pathology* 100, 245-58, 1989

Parton K, Bruère AN, Chambers JP. *Veterinary clinical toxicology*, Publication No. 249. VetLearn Foundation, Massey University, Palmerston North, New Zealand, 2006

Smart J. Sudden death in housed Merinos. *Proceedings of the 34th Annual Seminar of the Society of Sheep and Beef Cattle Veterinarians, New Zealand Veterinary Association*, 217-20, 2004

Smith BL, Towers NR. Mycotoxicoses of grazing ruminants in New Zealand. *New Zealand Veterinary Journal* 50 (Suppl.), 28-34, 2002

Surveillance

(1974) 2: 20	Nervous diseases of sheep
(1976) 3: 20	Listeriosis in Perendale
(1977) 3: 17	Parapituitary abscess in rams
(1978) 5(3): 18	FSE in sheep
(1978) 5(1): 18	Ataxia in lambs
(1980) 7(3): 12	Listeria on the increase
(1981) 8(2): 21	Listeria in sheep, rabbits and man
(1982) 9(3): 22	Nervous diseases of sheep
(1983) 10(2): 21	Axonal degeneration in sheep
(1987) 14(3): 7-8	Listeriosis: An emerging concern

(1990) 17(2): 7-13	Listeria monocytogenes in meat and meat products — an unwanted Cinderella or a real menace
(1990) 17(3): 29	Neuraxonal dystrophy
(1991) 18(1): 3	Daft lamb disease
(1991) 18(1): 3	Neuraxonal degeneration in lambs
(1992) 19(4): 15	FSE: Still an important disease
(1994) 21(4): 3	Cerebral listeriosis and silage feeding
(1995) 22(1): 3-5	Neuroaxonal dystrophy in Merino sheep
(1995) 22(4): 4	Listeriosis in silage fed sheep, 80/600 dead
(1997) 24(2): 22	Polioencephlomalacia in sheep, 15/700 deaths
(1997) 24(4): 12-13	Listerial infections of animals and birds in New Zealand
(1997) 24(4): 16-17	Monitoring the disease status of sheep and goats in New Zealand
(1998) 25(2): 3-5:	Perennial ryegrass staggers
(1998) 25(3): 17	Phalaris staggers in sheep
(1998) 25(3): 15	Cerebellar abiotrophy in Corriedale sheep
(1999) 26(3): 16	Encephlopathy of Poll Dorsets
(1999) 26(3): 18	Ovine segmental axonopathy in Merino sheep
(2000) 27(3): 19	Ceroid lipfuscinosis in Hampshire sheep
(2000) 27(1): 13	Swayback in lambs
(2001) 28(3): 19	Listeriosis; nervous and enteric signs
(2005) 32(1): 11-15	Enzootic ataxia
(2005) 32(2): 28-32	Ram lambs listeriosis
(2005) 32(4): 14-19	FSE in sheep

Thompson KG, Lake DE, Cordes DO. Hepatic encephalopathy associated with chronic facial eczema. *New Zealand Veterinary Journal* 27, 221-3, 1979

West DM. Listeriosis. *Proceedings of the 12th Annual Seminar of the Society of Sheep and Beef Cattle Veterinarians, New Zealand Veterinary Association*, 339-41, 1982

Wilesmith JW, Gitter M. Epidemiology of ovine listeriosis in Great Britain. *Veterinary Record* 119, 467-70, 1986

Woodfield DR, Easton HS. Advances in pasture plant breeding for animal productivity and health. *New Zealand Veterinary Journal* 52, 300-10, 2004

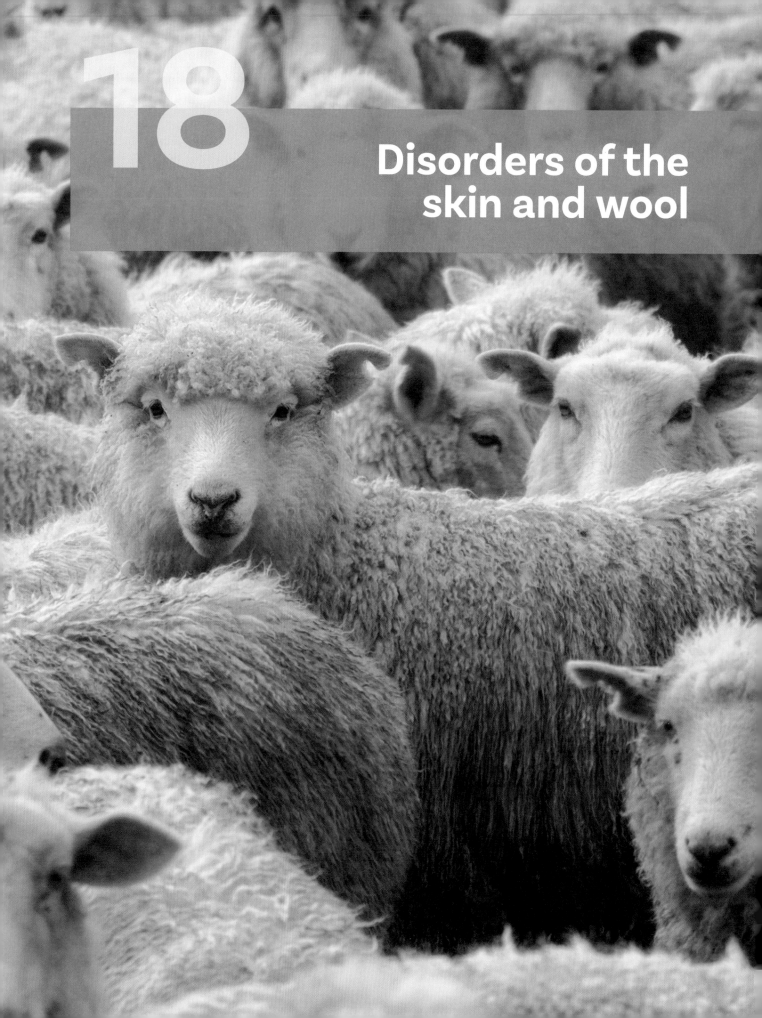

18

Disorders of the skin and wool

Disorders of the skin and fleece of sheep are common in New Zealand. Some, such as facial eczema, are severe and cause large production losses. Others are less dramatic and the effects of many of these conditions may be underestimated. This is because they do not necessarily result in death and may not appear to affect the health of the animal.

It would appear that the most common and important skin and fleece disorders of sheep are due to ectoparasites, scabby mouth, dermatophilosis and facial eczema (Familton, 1984). The skin conditions that are encountered in sheep in New Zealand are given in Table 18.1.

From a diagnostic viewpoint it is convenient to divide these into three groups. Group 1 comprises those disorders producing skin lesions that may or may not involve the wool fibre. Group 2 comprises those disorders that produce damage to the wool fibre. Group 3 comprises those disorders that cause abnormal colouration to the wool.

Many of these disorders require a predisposing factor before it can become established. Predisposing factors include fleece structure, body conformation, temperature and humidity. An open fleece structure allows air to circulate and drying to occur, which will not predispose to the growth conditions of some bacteria requiring moisture for development. Faults in body conformation such as a hollow back may allow the accumulation of water, leading to the development of certain disorders. The fleece and skin of sheep can be affected by several primary pathogens, and alterations in wool fibre structure can be recognised as a clinical sign in several disorders.

Group 1 disorders — those producing skin lesions

Photosensitisation

Skin lesions caused by the action of sunlight on photodynamic agents in the blood account for a large percentage of the skin problems seen in sheep in New Zealand. The pathological processes involve initial erythema, followed by oedema and later superficial skin necrosis of the affected parts. Facial eczema, which is by far the most important of this class of disease, is observed mainly during the late summer to autumn period.

Other conditions due to photosensitivity are:
- rape scald (from *Brassica napus*)
- photosensitivity from eating musky storksbill (*Erodium moschatum*)
- photosensitivity from eating blue lupin (*Lupinus angustifolius*)
- ngaio poisoning (from *Myoporum laetum*)
- St John's wort poisoning (from *Hypericum perforatum*)
- trefoil dermatitis (from various clover species)
- ergotism (from *Claviceps purpurea*)
- algal poisoning (blue-green algae)
- inherited defect in phylloerythrin excretion in strains of Southdown and Corriedale sheep
- ovine white liver disease.

A full description of these is given in *Veterinary Clinical Toxicology* by K Parton, AN Bruère and JP Chambers, Veterinary Continuing Education Publication No. 208, Massey University, but the following are comments relevant to a text on sheep diseases.

Facial eczema

In New Zealand, facial eczema is one of the most important diseases of sheep. Estimates of the annual losses to the sheep and beef industry due to facial eczema vary, but in some years the cost of losses is likely to reach the hundreds of millions of dollars. Not only can the disease cause severe production losses, but it also has serious animal welfare consequences. Its occurrence is seasonal, with most cases occurring during the autumn. The disease occurs in the lowland warm areas of the North Island but has been seen occasionally in the northern areas of the South Island. It also occurs in coastal areas of Australia, South Africa and South America.

	Condition	Incidence	Aetiology
Group 1 (with scab formation)	Photosensitisation	++++	Various agents
	Dermatophilosis	++++	*Dermatophilus congolensis*
	Contagious ecthyma	++++	*Parapoxvirus*
	Dermatitis	++	*Staphylococcus aureus*
		+	*Pseudomonas aeruginosa*
	Squamous cell carcinoma	rare	Skin exposure, injuries
	External parasites	++++	Various species
	Epidermolysis bullosa	rare	Inherited
	Cutaneous aesthesia	rare	Inherited
Group 2 (wool fibre damage)	Black fungus tip	+	*Peyronella glomerata*
	Pink rot	rare	*Bacillus* spp
	Steely wool	+	Copper deficiency
	Wool break	++++	Stress and disease
Group 3 (colouration faults)	Yellow banding	++	Gland secretions
	Scourable diffuse yellow	+++	Humidity
	Canary yellow	+++	High temperature
	Green and brown banding	++	*Pseudomonas aeruginosa*
	Blue banding	rare	*Pseudomonas indigofera*
	Apricot stain	rare	Unknown
	Purple stain	rare	Unknown
	Pink tip	++	Red yeast
	Stringy yolk	+	Skin gland abnormality
	Doggy wool	+	Follicle abnormality

Key: ++++ very common; +++ common; ++ occasional; + uncommon.

Table 18.1 Skin and wool conditions of sheep in New Zealand (modified after Familton, 1984).

Aetiology and pathogenesis

The disease is a hepatogenous photosensitisation caused by the toxin sporidesmin, which is produced by the saprophytic fungus *Pithomyces chartarum*. Under the warm, moist conditions of autumn *P. chartarum* proliferates on pasture litter, producing spores that contain the toxin sporidesmin which is consumed by ruminants, especially under close grazing conditions.

The sporidesmin is rapidly absorbed from the intestine, and is concentrated in the liver and hepatic bile. Here the molecule undergoes a glutathione-linked, copper-catalysed cycle of oxidation and reduction to produce the toxic free radical superoxide and other free radicals. The resulting liver injury, particularly of the biliary system, blocks the excretion of phylloerythrin, the breakdown product of chlorophyll. Endogenous porphyrins (e.g. haemoglobin and myoglobin) accumulate, producing the clinical condition of jaundice. The major liver enzyme change, used in the diagnosis of the disease and the quantitation of susceptibility or resistance in sheep, is gamma glutamyl transferase (GGT).

Conditions for fungal growth and toxin production

Pithomyces chartarum does not require special nutrients and appears to grow on a wide range of substrates. It has large characteristic spores, a feature invaluable in the recognition of dangerous pastures. The spores are produced most freely between 20°C and 24°C, especially when minimum night temperatures exceed 14°C and when humidities are close to 100%. As *P. chartarum* sporulates it produces sporidesmin. The amount of sporidesmin produced is directly proportional to spore numbers.

In the field, spore numbers commonly increase after a fall of at least 4 mm of rain followed by high minimum grass temperatures. A significant grass minimum of 12°C is often quoted but a higher minimum, e.g. 16–18°C for two or more nights, is more commonly associated with significant spore rises. Under such conditions, rapid and significant rises in spore numbers can occur within 48 hours. It is generally recognised that several such climatic periods are required before danger periods arise. These danger periods are recognised by pasture spore counting, a technique that appears to work in New Zealand where most field isolates are sporidesmin producers.

Monitoring spore counts is a very important part of assessing facial eczema risk and determining when to begin and stop facial eczema prevention programmes. Spore counts of 80,000–100,000 per gram of grass are often quoted as the dangerous level, but longer-term exposure to lower spore levels can also result in clinical disease as cumulative exposure is more important than an absolute spore count. Hence it is not possible to be absolute about the 'danger' level. Stocking rate, the closeness of grazing, the type of stock, the age of the spores, the length of time spent grazing the pasture and previous exposure to toxic spores are all important considerations. It should also be noted that there is large variation in spore counts both within and between farms; district spore counts, while very useful, should thus be used as a guide only. Ideally, individual farm monitoring of the paddocks to be grazed, along with consideration of the factors noted above, should be taken into account when deciding when to start and stop a facial eczema prevention programme. As a general recommendation, when spore counts are trending upwards and reach 20,000–30,000/g then control measures should begin. Faecal spore counting is also available but currently fewer data are available on how to interpret these.

Clinical features

The clinical features of facial eczema may be used as the example for all photosensitivity diseases of sheep; the following are the commonly seen features:

1. The areas of skin most affected are those exposed to light and those lacking protection of pigment, hair or wool. In sheep the ears, eyelids, face, lips, vulva and coronets are most affected.
2. The first signs seen are restlessness, shaking of the head and ears, rubbing or scratching of affected parts and seeking relief in shade (pruritis and photophobia).
3. Erythema and oedema develop rapidly and the ears of sheep may become so heavy with oedema in the first 24 hours that they show a characteristic drooped appearance. There is also intermandibular swelling and swelling around the nose and eyes with nasal discharge and lachrymation.
4. Oedema may be followed by seepage of serous fluid through the skin. The affected skin may become necrotic and rubbing leads to infection and scab formation. Necrosis is often first noticed at the tips of the ears which curl up.

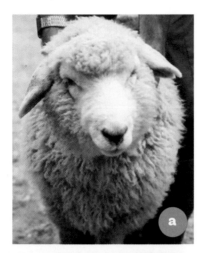

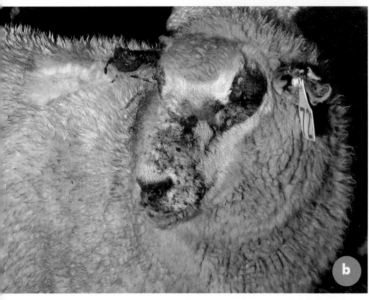

Figure 18.1 Characteristic drooping ears and swollen face of a sheep with photosensitisation. **(a)** In the early stages. (Photograph courtesy KG Thompson) **(b)** In the later stages.

5. Recently shorn sheep and open-fleeced breeds may show other signs of photosensitisation, including crouching as if to urinate and lying prostrate.
6. The nature and degree of the lesions depend on the amount and nature of the photosensitising substance and the intensity of the light and exposure time. In photosensitisation, usually the photodynamic action alone is not severe enough to produce rapid death. In severely affected animals, the systemic reactions resemble shock reactions from other causes and may be due to the release of toxic products (from the photodynamic destruction of skin cells) into the general circulation.

However, it is important to recognise that only a proportion of sheep with facial eczema show clinical signs of photosensitisation. For every sheep showing signs of photosensitivity many more will have liver damage, and while some liver regeneration may take place, a proportion will develop fibrosis of the liver ('chronic' facial eczema). In general, these sheep have reduced fertility and fecundity (ewes) or reduced growth rates (lambs). Ewes with liver fibrosis may become evident during stress periods such as pregnancy and lambing because they are more likely to lose body condition.

Breeds of sheep and individual sheep vary in their tolerance or susceptibility to sporidesmin. Of the sheep breeds, the Merino and Finn appear most resistant. The individual variation in tolerance is inherited and this is used to advantage commercially in breeding programmes.

Diagnosis and pathology

Diagnosis of facial eczema is usually straightforward based on the history and clinical signs. Some affected sheep may have jaundice in addition to photosensitivity. Affected sheep will have raised serum GGT levels. Postmortem examination of acute cases may reveal enlargement and mottling of the liver, and sometimes a jaundiced carcass. In chronic cases there is atrophy of the liver, particularly of the left lobe, and fibrosis. Less severely affected areas may be hypertrophied, giving the liver an almost nodular appearance.

Treatment

It is essential that affected sheep are provided with shade.

Trees, sheds and the use of topical zinc cream can be used, but the most effective method is to keep affected sheep in the woolshed during the day with the windows covered. The use of black polythene to create a 'tent' around the pen in which affected sheep are kept has also proven effective. While in the woolshed, sheep should be provided with water and hay. They may be let out at night to graze, but it is important that they are grazed on safe pasture. Severely affected cases should be euthanased.

Control

There are a number of options for the control of facial eczema and often a combination of these is used. It is important to recognise that in the face of severe challenge some animals may still become affected despite control measures being utilised.

Management of animals and prediction and identification of danger periods

Some habitats are more favourable for *P. chartarum* and produce higher spore counts than others. Risk areas include warm, north-facing slopes and sheltered paddocks or areas in the lee of trees, etc.; exposed, windy hillsides or cool, shady south-facing slopes tend to have lower spore counts. Similarly, pastures such as ryegrass-dominant pastures have higher levels of spores than pastures containing a high clover, lotus or chicory content. Pastures with a large amount of litter due to lax grazing in the spring/summer period, or following tupping, are higher risk. Farmers may use spore counting to identify safe and dangerous paddocks on their farms.

Spore counting on a regional basis can identify danger periods. Many veterinary practices do regular spore counts around the district during the late summer/autumn period and this monitoring can show trends in spore counts from week to week. A knowledge of habitats known to produce high spore counts on a farm, and weather conditions favouring *P. chartarum* growth, can help to identify dangerous locations and periods.

Thus danger periods should be recognised by spore counting and, during these periods, where possible stock should be grazed on 'safer' paddocks. Hard grazing during the danger period should be avoided as spores tend to be concentrated towards the base of the sward. Hay, silage or crops can be used during the danger period as these are relatively safe fodders as far as facial eczema is concerned. Non-capital stock (e.g. lambs, cull ewes) should be sold early, prior to the facial eczema season.

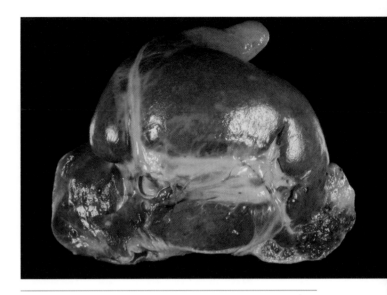

Figure 18.2 A nodular, fibrosed liver following damage during facial eczema. (Photograph courtesy KG Thompson)

Spraying pastures with fungicides to prevent fungal growth

On some high-risk farms, especially where valuable stock are grazed, the toxicity of pasture can be reduced by spraying pastures with fungicides. The fungicides commonly used include carbendazim or thiophanate methyl. Efficacy may be improved by applying a wetting agent at the same time. Clean water must be used to distribute the ingredient using a boom and nozzle and applying either by ground application or helicopter. It is usual to spray sufficient pasture to last livestock for 7 days. Sprayed pastures can remain safe for 6 weeks. Re-spraying must be carried out if heavy rain occurs within 3 days of spraying.

Ideally, fungicides should be applied before spore counts become high. They may make dangerous pastures safer, but 5 days should be allowed before they are grazed by stock. Spore counting should be carried out to check the safety of pastures. Other methods of control can be combined with this method.

Zinc administration for the prevention/control of facial eczema

Administration of zinc salts before sheep are exposed to pasture with high spore counts will reduce the amount of liver injury and hence the number of animals affected by facial eczema. The dose rates of zinc required to prevent facial eczema are high. Zinc does not prevent facial eczema if given after the sporidesmin challenge, nor does it appear to have a therapeutic effect when given orally to animals with the photodermatitis of facial eczema. The protective effect increases with increasing dose rates of zinc but at a diminishing rate. Ideally, dosing should begin 2 weeks prior to the danger period. It should be noted that zinc is potentially toxic in overdose.

There are several administration methods, outlined below:

1. Zinc sulphate in drinking water

This method has been shown to be particularly effective in preventing facial eczema in cattle, especially dairy cows that consume a large amount of water. It is usually administered via an in-line dispenser. Due to inconsistent water intake, this method does not work as effectively for sheep. Additives can be used to make treated water more palatable, but it is not recommended as a sole prevention method for facial eczema in sheep.

2. Drenching with a zinc oxide slurry

This method has given effective control of facial eczema in sheep. The problem with sheep has been that while weekly dosing of zinc oxide has given effective control of facial eczema, it is not popular because of the impracticability of mustering and handling sheep at such frequent intervals. Frequent mustering and yarding also increases the likelihood of pneumonia (Chapter 6). Increasing the interval between doses to 2 weeks has given inconsistent results, and at dose rates beyond this hypocalcaemia is a risk. In conditions of stress, salmonellosis may occur.

The slurry is made by mixing zinc oxide and water to such a consistency that it will pass through a drenching gun but not such that it will settle out too quickly. Settling out and flowability problems can be improved by adding seaweed fertiliser to the mixture; this is often referred to as a stabilised mixture.

- For stabilised mixtures, 1 kg of zinc oxide, 1 litre of water and 0.2 litre of stabiliser should be mixed and given at a rate of 0.5 ml/10 kg liveweight x number of days between doses.
- For unstabilised mixtures, 1 kg zinc oxide and 2.5 litres of water should be mixed and given at a rate of 1 ml/10 kg liveweight x number of days between doses.

Sheep should be dosed for 2 weeks prior to, and during, the danger period.

3. Zinc oxide intra-ruminal boluses

Slow-release zinc oxide capsules are available for lambs, adult sheep, calves and larger cattle. In sheep they pay out over a 6-week period and should ideally be given 2 weeks before the danger period. Care must be exercised during administration to ensure that damage to the pharynx, larynx or oesophagus does not occur. Provided they are not regurgitated, they provide a fairly reliable method of protection and negate the necessity for regular yarding for zinc dosing. However, as they only last for 6 weeks, in protracted facial eczema seasons sheep may need to be re-treated after the first bolus has paid out.

Breeding for tolerance

The heritability for susceptibility to facial eczema in sheep has been calculated to be 0.45 ± 0.03, which is high compared with other heritable traits for which selective breeding is undertaken. A practical long-term solution to facial eczema control in sheep is to breed animals with greater tolerance to the disease. A number of pedigree ram breeders are breeding for tolerance, and commercial farmers can purchase sire rams from these flocks to breed ewe replacements. Along with production traits, facial eczema tolerance is included in Sheep Improvement Ltd (SIL) indexes.

A performance test for facial eczema tolerance in rams has been available since 1985. As an example of the genetic gains that can be made, a group of Romney breeders who have been breeding for tolerance for some years have shown a 2% genetic gain per year. Potential sires must be grazed on safe pasture before the test challenge commences. Blood samples from each ram are collected before testing commences for GGT analysis. Rams are then challenged with small individually calculated doses of a commercially prepared sporidesmin preparation

(Ramguard) and subsequent liver injury measured by examining serum GGT levels 21 days later. Tolerant rams show little or no elevation in serum GGT. The welfare aspects of this procedure need to be carefully watched and rams that are under test must be provided with adequate shade, water and good feed. Research is being undertaken to identify a genetic marker for tolerance to facial eczema.

It should be noted that in severe facial eczema seasons, some disease will still occur in tolerant flocks and additional facial eczema prevention methods may be required.

Rape scald (*Brassica napus*)

Rape scald is seen when *Brassica* crops such as rape are fed in the immature state. Rape should be fed when the leaves have a blue tinge and for only ½–1 hour at a time until lambs become used to it. Clinical signs include a marked oedema of the ears and neck and sometimes along the midline of the back with eventual necrosis and loss of skin. There is no liver damage. There may be haemoglobinuria. Recovery is rapid when the lambs are taken off the crop and put into the shade. It is preferable to hold severe cases in a darkened woolshed and allow animals to feed and water at night, until the signs have subsided. Rape scald can predispose to severe outbreaks of dermatophilosis affecting the back wool of sheep (see later).

Storksbill poisoning (*Erodium spp*)

Typical photosensitisation has been seen in lambs grazing on herbage that was mainly storksbill, both in Australia and New Zealand (North Canterbury and Hawke's Bay).

Lupinosis

Phomopsis leptostromiformis is a parasite of the *Lupinus* species and produces the mycotoxin phomopsin, which produces progressive liver damage and ultimately may lead to photosensitisation of affected animals in the same manner as facial eczema.

Ngaio poisoning

Myoporum laetum is one of the most poisonous of the native plants in New Zealand. Poisoning most often occurs in cattle and has been recorded in sheep. Poisoning usually occurs when the branches of trees are brought down in a storm. The toxic principle is believed to be ngaione and the leaves are the most toxic part of the plant.

Hypericism

Various species of *Hypericum* (St John's wort) give rise to photosensitisation in animals eating them. This plant grows in waste places, pastures and road-sides in both the North and South Islands. The photodynamic agent hypericin is a red-fluorescent pigment found in semi-solid state in the black dots that are scattered over the surface of the leaves, stems and petals. Hypericin is present in the plant at all times and even persists when the plant is dried. Sheep, cattle and horses may be affected (sheep most commonly).

In addition to signs of photosensitisation, extreme hyperaesthesia to touch or contact with cold water has been noted. Fording a stream or dipping causes acute and violent convulsions in sheep. Note that other forms of photosensitisation, e.g. facial eczema, cause only mild reactions of this kind.

Trefoil dermatitis

Trefoil dermatitis is a photosensitivity disease of unknown aetiology and of sporadic and transitory occurrence in horses, cattle, sheep and pigs. It has been reported in New Zealand following ingestion of birdsfoot trefoil (*Lotus corniculatus*), in Australia following the ingestion of bur medick (*Medicago polymorpha*) and in the United States following the ingestion of hay made from flood-damaged lucerne (*Medicago sativa*).

Algal poisoning

The ingestion of fresh-water blue-green algae has caused deaths and, in less acute cases, liver damage, jaundice and photosensitisation in animals in all parts of the world.

Congenital photosensitivity

This unusual photosensitisation is seen in lambs of the Southdown, Corriedale and Dorset breeds and their crosses in New Zealand and the United States. Lambs are normal at birth but become clinically affected when they start to graze at 3–7 weeks and are photosensitive for the rest of their lives. The condition is fatal unless shade is provided. The disease is inherited as a single recessive gene; it is caused by a congenital defect in the excretion of biliary pigment, allowing phylloerythrin to accumulate in the blood and become the photodynamic agent.

Ovine white liver disease

Photosensitisation is sometimes a feature of this disease along with poor growth rates in lambs and hoggets. It is believed to be a mycotoxicosis that only causes lesions and disease in cobalt-deficient areas. It has mainly been recorded in the northern parts of New Zealand. At necropsy the main feature is a fatty, swollen liver.

Dermatophilosis (mycotic dermatitis, lumpy wool)

Dermatophilosis is a naturally occurring disease of a wide variety of species including sheep, cattle, pigs, horses, goats, deer, humans and a number of wild species. It is a worldwide disease of sheep and can be both clinically and economically important.

Aetiology

The disease is caused by the bacterium *Dermatophilus congolensis* which can occur in either of its two morphological entities. Hyphal filaments form during the active stage of the disease, and these produce pockets of Gram-positive cocci that when released and exposed to moisture develop long flagellae. Infection occurs when these motile forms (zoospores) invade the skin, and hyphal penetration of the skin follows (Figure 18.3).

The effects of the disease

The lesion caused by dermatophilosis results in an accumulation of exudate, which binds the wool fibres together as a scab colloquially known as lumpy wool. It was believed previously that wool with dermatophilosis scabs could be cleaned effectively at scouring, carding and combing. Edwards (1985) has drawn attention to this misconception — the scab is not removed from the fleece during laboratory or commercial scouring under standard conditions. Considerable price penalties are associated with sale wool containing dermatophilosis scab.

The fate of the scab and its effect on the wool during subsequent carding, gilling and blending is still unknown. It is assumed that most scab is removed during the above processes, but it is unknown whether quality of the top suffers as a result of processing wools containing scab because of decreased mean fibre length, increased neps (small entanglements of fibres that cannot be unravelled) and noils (short fibres removed from wool during combing) and residual scab flakes in the top.

The sale value of sheep affected with dermatophilosis is also reduced. This is particularly so for ram hoggets that are being prepared for a particular sale schedule. In some cases the back wool may be so severely affected that rams may be rendered unsaleable in that season.

Very extensive lesions are often seen in young lambs.

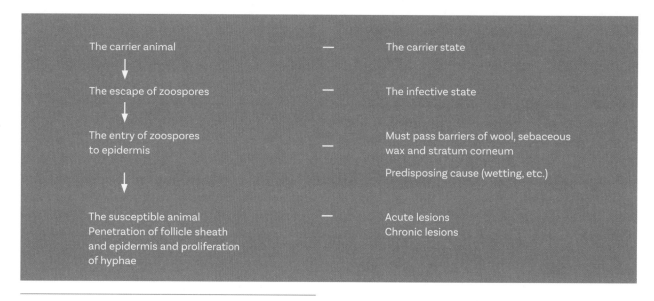

Figure 18.3 The development of dermatophilosis.

It takes up to 5 weeks from birth for the sebaceous film on the skin of lambs to become complete and thus fully protective. In addition, the wet skin at birth is especially susceptible to infection by *D. congolensis*. Hence losses of lambs carrying severe lesions have been reported. It is assumed that the severe dermatophilosis renders the wool's normal insulating properties ineffective.

Dermatophilosis is an important predisposing factor to flystrike and may make the fleece attractive to the primary strike flies, particularly when the lesions are in the acute phase.

In Australia in particular, dermatophilosis can cause difficulty in shearing affected sheep. The degree to which this involves the alteration of shearing arrangements varies considerably, and so too does the expense caused to owners to avoid it. In New Zealand damage to lamb pelts has been reported during the liming process following slaughter. The damage has been attributed to earlier skin infection with *D. congolensis*.

Epidemiology and predisposing factors

Edwards (1991) has demonstrated that the spread of dermatophilosis infection in sheep requires a 'close contact wetting event', which is summarised as follows:
1. The presence of sheep in the flock with lesions of dermatophilosis in the fleece or on the ears or nose as a source of infection.
2. The presence of sheep that have not been infected previously.
3. Wetting to permit the release of *D. congolensis* zoospores from the lesions. Any event that results in wetting of the surface of scabs is suitable, e.g. rainfall, jetting and dipping.
4. Mechanical transfer by close contact between sheep can occur from 30 minutes after the commencement of wetting. The times when sheep are most likely to be in close contact are during yarding, droving or trucking. Close contact may also occur in the paddock when sheep congregate while they are feeding, drinking or in shelter.

It is now believed that the spread of the disease by insects is unimportant and that the main spread of dermatophilosis is from infected sheep either on the farm or introduced to the farm from another source. Severe outbreaks of dermatophilosis may also occur in lambs grazing brassica crops, and this is probably predisposed to by the wetting effects of the crop and mild photosensitisation caused by rape scald (see previously).

Clinical features

The lesion of dermatophilosis is essentially a dermatitis resulting in an accumulation of exudate containing purulent and epithelial material. Its appearance and clinical effects vary according to the duration, location on the sheep and the stage of infection.

The lesion begins as a small area of hyperaemia lasting for a week or more and is followed by exudation and encrustation. This stage is referred to by some observers as the acute or active lesion. As exudation continues by lateral extension of the lesion, cornification occurs and there is separation of the scab material from the underlying epidermis. If conditions are suitable, re-infection takes place in the newly formed epidermal layer and the process is repeated. As the lesion becomes more chronic the crust separates from the skin and is contained in the surrounding wool fibres as a conical mass. Such masses may vary in size from a few millimetres to large coalesced masses several centimetres across.

If the scab is removed from the lesion in the early stages,

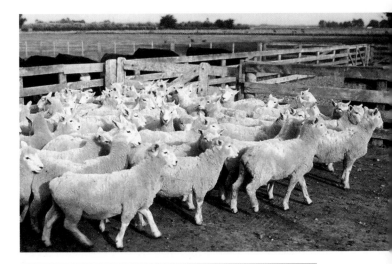

Figure 18.4 Midline *Dermatophilus congolensis* infection of a group of hoggets that had been grazing on a brassica crop. Note loss of back wool in all sheep.

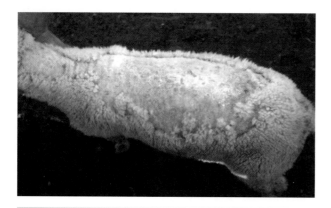

Figure 18.5 Severe *Dermatophilus congolensis* infection.

it will show a typical concave base and the underlying skin is moist and haemorrhagic. In the case of the more chronic lesions no exudation is seen if the scab is removed. Generally the lesions are not pruritic, which is a helpful point in the differential diagnosis of the disease. In natural cases, lesions may last from days to several months and in the case of lumpy wool the lesions remain until removed at shearing.

Although lesions occur on most parts of the sheep, they characteristically occur in the woolled areas as many hard masses of crust or scab. These bind wool fibres together and are scattered irregularly over the back, flanks, limbs and upper surface of the neck. The lesions may be isolated or found as groups of lesions that coalesce to form a sheet of scab. In the most extreme cases the whole skin surface may be covered with scabs. The lesions are basically similar, but the degree of covering of wool or hair affects the appearance of the lesions. Woolled areas tend to have lesions that are concealed under the mass of fleece and are often not noticed until the sheep are handled. Lesions on the haired parts of the sheep are more noticeable and tend to attract attention.

In New Zealand, back lesions are most commonly reported but lesions on the hair-covered areas of the head, especially the ears, commissures of the lips and the hair over the nasal bones also occur. Lesions on the scrotum of the ram may also be seen. This latter is frequently referred to as dermatitis and must be differentiated from chorioptic mange.

Diagnosis

Diagnosis usually presents little difficulty as the clinical lesions are quite distinctive. Confirmation can be obtained from stained smears made from the surface of active lesions. Culture isolates and experimental transmission would confirm a diagnosis but are usually unnecessary.

Treatment and control

The organism is so widespread that eradication from a flock is impractical. Also, under New Zealand conditions it is difficult to prevent natural trauma and wetting, which are important predisposing causes. It must be emphasised that infected sheep must not be yarded in wet conditions and the yarding of non-infected sheep with affected animals should also be avoided, particularly if they are wet. Sheep grazing brassica crops should be checked regularly for signs of dermatophilosis and/or photosensitisation. In Australia where rainfall areas are generally more predictable, it may be possible to change some husbandry procedures such as time of shearing to avoid wetting of sheep until the sebaceous layer has re-established on the skin. However, the value of changing husbandry procedures is limited. Nevertheless, since up to 70% of 'clean sheep' may become infected following dipping it is advisable to separate actively infected animals and dip these separately.

A variety of dip solutions have been recommended for treating infected sheep. These include the following:

Zinc sulphate

Solutions of zinc sulphate used at 1% have been recommended for treating sheep immediately after shearing to prevent infection of cuts. Such solutions can be sprayed on to the sheep or used as a dip material, but care must be taken that the solution does not interfere with the mechanical parts of shower-dips or spraying machines. Many dips now have compatibility advice on the container.

Potassium aluminium sulphate

May be used either as a 1% spray or dip solution or as a dusting powder, mixed with an appropriate vehicle. Potassium aluminium sulphate has given protection to shorn sheep for up to 70 days when applied by either of these means. It must be emphasised that it cannot be mixed with other insecticides at dipping as it is incompatible with most of these materials. The disadvantage of using potassium aluminium sulphate is that it strips out from dip material fairly readily and thus constant dip replenishment is necessary (2 kg of potassium aluminium sulphate should be used for every 50 sheep with 5 cm of wool. This could be reduced for shorter fleece length).

Neither zinc sulphate nor potassium aluminium sulphate will affect the chronic lesions, but they are useful as preventive measures and will destroy zoospores, causing flagellae to coagulate, in the active lesions.

Antibiotics

A number of antibiotics have been suggested for the treatment of dermatophilosis, including procaine penicillin injected intramuscularly for 3 days, intramuscular oxytetracycline (20 mg/kg) or high doses of streptomycin or streptomycin/penicillin (70 mg/kg of streptomycin). If using this last option it is essential that appropriate meat withholding periods are adhered to.

The culling of infected sheep is of little value in preventing the disease because of the ubiquitous nature of the organism and the low heritability of resistance (h^2 = 0.1–0.15).

Scabby mouth (contagious ecthyma, contagious pustular dermatitis, orf)

Scabby mouth is a highly infectious viral disease affecting sheep, goats, deer, tahr, chamois, possibly other ungulates, and dogs, and is transmissible to humans (orf). It is very common in New Zealand and mainly infects young lambs and hoggets, but older sheep can be infected. The disease is common and occurs throughout the year (Figure 18.6).

Aetiology and epidemiology

The scabby mouth virus is a parapoxvirus, a member of the *Poxviridae*. Scabby mouth is a self-limiting disease with a fairly defined course. The incidence within a flock may be as high as 90%. Mortalities are usually very low, and usually occur in lambs that are unable to suckle or become flystruck on their lesions.

The virus can remain viable in scab material for very long periods of time, and it was formerly believed that such material was the cause of the annual epizootics which tend to occur on severely affected properties. However, it has been demonstrated that much of the virus in scab

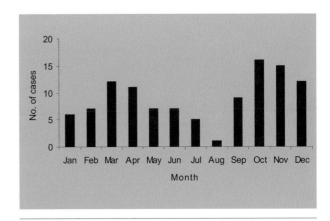

Figure 18.6 Annual distribution of scabby mouth cases (AHL — 11 years of results).

material is destroyed by low temperatures, ultraviolet light and wetting by rain. This suggests that carry-over of the virus from year to year on pasture is unlikely but carry-over may occur in buildings. Carrier animals, in which low-grade infection may persist for some time, are probably an important source of the virus and contribute to the continued reappearance of the disease within a flock. This is supported by evidence that apparently uninfected flocks grazing pastures abundant in thistles on which no sheep have grazed for some years still get scabby mouth. It is well recognised that the trauma caused by thistles is one of the main factors that allow the virus to proliferate and cause the disease. Other abrasive plants may also have the same effect as thistles.

Under New Zealand conditions the carrier-animal means of spread would appear to be the more likely, since from Figure 18.6 it can be seen that isolations of the virus may be made from some sheep at any stage of the year.

Importance

On many farms the disease will make its appearance regularly. The lesions, although only temporary, can severely affect the growth of suckling lambs and hoggets. In the case of lactating ewes, scabby mouth of the udder may predispose to mastitis and lamb starvation. If a flock is heavily infected, the disease is particularly troublesome as it may interfere with shearing and crutching. Shearers do not relish handling sheep infected with scabby mouth

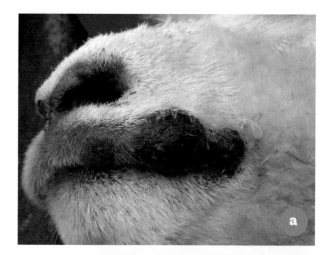

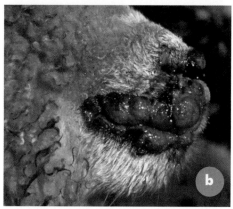

Figure 18.7 Characteristic proliferative scabby mouth lesions around the nose and lips of a lamb. **(a)** Note the circular raised nature. **(b)** Note how the lesions coalesce into proud flesh.

as it is readily transmitted to humans. Meatworkers, farm workers and other people handling affected sheep are also at risk.

Transmission and pathogenesis

It would appear that trauma aids the establishment of the virus. Any break in the skin caused by such things as thistles, matagouri and tooth eruptions will allow virus to enter the epidermal cells.

After the abrasion, three separate epidermal layers of the skin appear to be involved in the development and resolution of the lesions, with only one actually supporting virus replication. These are keratinocytes, which are the target cells for viral replication and are the basic requirement for infection. It is the proliferation of the keratinocytes, associated with the repair process, that produces the typical proliferative lesions of scabby mouth.

The incubation period ranges from 4 to 8 days. The infection is localised with no evidence of a viraemia. The affected epidermal cells soon undergo vacuolation, swelling and shrinkage of the nuclei. Over the next 3–4 days these cells become necrotic; at this stage, structures resembling intra-cytoplasmic inclusion bodies may be seen. Usually there is no development of vesicles at this stage. Over the next few days the dermis becomes infiltrated with neutrophils. Pustules then develop and rupture to form thick, typical scabs about 8 days after infection. The scabs may remain for up to a month after the initial infection and when damaged, bleed profusely and form large amounts of granulation tissue.

Clinical features

The lesions (dry scabs and granulomatous proliferations) may be found on the lips, particularly at the lip margin. They may also extend inside the mouth and even affect the tongue. Occasionally they may become more generalised and cover the entire muzzle, head and ears. Lesions may also be found between the digits and behind the fetlock and around the coronet. In ewe hoggets lesions are frequently found in the vulva, while lesions of the udder are common in lactating ewes. The lesions are self-limiting and generally resolve within a few weeks, but in some cases secondary bacterial infection may occur.

Under field conditions, sheep usually develop a protective immunity that may effectively last for several months. However, scabby mouth virus may re-establish in recently recovered sheep, although the intensity and duration of the response will be reduced in relation to the previous infection.

In a typical scabby mouth epizootic the clinical features described above are characteristic and diagnosis is relatively easy.

Prevention and treatment

It is often not worthwhile attempting treatment of scabby mouth in adult sheep and hoggets. Usually, by the time the disease is recognised it is already widespread in a flock and many animals will be recovering. However, where secondary bacterial infection has occurred, topical antibiotic treatment may assist recovery. It is usually recommended that antiseptic and glycerine, or glycerine (1 part), water (3 parts) and iodine be sprayed onto the scabs. Parenteral antibiotics may occasionally be required for sheep with severe secondary bacterial infections.

Vaccination

On farms where the condition is endemic and suckling lambs are at risk of infection, vaccination may be recommended. Prevention by vaccination is practical and generally quite successful. The immunity produced may not be lifelong, but the success of vaccination is possibly due to the continual challenge from the environment which boosts the immunity.

In New Zealand, live vaccines are available. A single dose of the vaccine is given, usually at docking time. The vaccines have a wire applicator and are given to the lambs by firmly scratching the inside of the thigh or axilla twice. The scratches should not be so deep as to cause bleeding as this could wash the vaccine away. The prongs of the needle should be checked regularly, as a build-up of grease and wool will reduce the dose of vaccine given. At the site of inoculation a small scab lesion develops. The inside of the thigh is a safe position to select as it is difficult for lambs to lick the area and infect their mouths. It is wise to inspect the inoculation site on about 20 lambs 5–7 days later to check that the vaccine has taken. Care needs to be taken in handling the vaccine as it is inactivated by disinfectants. Particular care must be taken when treating lambs for flystrike at docking using a spray-on ectoparasiticide containing an antiseptic. Accidental self-vaccination should be avoided.

Where paddocks that are to be used to graze ewes and lambs are heavily infested with thistles, efforts should be made either to avoid these or control the thistles.

Dermatitis caused by *Staphylococcus aureus*

Staphylococcal infections occur in sheep as well as most other animals and humans. In sheep, two separate conditions have been described.

A severe necrotising dermatitis characterised by thick black scabs covering deep areas of ulceration are

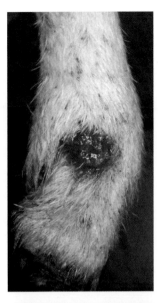

Figure 18.8 A scabby mouth lesion on the lower leg of a lamb.

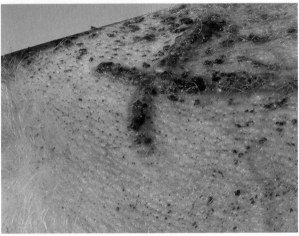

Figure 18.9 The characteristic vaccination reaction at 7 days.

commonly seen. This condition affects mainly older sheep but it can also occur in lambs. It is generally found in the facial region, but can be found on any non-woolled areas as well. The cause is a coagulase-positive, haemolytic strain of *Staphylococcus aureus* which produces both α, β and frequently γ haemolysins. By comparison a folliculitis found in lambs, with transient pustule formation, is caused by β-haemolytic, coagulase-positive staphylococci but seldom causes epizootics in New Zealand and individual cases usually heal spontaneously in 4–6 weeks. The staphylococcal dermatitis lesions can be recognised by an area of alopecia around the lesion and by the cream colour of the pus. A secondary complication of any staphylococcal infection in ewes is the possibility of spread to the udder. In the United Kingdom the disease is seen in ewes closely confined for trough feeding.

Treatment, if required, involves the use of parenteral antibiotics.

Dermatitis caused by *Pseudomonas aeruginosa*

In 1975 the Lincoln Animal Health Laboratory reported an outbreak of severe progressive dermatitis in a flock of Romney sheep. The disease began as thick scabs on the sheep's back which increased in size and in some cases spread to the internal organs. Affected animals became very thin and died or were slaughtered. In that outbreak 26% of the flock (344/1400) died. Since that first occurrence, the disease has been reported on a number of occasions. The colonisation of the skin by *Pseudomonas aeruginosa* is favoured by constant wetting, particularly after shearing (see dermatophilosis). Most of the cases reported in New Zealand have been in the wetter parts of the South Island (Reefton, Westport, Greymouth, Kotuku, although cases have also occurred in Canterbury), 1–2 months after shearing.

Clinical features

In severe cases 5-mm to 200-mm-diameter skin ulcers with crusty scabs are formed. These have a greenish scab base and greenish ulcer floor, usually surrounded by a red weal. They all have an offensive smell. Lesions are found mainly along the back, flanks and chest and occasionally on the neck, head and feet. Lymph nodes draining the skin areas are enlarged and inflamed. These lesions may go unnoticed under the cover of wool unless the sheep are handled. Affected animals may die and at necropsy have greenish abscesses up to 20 mm in diameter which may be found in body organs, frequently the lungs. Mild cases may resolve over 2 months but severe cases usually die, despite antibiotic treatment.

Diagnosis

Laboratory specimens from abscesses and scabs, fresh and fixed lesions should be collected for culture and histological examination.

Treatment and control

There is little information about treatment. Once the disease is established, treatment with systemic antibiotics is largely unsuccessful, but 1% zinc sulphate solution sprayed along the back of sheep after shearing may prevent infection. Affected sheep should not be sent to slaughter but destroyed on the farm if debilitated.

Squamous cell carcinoma

Superficial or skin cancers of various types are not uncommon in animals. One of the more common skin cancers of sheep is squamous cell carcinoma, which is reported frequently in Australia but only occasionally in New Zealand.

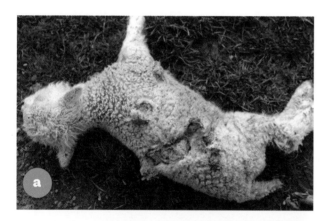
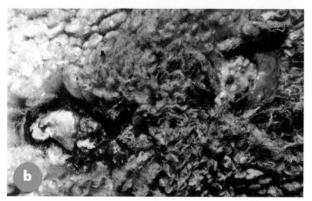

Figure 18.10 (a) A dead lamb with *Pseudomonas dermatitis*. **(b)** Close-up of *Pseudomonas dermatitis* skin lesions.

Clinical features

In Australia, squamous cell carcinoma occurs mainly on the vulva of the ewe and on the perineal skin of wethers and ewes that have been mulesed. Lesions are occasionally seen on other non-woolled parts of the body, in particular the ears. In New Zealand, most reported cases of squamous cell carcinoma are seen on the ears.

The cancer usually appears as a skin thickening on the edge of the ear, and over several months grows until in some cases it may measure several centimetres in diameter. These are frequently damaged, and bleed and develop granulation tissue with cauliflower-like growths. They are ideal sites to attract flies. Severely affected sheep should be destroyed.

It is believed that the condition is caused by skin exposure to direct sunlight and that short tail docking and extensive mulesing are contributing factors.

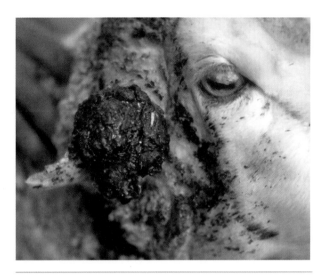

Figure 18.11 Squamous cell carcinoma on the ear of a ram.

Treatment and prevention

Severely affected sheep must be destroyed. In Australia where rear-end cancer is common, it is recommended that tails be left at docking, sufficient to cover the vulva, and a modified V mules operation be performed. This operation removes wool from the side of the tail but leaves a strip of wool along the top to shade the perineal region. Other features to be addressed include the provision of shade and reducing the culling age of ewes if the disease is a serious problem.

Epidermolysis bullosa ('red foot')

An inherited skin disease of sheep called epidermolysis bullosa has been described in several breeds of sheep in New Zealand, Britain and Norway. The disease is characterised by the formation of bullae and shedding of the epidermis and exposed parts of the skin together with partial separation of the hooves.

Clinical and pathological features

In New Zealand the disease has been reported in Suffolk, South Dorset Down and Romney sheep. It has also been reported in Romney sheep in Scotland, and Norwegian sheep. The disease closely resembles a skin-fragility syndrome seen in Hereford calves and calves of Belgium breeds and is similar in some clinical aspects to familial acantholysis described in Angus calves. The disease in Britain has been referred to as 'red foot'.

The skin lesions are generally recognised at birth or soon after. Lambs are usually lame and often unable to stand. There is usually separation of the hoof from the corium. In addition mouth lesions are seen, with lifting of the gingival epithelium and epithelial erosion of the hard palate and tongue. The skin is fragile, and lambs that survive a few weeks often have skin loss, particularly on the limbs. The disease is relatively rare and is believed to be inherited.

A condition reported in New Zealand Romney lambs which is probably a collagen deficiency disorder similar to epidermolysis bullosa has occurred on occasions. In this condition large loose folds of skin over the body and legs occur and in handling these are easily torn or form blood-filled pouches. This disease has been likened to Ehlers–Danlos syndrome in humans.

Cutaneous aesthesia

This is a hereditary collagen dysplasia disease which causes fragility and hyperextensibility of the skin. It is characterised by large, sagging skin folds with 'unattached' skin over the legs and back. It has been reported in Perendale lambs in New Zealand but is rare.

Ringworm

Ringworm of sheep is rare. *Trichophyton verrucosum* has been reported in the United Kingdom as a cause of crusty wart-like lesions accompanied by severe irritation. It has also been reported in Dorper sheep in South Africa. These lesions are mainly confined to haired areas such as the face and ears, but can occur on the back. Treatment is generally not required as resolution occurs within 4–6 weeks.

External parasites

External parasitism is mentioned here because it is an important inclusion in the differential diagnosis of skin lesions (see Chapter 19 for information on external parasites).

Group 2 disorders — those causing fibre damage

Black fungus tip

The abnormal black colouration associated with this fault is confined to the upper 1.5 cm of the staple tip. It is found in all types of sheep and occurs in both high- and low-rainfall areas, although it is found more commonly in high-rainfall areas. The condition is the result of infection of the wool fibres with a fungus, *Peyronella glomerata*. It would appear that this fungus only attacks wool that has been damaged previously by producing enzymes which break down the compounds cementing the cortical cells, allowing hyphal penetration and fungal development within the wool fibre. The cuticle is subsequently ruptured by developing fruiting bodies. The black pigment produced by the fungus is not soluble and produces the most permanent discolouration seen in wool. It is indeed fortunate that only a small proportion of the fibre is affected and this is normally lost in the scouring process. The fungus is a widespread contaminant and has been isolated from a number of organic materials which it decomposes. No control or treatment measures have been advocated.

Pink rot

Pink rot is a condition found in many breeds and wool types, and depends on a period of prolonged wetting for its occurrence. Fibres are bound together in a creamy-pink mass in the middle of the staple. The bacterium responsible belongs to the *Bacillus* species and is capable of breaking down wool fibre by the enzymes it secretes. The condition is rare and no control measures have been devised.

Steely wool

Wool can be affected by copper deficiency in two ways. First by loss of crimp, particularly in the fine-woolled breeds, as a result of the failure of formation of disulphide linkages in the keratin structure and the misorientation of keratin fibrillae within the wool fibres. This gives the wool of copper-deficient animals its steely or stringy appearance. Second, the wool of black sheep turns grey-white during periods of copper deficiency due to the lack of the copper-containing enzyme polyphenoloxidase, which converts tyrosine to melanin.

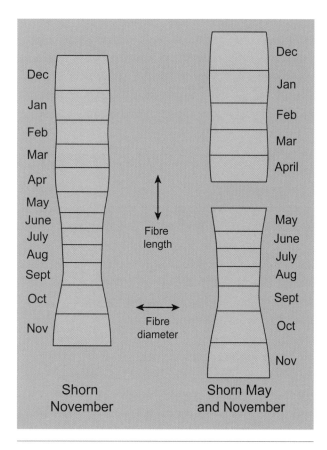

Figure 18.12 Diagrammatic presentation of summer- and winter-shorn wool (from Sumner, 1984).

Wool break

Wool break, or tenderness, can be recognised as a localised weakness in the tensile strength of the fibre. It is difficult to estimate the economic significance of wool break. Much of the wool in lower grades is not reduced in value by the condition, probably because such wool has many alternative uses.

There are three possible causes of wool break. Decrease in the cross-sectional area of the fibres is probably the most important. Second, shedding occurs where a variable number of the fibres cease growing (where fibres shed from the skin and become grossly entangled, cotts may form) and the tensile strength of the staple depends on fewer fibres. The third occurs where the fibre has normal diameter but is structurally weak (e.g. as in copper deficiency).

Wool growth and fibre diameter are affected by seasonal changes. During the winter months wool growth in both Romney and Corriedale sheep is approximately one-third of that which occurs in the February–March period.

Other factors apart from the seasonal and the photoperiodic effects are stress, level of nutrition, pregnancy, lactation and disease. A classical disease effect is that produced by pregnancy toxaemia, where wool break is a diagnostic feature of the disease.

Group 3 disorders — those causing wool discolouration

Group 3 disorders are responsible for many of the abnormal colour effects and other disorders in the fleece where no skin lesions or fibre faults are noted.

Normal fleeces can contain up to 400,000,000 bacteria per gram and up to 4000 fungal organisms per gram. Whether some of the bacteria cause problems or not is largely dependent on the micro-climate within the fleece. In other words, most of the problem bacteria are those that require a high relative humidity at the base of the staple. The rate of drying of the fleece is important. Those animals with an open fleece structure will be less susceptible to these conditions than those with a confused mass of fibres which allows little ventilation. This is a very simplified explanation. In reality, susceptibility to discolouration depends on the ratio of wax to suint and climate, as well as fleece humidity.

Pseudomonas aeruginosa is responsible for most of the abnormal colouration that occurs in wool under New Zealand conditions. For abnormal colouration to develop, relative humidity within the fleece must remain high for several days. Constant wetting and an inability of the fleece to dry out completely are required. Since dermatophilosis

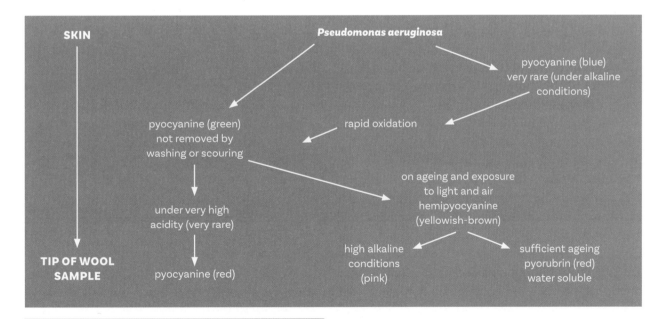

Figure 18.13 Possible pathway of pigments produced by *Pseudomonas aeruginosa* in wool (after Henderson, 1968).

requires just such conditions, these pigment-producing bacteria may be opportunists superimposed on a mild infection of dermatophilosis, and the measures advocated for the control of dermatophilosis may also reduce the incidence of fleece discolouration.

Following is a list of these Group 3 conditions, with short notes on each.

Canary yellow

This diffuse unscourable yellow stain is the most serious of the yellow discolourations. It occurs after periods of high temperature and humidity, following wetting of the fleece, and is found in the lower regions of the fleece of the sheep. The two factors probably associated with its development are a high suint content associated with high alkalinity, and lanaurin, an insoluble yellow pigment found associated with suint.

Scourable diffuse yellow

Within breeds of sheep, particularly the long-woolled varieties, there are strains in which the fleece, especially the yolk, has an obvious yellow colour. This diffuse yellow discolouration is of a seasonal nature and is variable in incidence within flocks. Pigments secreted by the skin glands are thought to be responsible, and there appears to be variation between animals in their ability to remove these pigments and their metabolites from the body. Scourable diffuse yellow appears to be a highly inherited condition. Scouring will remove the fault as long as the wool has not been stored for sufficient time to allow polymerisation of the pigment(s) to occur.

Yellow banding (or fleece rot)

It is unusual for fibre damage to be present in yellow banding, so the colloquial name fleece rot is a misnomer. The condition probably depends on the development of a moist eczema at the skin surface. It is of short duration in the majority of cases. The yellow banding produced grows up in the staple as a band effect, in comparison with dermatophilosis where the scab in severe cases is more permanent and produces a perpendicular effect within the staple above the scab. Provided that the fleece is opened before scouring, the colour and foreign material can be removed.

Green and brown banded stains

Wool affected with this fault is generally on the back or flank area. The condition is due to pigments from *Pseudomonas aeruginosa* and is very common. The green colour, caused by pyocyanine, is insoluble in water and the hemipyocyanine (brown) is only sparingly soluble. Other colours can be produced by variable pH effect and ageing.

Blue banding

The incidence of this stain is low. It occurs as a bright blue horizontal band within the staple and is caused by *Pseudomonas indigofera*. The pigment involved is insoluble in water.

Apricot stain

This diffuse yellow-red or apricot-coloured stain is confined to the lower parts of the fleece, which are continually wet when sheep graze long, damp pastures. The cause is unknown and the stain is only partially scourable. It has been postulated that it may be a combination of several effects.

Purple stain

This can vary from reddish-purple to dark purple but is uncommon. It is usually found during a very wet season. The problem with this stain is the residual pink colour that is left after the scouring process.

Pink tip

Pink tip, which is commonly seen, produces a red or light pink colour and affects the distal end of staple, particularly over the back of the sheep. The condition is due to a non-fermenting red yeast and occurs during cold, damp seasons. The affected wool is cleaned during the scouring process and the condition is of little commercial significance.

Stringy yolk

Affected wool with this fault has long strings of yellow greasy material incorporated with the fibre. These strings are about 0.5 cm in diameter and stretch vertically from the skin level to the tip of the staple. In small isolated patches of skin, yolk production may be trebled and suint production increased by 50%. It has a genetic basis, but due to the low incidence control measures are not usually warranted unless the fault is in a ram used for breeding replacements.

Doggy wool

This condition is seen only in Merino sheep or sheep with Merino ancestry. Doggy wool has a poor crimp and in some cases a lustrous appearance. In addition such wool has an abnormal amount of yolk present. As sheep age their fleeces generally tend to become coarser. With doggy wool the fault does not appear to be age-related, but rather to be associated with the development of cystic structures at the base of wool follicles. No cause has been found. The fleece is downgraded mainly because of its appearance.

Pelt defects

New Zealand exports large quantities of animal hides and the value of these is substantial. For example, in 2016 exports of hides and skins were worth almost 230 million dollars. Pelt defects result in decreased quality and value of pelts. A range of defects can occur on sheep pelts including seed damage, cockle, ribbing, shearing scars, flystrike, whitespot and butcher damage. Of these, shearing scars are the most common and are estimated to affect 20–25% of lamb pelts and 60–80% of adult sheep pelts.

Cockle

Cockle is thought to be due to a hypersensitivity reaction in response to the biting louse *Bovicola ovis* (Chapter 19). It causes small, hard nodules in the pelt that cannot be detected in the live animal but are visible in the pickled pelt and finished leather. This renders the leather unusable for most types of clothing and for suede. Not all sheep infested with lice will develop cockle, but in some lines the incidence is very high. The severity of cockle appears to be related to the louse burden and can be reduced by treating the sheep for lice well before slaughter.

REFERENCES

Alley MR, O'Hara PJ, Middelberg A. An epidermolysis bullosa of sheep. *New Zealand Veterinary Journal* 22, 55-9, 1974

Alley MR, Halligan G, Passman A. Dermatophilosis as a cause of pelt defects in lambs. *New Zealand Veterinary Journal* 35, 180, 1987

Allworth MB, West DM, Bruère AN. Ovine dermatophilosis in young sheep associated with grazing of *Brassica* spp crops. *New Zealand Veterinary Journal* 33, 210, 1985

Allworth MB, West DM, Bruère AN. Salmonellosis in ram hoggets following prophylactic zinc dosing. *New Zealand Veterinary Journal* 33, 212, 1985

Amyes NC, Hawkes AD. Ramguard — increasing the tolerance to facial eczema in New Zealand sheep. *Proceedings of the New Zealand Society of Animal Production* 74, 154-7, 2014

Anon. Facing up to facial eczema version 2. Beef and Lamb New Zealand, http://beeflambnz.com/Documents/Farm/Facing-up-to-facial-eczema.pdf 2016, accessed 8 August 2017

Brightling A. Skin cancer. *Diseases of Sheep*, pp 116-17. Inkata Press, Melbourne, Sydney, 1988

Cooper BS, Lynch RE, Marshall PM. An outbreak of contagious pustular dermatitis associated with *Dermatophilus congolensis* infection. *New Zealand Veterinary Journal* 18, 199-201, 1970

Cooper SM. Skin and hide faults — strategies for prevention. *Proceedings of the 23rd Annual Seminar of the Society of Sheep and Beef Cattle Veterinarians, New Zealand Veterinary Association*, 43-50, 1993

Edwards JR. Studies of the epidemiology of ovine dermatophilosis. *PhD Thesis*, Murdoch University, Western Australia, 1991

Edwards JR, Gardner JJ, Norris RT, Love RA, Spicer P, Bryant R, Gwynn RV, Hawkins CD, Swan RA. A survey of ovine dermatophilosis in Western Australia. *Australian Veterinary Journal* 62, 361-5, 1985

Familton AS. Diseases of skin and wool of sheep. *Proceedings of the 14th Annual Seminar of the Society of Sheep and Beef Cattle Veterinarians, New Zealand Veterinary Association*, 79-91, 1984

Grace ND, Munday R, Thompson AM, Towers NR, O'Donnell K, McDonald M, Stirnemann M, Ford AJ. Evaluation of intraruminal devices for combined facial eczema control and trace element supplementation in sheep. *New Zealand Veterinary Journal* 45, 236-8, 1997

Hart CB. Mycotic dermatitis in sheep. I. Clinical observations in Great Britain. *Veterinary Record* 81, 36-47, 1967

Hart CB, Tyszkiewicz K. Mycotic dermatitis in sheep. III. Chemotherapy with potassium aluminium sulphate. *Veterinary Record* 82, 272-81, 1968

Hart CB, Tyszkiewicz K, Rogers BA, Kane GJ. Mycotic dermatitis in sheep. II. *Dermatophilus congolensis* and its reactions to compounds in vitro. *Veterinary Record* 81, 623-31, 1967

Hawkins CD, Swan RA, Chapman HM. The epidemiology of squamous cell carcinoma of the perineal region of sheep. *Australian Veterinary Journal* 57, 455-7, 1981

Heath ACG, Cooper SM, Cole DJW, Bishop DM. Evidence for the role of the sheep biting-louse *Bovicola ovis* in producing cockle, a sheep pelt defect. *Veterinary Parasitology* 59, 53-8, 1995

Heath ACG, Cole DJW, Bishop DM, Pfeffer A, Cooper SM, Risdon P. Preliminary investigations into the aetiology and treatment of cockle, a sheep pelt defect. *Veterinary Parasitology* 56, 239-54, 1995

Heath ACG, Bishop DM, Cole DJW, Pfeffer AT. The development of cockle, a sheep pelt defect, in relation to size of infestation and time of exposure to *Bovicola ovis*, the sheep-biting louse. *Veterinary Parasitology* 67, 259-67, 1996

Henderson AE. Microclimate of the fleece. *New Zealand Veterinary Journal* 13, 86, 1965

James PJ, Warren GH. Effect of disruption of the sebaceous layer of the sheep's skin on the incidence of fleece-rot. *Australian Veterinary Journal* 55, 335-8, 1979

Lambert MG, Clark DA, Litherland AJ. Advances in pasture management for animal productivity and health. *New Zealand Veterinary Journal* 52, 311-19, 2004

Lewis CJ. Update on orf. *In Practice*, 376-81, 1996

Lipson M. The significance of certain fleece properties in susceptibility of sheep to fleece rot. *Wool Technology and Sheep Breeding* 26, 27-32, 1978

Litherland A, Deighton L, Boom C, Knight TW, Hyslop M, Lambert G, Cook TG. Ill-thrift and Q-graze. *Proceedings of the 37th Annual Seminar of the Society of Sheep and Beef Cattle Veterinarians, New Zealand Veterinary Association*, 109-12, 2007

McKeever DJ, Reid HW. Survival of orf virus under British winter conditions. *Veterinary Record* 118, 613-14, 1986

McKeever DJ, McEwan Jenkinson D, Hutchison G, Reid HW. Studies of the pathogenesis of orf virus infections in sheep. *Journal of Comparative Pathology* 99, 317-28, 1988

Merrit GC, Watts JF. The changes in protein concentration and bacteria of fleece and skin during the development of fleece-rot and body strike in sheep. *Australian Veterinary Journal* 54, 517-20, 1978

Morris CA, Smith BL, Hickey SM. Relationship between sporedesmin-induced liver injury and serum activity of gamma-glutamyl transferase in Romney lambs sired by facial eczema-resistant and control rams. *New Zealand Veterinary Journal* 50, 14-18, 2002

Morris CA, Towers NR, Hohenboken WD, Maqbool N, Smith BL, Phua SH. Inheritance of resistance to facial eczema: A review of research findings from sheep and cattle in New Zealand. *New Zealand Veterinary Journal* 52, 205-15, 2004

Mulcock AP. The fleece as a habitat for micro-organisms. *New Zealand Veterinary Journal* 13, 87-93, 1965

Munday R, Thompson AM, Fowke EA, Wesselink C, Smith BL, Towers NR, O'Donnell K, McDonald RM, Stirnemann M, Ford AJ. A zinc-containing intraruminal device for facial eczema control in lambs. *New Zealand Veterinary Journal* 45, 93-8, 1997

Nandi S, De UK, Chowdhury S. Current status of contagious ecthyma or orf disease in goat and sheep — a global perspective. *Small Ruminant Research* 96, 73-82, 2011

Parton K, Bruère AN, Chambers JP. *Veterinary clinical toxicology, 3rd edition.* Foundation for Veterinary Continuing Education of New Zealand Veterinary Association, Massey University, 2006

Pfeffer A, Cole DJW, Bishop DM, Heath ACG, Phegan MD. Detection of dermatophilosis and lice (*Bovicola ovis*) on flayed pelts and cockle on the skin of live lambs. *New Zealand Veterinary Journal* 44, 121-5, 1996

Reid TC, Urquhart RA. Can dipping sheep and zinc sulphate reduce wool yellowing? *Proceedings of the New Zealand Society of Animal Production* 63, 164-8, 2003

Reid TC, Urquhart RA. Zinc dipping can help reduce wool yellowing. *Proceedings of the New Zealand Society of Animal Production* 64, 277-81, 2004

Roberts DS, Graham NPH. Control of ovine cutaneous actinomycosis. *Australian Veterinary Journal* 42, 74-8, 1966

Robinson AJ, Petersen GV. Orf virus infection of workers in the meat industry. *New Zealand Medical Journal* 96, 81-5, 1983

Scheie E, Smith BL, Cox N, Flaoyen A. Spectrofluorometric analysis of phylloerythrin (phytoporphyrin) in plasma and tissues from sheep suffering from facial eczema. *New Zealand Veterinary Journal* 51, 104-10, 2003

Smith BL, Briggs LR, Embling PP, Hawkes AD, Towers NR. Urinary excretion of immunoreactive sporedesmin metabolites in sheep in relation to factors influencing susceptibility to sporedesmin intoxication. *New Zealand Veterinary Journal* 47, 13-19, 1999

Smith BL. Effects of low dose rates of sporedesmin given orally to sheep. *New Zealand Veterinary Journal* 48, 176-81, 2000

Smith BL, Towers NR. Mycotoxicoses of grazing animals in New Zealand. *New Zealand Veterinary Journal* 50, 28-34, 2002

Stafford KJ, West DM, Alley MR, Waghorn GC. Suspected photosensitisation in lambs grazing birdsfoot trefoil (*Lotus corniculatus*). *New Zealand Veterinary Journal* 43, 114-17, 1995

Stewart GH. Dermatophilosis: A skin disease of Animals and Man. Part I. *Veterinary Record* 91, 537-44, 1972

Stewart GH. Dermatophilosis. A skin disease of Animals and Man. Part II. *Veterinary Record* 91, 555-61, 1972

Sumner RMW. Sheep management and wool production. *Proceedings of the 14th Annual Seminar of the Society of Sheep and Beef Cattle Veterinarians, New Zealand Veterinary Association*, 67-78, 1984

Sumner RMW, Craven AJ. Relation between skin structure and wool yellowing in Merino and Romney sheep. *Proceedings of the New Zealand Society of Animal Production* 65, 197-202, 2005

Surveillance

(1974) 4: 20	'Red foot' in lambs
(1974) 4: 26	Skin fragility in sheep
(1975) 1: 20	Contagious ecthyma — goat, ram, chamois
(1975) 3: 4	*Epidermolysis bullosa* suspected as a scheduled disease

(1975) 4: 7	*Epidermolysis bullosa* and familial acantholysis
(1975) 5: 22-3	Crutcher's nightmare
(1975) 5: 8	Scabby mouth lesions suggestive of 'strawberry foot rot'
(1977) 3: 17	Specimens for scabby mouth
(1978) 1: 16	Scabby mouth in lambs at meatworks
(1982) 4: 19-20	*Pseudomonas* dermatitis in sheep
(1998) 25(4): 14	*Pseudomonas* dermatitis in Corriedale ewes
(1997) 24(4): 17	Osteogenesis imperfecta in Romney lambs
(1998) 25(2): 15	Cutaneous aesthesia of Perendale lambs
(2000) 27(1): 3	Inherited photosensitivity of Dorset lambs

Watts JE, Merrit GC. Leakage of plasma proteins onto the skin surface of sheep during the development of fleece-rot and dody strike. *Australian Veterinary Journal* 57, 98, 1981

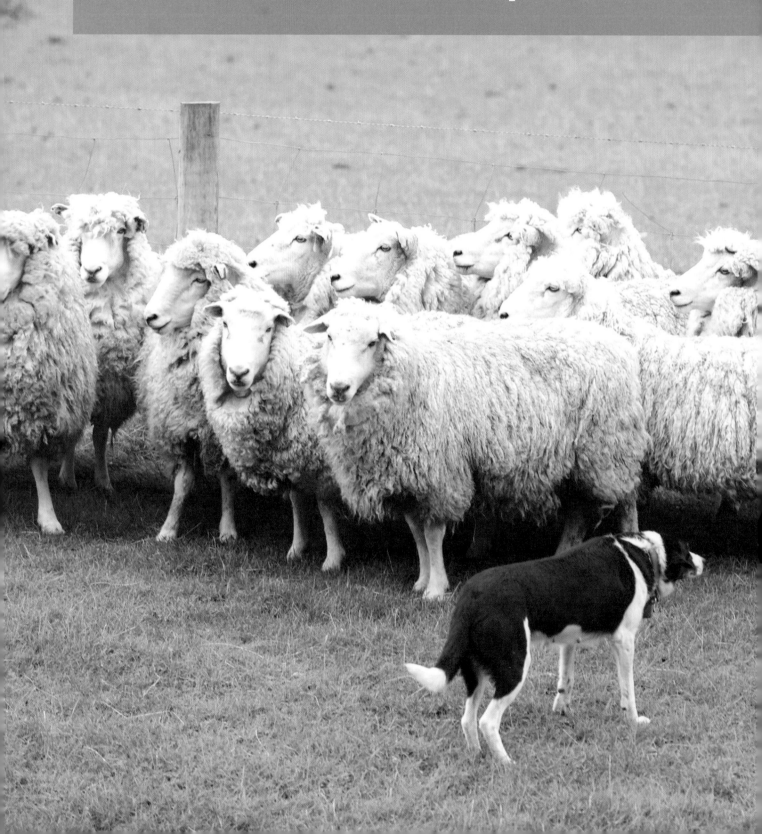

19

External parasites

External parasites cost the sheep industry tens of millions of dollars each year in production losses, chemical costs and time spent in prevention and control. Not only can they result in considerable production losses, but the animal welfare consequences of flystrike in particular are also of grave concern. With increasing pressure to reduce the amount of chemical use because of concern about dip residues in wool and the environment, and with increasing levels of resistance to the currently available chemicals, the control of ectoparasites presents a major challenge to the sheep industry.

There is no simple solution for the control of ectoparasites and therefore a good understanding of the parasites involved and the options for control are required to develop a suitable control programme for each individual property.

Blowflies

Flystrike is the most important ectoparasitic disease of sheep in New Zealand. In some seasons, particularly on large stations, flystrike can occur so quickly that many sheep may die before detection. In others it causes serious weight loss and damage to the fleece.

There are three species of blowfly that can initiate flystrike in sheep:
- *Lucilia sericata* — common green blowfly
- *Lucilia cuprina* — Australian green blowfly
- *Calliphora stygia* — brown blowfly
- In addition, *Chrysomya rufifacies* (sometimes called the hairy maggot fly) and other *Calliphora* spp are secondary invaders.

The main flystrike challenge normally occurs from November through to March during the warm, humid climatic conditions that are ideal for a rapid increase in blowfly populations. The flystrike challenge varies seasonally and regionally and it is important to know when it is likely to occur in a given area. In some years and in some districts the challenge can occur from October through to May or longer.

Blowflies overwinter either as adults or as pupae. As temperatures rise in springtime and soil temperatures exceed about 12°C, the adults that have overwintered become active, and pupae that have overwintered hatch. Flies lay their eggs on parts of the sheep where there is warmth, moisture and a food supply. Within about 12 hours the eggs hatch and the first-stage maggots feed on the surface of the skin before moulting to second-stage maggots. These have hook-like mouth-parts and feed by scraping the skin and secreting enzymes to liquefy the skin. The maggots continue to feed and develop through to third-stage larvae, after which they drop onto pasture and burrow into soil where they pupate and emerge in 1–2 weeks as an adult fly. During feeding, the maggots cause considerable damage to the sheep and the wound attracts more flies, exacerbating the problem.

The earliest signs of flystrike are obvious irritation which is seen as stamping, tail twitching, rubbing and biting the affected area. After a few days affected sheep stop eating, seek shade and appear depressed. As the wound enlarges, fluid is lost through the open wound and affected sheep become dehydrated. Severely affected untreated sheep almost invariably die and this is due to loss of protein, fluid and electrolytes as well as the toxaemia that occurs following tissue damage. Treated sheep may take up to 6 weeks to recover lost weight, with up to 8 months for the fleece to recover.

Flies must be attracted to lay their eggs on sheep, and the following factors predispose sheep to flystrike:

- Faecal and urine stain around the crutch region, especially in lambs (breech strike). The majority of strike occurs in the breech region. In lambs from 17 flocks, the mean incidence rate of flystrike per farm was 1.76–2.54% and 88% of these strikes occurred on the breech.
- Fleece rot and *Dermatophilus* infection of the wool predisposes sheep to body strike.
- Footrot may indirectly result in body strike where exudate from the feet is rubbed off on the thorax or abdomen when the sheep lies down. In addition the footrot lesion itself may be struck.
- Wethers with balano-posthitis may be struck on the prepuce and ventral abdomen, or occasionally urine staining may be sufficient on its own to attract flies.
- Rams may be struck on the head if injured through fighting (poll strike).
- The wrinkled skin of the crutch region of some Merino strains predisposes them to flystrike.

However, at times sheep will be struck on other parts of the body for no apparent reason.

Treatment of flystrike

When treating crutch and tail strike, the wool immediately around the affected area should be removed because this contains exudate attractive to flies, but avoid clipping to skin level because exposing the area may result in sunburn which will retard healing. Ideally, destroy the clippings so that the maggots cannot crawl away and

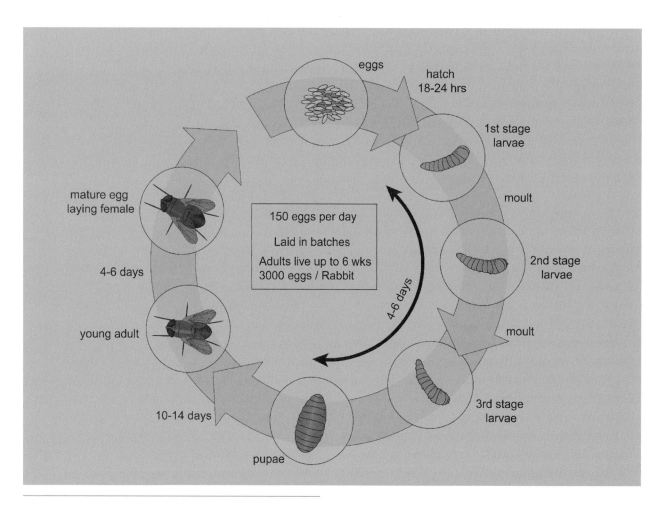

Figure 19.1 Blowfly life cycle.

pupate. Insecticide dressing can be applied liberally to the flystruck area and the fleece around it. Commercially available fluids that contain insecticides and healing materials can be used for this purpose, or standard dip liquid can be used. Organophosphates or combination products containing ectoparasiticides that kill maggots (e.g. imidacloprid) are the chemicals of choice as they act instantly, but other products are also available for dressing individual flystruck sheep. Clearly, prevention of flystrike is preferable to treatment. In more advanced or valuable cases treatment with topical or parenteral broad-spectrum antibiotics and pain relief may be useful. Severely affected cases should be euthanased.

Prevention of flystrike

The use of chemicals for the prevention of flystrike will be discussed later in the chapter, but other prevention strategies involve:

1. Anticipate the start of the flystrike season using monitor flytraps and assessing weather conditions.
2. Crutching and dagging to remove soiled wool are standard precautionary measures. Ensure that lambs' tails are docked to the correct length and maintain a good parasite control programme to reduce soiling of the perineal region.
3. In Australia the practice of 'mulesing' Merino lambs has been used to reduce the incidence of flystrike but is no longer considered acceptable on humane grounds.
4. Shearing is effective at preventing flystrike for a few weeks, because the eggs and maggots desiccate (note that severe shearing wounds may get flystruck). While every property has a different shearing policy, and different mobs of sheep on the same property may have different shearing times, shearing during the problem time can be an important short-term flystrike prevention strategy and it also allows a rational dip programme of dipping with 4–6 weeks of fleece (see later).
5. When saturation-dipping sheep, ensure that the correct procedure is used and that the time of application is suitable with regard to wool length and time of expected challenge.
6. Some areas have a particularly high fly challenge — these include areas that are warm and sheltered such as scrub-filled gullies, bush margins and in the lee of shelterbelts. During periods of high fly pressure it is preferable to keep sheep out of these areas/paddocks. Windy exposed paddocks are less favourable to flies.
7. Dispose of dead sheep carcasses quickly to reduce sites where flies multiply.
8. Flytraps are a possible means of reducing the blowfly challenge.
9. There appears to be an inherited susceptibility to breech strike, with New Zealand-based heritability estimates ranging from 0.18 to 0.32. It has also been reported that dag score is correlated with flystrike susceptibility and is also heritable; hence selection on dag score could be useful as an indirect selection tool for breech strike resistance.

Lice

There are three species of lice that infest sheep in New Zealand:
- *Bovicola ovis* (formerly *Damalinia ovis*) — body or biting louse
- *Linognathus pedalis* — foot louse (sucking)
- *Linognathus ovillus* — face louse (sucking).

Bovicola ovis, the body louse, can have serious effects on the sheep. It can reduce fleece quality and quantity, and in fine-woolled breeds in particular lice are considered to be a major factor affecting fleece quality. Lice also cause cockle, which is a serious defect in sheep pelts and downgrades their quality (see Chapter 18). Cockle is thought to be due to a recurrent Type I hypersensitivity reaction to *Bovicola ovis*. In comparison, the two species of sucking lice are considered to be very rare in New Zealand and are seldom of clinical significance.

Until the 1980s it was compulsory to dip all sheep for lice at least once a year, but this legislation no longer applies.

Life cycle

The entire life cycle is spent on the sheep and therefore the key to preventing lice is to break the life cycle on the sheep's body. The adult louse is about 2 mm long, light brown in colour and feeds by biting at the skin surface. They readily move up and down the wool staple. Lice can thus spread from sheep to sheep by close contact such as during yarding,

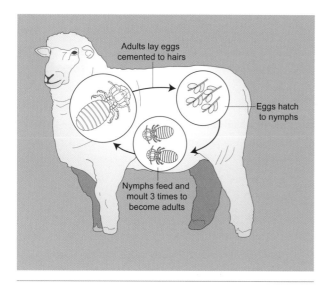

Figure 19.2 Life cycle of *Bovicola ovis*, which is completed in 22 days.

in sheep camps and from ewe to lamb contact.

Each female louse lays between 10 and 30 eggs over her lifetime of up to 30 days. Louse populations usually build up in autumn, reaching a peak in winter and then declining in spring and summer.

Detecting lice and estimating the burden

Sheep lightly infested with *B. ovis* may show no clinical signs. However, as lice numbers increase the sheep begin to rub against fences and other objects and bite and pull at their wool. Observation of the mob in the yard for several minutes will allow selection of any sheep with pulled wool or any that are rubbing or biting. These sheep should be caught and examined. At least 10 sheep per mob should be examined by holding them with the side to be examined facing the light and parting the wool so that a length of approximately 10 cm of skin is exposed. Lice are sensitive to light and will move away when the fleece is parted. As lice tend to congregate in colonies and are not evenly distributed over the body, thorough lice detection requires more than one or two partings of the fleece. At least 10 and up to 20 partings are recommended per side of the sheep, beginning at the neck and working down the side to the flank. An estimate of the burden can be made from this careful examination.

Because of the relatively slow reproductive rate of lice, it can take 2–3 months for a light infestation to build up to levels where they become obvious.

Control of lice

As already stated, the entire lice life cycle is spent on the sheep and it is theoretically possible to eradicate lice from a property or reduce them to very low levels by removing all lice from the existing sheep and avoiding introduction of lousy sheep. The use of dip chemicals will be discussed later, but other strategies for lice control include:

1. Check for lice early. Because numbers build up during autumn and winter, if lice are present in summer it is likely that there will be a large number present in winter.
2. Shearing removes many lice and exposes the remainder to the deleterious effects of the sun, reduced humidity and rain.
3. Ensure that boundary fences are secure to prevent neighbouring sheep entering.

Level of infestation	Average number lice/parting	Total number of lice
Light	Less than 1	Less than 5000
Medium	1–5	5000–250,000
Heavy	More than 5	More than 250,000

Table 19.1 Guide to estimating burden of *Bovicola ovis*.

4. Where possible, encourage neighbours to dip their flocks at the same time to minimise the risk of re-infestation.
5. When dipping sheep, ensure that the correct procedure is used and the time of application is suitable with regard to wool length and time of expected challenge.
6. When dipping for lice, all sheep on the farm should be treated.
7. Ensure that all bought-in sheep are free from lice.

Sheep ked

The sheep ked *Melophagus ovinus* has been largely controlled by regular annual dipping for lice and it is unlikely to be a significant parasite in the future. It used to be of some importance, particularly in fine-woolled sheep, as its faeces readily stain wool and are difficult to scour out. Control procedures are similar to those for lice and it will not be considered further in this publication.

Cattle tick

The cattle tick *Haemaphysalis longicornis* is mainly found in the northern half of the North Island and in the coastal regions of East Coast and Taranaki, although it has also been reported in the southern North Island and Nelson region. Sheep and lambs can be affected causing skin irritation in the non-woolled areas of the head and crutch. Tick infestations can cause clinical disease, especially in lambs, but such cases tend to be sporadic and are generally associated with farms where there is unimproved, rank (paspalum) pasture or secondary regrowth of scrub. This provides shelter for ticks and ready access to and from the host. Ticks also affect deer and may cause severe anaemia of young deer calves and damage to velvet antler. They are of particular importance in cattle due to their role in transmitting *Theileria orientalis*.

Mites

Itchmite

Psorobia (Psorergates) ovis is mainly confined to Merino and Merino-crossbred sheep in areas of the South Island high country.

The entire life cycle of *P. ovis* is completed on the host, and mite numbers only increase gradually due to the relatively long generation interval and the low rate of egg production. Most transfer from sheep to sheep occurs soon after shearing and mite numbers peak in winter.

It is thought that as sheep become infected, most develop skin irritation but the majority become desensitised within a short period of time. A small proportion of sheep do not become desensitised and develop a hypersensitivity reaction to the mite with severe irritation and fleece derangement. Fleece derangement is usually confined to the sides, an area that the sheep can most readily nibble.

Confirmation of the diagnosis by demonstrating the presence of the mite in skin scrapings is difficult, especially in lightly infested animals. Scrapings do not have to be deep and it is more important to take scrapings from as large an area as possible. While organophosphate dips have given disappointing results in control, injectable formulations of ivermectin and moxidectin have been shown to eradicate the mite following a single treatment at the normal dose of 0.2 mg/kg.

Scrotal mange mite (*Chorioptes bovis*)

Scrotal mange and its control are discussed in Chapter 2.

Sheep scab (*Psoroptes ovis*)

Sheep scab and its control are covered in Chapter 21.

Prevention of flystrike and lice

Achieving effective control of flystrike and lice requires a combination of good farm management and the correct use of chemicals. The important farm management practices have been mentioned under each condition and, with increasing pressure to reduce chemical use, they are a very important part of an ectoparasite control programme.

The chemicals used for flystrike and lice control

There is a wide range of chemical types available for the control of flystrike and lice in sheep. These include the organophosphates, synthetic pyrethroids, insect growth regulators (IGR), ivermectin and spinosad.

1. Organophosphates (OP, e.g. diazinon, propetamphos)

The organophosphates can be used to control both lice infestations and flystrike, but their use has declined markedly in recent years. They are still useful for treating individual cases of flystrike as they kill the maggots rapidly and are relatively cheap, but they do not give reliable long-term protection. Resistance to them by blowflies is common and shows as a shorter period of protection than expected.

The organophosphates act by inhibiting cholinesterase and can prove toxic to human operators if used incorrectly. Features of OP toxicity include dizziness, headache and coma. Because of operator safety concerns their use has been curtailed in some countries.

A disadvantage of the organophosphates is that many of them strip in dips, being taken up selectively by wool and grease, and thus their concentration in the dip wash reduces as dipping proceeds. It is important that to be effective, the OPs should saturate the fleece to the skin.

2. Synthetic pyrethroids (SP, e.g. cypermethrin, deltamethrin)

The synthetic pyrethroids are used primarily to control lice, although cypermethrin can be used to deter oviposition by striking flies. They are nerve poisons (sodium-channel modulators) but have a relatively high level of human safety, although allergic reactions to them have been reported. However, they are very toxic to fish, and dip wash and containers must not be disposed of in waterways after use.

They are most effective against lice when applied immediately after shearing (within 12 hours), although some products have label claims for use on sheep with longer wool. Pour-on synthetic pyrethroid products are spread slowly around the sheep through the wool and body grease, so it may take from 4 to 6 weeks to achieve maximum kill of lice. Resistance of lice to the synthetic pyrethroids has been reported frequently in Australia, but has also occurred in New Zealand and is shown as a more rapid build-up of louse numbers than would normally be expected.

3. Insect growth regulators (IGR)

These work by affecting the moulting process and development of larvae. With regard to operators and stock they are safe to use, do not strip from saturation dips, have very good residual effects and are virtually non-toxic to mammals. Most are available as jetting fluids and/or low dose pour-ons.

There are two distinct groups of IGR:

- The benzoyl phenyl ureas (diflubenzuron, triflumuron) are effective against both flies and lice, but because IGRs only affect the insect moulting process they do not kill adult lice which must die out naturally and may take several weeks to do so. There are reports from both Australia and New Zealand about tolerance, especially by blowflies, to the benzyl phenyl ureas. This results in a reduction in the expected period of protection.
- The triazine and pyrimidine derivatives cyromazine and dicyclanil provide flystrike protection only, with no activity against lice. These compounds have a completely different IGR mode of action to the benzoyl phenyl ureas. While there is some evidence of reduced *in vitro* susceptibility by some New Zealand *Lucilia* populations to dicyclanil, as yet this does not seem to have resulted in reduced field efficacy. Depending on the formulation and application method used, they can provide up to 12 weeks of protection (cyromazine) or up to 18 weeks of protection (dicyclanil), and appear to be the products of choice where the fly challenge is prolonged and severe.

4. Spinosad

Spinosad has a novel mode of action at the nicotinic acetylcholine receptors. It is primarily used for lice control in saturation-dipping systems, but will also give short-term fly protection. Its efficacy against lice, even in Merino sheep, is very good but it does strip so constant replenishment of dips is necessary. The withholding times for meat, wool and milk are nil. A low-volume pour-on for louse control is also available.

5. Combination products

Several products are available that contain combinations of chemicals, such as an SP combined with spinosad or an SP combined with an IGR. Imidacloprid is sometimes included with an IGR to provide treatment of active flystrike in addition to longer-term protection.

6. Ivermectin

Ivermectin is better known as an oral drench for internal parasites in sheep, but is also effective when used as a jetting fluid for the control of flystrike and lice infestations. It can also be used as a local treatment for flystrike in sheep. However, ivermectin is not currently available as an ectoparasiticide for sheep in New Zealand.

Choice of chemical

The choice of dip chemical selected will depend upon a range of factors, such as:

- species to be prevented (fly, lice, or fly and lice)
- required period of protection
- dipping equipment available and preferred method of application
- cost
- shearing date and wool length
- likelihood of resistance
- withholding periods for meat and wool.

There are many products available for the treatment and prevention of external parasites. They come in a range of formulations including dips intended for saturation dipping, jetting, pour-on products and spray-on products. Regardless of the type of chemical chosen and the application method, it is essential that products are used appropriately to ensure optimal results (see later).

Wool withholding periods

It is generally recommended that there is a minimum of 60 days between application of ectoparasiticides and shearing, and in mid-micron and fine-wool sheep at least 90 days is preferable. It is important to note that animal welfare concerns are paramount; for example, if animals are facing a severe flystrike challenge within 60 days of shearing, a preventative treatment should be applied.

Time of dipping

The time of dip application is an essential component of achieving effective ectoparasite control. However, it is a very complex issue because time of challenge, shearing dates and impact on wool residue levels all need to be taken into consideration. For this reason, fly and/or lice prevention strategies are likely to vary between farms.

Some important factors to consider:

- Dipping long-woolled sheep is unlikely to be effective. The fleece acts as a natural raincoat and achieving saturation to skin level is very difficult.
- The ideal time to saturation dip for flystrike is 6 weeks after shearing. At this time there is enough fleece to bind the chemical and give long-term protection, but not so much fleece that full saturation is not achieved.
- For low-volume IGR spray-ons and pour-ons applied to prevent flystrike, the optimum time to treat is before any flystrike pressure occurs. This is generally determined by farmer experience and knowledge of the farming region, class of stock to be treated, wool length, etc. Product labels should be checked to ensure that the appropriate product is used for the wool length to be treated.
- The ideal time to saturation-dip for lice is 3–4 weeks after shearing.
- The ideal time to use back-line lice products is on the day of shearing. However, some fine-wool farmers have not achieved good lice control using this method and it is possible that a combination of shearing with a snow or cover-comb, thus leaving a small amount of wool still on, and increasing lice resistance to synthetic pyrethroid products may be contributing to this.

Methods of insecticide application

Applying insecticides to sheep is probably the most complex animal health procedure undertaken by farmers, and the results are frequently disappointing. Poor dipping procedure is one of the main reasons for poor fly and lice control, and it is appropriate to briefly review the methods used and to comment on the problems that may arise and the aspects that require particular attention. Regardless of what chemical and method is used, it is imperative that the product label instructions are carefully read and followed and that the appropriate equipment is used.

There has been an almost complete shift in recent years away from saturation-dipping using showers or plunge-dipping to lower-volume methods such as jetting races and spray-ons. The use of low-volume techniques results in lower overall chemical loading of the fleece and the environment, as clean dip is applied to specific areas of the fleece such as the breech and there is no dip wash left to dispose of. Regardless of the method of application, operator safety is paramount and appropriate protective equipment should be used.

The following methods are available for applying insecticide:

1. Direct methods of application to body areas most at risk:
    (a) jetting (spray) races
    (b) jetting wands
2. Pour-on and spray-ons (back-line treatments)
3. Saturation systems (note these are rarely used now):
    (a) plunge-dips
    (b) shower-dips.

Automatic jetting (spray) races

Automatic jetting races are very convenient to use, as the sheep run through a short race and a small amount of clean chemical is sprayed onto those areas considered most at risk (back and breech). There are a range of spray races on the market and some are more effective than others. With the poorer systems the contact time can be very short, which limits the uptake of insecticide and saturation of the fleece is seldom achieved; such spray races provide limited protection against heavy challenge of flystrike. However, well-designed spray races appear very effective and large numbers of sheep can be treated in a short time.

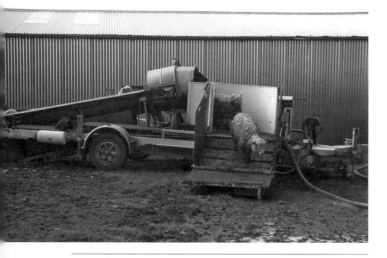

Figure 19.3 Automatic jetting race dipping. (Photograph courtesy C McKay)

As with any dipping system, it is important that sheep are dipped with the correct wool length (not more than 6–8 weeks). Following treatment, a number of sheep should be checked for the level of saturation using an indelible pencil or absorbent paper.

Jetting wands

Jetting wands allow application of dip chemicals directly to the area most at risk. Using a specially designed wand, clean dip wash can be applied directly to the desired target areas and the amount of dip wash applied can be carefully controlled (Figure 19.4). Sheep with longer wool that would be difficult to saturate using other methods can be treated successfully.

Before jetting, the equipment should be checked to ensure that it is working properly. If the pump, hoses and reservoir have been used for other purposes such as weed spraying, it is essential to clean them thoroughly to remove the herbicide and the indicatory dye that it may contain. This dye is not scourable. The correct amount of dip material is pre-mixed in a bucket and then thoroughly mixed in the reservoir. The wand should be calibrated to determine how many seconds are required to deliver the required amount of dip wash to each sheep. Having determined the sites of application for the sheep being treated, the wand is combed through the fleece applying the dip wash at skin level. Because the operator is in prolonged close contact with the sheep and chemical, waterproof leggings, coat and gloves should be worn.

Jetting wands use less dip chemical than jetting races, and if done properly it can be ensured that the back line of each sheep is fully saturated. However, it is laborious and requires well-designed facilities and proper jetting equipment. Hand jetting is only a supplementary treatment for lice, as total body coverage is difficult to achieve.

Some farmers use a gorse gun (gun designed to spray gorse and other weeds) to apply dip, rather than a specifically designed hand jetting wand. This is not recommended, because with their small diameter it takes a long time to deliver an adequate dose and it is difficult to control where the dip is being applied. If they are used, the gun should be first calibrated to determine the seconds required to deliver the desired amount of dip wash. Following treatment, a number of sheep should be checked for the level of saturation using an indelible pencil or absorbent paper.

Pour-ons and spray-ons (back-line treatments)

The terms 'pour-on' and 'spray-on' are often interchangeable and are used to describe low-volume treatments. It is important to note that the application pattern and dose rate may differ for louse and flystrike treatments. An obvious advantage of these products is that little equipment is required, additional water is not required, and chemical is not wasted. They are, however, relatively expensive.

While some back-line treatments have efficacy claims for long wool they all work better on short wool, and in the case of SP back-line treatments for lice they should preferably be used on the day of shearing. While some have claims for efficacy in long-woolled sheep, they are unlikely to eradicate lice infestations in such circumstances. However, they do reduce lice infestations and minimise wool damage until shearing. It must be appreciated that some lice may survive for 5–6 weeks after treatment and ewes should not be treated within 8 weeks of lambing to ensure that there is sufficient time for the treatment to work before the lambs are born. Otherwise the lice may transfer to the lambs and then re-infect the ewes.

Care is required to ensure that the treatment is applied properly, and that it is applied at the correct dose. It is important to ensure that the correct applicator is used for the product and that the label directions are followed. If the dose is not administered along the centre of the back from the poll to the tail, the sheep should be re-treated. In the case of flystrike, only the treated areas will be protected. Thus the back and crutch regions are the main target areas, although in rams and wethers the pizzle region may also need to be treated. For protection against flystrike they are most effective when applied about 4 weeks after shearing. Spray-on formulations have also been specifically designed for treating lambs at the time of docking or tailing, at the beginning of the flystrike challenge. The IGR products (cyromazine, dicyclanil, diflubenzuron, triflumuron) are the most commonly used. Water-based products are preferable to flammable-solvent-based products if tailing is being done with a hot iron.

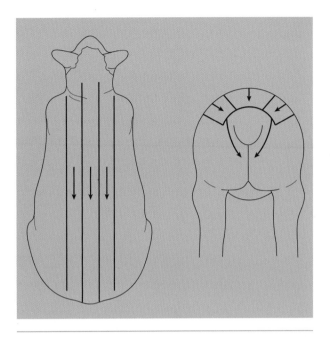

Figure 19.4 How to apply a jetting wand — three strokes down the back and two around the tail.

Plunge-dips and saturation showers

In the past, full-immersion dipping systems consisting of either plunge-dips or shower-dips were used. They are seldom used nowadays due to a range of issues including disposal of dip chemical and the difficulty in using them effectively. If they are used, then great care is required to ensure that the appropriate concentration of chemical is applied to each sheep and, particularly in the case of shower-dipping, that the sheep are saturated down to skin level.

For shower-dipping it is recommended that sheep should spend at least 1 minute in the shower for every week off-shears, to a maximum of 9 minutes, although it is recommended that sheep should be treated 6 weeks off-shears for flystrike. The dip wash should be disposed of carefully and should not be allowed to contaminate waterways. Plunge-dips have the potential to spread infections such as *Erysipelothrix rhusiopathiae* (post-dipping lameness; see Chapter 11) if the correct procedure is not followed. In addition, plunge- and shower-dipping is stressful to sheep and to the operators, and the dips pose a hazard to children and dogs.

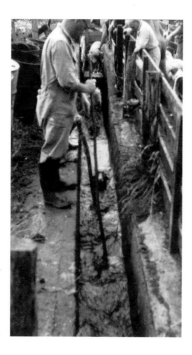

Figure 19.5 Plunge-dipping. (Photograph courtesy C McKay)

Other potential control options

Biological control of flies using bait bins and parasitoid wasps may help reduce the local fly population. Genetic tolerance to flystrike is also being investigated, particularly in Australian Merinos. Grazing lambs on forage that reduces the incidence of dags is likely to result in a decreased incidence of flystrike.

Stock problems associated with dipping

A number of diseases can be enhanced or spread during dipping, although these are less likely to be an issue now that plunge- and shower-dipping is rarely practised. They include:

- Pneumonia (see also Chapter 6). The stress of mustering and yarding may precipitate pneumonia. Less commonly, inhalation of dirty dip wash occurs.
- Post-dipping lameness (see also Chapter 11). This is caused by the proliferation of *Erysipelathrix rhusiopathiaea* in contaminated dip wash and can be prevented by the correct use of bacteriostats.
- Clostridial infections of exposed wounds (see also Chapter 15). Sheep should not be showered or plunge-dipped off-shears before shearing cuts have healed. Sheep can be vaccinated against clostridial diseases and contaminated dip wash should be avoided.
- Dermatophilosis (see also Chapter 18). Dips can spread *Dermatophilus* infection, and zinc sulphate (1%) is sometimes added to the dip to help prevent dermatophilosis developing.
- Fleece rot (see also Chapter 18). The multiplication of some bacteria in the fleece (*Pseudomonas aeruginosa*) can be enhanced by dipping, especially if the dip wash is dirty and if there is slow drying after dipping. This is difficult to prevent.
- Caseous lymphadenitis (see also Chapter 13). *Corynebacterium pseudotuberculosis* can survive in dip wash and may infect exposed wounds. Shower- or plunge-dipping within 2 weeks of shearing should be avoided. A vaccine is available.

The investigation of dipping failure

Dipping is a very complex procedure and the many dips and methods available to the farmer can be confusing. Veterinarians should establish a sound programme suitable for their clients and be prepared to investigate instances where label claims are not achieved.

Establishing the reasons for parasite control failure can be a challenge, especially as the complaint is usually lodged weeks or months after the dipping event. Obtaining an accurate history is then difficult, but it is usually possible to identify areas of weakness regarding dipping technique and these can be modified. The following checklist covers many of the aspects that should be considered. Not all will apply to every investigation.

1. Confirm that the problem is present and the extent of the problem. Flystrike is very obvious and most farmers are adept at identifying lousy sheep.
2. Enquire as to the dip product used and batch number.
3. Calculate the total amount of dip that should have been used and compare this with the amount actually used.
4. Determine whether it rained before or after dipping.
5. For saturation products:
    * check the dilution of the dip was appropriate
    * assess when the sheep were shorn in relation to dipping — was the wool length appropriate?
    * assess whether all sheep were dipped with the same wool length
    * determine whether the degree of saturation was assessed and if so, how

* estimate the likely level of contamination of the dip (plunge- or shower-dips).
6. For low-volume spray-/pour-on products applied for flystrike and/or lice protection, check that:
   * the correct applicator was used
   * the correct dose rate was used (were animals weighed?)
   * the correct application pattern was applied
   * check shearing date/wool length of animals.
7. For lice, the possibility of re-infection should be investigated, but failing to eradicate lice is a more common problem.
   * Were all sheep on the farm dipped?
   * When did the neighbours dip?
   * Has there been any contact with other sheep since dipping?
8. Contact the manufacturer.
9. Sampling. In some instances it may be appropriate to sample wool to assess the concentration of insecticide, although this usually only confirms what is already obvious — the levels of insecticide are too low. Before sampling, confer with the dip manufacturer about measuring the level of insecticide. Wool samples from the mid-back, flank and ventral neck regions can be collected from at least three sheep, labelled and packed in paper before despatch.

REFERENCES

Bishop DM. Subspecies of the Australian green blowfly (*Lucilia cuprina*) recorded in New Zealand. *New Zealand Veterinary Journal* 43, 164-5, 1995

Charleston WAG. (Ed) *Ectoparasites of sheep in New Zealand and their control*. Occasional publication of the Society of Sheep and Beef Cattle Veterinarians, New Zealand Veterinary Association, Palmerston North, New Zealand, 1985

Edwards S. Wools of New Zealand approach to dip residue management. *Proceedings of the Society of Sheep and Beef Cattle Veterinarians, New Zealand Veterinary Association* 28, 1-8, 1998

Edwards S. Lice management and fine wool sheep. *Proceedings of the Society of Sheep and Beef Cattle Veterinarians, New Zealand Veterinary Association* 31, 67-73, 2001

Edwards S. The ELISA test for the detection of sub-clinical lousiness in sheep. *Proceedings of the Society of Sheep and Beef Cattle Veterinarians, New Zealand Veterinary Association* 33, 91-9, 2003

Heath ACG, Bishop DM. Flystrike in New Zealand. *Surveillance* 22, 11-13, 1995

Heath ACG, Levot GW. Parasiticide resistance in flies, lice and ticks in New Zealand and Australia: Mechanisms, prevalence and prevention. *New Zealand Veterinary Journal* 63, 199-210, 2015

Kettle PR. External parasites of sheep in New Zealand — epidemiology and damage caused. *Proceedings of the Society of Sheep and Beef Cattle Veterinarians, New Zealand Veterinary Association* 4, 3-14, 1974

Nottingham RM. Investigating apparent breakdowns in fly control. *Proceedings of the Society of Sheep and Beef Cattle Veterinarians, New Zealand Veterinary Association* 20, 87-96, 1990

Pickering NK, Blair HT, Hickson RE, Johnson PL, Dodds KG, McEwan JC. Estimates of genetic parameters for breech strike and potential indirect indicators in sheep. *New Zealand Veterinary Journal* 63, 98-103, 2015

Smart JA. Investigating apparent breakdowns in lice control. *Proceedings of the Society of Sheep and Beef Cattle Veterinarians, New Zealand Veterinary Association* 20, 75-86, 1990

Waghorn TS, McKay CH, Heath ACG. The *in vitro* response of field strains of sheep blowflies *Lucilia sericata* and *L. cuprina* (Calliphoridae) in New Zealand to dicyclanil and triflumuron. *New Zealand Veterinary Journal* 61, 274-80, 2013

Wilson JA, Heath ACG, Stringfellow L, Haack NA, Clark AG. Relative efficacy of organophosphates against susceptible and resistant strains of the strike blowfly *Lucilia cuprina* (Calliphoridae) in New Zealand sheep. *New Zealand Veterinary Journal* 44, 185-7, 1996

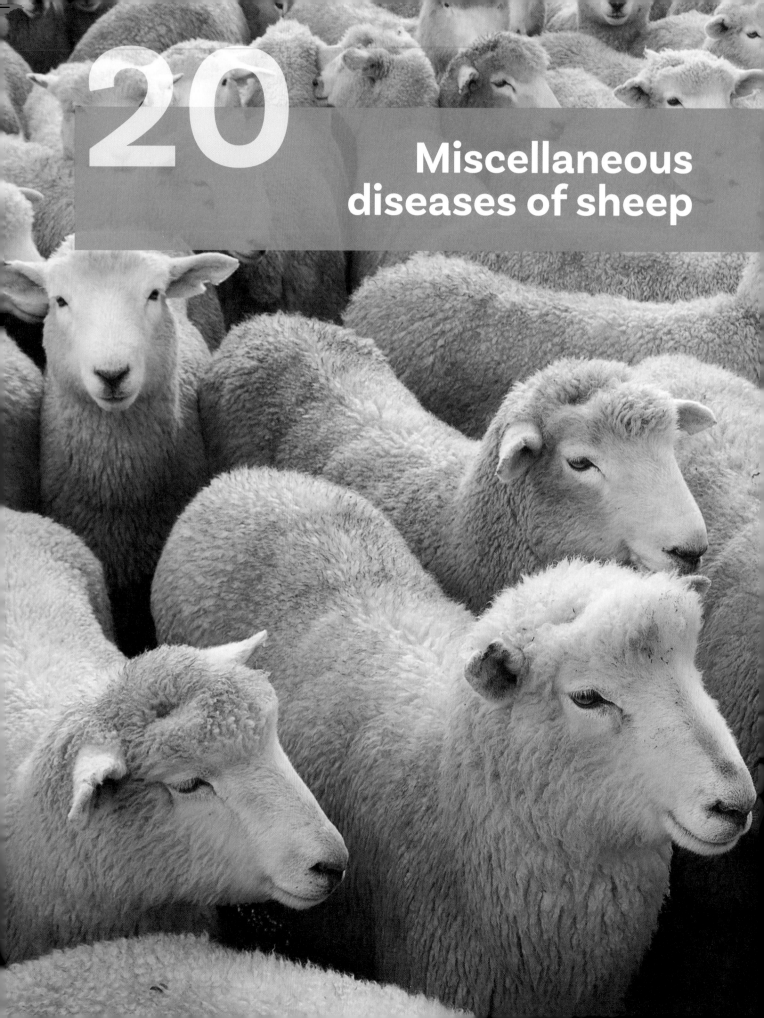

20
Miscellaneous diseases of sheep

Vaginal prolapse (bearings)

Prolapse of the vagina occurs in pregnant and occasionally in non-pregnant ewes. Under certain conditions the disease may assume epizootic proportions, with its highest incidence during the terminal stages of pregnancy. Records of the disease in New Zealand show incidences of as high as 10–12% of a given ewe flock, but more usually it affects 0–2% of the flock. The prevalence appears to vary from season to season but the exact causes are unknown. While vaginal prolapse generally only affects a small proportion of sheep in each flock, affected ewes are distressing for farmers and veterinarians are frequently asked about the causes and prevention of this condition.

Clinical features

The disease usually occurs during the last month of pregnancy and affected ewes are usually carrying multiple lambs. The first sign is the appearance of some part of the vaginal mucosa between the lips of the vulva. In the early stages this may happen only when the ewe is lying down. Later it fails to return when the sheep stands up, and if the condition progresses then more and more of the vaginal wall becomes everted until the vagina is turned completely inside out (Figure 20.1).

As passive congestion of the everted vagina develops, the wall becomes thickened and the colour changes through deep red to purple-blue and finally black. If not treated and after prolonged exposure, the mucous membrane dries, becomes rough and cracks develop, which may haemorrhage. In extreme cases necrosis, suppuration and gangrene may develop. The organ also becomes contaminated with faecal material.

The ewe shows great discomfort and may rise and lie down frequently. Each time it rises it may attempt to urinate, but will usually only pass scant amounts of urine as the urethra is closed, being folded on itself as a result of the eversion of the vagina. The ewe usually separates from the flock.

Occasionally some mild cases may recover spontaneously but more usually, unless treated, death occurs often as a result of the ewe being unable to lamb, or in most cases as a result of uraemia and rupture of the over-extended bladder.

Acute cases also occur. In these, severe and almost continuous straining develops within 24 hours. The prolapse is large, 15–20 cm in diameter, with a bright red mucosa. These cases often progress to rupture of the bladder, tearing of the vaginal wall with profuse haemorrhage and the descent of variable amounts of large and small intestine. Death is usually from haemorrhage.

In epizootics of the condition, the mortality rate of affected ewes is usually greater than 50%, particularly if treatment is delayed.

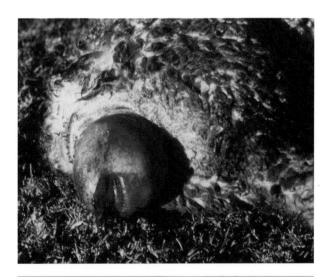

Figure 20.1 Prolapse of the vagina.

Aetiology

While a large number of theories have been proposed as to the aetiology of vaginal prolapse in sheep, few of these are backed by good scientific evidence and the aetiology of the condition in New Zealand is not well understood. Whatever the exact aetiology of the disease, three principal factors seem to be associated with its occurrence. These are a full and dilatable condition of the vaginal wall, a relaxed state of the vulva and vestibule, and the existence of positive intra-abdominal pressure.

The first descriptions of the disease in New Zealand by Gilruth describe the conditions under which the disease is sometimes seen: 'The eversion occurs suddenly and almost invariably within a week or fortnight before lambing. In most cases the ewe is carrying twins. She is in gross condition and may have an excessive quantity of fat in the abdominal cavity. Food is plentiful, and this, together with the natural tendency of a heavy ewe in advanced pregnancy, leads her to taking minimum exercise. The tendency is to be down for long periods, and while doing so the bladder becomes distended with urine to a degree that difficulty is found in urination when eventually she rises to her feet. Straining is thus induced, the result of which is to force the gravid uterus back over the bladder into the pelvis and as the pressure is continued forcing the vagina to the exterior.'

However, the disease does not always occur in fat, well-fed ewes and earlier authors including Leslie (1938) describe the condition in poor-conditioned ewes fed turnips and hay. He concluded that the poor diet led to loss of muscle tone and the prolapse of the vagina.

A two-year study of the epidemiology of vaginal prolapse on 201 farms involving over 300,000 ewes in the Hawke's Bay and Southland districts of New Zealand in 2001–2002 (Jackson et al., 2014) reported an overall incidence of 1.05 cases per 100 mixed-age ewes, with a range from 0 to 5.9. The risk of prolapse was 11.3 times higher in ewes carrying triplets and 5.3 times higher in those carrying twins, relative to those carrying single lambs. The risk was increased with increased weight gain from the start of mating to pregnancy diagnosis and also for ewes farmed on moderate to steep terrain. The latter had also been observed by previous authors. McLean (1957) noted a striking increase in incidence of the disease in ewes grazed on sloping country when compared with those grazed on flat land. He also noted a tendency for heavy ewes to be facing uphill, presumably to reduce the extra abdominal pressure on the diaphragm.

Jackson et al. (2014) reported that the risk was increased in ewes with access to salt or being fed swedes in the latter stages of pregnancy and suggested this may be due to high levels of water intake. Other authors have suggested that distended bladders may lead to excessive straining during urination, which may promote vaginal prolapse. Jackson et al. (2014) also reported that shearing in the 3 months before mating, or within the second half of pregnancy, appeared to be protective. No associations were found between vaginal prolapse and body condition score of the ewes, weight change in late pregnancy, culling of ewe lamb offspring of affected ewes, or ewe tail length.

It has been suggested that heredity may be a contributing factor to vaginal prolapse and as a consequence some farmers cull the offspring of affected ewes, although the evidence for this is scant. The disease is often associated with the sudden introduction of pregnant ewes to new and lush feed. In addition, various nutritional factors have been investigated including the oestrogenic activity of *Fusaria* and the association of vaginal prolapse with subclinical hypocalcaemia. However, it has been suggested that hypocalcaemia is probably a consequence of vaginal prolapse rather than a cause.

In Australian sheep, the ingestion of highly active oestrogenic substances during prolonged grazing on subterranean clover pastures may produce prolapse of the vagina. It also commonly produces an eversion of the uterus and vagina. However, this is a distinct entity from the vaginal prolapse of ewes reported commonly in New Zealand (McLean, 1956).

Treatment and prevention

The earlier treatment is attempted, the greater the chance of success. Severe cases, or those where the tissue is damaged or becoming gangrenous, should be euthanased and this may also apply to habitual cases when the ewe repeatedly forces the prolapse to occur. A further consideration is whether the ewe is close to or attempting to lamb through the prolapsed vagina.

Early treatment involves careful cleaning of the vagina with suitable disinfectant and gently raising it to allow the ewe to pass urine. This is very important, as the bladder is invariably full and any attempt to return the vagina before this is done may cause a rupture of the bladder and the vagina.

The operation of returning the vagina is helped if the hindquarters of the ewe can be slightly raised from the ground to reduce the pressure in the pelvis. Epidural anaesthesia using 0.2 ml 2% xylazine and 1–2 ml lignocaine will aid in returning the prolapse and prevent straining for approximately 24 hours. With careful manipulation the swollen vagina can usually be returned to the pelvis. Care must be taken to only handle the tissue with the flats of the hands to avoid perforating it. Retention is necessary, and various devices and methods have been used. These include harnesses that prevent the ewe from straining, plastic retaining devices and safety pins. These latter two can be potentially damaging and should be used with care. Alternatively the lips of the vulva can be sutured with a purse-string suture using strong suture material or umbilical tape, ensuring that the ewe is still able to urinate. Sutures should not penetrate the vaginal mucosa but must be deeply placed in the perivulvar subcutaneous tissue in order to resist the straining that may ensue for some time until the vagina reduces in size.

Non-steroidal anti-inflammatory drugs (NSAIDs) are recommended to reduce inflammation and treat endotoxaemia. If sutures are used, it is recommended that antibiotics are also administered.

Ewes need to be marked and watched carefully as they will frequently need assistance at lambing, and if sutures or retainers have been used these will need to be removed.

Ewes that recover and lamb normally should be identified clearly and culled.

Prolapse of the rectum

Prolapse of the rectum is seen occasionally in sheep. In New Zealand it has been reported in ram and ewe hoggets in which the tail docking has been too short, possibly resulting in some loss of control of the anal sphincter muscles (Figure 20.2).

In Australia the condition is reported in wethers grazing pastures, particularly of subterranean clover.

The importance of the length of the tail left after docking and its relationship to rectal prolapse has been highlighted from an extensive American trial. A total of 1227 lambs from six farms were randomly allocated to two or three docking lengths of tail: (1) short-tail, removed as close to the body as possible; (2) medium-tail, removed at a point midway between the attachment of the tail to the body and the attachment of the caudal folds to the tail; and (3) long-tail, removed at the attachment of the caudal folds to the tail.

The short-docked lambs had an incidence of rectal prolapse of 7.8%, the medium length 4.0% and the long length 1.8%. Ewe lambs had a higher incidence of rectal prolapse than ram lambs. As the half-sib estimate of the heritability for the incidence of rectal prolapse was low (0.14), it was concluded from this study that short dock length is strongly implicated in the occurrence of rectal prolapse.

Treatment and prevention

The condition may be treated surgically. The everted tissue is cleaned and carefully returned to the pelvis. A purse-string suture is then placed around the anal sphincter. The sutures should be removed after about 7 days. Care should be taken in docking lambs, particularly when using rubber rings, to ensure that the tail is removed below the fifth coccygeal vertebra so that about 5 cm of tail remains.

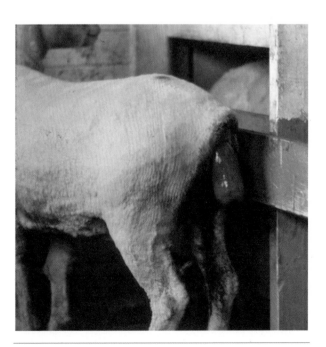

Figure 20.2 Prolapse of the rectum.

Hereditary chondrodysplasia (spider lamb syndrome)

Hereditary chondrodysplasia is a genetic disease of Suffolk and Hampshire sheep caused by an autosomal recessive gene. Lambs with the homozygous recessive genotype have a crippling congenital osteopathy, with the most striking feature being very long, bent limbs; hence the name 'spider'. The disease was introduced to the New Zealand Suffolk breed following the importation of North American blood-lines. Because it is a recessive gene, the disease is only likely to occur in pure-bred Suffolk sheep in New Zealand.

Clinical findings and diagnosis

The most striking clinical feature is an outward bending of the forelimbs from the carpi. Angular deformities of the hind-limbs generally are present, but the nature and extent of these are more varied than those of the forelimbs. The limbs are extremely long and fine-boned. Curvature of the spine in the thoracic region is often found in affected animals and the ribs and sternum are also deformed. The heads of affected lambs, when viewed laterally, are often shorter and more convex from the poll to the nostrils than those of normal lambs, and this may give a 'Roman nose' appearance. In severely affected lambs, many of these abnormalities are obvious at birth and may be lethal. Others do not develop characteristics of the disease until 4–6 weeks of age. The mortality among affected lambs is high.

Affected ram lambs have very small testes and poor semen quality, and ewe lambs are invariably infertile although occasionally some have conceived. There is no treatment.

Diagnosis of affected animals is based on the classical clinical findings, although the deformities present vary from lamb to lamb. The most useful method of confirming a diagnosis is by radiography. The best view is a lateral thoracic radiograph that includes the shoulder and flexed elbow joints. The characteristic finding is a mottled, irregular ossification pattern and uneven width of growth plates. In addition, blood testing of genotype is possible (see below).

Control

A DNA test to identify whether sheep have the hereditary chondrodysplasia gene is available from the Equine Blood Typing and Research Centre, Massey University, New Zealand. Suffolk breeders have agreed to test all rams that are sold between Suffolk breeders. Breeders may choose to only test sire rams to ensure that they are not carriers of the gene, or they may also test stud ewes.

Two full tubes of blood should be collected into EDTA anticoagulant tubes, ensuring that clotting does not occur. A new needle should be used for each sheep as it is essential that no blood contamination occurs between animals. It is also essential that samples are correctly identified for each animal. Because DNA quality decreases with time, the samples should be despatched to the laboratory as soon after collection as possible.

Another option to identify rams carrying spider syndrome is to test-mate the ram to sufficient numbers of his daughters, but this is a time-consuming, costly and impractical method.

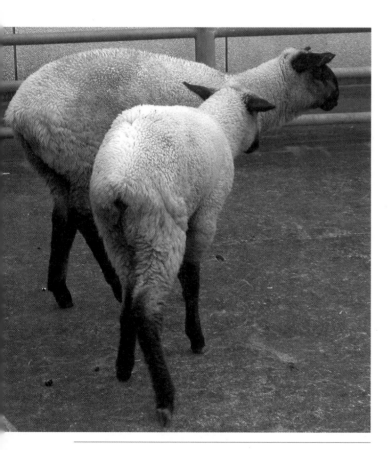

Figure 20.3 Spider lamb syndrome.

Leptospirosis

Leptospirosis has been recognised as a disease affecting most domestic animals. The organism is prevalent on New Zealand livestock farms, including sheep farms. A large serological survey conducted in 2010 showed 91% and 74% of sheep flocks had a least one adult sheep seropositive to *Leptospira borgpetersenii* serovar Hardjobovis (*L.* Hardjo) and *Leptospira interrogans* serovar Pomona (*L.* Pomona), respectively; 43% and 14% of individual sheep were seropositive to *L.* Hardjo and *L.* Pomona, respectively. Epidemiological studies have shown that seroconversions in young sheep mainly occur from late autumn to early summer.

Clinical disease due to *Leptospira* spp has been reported commonly in pigs and cattle in New Zealand. In sheep, *L.* Pomona has been associated with sporadic deaths in lambs and hoggets, and it has occasionally been associated with foetal losses in hoggets. Interestingly, it was first diagnosed in sheep in New Zealand in 1952, almost at the same time as its confirmation in calves. The field diagnosis in calves was made in 1951 and its association with human disease was made simultaneously. These early and somewhat dramatic cases were due to *Leptospira pomona*, later renamed *Leptospira interrogans* serovar Pomona. The widespread existence of leptospirosis in dairy cattle and pigs, and the common occurrence of severe and debilitating disease in humans, led to extensive research at Massey University and the development of vaccines, particularly for use on dairy farms.

Since the introduction of preventive vaccination of dairy cattle against *Leptospira*, the incidence of human leptospirosis has diminished significantly. However, meat-processing workers, including those working in sheep-only slaughter plants, have now become those at greatest risk of contracting the disease. In a slaughterhouse study conducted on lambs (<1 year of age), leptospires were isolated from the kidneys of approximately 20% of seropositive lambs and 1% of seronegative lambs. Given the number of carcasses they handle each day, this emphasises the potential risk that sheep carcasses pose to meatworkers.

L. Hardjo and *L.* Pomona appear to be the most common infections of meatworkers and non-dairy workers. However, these serovars are also associated with contact with pigs, sheep, beef cattle and deer, so it is difficult to delineate the precise role that sheep play in the transmission of the disease to humans.

The importance of sheep as a maintenance host for *L.* Hardjo is not yet clearly defined. A number of clinical outbreaks of leptospirosis in sheep have been associated with field contact with pigs, and *L.* Pomona has been confirmed in affected sheep but not all reported cases had a history of pig contact.

Aetiology

There are more than 150 serovars of *Leptospira* spp described, of which six are found in New Zealand. *L.* Hardjo and *L.* Pomona are the two serovars frequently encountered. *L.* Hardjo is maintained in cattle, while pigs are the natural host for *L.* Pomona. Serological surveys of sheep have shown that *L.* Hardjo is a common serovar, with greater than 90% of flocks having serum antibodies to this serovar. Studies investigating the clinical effects of *L.* Hardjo on sheep suggest that infection of sheep is usually asymptomatic, with minimal or no effects on growth rates and reproductive performance.

Similarly, infection with *L.* Pomona, while less common than *L.* Hardjo, appears relatively common in New Zealand. It has occasionally been associated with clinical disease, as outlined below.

Epidemiology

Outbreaks associated with *L.* Pomona in sheep have usually been preceded by exceptionally heavy rainfall, with surface water accumulating in the paddocks grazed by the affected sheep. In most cases lambs are affected and infection may sometimes, but not always, be associated with the presence of pigs either on the same or a neighbouring property.

Clinical features

Usually losses are seen following heavy rain. In an outbreak of leptospirosis in sheep, a few animals may be found dead while others are showing signs of malaise. This is usually characterised by anorexia, disinclination to move and in some cases a red urine stain of the wool of the crutch and hind legs may be seen. Careful observation of urinating animals will reveal haemoglobinuria. Close examination of affected animals usually reveals pale to muddy coloured mucous membranes with jaundice.

Leptospira Pomona has also occasionally been associated with mid-gestational foetal losses in ewe hoggets.

Pathology

Affected animals may be in good body condition and the carcass is usually jaundiced. The liver is pale and the kidneys are a dark grey/black colour with haemorrhagic and pale areas present on the surface. Blood-tinged fluid may be seen in the thoracic cavity. There is haemoglobinaemia and haemoglobinuria. Postmortem examination must be undertaken with extreme caution as leptospirosis is a highly contagious zoonosis and is readily transferred from infected body excretions and contaminated carcasses.

Diagnosis

A diagnosis can be confirmed by the collection of blood samples from several (10) sick or in-contact animals for *L.* Pomona serology. On occasion leptospirae may be observed in the serum or aqueous humour of affected animals by using darkfield microscopy, but leptospiruria is not a common feature of *L.* Pomona infection in sheep, as in cattle. Histologically, there may be a non-suppurative interstitial nephritis with leptospirae visible using silver stain, and centrilobular necrosis of hepatocytes.

Treatment and prevention

In an outbreak of leptospirosis in sheep, the immediate injection of any clinically sick animals with streptomycin at the rate of 20 mg/kg liveweight is recommended. This usually results in rapid recovery of the animals. In addition, all sheep that are at risk of infection should be vaccinated with a bivalent vaccine containing serovars *L.* Pomona and *L.* Hardjo. Investigation should also proceed to identify the source of infection to prevent further occurrences.

While the routine vaccination of sheep with a vaccine containing *L.* Hardjo and *L.* Pomona would be desirable for protection of human health, the rarity of clinical or subclinical effects from these organisms make this difficult to justify from an economic perspective.

Laryngeal chondritis

Chronic ovine laryngitis, also called laryngeal chondritis, is an obstructive upper respiratory tract disease of sheep and other species characterised by severe oedema of the larynx, dyspnoea, and usually death. Chronic suppuration of the arytenoid cartilages of the larynx usually follows the initial oedema, causing occlusion of the lumen and death of the animal by suffocation.

History

Laryngeal chondritis has been described in a number of sheep breeds from different countries since 1943. In New Zealand, the disease was first reported by Salisbury in 1956 in Southdown rams and ewes. The disease has now been reported in a variety of breeds including Hampshires, Suffolks, Corriedales, Romneys, Texels and East Friesians. Most recent literature has named the disease laryngeal chondritis, so to avoid confusion in this text the latter

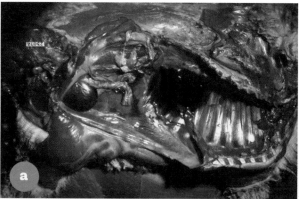

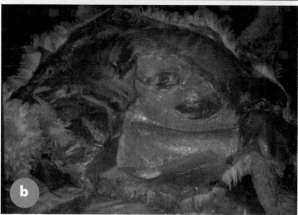

Figure 20.4 (a) Jaundiced lamb carcass with blood-tinged fluid in the chest cavity and dark-coloured urine in the bladder, from a case of leptospirosis. **(b)** Jaundiced lamb carcass with yellow fat from a case of leptospirosis (*L.* Pomona).

name is used rather than chronic ovine laryngitis as used by Salisbury (1956).

Clinical features

The occurrence of the disease is relatively sudden. There is extreme respiratory distress with cyanosis, even at rest, and a marked thoracic inspiratory lift with sinking flanks. On expiration the thorax collapses and the flanks become ballooned. Any handling of the sheep, particularly the head or throat, causes further distress. There is usually no temperature elevation. In cases where tracheotomy has been performed there is usually a noticeable respiratory relief and thoracic excursions returned to normal. In some mild cases of the disease, and with treatment, recovery has been reported, but in most cases respiratory distress increases until the sheep either suffocates or is destroyed on humane grounds.

Pathology

There are a number of reports on postmortem findings in sheep of different breeds, but the main features include oedema of the laryngeal folds, often with complete stenosis. In most advanced cases there is an abscess involving one or more cartilages, with necrosis of the cartilage or hyoid bone and enlargement of the regional lymph node. In the majority of cases there is no involvement of the lungs. The primary lesion is in the larynx, and death is invariably shown to be due to laryngeal stenosis.

Fusobacterium necrophorum is almost invariably recovered by bacteriological examination of the laryngeal lesions.

Predisposition and aetiology

The cases of laryngeal chondritis reported in Southdowns by Salisbury (1956) occurred mainly in rams of mixed ages from two-tooth to full-mouth sheep, but the majority were two-tooths. Some ewes were also affected. Salisbury claimed a strong hereditary predisposition to the disease, associated with the strong muscular development of the head, neck and shoulders of the Southdown sheep. This is similar to the Texel breed, in which numerous cases of the condition have been reported.

To support his suggestion, Salisbury cited one breeder who lost 40 ram hoggets over a period of 12 months. However, other cases seen and reported have been sporadic and difficult to explain on a hereditary basis.

Various other causative factors have been suggested, including feeding dry grain and trauma from drenching procedures. A more recent suggestion proposes that the oedema of the glottis leads to the development of excess granulation tissue because the mucoperichondrium of the vocal process is firmly adherent to the underlying cartilage. The epithelium is therefore relatively immobile and any pressure will result in erosion and ulceration of the laryngeal cartilage.

Treatment

The prospects of successful treatment of this condition are probably no better than described in earlier reports. Tracheotomy offers temporary relief but has little merit as a treatment. Recent authors suggest that the chronic lesions are irreversible and treatment is difficult.

Successful treatments have nevertheless been reported following prompt diagnosis of the condition, which requires an alert stockperson. The best responses have been when a single dose of corticosteroid is given initially to reduce laryngeal oedema, along with treatment with a broad-spectrum antibiotic for at least 7–10 days. Sheep must also be rested and not disturbed unnecessarily. It is emphasised that severely distressed sheep should be euthanased on humane grounds.

Tuberculosis in sheep

Occasional discoveries of tuberculosis have been made in sheep slaughtered in New Zealand abattoirs. The frequency of these discoveries has been low; however, there are at least two documented reports of tuberculosis in sheep where a number of animals were infected in each flock. In the first, a flock of nearly 600 mixed-age ewes on a farm in the Buller area was found to have 108 reactors to the intradermal tuberculin test. Of these, gross lesions resembling tuberculosis were found in 43 sheep. The second case involved a flock of 15,000 mixed-age Romney and Romney-cross ewes. A sample tuberculin test on 281 sheep gave 31 reactors, of which 30 had tuberculous lesions.

Pathology

In most cases the lesions have been found in the respiratory system, including the lungs and thoracic cavity. Lesions have also been seen in the retropharyngeal and mediastinal lymph nodes. The majority of lesions consisted of firm, enlarged lymph nodes which on incision contained one or more areas of yellow-grey caseous necrosis, well encapsulated by fibrous tissue and containing foci of calcification detectable by palpation and grittiness. In the most severely affected cases, multiple well-encapsulated nodules 5–20 mm in diameter were found in the lungs and were distributed mainly in the dorsal portions of the caudal lobes.

Direct microscopic identification of *Mycobacterium bovis* from lesions may prove difficult and in the cases reported in New Zealand culture methods were used to confirm the diagnosis.

Prevalence in sheep

The apparent marked difference in measured prevalence of tuberculosis in the overall sheep population when compared with cattle and deer is probably due to the following factors.

1. Sheep are inherently more resistant to contracting the disease, i.e. they require a much higher infective dose than cattle before infection can become established.
2. Grazing behaviour of sheep is different from cattle. Cattle tend to graze more frequently at night, and because of their inquisitive behaviour it is believed that contact with possums is considerable. Further, it is believed that much cattle infection is the result of the inhalation of aerosols of organisms generated during this mutual grazing of pasture by cattle and possums. Because of the grazing patterns of sheep, the potential contact with possums is reduced. Sheep grazing is mainly confined to daylight. At night sheep tend to 'camp' and to spend the night ruminating, which would keep them away from grazing possums. Further, sheep do not exhibit the same degree of curiosity as cattle and are more likely to avoid any possum rather than approach it.
3. Pasture management with sheep farming tends to produce a sward that is more closely grazed than cattle pasture, and this may not be as attractive to possums. It would also affect the length of time the organism could survive on the pasture.

It is most likely that the collective effect of these factors and others not yet defined is the main reason that tuberculosis is present at very low levels in the New Zealand sheep population.

Urolithiasis

The aetiology and pathogenesis of urolithiasis in sheep is complex and, while it is a serious disease of sheep in some countries such as Australia, its occurrence in New Zealand is sporadic and usually affects only a few or individual sheep, mainly rams. In Australia it may cause mortalities of up to 10% in some mobs of rams and wethers.

Aetiology and pathogenesis

Under certain circumstances, oversaturation of the urine with a particular solute or solutes may lead to precipitation of solids. The precipitate, in the form of a sludge or aggregate, may be flushed from the renal pelvis into the ureter or from the bladder into the urethra and cause obstruction of the urine flow. The blockage may be partial or complete, and uraemia and death occur if the obstruction is not removed. Urinary calculi found in sheep may contain:

- phosphate — magnesium ammonium phosphate, calcium phosphate
- silica — pure silica and/or organic matter
- calcium carbonate — mixed silica containing in part calcium oxalate or calcium carbonate
- organic complexes — calcium oxalate, cystine and xanthine.

Phosphate calculi

Calculi associated with feeding concentrate diets are caused by the precipitation of calcium and magnesium phosphate complexes from urine. Sheep normally excrete alkaline urine, which favours the precipitation of calcium and magnesium phosphates. Cereal grains are low in calcium and high in phosphorus, leading to an increased urinary output of phosphorus and the formation of insoluble phosphates and urinary calculi. Probably most of the cases of urolithiasis seen in display rams in New Zealand are due to this type of calculus.

Silica calculi

Silica calculi are the most common type of calculi seen

in the sheep from the wheat-belts in parts of Australia. Cereals contain high levels of silica, as do some native grasses. Some of the ingested silica is dissolved in the reticulo-rumen to form monosilicic acid, part of which is absorbed into the blood. Reabsorption of water in the kidneys results in high concentrations of silicic acid and precipitation of silica may occur.

Calcium carbonate calculi
Calcium carbonate calculi are most commonly found in sheep that have grazed plants such as mulga, *Portulaca* spp and parakeelya. Such plants are often eaten by sheep grazing in parts of Australia, particularly Queensland, and contain high levels of calcium oxalate. The reason why calcium carbonate and not calcium oxalate uroliths are formed is not known.

Organic complexes
Phyto-oestrogen-induced calculi may occur in sheep grazing high-oestrogen subterranean clovers. The high phyto-oestrogen intake causes epithelial metaplasia and the debris is deposited in the urethra as a sludge. Precipitates may also be seen filling the renal pelvis and sometimes in the bladder.

Other calculi caused by organic complexes such as oxalate calculi and cystine and xanthine calculi appear to be rare in sheep.

Clinical findings
Animals that develop urolithiasis are commonly housed and fed concentrates or may have been grazing stubble or clover pastures. The clinical picture may vary depending on the position of the obstruction and whether it is complete or partial. Most cases of urolithiasis in sheep are associated with urethral obstruction. Sites of obstruction include the sigmoid flexure, ischiatic arch, glans penis and the urethral process.

In partial obstruction the following features may be seen:
- anorexia
- twitching of the penis, discomfort and evidence of abdominal pain
- excretion of small amounts (dribbles) of urine, which may be blood-tinged.

In total obstruction the following may be seen:
- severe depression and anorexia
- apparent temporary improvement in the animal's condition as a result of bladder rupture leading to post-renal azotaemia
- distended abdomen due to urine in the abdominal cavity
- swelling of the ventral abdominal wall and prepuce as a result of urine leakage into the subcutaneous tissues; in extreme cases the skin may slough, allowing drainage of the urine
- contrast radiography may be of use in valuable rams to aid the diagnosis.

If the obstruction is not relieved and, in most cases, the bladder or the urethra has ruptured, death occurs within a week, usually due to uraemia.

Clinical pathology
Urine samples, if obtainable, may be helpful in reaching a diagnosis in individual animals. Blood samples may also be useful in monitoring valuable animals for azotaemia. If urinary calculi can be obtained they may be sent to a diagnostic laboratory for analysis.

Pathology
Hydronephrosis may be seen as a result of back pressure of urine into the kidney. Part of the urinary tract may rupture. If the bladder has ruptured, the abdominal cavity may contain large quantities of urine. Calculi may be found in the urethra, bladder and kidneys and rarely the ureters. In cases of rupture of the urethra, urine may have pervaded the subcutaneous tissue of the preputial region and may even have filled the scrotum in rams.

Treatment
If the calculus is lodged in the urethral process then amputation of this is straightforward. If the blockage is further up the urethra, in most cases euthanasia is recommended. In valuable sheep sub-ischial urethrostomy can be considered, but the difficulty in performing this procedure and the costs involved precludes it in most cases. A reported complication is ascending infection resulting in cystitis or pyelonephritis 4–6 weeks after surgery.

Prevention
Once the problem has developed, the prevention of further

urinary calculi forming may be difficult and requires persistence. However, the following suggestions may prove helpful:

- Lower urinary phosphate levels by adding calcium carbonate to the diet. The addition of 1.5–2% of ground limestone to a grain ration will correct the Ca : P imbalance. In addition, increasing the roughage in the diet or growing more good-quality forage will also help to improve the Ca : P balance.
- Acidification of the urine, by feeding acid-forming salts, helps to prevent the precipitation of calcium phosphate and magnesium ammonium phosphate crystals. Acidification of the urine can be achieved by feed withdrawal for 24 hours or dosing sheep at the rate of 7–10 g/day of ammonium chloride in solution. Free access to water is essential at all times.
- Increasing urine volume by the addition of sodium chloride to the diet (4% of the ration) for short periods of time may help to increase water consumption.
- Changing the diet of the sheep and removal from feeds that induce calculi is also an obvious move, but may be difficult when alternative feeds are hard to supply.

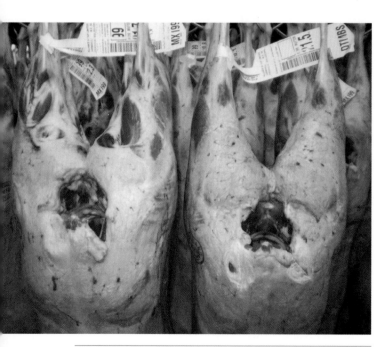

Figure 20.5 Yellow fat in sheep. (Photograph courtesy R Tecofsky, AgResearch)

Yellow fat in sheep

Throughout New Zealand a number of lambs and ewes are condemned at slaughter because of yellow fat, which makes the carcass aesthetically unacceptable. Affected carcasses cannot be exported and are sold locally for use in inferior products, thus markedly reducing the cash return to the producer. Although the condition occurs at low overall incidence it is usually associated with particular flocks, where incidence levels of 0.1% for lambs and 0.5% for ewes have been reported. In some individual mobs higher frequencies of up to 8.0% have occurred.

The condition is seen internationally and is believed to have come from Icelandic sheep into Britain centuries ago to eventually be passed to the Cheviot breed, hence the reported more common occurrence in the Perendale breed in New Zealand, although it is seen in Romneys and other sheep on occasion.

Aetiology

The condition is mainly caused by a recessive gene that blocks the normal breakdown of xanthophylls. Xanthophylls are chemically distinct carotenoids found in all pasture species ingested by sheep and cattle and include lutein, zeaxanthin and auroxanthin, all of which are directly responsible for the yellow fat condition. In normal sheep these are broken down and the fat remains white, while in sheep affected by yellow fat they are stored at high levels in adipose tissue, resulting in fat discolouration. As the sheep ages the colour intensifies.

It should be noted that some breeds of cattle, notably the Jersey, also have a condition similar to yellow fat. The gene causing yellow fat colouration in cattle has been linked to the β-carotene pathway, resulting in a similar effect as seen in sheep.

Prevention

A test has been used to check for chromogen (xanthophyll) levels in clotted blood. It is carried out on rams and may detect homozygous carrier sheep. It does not identify heterozygous animals. The blood should be shielded from UV light as this rapidly degrades the chromogen. The test has mainly been used for research purposes, and is not regularly available as a routine diagnostic test. Possible users should either contact an Animal Health Laboratory or AgResearch for information.

REFERENCES

VAGINAL PROLAPSE

Bruère AN. The treatment of bearing trouble. *New Zealand Veterinary Journal* 4, 170, 1956

Jackson R, Hilson RPN, Roe AR, Perkins N, Heuer C, West DM. Epidemiology of vaginal prolapse in mixed-age ewes in New Zealand. *New Zealand Veterinary Journal* 62, 328-37, 2014

Hosie BD, Low JC, Bradley HK, Robb J. Nutritional factors associated with vaginal prolapse in ewes. *Veterinary Record* 128, 204-8, 1991

Leslie A. *Diseases of Breeding Ewes.* Whitcombe & Tombs, Christchurch, New Zealand, 1938

McLean JW. Vaginal prolapse in sheep. Parts I & II. *New Zealand Veterinary Journal* 4, 38-55, 1956

McLean JW. Vaginal prolapse in ewes. Part III. The effect of topography on incidence. *New Zealand Veterinary Journal* 5, 93-7, 1957

McLean JW. Vaginal prolapse in ewes. Mortality rate in ewes and lambs. *New Zealand Veterinary Journal* 7, 137-9, 1959

McLean JW, Claxton JH. Vaginal prolapse in ewes. Part IV. Cyclic changes in the vulva, vestibule and vagina during the year. *New Zealand Veterinary Journal* 6, 133-7, 1958

McLean JW, Claxton JH. Vaginal prolapse in ewes. Part V. Seasonal variation in incidence. *New Zealand Veterinary Journal* 7, 134-6, 1959

McLean JW, Claxton JH. Vaginal prolapse in ewes. Part VII. The measurement and effect of intra-abdominal pressure. *New Zealand Veterinary Journal* 8, 51-61, 1960

Scott PR, Gessert M. Management of ovine vaginal prolapse. *In Practice* 20, 28-34, 1998

PROLAPSE OF THE RECTUM

Abstract from the *Journal of Animal Science* (2003) 81: 2725-32, cited in *Australian Sheep Veterinary Association Newsletter*

HEREDITARY CHONDRODYSPLASIA

Matthews M. Spider lamb syndrome (inherited chondrodysplasia) — a case study. *Proceedings of the 30th Annual Seminar of the Society of Sheep and Beef Cattle Veterinarians, New Zealand Veterinary Association,* 133-6, 2000

Rook JS, Trapp AL, Krehbiel J, Yamini B, Benson M. Diagnosis of hereditary chondrodysplasia (spider lamb syndrome) in sheep. *Journal of the American Veterinary Medical Association* 193, 713-18, 1988

Thompson KG, Piripi SA, Dittmer KE. Inherited abnormalities of skeletal development in sheep. *Veterinary Journal* 177, 324-33, 2008

Vanek JA, Alstad AD, Berg IE, Moore BL, Limesand W. Spider syndrome in lambs: a clinical and postmortem analysis. *Veterinary Medicine* 81, 663-8, 1986

Vanek JA, Walter AD, Alstad AD. Comparing spider syndrome in Hampshire and Suffolk sheep. *Veterinary Medicine* 82, 430-7, 1987

West DM, Burbidge HM, Vermunt JJ, Arthur DG. Hereditary chondrodysplasia ('spider syndrome') in a New Zealand Suffolk lamb of American origin. *New Zealand Veterinary Journal* 43, 118-22, 1995

LEPTOSPIROSIS

Bahaman AR, Marshall RB, Blackmore DK. Isolation of *Leptospira interrogans* serovar *hardjo* from sheep in New Zealand. *New Zealand Veterinary Journal* 28, 171, 1980

Baker M. The changing epidemiology of human leptospirosis in New Zealand. *Proceedings of the 34th Annual Seminar of the Society of Sheep and Beef Cattle Veterinarians, New Zealand Veterinary Association,* 27-34, 2004

Blackmore DK. Current view on the epidemiology of leptospirosis in New Zealand. *Antech* 2, 21-34, 1981

Blackmore DK, Bahaman AR, Marshall RB. The epidemiological interpretation of serological responses to leptospiral serovars in sheep. *New Zealand Veterinary Journal* 30, 38-42, 1982

Bowsher H, Reichel MP. Leptospirosis deaths in sheep. *Society of Sheep and Beef Cattle Veterinarians, New Zealand Veterinary Association — Newsletter* 33, 12-13, 2008

Bruère AN. An association between leptospirosis in calves and man. *Australian Veterinary Journal* 28, 174, 1952

Dorjee S, Ridler AL, Collins JM, Midwinter A, West DM, Heuer C, Jackson R. Leptospirosis in sheep in New Zealand. *Proceedings of the 35th Annual Seminar of the Society of Sheep and Beef Cattle Veterinarians, New Zealand Veterinary Association,* 19-31, 2005

Dorjee S, Heuer C, Jackson R, West DM, Collins-Emerson JM, Midwinter AC, Ridler AL. Prevalence of pathogenic *Leptospira* spp. in sheep in a sheep-only abattoir in New Zealand. *New Zealand Veterinary Journal* 56, 164-70, 2008

Dorjee S, Heuer C, Jackson R, West DM, Collins-Emerson JM, Midwinter AC, Ridler AL. Assessment of occupational exposure to leptospirosis in a sheep-only abattoir. *Epidemiology and Infection* 139, 797-806, 2011

Dreyfus A. Leptospirosis in humans and pastoral livestock in New Zealand. PhD Thesis, Massey University, Palmerston North, New Zealand, 2013

Dreyfus A, Benschop J, Collins-Emerson J, Wilson P, Baker MG, Heuer C. Sero-prevalence and risk factors for leptospirosis in abattoir workers in New Zealand. *International Journal of Environmental Research and Public Health* 11, 175-75, 2014

Gordon, LM. Isolation of *Leptospira interrogans* serovar hardjo from sheep. *Australian Veterinary Journal* 56, 348-9, 1980

Hartley WJ. Ovine leptospirosis. *Australian Veterinary Journal* 28, 169-70, 1952

Heuer C. Human health and leptospirosis. *Proceedings of the 35th Annual Seminar of the Society of Sheep and Beef Cattle Veterinarians, New Zealand Veterinary Association*, 19-31, 2005

Heuer C, Davies PR. Leptospirosis in sheep — a human health hazard in New Zealand. *Proceedings of the 34th Annual Seminar of the Society of Sheep and Beef Cattle Veterinarians, New Zealand Veterinary Association*, 21-5, 2004

Hilson R. Leptospirosis in slaughter lambs — to vaccinate or not to vaccinate, that is the question. *Proceedings of the 36th Annual Seminar of the Society of Sheep and Beef Cattle Veterinarians, New Zealand Veterinary Association*, 137-40, 2006

Hodges RT. Some observations on experimental *Leptospira* serotype *pomona* infection in sheep. *New Zealand Veterinary Journal* 22, 151-4, 1974

Kirschner L, Millar TF, Garlick CH. Swineherds disease in New Zealand. Infection with *Leptospira pomona* in man, calves and pigs. *New Zealand Medical Journal* 51, 98-108, 1952

Marshall RB, Manktelow BW. Fifty years of leptospirosis research in New Zealand: A perspective. *New Zealand Veterinary Journal* 50 (Suppl.), 61-3, 2002

Matthews M, Collins-Emerson J, Marshall R. Leptospirosis in beef herds in Hawkes Bay. *Proceedings of the 30th Annual Seminar of the Society of Sheep and Beef Cattle Veterinarians, New Zealand Veterinary Association*, 165-6, 2000

Millar KR, Hodges RT, Sheppard AD, Hammington MW. Clinical and biochemical changes in sheep inoculated with *Leptospira interrogans serotype pomona*. *New Zealand Veterinary Journal* 25, 20-37, 1977

Moffat JR. Leptospirosis in sheep in New Zealand — an update. *Proceedings of the 37th Annual Seminar of the Society of Sheep and Beef Cattle Veterinarians, New Zealand Veterinary Association*, 147-54, 2007

Morse EV, Morter RL, Langham RF, Lundhberg AM, Ullrey DE. Experimental ovine leptospirosis, *Leptospira pomona* infection. *Journal of Infectious Diseases* 101, 129-36, 1957

Oswald A. Acute deaths in hoggets grazing in forestry blocks. *Proceedings of the 35th Annual Seminar of the Society of Sheep and Beef Cattle Veterinarians, New Zealand Veterinary Association*, 159-65, 2005

Ridler AL, Vallee E, Corner RA, Kenyon PR, Heuer C. Factors associated with fetal losses in ewe lambs on a New Zealand sheep farm. *New Zealand Veterinary Journal* 63, 330-4, 2015

Ris DR. Serological evidence for infection of sheep with *Leptospira interrogans* serotype *Hardjo*. *New Zealand Veterinary Journal* 23, 154, 1975

Smith BP, Armstrong JM. Fatal hemolytic anemia attributed to leptospirosis in lambs. *Journal of the American Veterinary Association* 167, 739-41, 1975

Surveillance

(2000) 24: 17   Leptospirosis in ewes and lambs

(2006) 33(1): 11-16   Leptospira in milk lambs

(2006) 33(4): 18-23   Leptospira abortion in ewe hoggets

(2008) 35(1): 11-15   Leptospira in ewe lambs and pigs

Thornton R. Leptospirosis in New Zealand sheep. *Surveillance* 21, 13-4, 1994

Vallee E, Heuer C, Collins-Emerson J, Benschop J, Wilson P. Update on research into the effects of *Leptospira* serovar Hardjo and Pomona on sheep and beef cattle growth and reproduction. *Proceedings of the Society of Sheep and Beef Cattle Veterinarians, New Zealand Veterinary Association*, 29-34, 2014

Vallee E, Heuer C, Collins-Emerson JM, Benschop J, Wilson PR. Serological patterns, antibody half-life and shedding in urine of *Leptospira* spp. in naturally exposed sheep. *New Zealand Veterinary Journal* 63, 301-12, 2015

Vermunt JJ, West DM. Leptospirosis in a lamb. *New Zealand Veterinary Journal* 42, 155, 1994

Vermunt JJ, West DM, Cooke MM, Alley MR, Collins Emerson Y. Observations on three outbreaks of *Leptospira interrogans serovar pomona* infection in lambs. *New Zealand Veterinary Journal* 42, 133-6, 1994

Webster WM, Reynolds BA. Immunisation against *Leptospira pomona*. *New Zealand Veterinary Journal* 3, 47-59, 1955

LARYNGEAL CHONDRITIS

Faull WB, Scholes SFF. Laryngeal chondritis in Texel sheep. *Veterinary Record* 123, 155, 1987

Gill JM. Diseases of East Friesian sheep. *Surveillance* 26, 2, 1999

Lane JG, Brown PJ, Lancaster ML, Todd JN. Laryngeal chondritis in Texel sheep. *Veterinary Record* 121, 81-4, 1987

Salisbury RM. Chronic ovine laryngitis. *New Zealand Veterinary Journal* 4, 144-6, 1956

TUBERCULOSIS

Cordes DO, Bullians JA, Lake DE, Carter ME. Observations on tuberculosis caused by *Mycobacterium bovis* in sheep. *New Zealand Veterinary Journal* 29, 60-2, 1981

Davidson RM, Alley MR, Beatson NS. Tuberculosis in a flock of sheep. *New Zealand Veterinary Journal* 29, 1-2, 1981

Surveillance (1988) 15: 8-9: Tuberculosis in sheep — a very rare disease

UROLITHIASIS

Chapman HM, Sutherland RJ. Urolithiasis of sheep. *Sheep Medicine*. Proceeding 141, 33-41. Postgraduate Committee in Veterinary Science, Sydney University, 1990

Hay L. Prevention and treatment of urolithiasis in sheep. *In Practice* 12, 87-91, 1990

YELLOW FAT

Baker RL, Steine T, Vabeno AW, Breines D. The inheritance and incidence of yellow fat in Norwegian sheep. *Acta Agriculturae Scandinavica* 35, 389-97, 1985

Kirton AH, Belton DJ. Yellow fat inherited? *New Zealand Journal of Agriculture*, Dec, 8-9, 1981

Prache S, Priolo A, Grolier P. Effect of concentrate finishing on the carotenoid content of perirenal fat in grazing sheep: Its significance for discriminating grass-fed, concentrate-fed and concentrate-finished grazing lambs. *Animal Science* 77, 22533, 2993

Surveillance (1988) 15(2): 13 Yellow fat survey

Tian R, Pitchford WS, Morris CA, Cullen NG, Bottema CDK. Molecular genetics of beef fat colour. *Plant and Animal Genomes XVII Conference*, 2009

Yang A, Larsen TW, Tume RK. Carotenoid and retinol concentrations in serum, adipose tissue and liver and carotenoids tgransport in sheep, goats and cattle. *Australian Journal of Agricultural Research* 43, 1809-17, 1992

21

Exotic diseases

In these sections a brief description is given of several exotic diseases of sheep that are very important internationally. Some of these present very little risk to the New Zealand sheep industry but nevertheless are of particular significance to the countries where they occur. As New Zealand veterinary students are trained to meet international requirements for the profession it is very important that these diseases are well understood. Should the sad day arrive when one of them may appear in our sheep population, it is hoped that it would be recognised promptly and appropriate action taken to eliminate it.

Transmissible spongiform encephalopathies (TSEs)

Scrapie disease of sheep is probably the longest recognised of the spongiform encephalopathy diseases. It is a transmissible neurological disease that occurs in most breeds of sheep of either sex. Because of its inherently long incubation period (as with other TSEs), it is mainly seen in sheep between 2 and 5 years of age. Scrapie also affects goats, often as a result of exposure to sheep affected with the disease. The disease is progressive and the aetiology is complex. It is a significant stigma for countries with infected sheep populations, and a major restrictive factor in the international trade of live sheep.

With the recognition of bovine spongiform encephalopathy (BSE) in cattle in the UK in 1986 and its subsequent association with cases of variant Creutzfeldt-Jakob disease in humans, an enormous amount of research was generated into the mammalian spongiform encephalopathies. Further, their occurrence has now been recorded in a wide variety of species, as shown in Table 21.1. While scrapie is the oldest, and until recently the most significant, of these, because of their unique characteristics some of their features are discussed collectively.

In humans	
Creutzfeldt-Jakob disease (CJD)	(Sporadic Iatrogenic)
Kuru	(Transmissible — sporadic)
Gerstman Sträussler Scheinker	(Familial)
Fatal familial insomnia	(Familial)
Variant Creutzfeldt-Jakob disease (vCJD)	(Genetic susceptibility)
In animals	
Scrapie	Sheep and goats
Transmissible mink encephalopathy	Mink
Chronic wasting disease (CWD)	Mule-deer, elk, white-tailed deer
Bovine spongiform encephalopathy (BSE)	Cattle, exotic species, experimentally sheep

Table 21.1 Transmissible spongiform encephalopathies of humans and animals.

Spongiform encephalopathy attributed to BSE has been identified in a number of species, including cattle, nyala, gemsbok, eland, Arabian Oryx, Scimitar-horned Oryx, kudu, domestic cats, moufflon, puma, cheetah, ostrich and lion.

Nature of the causative agents

Because of its long incubation, scrapie was originally described as a slow virus disease by Sigurdsson (1954) but its true nature defied understanding for many years. Increasingly, research is confirming the hypothesis suggested by Prusiner that the infective agents causing scrapie and the other transmissible encephalopathies are abnormal distorted prions. A prion (PrP) is a small glycosylated protein molecule found in the brain-cell membrane. It is not 'live', as for example a virus is; it has no associated nucleic acid. Prion is a generic term. Different species of animals have brain-cell prion protein of different compositions. For example, the amino acid sequence of the human prion differs at more than 30 positions from that of the cattle prion, whereas sheep and cattle differ at only 7 positions.

Protein molecules have three-dimensional folded shapes. An infective prion is one whose shape has become distorted and is protease-resistant so is not broken down into amino acids in the digestive system. It is suggested that when a distorted prion molecule reaches the prions in the brain-cell membrane of a susceptible host, the distorted molecule acts as a template causing more distorted prions to be formed. Because only small quantities of brain-cell prion are produced, the process takes time, and hence the long incubation period of the encephalopathies.

Ultra-structural examination of highly purified biologically active scrapie material has revealed clusters of rod-like structures not seen in control materials. These have been termed 'scrapie-associated fibrils'. Evidence has accumulated to suggest that the fibrils may be composed substantially of prion protein and could possibly represent the scrapie agent.

The stability of TSE prions

Prions are very resistant to the usual methods of sterilisation. They are able to withstand boiling, UV light, ionising radiation, formalin, ultra-sonification, freezing, drying, autolysis, organic solvents and detergents. They are very heat-resistant, but exposure to 20,000 ppm available chlorine for 1 hour is believed to be effective decontamination.

A classical demonstration of resistance to destruction of the scrapie agent was its inadvertent transmission through formalised louping ill vaccine produced at the Moredun Institute in Scotland in 1935. One of three batches of the vaccine also contained the scrapie agent, with the result that 7% of the recipients of the 18,000 doses of that batch of vaccine developed scrapie.

The inactivation of TSE agents has been reported by Taylor et al. (1994) and reviewed by Taylor (2000). It is evident that procedures that were once thought to be effective do not reliably decontaminate all infection, especially of some strains of agent. Initially it had been found that 50 mg samples of brain tissue containing mouse-passaged scrapie strains were inactivated by exposure to porous-load autoclaving at 136°C for 4 minutes, and it was consequently recommended that one cycle of 134–138°C for 18 minutes or six cycles of 3 minutes should be used to inactivate the human form, Creutzfeldt-Jakob disease (CJD).

However, it was recommended that instruments used in brain or eye surgery of CJD patients or other high-risk groups be discarded after use. Subsequently it has been shown that the BSE agent, and some scrapie agents, were not inactivated completely by porous-load autoclaving cycles of up to 1 hour at 134–138°C (the standard procedure for autoclaving surgical instruments).

Further studies have confirmed that mouse-passaged BSE can survive exposure to 138°C for 1 hour. The data also suggested that for some strains the survival was enhanced at higher temperatures and that simply increasing porous-load autoclaving temperatures and holding times would not necessarily be effective in achieving a reliable decontamination of TSE agents.

Further concerns about the difficulty of decontamination of TSE agents have been raised by Brown et al. (2000), who demonstrated that infectivity remained in 1 g samples of hamster brain infected with the 263K hamster-passaged strain of scrapie agent when exposed to 600°C. The brain samples were completely ashed but when reconstituted with saline to their original weights, transmitted disease to 5 of 35 inoculated hamsters. No transmission occurred after exposure to 1000°C.

Genetic control of susceptibility and incubation period

Experimental work with mice has shown that the incubation period and the distribution of lesions within the brain are functions of the dose, route of administration, 'strain' of scrapie agent and mouse genotype. In experimental mice the Sinc gene (scrapie incubation period) has two alleles, p7 and s7, so called because homozygous s7 mice inoculated with the ME7 strain of the scrapie agent develop scrapie with a short incubation period, whereas the incubation period is prolonged in homozygous p7 mice. Changing the genotype but keeping the other variables constant has a profound effect on the incubation period. Indeed, in mice it is possible to manipulate these variables to produce an infection with scrapie, the incubation period of which exceeds the life span of the host.

In sheep, a similar situation has been defined by breeding studies designed to create 'susceptible' and 'resistant' lines of sheep by selective breeding of a foundation flock according to the response of related animals to inoculation with SSBP/1 (Sheep Scrapie Brain Pool/1). The incidence of experimentally induced scrapie in selected lines of Cheviot and Herdwick sheep suggested that susceptibility to inoculation with SSBP/1 was controlled by a single gene known as Sip (Short incubation period). The Sip gene has two alleles, sA and pA, and the sA allele is dominant for susceptibility to disease after inoculation with SSBP/1.

It is now known that the Sip gene of sheep is either closely linked to or identical to the PrP gene that has been extensively characterised by molecular genetics. Polymorphic variants of the PrP gene have been associated with the incidence of both experimental and natural scrapie in sheep and goats and TSE in human beings. The incidence of natural scrapie in sheep is now believed to be associated with polymorphisms of the PrP gene, particularly those at codons 136, 154 and 171. In many breeds of sheep the PrP allele encoding valine at codon 136 confers an extremely high risk of scrapie, but in Suffolk sheep, a breed with a known high incidence of scrapie, this allele is extremely rare. In a closed flock of Suffolk sheep in Scotland, scrapie was found to occur primarily in animals that were homozygous for glutamine at codon 171, a genotype which was significantly less frequent in healthy flockmates. These findings have suggested that breeding for increased resistance to scrapie in Suffolks by the selection of animals according to their PrP genotype may be possible.

As well as Suffolk sheep, polymorphism of the PrP gene has been defined in Cheviots. If the latter breed of sheep is injected with SSBP/1, the incubation period is varied as shown in Table 21.2.

However, susceptibility of Cheviots challenged with a different strain (CH1641) is not associated with variations of codon 136, but instead depends on codon 171. Cheviots homozygous for glutamine at codon 171 are susceptible. The genotypes of both Cheviot and Suffolk sheep in New Zealand, Australia and the United Kingdom have been compared. The results reveal that both New Zealand and Australia have sheep with scrapie-susceptible genotypes that could be susceptible to scrapie disease were it to gain entry to these countries. The fact that New Zealand has scrapie-susceptible sheep but no overt evidence of the disease strengthens our argument for scrapie freedom.

Transmission of the scrapie agent

In natural scrapie in sheep, it is generally accepted that lateral spread of infection from the environment and maternal spread from dam to lamb are the main means of transmission. The ram probably plays little or no part in the transmission of the disease. Historical evidence from the spread of scrapie in Iceland suggested that environmental contamination is important. In the latter example, on areas de-stocked during the Icelandic maedi-visna eradication programme, a high incidence of scrapie occurred in sheep returned to these areas even though they had been free of sheep for several months.

	Sheep codon	Incubation period
Homozygous valine	VV136	167 days
Heterozygous	VA136	322 days
Homozygous alanine	AA136	Resistant

Key: V = Valine, A = Alanine.

Table 21.2 Incubation period for Cheviot sheep of differing genotypes.

Previous work conducted in Edinburgh indicated that scrapie may be transmitted via unwashed embryos. Six of 20 lambs born following embryo transfer from donors experimentally infected with scrapie were of a susceptible genotype, and 5 of the 6 subsequently developed scrapie. However, no controls were included and it was possible that the disease could have been transmitted after embryo transfer, perhaps at lambing. The trial was repeated using known susceptible and resistant genotypes and included controls. Susceptible genotypes developed scrapie in spite of whether embryos were washed or unwashed or whether donor ewes were experimentally infected with scrapie or not. Because the controls also got scrapie, it appears that the experiment was contaminated and that despite the precautions taken, susceptible genotypes became infected after the lambs were born. A large embryo transplant experiment conducted in the USA and reported in 2001 concluded that scrapie was not transmitted to offspring via the embryo, nor was the infective agent transmitted to recipient ewes during embryo transfer procedures. The embryos were collected from 38 donor Suffolk ewes and the transfer procedure (embryo washing) was as recommended by the International Embryo Transfer Society. Although embryo transfer is otherwise excellent for importing new genetic material into New Zealand, its absolute safety as a means of ensuring the non-entry of scrapie from known infected countries is still in question. Extensive experimental work has failed to resolve the question, so that in the meantime New Zealand authorities have taken a conservative view on the use of this method of importing new genetic material from countries where scrapie exists.

A further possible vector of scrapie may be hay mites, of which there are several species. Researchers in Iceland sent mites from five known scrapie-infected farms to a laboratory in the USA for examination. Of 71 mice injected with mite samples, 10 were clinically positive for scrapie and the immunoblotting technique was used to detect PrP (scrapie) in 10 brain samples from these mice. The researchers emphasised the precautions taken to prevent contamination of the samples and suggested that the scrapie agent may have replicated in the mites because of an abnormal form of prion protein detected in the mite samples. It was suggested that this might be a plausible explanation for the reappearance of scrapie on some farms after a 3-year period of de-stocking. The importance of this observation in the natural transmission of scrapie is as yet undetermined.

Natural infection of the lamb occurs via the alimentary tract during or shortly after birth. Using mouse inoculation it has been possible to recover scrapie agent from the tonsils, retropharyngeal and mesenteric lymph nodes of clinically normal lambs from a Suffolk scrapie flock at 10–14 months of age. Infection of central nervous system tissues was not evident until 25 months of age.

Suffolks % genotypes

	UK	NZ	AUS
Susceptible 1 VV136 RR154 QQ171	0	0	4
Susceptible 2 VA136 RR154 QQ171	14	17	9
Resistant AA136 RR154 RR171	19	12	9

Cheviots % genotypes

	UK	NZ	AUS
Susceptible AA136 RR154 QQ171	13	39	53
Resistant AA136 RR154 RR171	33	8	3

Key: A = Alanine, R = Arginine, Q = Glutamine, V = Valine.

Table 21.3 Suffolk and Cheviot sheep compared for susceptibility and resistance in New Zealand, Australia and the United Kingdom.

Breed of sheep or goat	No. exposed to scrapie	No. developing scrapie	Reference*
Blackface	7	3	1
Blackface	75	21	2
Rambouillet	111	15	3
Targhee	101	19	3
Hampshire	23	2	3
Suffolk (NZ)	23	9	3
Suffolk (USA)	5	1	3
Angora	23	6	3
Dairy goats	72	44	3
Goats (various)	17	10	1

*References: 1 Brotherston et al. (1968); 2 Dickinson, Stamp & Renwick (1974); 3 Hourrigan et al. (1979).

Table 21.4 Lateral spread of scrapie to sheep and goats given long-term exposure to natural cases.

1. Lateral transmission

Under natural conditions, scrapie may spread laterally (Figure 21.1 and Table 21.4). After the scrapie agent has gained entry to the body it is mainly contained in lymphoid organs and the brain. Body fluids, such as blood, urine, milk and saliva, have very low levels. It is the placenta that contains a particularly large amount of scrapie agent and is likely to be the main source of infection to the lamb. Other possible sources of scrapie agent are cells that may slough from mucous membranes and from skin damaged by constant rubbing.

Experimentally, infection can be achieved by oral dosing, scarification and via the conjunctiva, all of which are likely to be routes of infection in natural scrapie.

Direct infection may occur when sheep either eat or lick placentae from natural cases at lambing. It is possible that scrapie infection could be transmitted by the use of docking knives or the same needle for mass inoculations of sheep flocks, but there is no direct evidence for this.

There is evidence that sheep may become infected indirectly from contaminated pasture, or from infected buildings, feeding troughs and so on. Since the scrapie agent is highly resistant to adverse conditions, infection from a contaminated environment could be quite important.

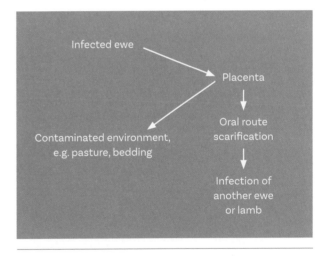

Figure 21.1 Lateral transmission of scrapie agent.

2. The role of the ewe in transmission

The probability of a lamb eventually developing scrapie depends more on the scrapie status of the ewe than that of the ram. This bias indicates the relative importance of the ewe in the transmission of scrapie infection. In part this may occur post-natally during the weeks of intimate contact between the ewe and its lamb (Figure 21.2). In addition there may be vertical transmission of the agent prenatally, but this has not been confirmed.

Scrapie agent is present in the extraneural tissues of sheep for a long time before clinical signs develop. Therefore, it is suggested that a ewe infected from birth could be a source of infection to her lambs and possibly to other sheep for much of her life. However, the exact importance of the ewe in the transmission of scrapie to the offspring is a very difficult problem to confirm. Although the agent is no doubt discharged from an infected ewe into the environment, particularly via the placenta, the weight of evidence suggests that the increased risk of disease in the offspring of infected ewes is largely the result of increased genetic susceptibility; the majority of cases occurring in the lambs of 'high-incidence' flocks is probably the result of the lateral transmission of infection.

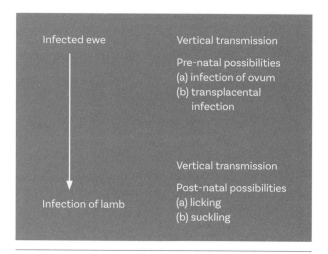

Figure 21.2 The role of the ewe in the transmission of scrapie.

3. The role of the ram

The role of the ram in transmitting the scrapie agent, either in semen or by other means, is unknown. However, it has often been reported that an outbreak of scrapie may follow the extensive use of a new ram. This could mean that the ram was the source of infection, but it is more likely that the infection was already in the flock and that the ram introduced susceptible genotypes into the flock that allowed the disease to be manifest.

Clinical signs of scrapie

The clinical signs of scrapie appear insidiously, with non-specific behavioural changes. It is reported that in some cases the fleece colour changes from white to a pale coffee colour prior to the onset of clinical signs. The initial signs include intermittent bouts of hyperaesthesia, often accompanied by an apprehensive or 'far away' appearance. Affected sheep may either lead or trail a mob that is being driven. As the disease develops two forms emerge.

1. Pruritis

There is extensive loss of wool caused by scraping or rubbing against fixed objects and by nibbling. The compulsive nature of this behaviour can often lead to the appearance of skin lesions. Rubbing sheep frequently show rapid jaw movements with flicking of the tongue — the so-called nibble reflex.

2. Incoordination

Affected sheep usually have an exaggerated and incoordinated gait. Some sheep exhibit a high-stepping (trotting) movement of the front legs, but mostly there is ataxia in the hind-limbs with much stumbling of the animal if driven. When at rest, an affected sheep may stand awkwardly with its hindquarters leaning against a fence, or it may be seen to sway drowsily and even lose its balance. As the disease progresses there is a marked loss of condition leading to emaciation.

Characteristically, the clinical signs are progressive leading to incoordination and inability to stand. The duration of the clinical course is very variable, lasting from a week or so to several months, but the disease always ends in death.

It must be emphasised that there is a great variation in clinical signs seen in any one animal. This variation is probably due to differences between breeds of sheep, strains of agent and environmental factors. It is not uncommon to find affected animals with pruritis and no incoordination and *vice versa*. Many cases of scrapie probably go unrecognised, especially in poorly supervised flocks.

Pathology and histopathology of scrapie

There are no gross pathological lesions attributable to scrapie. Histological changes are detected only in the central nervous system, and consist of spongy changes in the neuropil, vacuolation of the cytoplasm of nerve cells, hypertrophy of astrocytes with proliferation of their processes and, in some instances, a congophilic angiopathy. The distribution and type of lesion varies with breed of sheep and possibly other factors, but usually neuronal changes with single or multiple cytoplasmic vacuoles are present in the vestibular, dorsal motor vagus and facial nuclei and the reticular formation of the medulla. In some cases, notably in obese Suffolk sheep, the medial and lateral nuclei of the thalamus show spongy changes. Similar status spongiosis may be present in the frontal and parietal cortex. Vascular changes, i.e. congophilic angiopathy, which has been a feature of the pathology of certain strains of experimental scrapie in mice, has recently been found also in some natural cases of sheep scrapie, usually in the cerebral and cerebellar cortices.

In addition to the presence of vacuoles within specific areas of the brain, the presence of scrapie-associated fibrils can be used to confirm a diagnosis. Scrapie-associated fibrils consist of a glycoprotein or prion protein that is deposited in the brain and peripheral organs of infected animals.

Other diagnostic tests

A number of diagnostic tests have been developed to detect or confirm scrapie and BSE. Some of these claim to detect infectivity 3–12 months before the development of clinical signs. Most are based on detecting abnormal prion protein. In the live animal lymphoid tissue is used, taken either from the tonsils by biopsy or from the third eyelid of sheep, where lymphoid tissue develops once sheep reach 14 months of age. At slaughter, tests such as Western immunoblotting and immuno-histochemistry can be

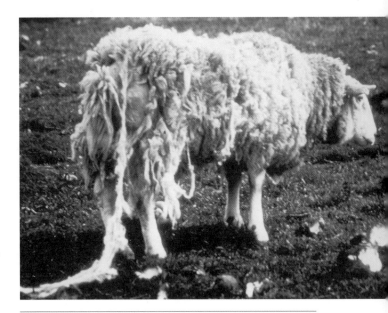

Figure 21.3 Scrapie sheep.

applied directly to brain tissue. It is proposed to use similar tests on a sample of slaughtered cattle in New Zealand to support the claim that New Zealand is free from BSE.

New Zealand-specific surveillance programme for TSEs

New Zealand has a specific surveillance programme to detect spongiform encephalopathies based on veterinarians identifying suspect cases. Although sheep and cattle in New Zealand are not affected with these diseases, any country that wants to trade as a free country must undertake an internationally accepted continuous TSE surveillance and monitoring programme that has been designed along the guidelines provided by the Office International des Epizooties (OIE). As part of this programme, the New Zealand Ministry for Primary Industries has to ensure that the brains from at least 300 cattle aged 30 months and over and sheep aged 2 years of age and older that are exhibiting clinical signs of progressive central nervous disease are screened annually for histopathological evidence of BSE and scrapie and found to be negative.

The laboratory requires:
- A good clinical history.
- Fixed brain (including brain stem). Brains should be

fixed in formalin in a bucket, then consigned to the laboratory in a plastic bag accompanied by a small amount of formalin or gauze pads soaked in formalin.
- A fresh 2-cm length of cervical spinal cord (this is required in case lesions are suspicious and material has to be referred overseas for additional testing). Sufficient fresh material can usually be obtained by severing the cord as far back from the brain as possible when removing the head from the atlas vertebra; the piece of cervical cord can then be cut from the medulla before the brain is fixed in 10% formalin.
- Where possible, a serum sample to allow the elimination of metabolic diseases from the diagnosis in cases where there are no histopathological lesions.

As well as BSE of cattle and scrapie of sheep and goats, all TSEs of New Zealand domestic animals are notifiable diseases and should they ever be suspected, MPI must be notified by calling 0800 809 966.

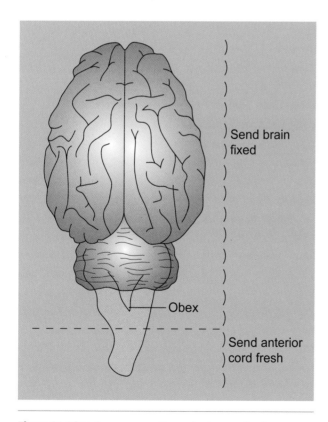

Figure 21.4 Specimen preparation — brain samples for TSE examination.

Control and prevention of scrapie

The best form of prevention of scrapie is to ensure that it is not introduced into a clean, secure environment. In a country where scrapie is endemic, such as the UK, once a farm has become contaminated then epidemiological considerations will determine which of two options, eradication or containment within economically acceptable limits, is viable. Eradication is feasible only where animals imported into a previously clean environment have been contained in the most stringent quarantine conditions.

It is difficult to advocate the duration of such quarantine, as incubation periods may be 8–10 years and could involve a number of generations. Environmental contamination is a further hazard. Icelandic experience indicates that keeping contaminated pasture free of sheep stocks for a number of years may be insufficient to eliminate infection.

Vigorous attempts to control scrapie have been made in the USA by slaughtering sheep in both affected flocks and source flocks. This policy has not brought scrapie under control, as new occurrences are reported annually and a relaxation of the policy would probably lead to an upsurge of cases.

In endemically affected countries the following procedures have been recommended in an attempt to reduce the incidence of scrapie.

1. Elimination of the affected flocks

This involves the total slaughter of an affected flock and its source flocks if these are known. However, this requires the payment of adequate compensation to sheep farmers; also, the infection may still be in the environment even after a period of decontamination (see the Icelandic experiences discussed above).

2. Culling of blood-line relatives

Selectively culling the blood-line relatives of scrapie cases can reduce the effects of maternal transmission of agent and remove some of the genetically susceptible sheep. In effect this means culling the progeny of affected ewes and the progeny of the female progeny. This requires good breeding records. In practice, this policy could lead to the destruction of the whole flock in instances where only one or two breeding rams have been used extensively.

3. Husbandry

The risk of introducing scrapie into a flock can be reduced by limiting the purchase of breeding rams and ewes to farms known to be free from the disease. Where this is not possible, the purchases should be limited to older ewes or the progeny of older ewes that are less likely to develop scrapie.

At lambing time, prompt removal of the afterbirth from the environment is helpful, as is avoiding the use of lambing pens and changing the lambing area each year.

The use of genetic screening and scrapie control

As it is possible to detect scrapie-resistant strains of sheep (see the section above on genetic control, and Table 21.3), the UK government introduced a voluntary ram genotyping plan aimed at pedigree ram breeders. Breeding rams (and sometimes ewes) were tested and those with scrapie-susceptible genotypes were culled or castrated. The government scheme ended in early 2009 but testing is still available to breeders through commercial providers. A blood sample is collected from screened sheep for genotyping and at the same time an electronic intra-ruminal device with a unique identification number is administered to the animal to ensure a permanent means of identification. Hence the animal and its genetic profile can always be identified.

Scrapie containment and elimination in New Zealand

It is sometimes forgotten that scrapie actually occurred in sheep in New Zealand that were not held in quarantine. It is indeed fortunate that those occurrences were controlled and that the disease did not become established and endemic to New Zealand. As the majority of New Zealand's stud sheep were derived from source flocks in the UK during the 19th century, it is important to review these earlier sheep importations.

1. Scrapie in the UK

Scrapie is still diagnosed in sheep in the UK, but since 2003 there has been a noticeable decline in the number of sheep testing positive for scrapie and particularly in the number of clinical cases.

The Suffolk, a 19th-century breed development from the Southdown crossed with the Norfolk Horn, became the UK's most widely used mutton sire and is associated with an apparently high prevalence of the disease. This latter point is emphasised by the fact that scrapie was spread to several countries in the world by this breed during the mid-20th century (Table 21.5).

2. New Zealand sheep imports

We will never know why both New Zealand and Australia remained free from scrapie in spite of importing many of their establishment sheep from the United Kingdom, particularly from the early 1840s to 1950.

Many of the large sheep importations to New Zealand were Australian Merinos, bred in that country and arriving in New Zealand following the serious 1850 droughts of New South Wales and Victoria. There is no evidence that any of the Australian Merinos ever developed scrapie, although Saxony Merinos from Germany were used extensively at that time.

Many British breeds, including the English Leicester, Border Leicester, Lincoln, Shropshire, Scottish Blackface, Cotswold, Ryeland and so on, were imported. It will be obvious from this list that some of these breeds were not suitable in their new environment and died out (Evans, 1969). From early records there is no evidence of scrapie occurring in any of these sheep.

The main development of the New Zealand sheep industry, therefore, was through Australian Merinos, and by 1871 some 10 million sheep, only 2 million of which were in the North Island, were being farmed. The introduction of the mutton trade through refrigeration in the late 19th century brought about a dramatic change in the New Zealand sheep population. Merino numbers declined and the Romney Marsh, and for a time the Leicester and the Lincoln, became our basic breeds. Through its extension into the Perendales and Coopworths, the New Zealand Romney has continued to enjoy a secure and dominant position in the New Zealand sheep industry. From what has been stated above, it is quite likely that the Romney Marsh breed in the UK was free of scrapie at that time. Indeed it will be important to know what its susceptibility/resistance genotype is eventually shown to be.

It is also important to emphasise that although the Suffolk sheep of the UK were known to have some flocks that were, and still are, scrapie-infected, the breed was never used to any extent in New Zealand until well into the 20th century. The Suffolk was not imported into New Zealand until 1903. However, there is no record of the fate of this single animal, so it is generally recognised that the first New Zealand Suffolk sheep stud flock was established in 1913 from the importation of one ram and four ewes. By 1940 there were only nine small, registered flocks, which must have been free from scrapie. The breed remained in small numbers until the 1970s. The first appearance of scrapie in New Zealand was in a Suffolk ram in 1952, which had been imported into New Zealand in 1950.

3. Scrapie in New Zealand

Following the diagnosis of scrapie in an imported Suffolk ram near Ashburton by KG Haughey and AR Campbell in 1952, inadequate follow-up and quarantine resulted in scrapie appearing in Southland in 1954. A serious containment exercise ensued, which lasted for three years until eradication was declared. It involved the destruction of 4339 animals and the listing and movement control of stock from 191 farms for these three years. There are many local tales of this period: tempers were frayed and unfortunately the then Department of Agriculture did not gain popularity.

In 1976 and 1977 two cases of scrapie were again diagnosed, one in a Finn sheep and the other in an East Friesian sheep, both of which were among the four exotic breeds being multiplied in quarantine on Mana Island. Subsequent events led to the total curtailment of this exercise, with the destruction of several thousand sheep in quarantine on Mana Island and Crater Farm at Rotorua.

The lessons learned from both this experience and those of 1952 and 1954 have been echoed by authorities of the disease many times — the rule being that if you wish to avoid scrapie, don't import sheep from a country in which the disease is endemic.

Historical examples all support this conclusion, particularly with the 1972 importations in which sheep were gleaned from 23 farms in the UK. Although all properties were reported free from scrapie, the assurances of the owners were, in hindsight, worthless.

Region	Date	Breeds affected
North America		
Canada — Ontario	1938	Suffolk, imported from the UK
USA — Michigan	1947	Suffolk, from the UK and Canada
— California	1952	Suffolk, imported
— Ohio	1952	Suffolk, imported from Canada
— Many states	1960	Mainly Suffolk; also Cheviot, Hampshire and Montadale
South America		
Colombia	1968–1971	Hampshire and Dorset Down, imported from the UK
Brazil	1977	Hampshire Down (same flock of origin as in Colombia)
South Africa	1964–1972	Hampshire Down, imported from the UK
East Africa — Kenya	1970	Hampshire Down, imported from the UK
Australia	1952	Suffolk, imported from the UK
New Zealand	1952–1954	Suffolk, imported from the UK
India — Himalayan foothills	1940	Local mountain breed, with imported Rambouillet stock

Table 21.5 Recorded occurrences of natural scrapie outside Europe, 1930–1980. (Modified after Parry, 1983)

4. Later importations

The risk of scrapie emerging as a result of the importation of sheep, as embryos from Denmark and Finland in 1985 and 1986, was considered to be minimal. Previous experiences were used to establish a much sounder animal health base than had been the case in the past. The preparation and investigation for the Danish and Finnish quarantine procedure was more detailed and covered a wider body of opinion with respect to veterinary input. In contrast, with the first Quarantine Advisory Committee set up for the 1972 New Zealand imports no veterinarian was appointed until a late stage and after scrapie had actually been diagnosed on Mana Island.

The key assurance that the exporting countries (Denmark, Finland and Israel) were free from scrapie was further covered by a 5-year quarantine and also the proviso that should there be any reason to extend this, action would be taken. In addition, mesenteric lymph nodes were collected from donor ewes and inoculated into the cerebrum of sentinel sheep or goats. These sentinel animals were monitored for the duration of the quarantine period. More-recent import protocols include the collection of brain and spinal cord from donor ewes in addition to lymphatic tissue for inoculation into sentinel animals.

Scrapie freedom assurance in New Zealand and Australia

New Zealand and Australia now operate scrapie freedom assurance programmes with respect to all imports of exotic breeds of sheep. The programmes are based on the following summarised principles:

1. Sheep may only be imported from low-risk countries. Examples of such countries are Denmark, Finland, Sweden and Israel, from which successful importations have taken place.
2. Flocks of origin in these countries must be assured as being 'historically' free from scrapie. Obviously this follows from the above, but some 'low-risk' countries have in place scrapie control programmes based on regular flock inspections and tissue sampling.
3. Donor animals must be held in quarantine for the collection of the embryos. The embryos must be collected and washed to international standards.
4. The donors are destroyed and samples of their brain, spinal cord and lymphatic tissue are collected and inoculated into sentinel goats. Goats are preferred sentinels but sheep (scrapie-free, of course) may be used.
5. The embryos and tissue samples are transported to a primary quarantine facility in New Zealand and the embryos are transplanted into recipient ewes. Sentinel goats are also injected with donor material.
6. All the progeny derived from the imported embryos are held in quarantine along with the sentinel goats (or sheep) for 3½ years after the birth of the last lamb. During this holding phase, the embryos and semen may be transferred to a secondary quarantine station to enable the multiplication of progeny.

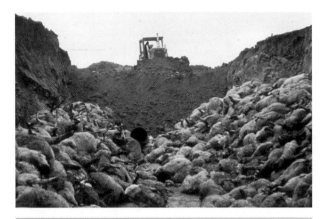

Figure 21.5 Burial of sheep on Mana Island following the diagnosis of scrapie while the sheep were in quarantine.

This assurance programme may be modified to suit the circumstances of specific countries, or changed in the light of new knowledge of the disease or the development of new diagnostic tests.

Norway 98/atypical scrapie

A different form of 'scrapie' was identified in Norway in 1998, and TSE surveillance programmes conducted by the European Union have confirmed the widespread nature of this form of scrapie. Many of the brain specimens diagnosed as positive have come from clinically normal sheep, which explains why the condition was previously undetected.

Norway 98/atypical scrapie differs from classical

scrapie in the following aspects:
- Age of onset — clinical cases of atypical scrapie are mainly over 5 years of age while some are up to 20 years old.
- The clinical signs are largely restricted to ataxia.
- There is no epidemiological information on its transmission and usually only 1 or 2 sheep are affected but in a large number of unrelated flocks.
- The histopathological changes in the brain have a different distribution.
- Unlike classical scrapie, sheep of 'scrapie'-resistant genotypes are susceptible to atypical scrapie (Table 21.6).

Based on clinical findings, pathology, biochemistry and epidemiology, it is considered that Norway 98/atypical scrapie is unrelated to classical scrapie. Instead it is considered to be a non-contagious, spontaneous degenerative condition of older sheep and occasionally goats (OIE, 2016).

Implications for New Zealand

Norway 98/atypical scrapie was diagnosed in Britain in 2007/08 in three sheep that had been derived from New Zealand and had been part of a closed flock used to study prion-type diseases. The sheep were in fact born in Britain but were descended from New Zealand stock. In 2009, the brain of a New Zealand sheep that was one of 200 sent to Europe to be used as scrapie-negative controls tested positive for Norway 98/atypical scrapie. Because this condition is considered to be unrelated to classical scrapie and there are no associated human health risks from it, the implications of this finding are considered minor.

Bovine spongiform encephalopathy

Origins of BSE and its transmission to cattle

After the first laboratory-confirmed cases of BSE were reported in 1986, an epidemiological study by Wilesmith of the first 200 cases indicated that the only factor common to all of them had been the feeding of commercial cattle feed concentrates containing meat and bone meal derived from slaughtered animals. This led to the possibility that BSE was caused by the sheep scrapie agent that had somehow been changed during the processing of the concentrate feed. It was suggested that this change to the agent may have begun in the late 1970s with an alteration to the food-processing system which was largely completed in 1981–1982. The alteration eliminated a solvent-extraction step and hence also eliminated a steam-stripping treatment. These conclusions led to a ban on feeding ruminant-carcass-based feeds to other ruminants.

There have been reservations about the hypothesis that sheep scrapie changed to BSE. Although the sheep scrapie prion and the cattle BSE prion differ at only 7 amino acid positions, the agent isolated from BSE cases in cattle and some other species has a different 'fingerprint' when inoculated into mice and compared with any of the known scrapie strains. Further, if scrapie-infected material is injected intracerebrally into cattle, a spongiform encephalopathy develops but the signs are not like those seen with BSE.

A view is also held that BSE in cattle may have existed

PrP genotype	No. of classical scrapie cases	No. of atypical scrapie cases
ARR/ARR	0	16
ARR/AHQ	0	40
ARR/ARH	0	1
ARR/ARQ	1	18
AHQ/AHQ	1	19
AHQ/ARH	0	3
AHQ/ARQ	4	31
ARH/ARH	0	0
ARH/ARQ	2	1
ARQ/ARQ	27	19
ARR/VRQ	40	0
VRQ/AHQ	0	0
VRQ/ARH	15	0
VRQ/ARQ	91	1
VRQ/VRQ	15	0

Table 21.6 Genotype profile of classical and atypical cases of scrapie detected from testing 205,677 active surveillance samples in the UK (as of December 2006).

for a very long time and at a clinically unrecognisable level, and that this infection was in some way exposed by the feeding of meat and bone meal.

Yet another possible explanation for the origins of the British BSE 'epidemic' has been given by the revelation that during the period 1970–1985 'thousands of tonnes' of African meat and bone meal were imported into the UK. It is possible that BSE might be a disease of a species such as the kudu which, on limited evidence, appears to be rather susceptible to BSE. Of eight kudu born at Regents Park Zoo in London since 1987, five have developed BSE. It may have been possible for an infected kudu carcass to have entered the animal food chain or have been included in meat and bone meal imported from Africa. This hypothesis is further supported by the argument that BSE will die out and cannot be sustained in cattle because it has a relatively low infectivity (an oral dose of about 1 g of terminally affected cattle brain is required for transmission), a low vertical transmission rate of about 10% (at worst) and an undetectable rate of horizontal transmission. Unfortunately, the source of the 1980s emergence of BSE may never be known for certain.

If the African meat and bone meal hypothesis is substantiated, it is a graphic example of the risk of trade in processed animal carcasses to be used as either feed or

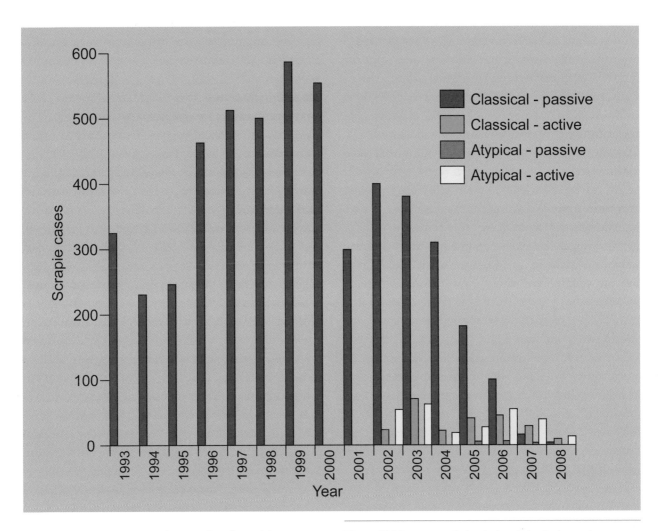

Passive surveillance: reporting and testing clinically suspicious cases. Active surveillance: testing cull animals at slaughter. This was introduced in 2002; the number of animals tested each year varies according to EU requirements so this affects the number of positive cases detected.

Figure 21.6 Summary of classical and atypical scrapie cases in sheep in Great Britain up to 31 December 2008, detected by passive and active surveillance. (Source: Veterinary Laboratories Agency)

fertiliser. In this respect it is worth remembering that meat and bone meal from India was reputed to have been the cause of anthrax in New Zealand in 1895 and later recrudescences of earlier infections from the bone dust source.

The transmission of BSE via cattle semen

Analysis of artificial insemination records of cattle in the UK show that there is no greater incidence of BSE among the offspring of bulls with the disease than among the offspring of healthy bulls. There was one case of BSE in every 156 offspring of BSE-infected bulls compared with one in every 126 offspring of non-infected bulls. These data were from 3889 progeny of diseased bulls and 23,319 progeny of healthy bulls.

In addition, BSE infectivity has never been demonstrated in semen using mouse bioassay (although mouse bioassay may be 500 times less sensitive than cattle bioassay). Further, BSE has occurred in a number of countries other than the UK, and there are no instances where this has been attributed to the use of semen imported from the UK. The Office International des Epizooties (OIE) now consider semen 'safe' for trade purposes.

The transmission of BSE via cattle embryos

An extensive experimental trial conducted over a 7-year period was completed in the UK in 2001. The trial aimed to test the possibility of the transfer of BSE infection via the embryo. In it, 167 cows with clinical BSE were artificially inseminated with semen from 13 bulls and 8 with clinical BSE. Later, 587 of the resultant viable embryos were transferred singly into 347 recipient heifers imported from BSE-free New Zealand; 266 live offspring were born of which 54% had a BSE-positive sire and a BSE-positive dam. Both the recipients and the offspring were monitored for clinical signs of BSE for 7 years after transfer: 27 of the recipients and 20 of the offspring died while under surveillance but showed neither clinical nor necropsy signs of BSE. In addition, extensive mouse inoculation experiments were conducted and all tests were negative for BSE infectivity. It was concluded that embryos are unlikely to carry BSE even if collected from animals at the end stage of the disease.

BSE incidence

BSE cases continue to fall as the ban on feeding ruminant protein to animals takes full effect.

From a peak of over 37,000 cases in 1992, there has been a large decrease in the number of cases of BSE in the UK such that in 2008 there were only 37 test-positive cattle — this figure includes clinical cases and non-clinical cases detected during active abattoir surveillance (Figure 21.7). In the 8 years from 2009 to 2016, 39 cases were confirmed via passive and active surveillance. The number of cases of BSE (excluding atypical BSE) in countries other than the UK, and the year the last case was detected, is detailed in Table 21.7.

From 1996 to 2008, schemes existed in the UK to prevent meat from cattle born before August 1996, and meat from older cattle, from entering the human food chain. These restrictions have now been lifted but active and passive surveillance testing is ongoing.

Clinical signs of BSE

Bovine spongiform encephalopathy is characterised by progressive neurological signs in affected cattle. The first sign is often a subtle mood change, with normally quiet cattle becoming noticeably more aggressive. Affected cows are hyperaesthetic and startle easily. This is followed by development of gait abnormalities and a progressive ataxia. High-stepping is a common feature combined with swaying of the hindquarters.

In the early stages BSE must be differentiated from hypomagnesaemia, the nervous form of ketosis and listeriosis. However, unlike metabolic diseases, BSE is progressive and signs will worsen despite treatment. In addition to the above it has been reported that non-responsive downer cows should also be considered as suspect BSE cases, especially if one or both hind legs are extended backwards.

It should be noted that the so-called 'typical' cases of BSE frequently shown on television are rare. The neurological signs fall into four categories:
- Changes in mental state, commonly seen as apprehension, aggression, nervousness, persistent licking of the flank or nose and teeth grinding.
- Abnormalities of posture and movement manifested as hind-limb ataxia, tremors and falling.
- Changes in sensation exhibited as hyperaesthesia to touch and sound.
- Non-responsive downer cows.

Variant Creutzfeldt-Jakob disease and BSE

From research published from October 1996 onwards, scientific evidence has been accumulating that BSE infectivity and vCJD infectivity carry the same 'fingerprint'. The evidence is consistent with the transmissibility of BSE infectivity to humans and, taken in conjunction with related circumstances such as the BSE epidemic in cattle, increases the likelihood of a causal connection.

Approximately 168 vCJD cases were reported between 1996 and 2008 in the UK. Predictions of the likely number of future cases is difficult because basic information such as the incubation period, infectious dose and even route of exposure are all unknown. An epidemiological investigation of a cluster of five cases in Queniborough, central England, indicated that people who developed vCJD were 15 times more likely to have eaten beef from a

Country	Total number BSE cases to end of 2016	Year in which last case was reported
Austria	6	2007
Belgium	133	2006
Canada	21	2015
Czech Republic	30	2009
Denmark	16	2009
Finland	1	2000
France	1021	2016
Germany	419	2009
Greece	1	2001
Ireland	1678	2015
Israel	1	2002
Italy	144	2009
Japan	36	2009
Liechtenstein	2	1998
Luxembourg	3	2002
Netherlands	87	2010
Poland	73	2013
Portugal	1083	2014
Slovakia	25	2010
Slovenia	8	2007
Spain	779	2011
Sweden	1	2006
Switzerland	464	2006

Table 21.7 Number of cases of BSE in countries other than the UK up to 31 December 2016, excluding atypical BSE cases. (Source: OIE website; www.oie.int)

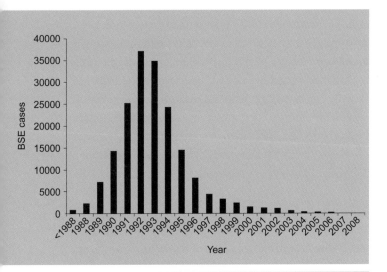

Figure 21.7 Number of cases of BSE in the United Kingdom detected by passive and active surveillance, up to 31 December 2008.

butcher who removed the cow's brain than were people in a population used as a control. It was suggested that the incubation period for vCJD in humans could be between 10 and 16 years.

Chronic wasting disease of deer

The emergence of BSE and other diseases in the TSE group raises the importance of chronic wasting disease (CWD) of elk and deer. Currently CWD exists in free-ranging Rocky Mountain elk, mule-deer, white-tailed deer and black-tailed deer. It is endemic in Colorado, Wyoming, southwestern Nebraska, South Dakota, Wisconsin and New Mexico in the USA and Saskatchewan in Canada. These states/provinces plus Oklahoma, Montana, Ontario, Alberta and Saskatchewan have seen cases of CWD in captive cervids. It has now also been confirmed in South Korea in captive deer imported from Canada. In 2016 it was identified in a small number of reindeer and moose in Norway.

The cause of CWD is currently unknown, but it is thought to be an infection of abnormal prions similar to other TSEs. Its mode of transmission is also uncertain, but in an outbreak in captive Rocky Mountain elk transmission appeared to be from animal to animal within a herd, without preference for spread by dam to offspring. It is thought that the CWD 'agent' is passed in saliva, faeces and/or urine and is transmitted by a faecal–oral route, and it is considered to be one of the most infectious of the TSE diseases. The disease has a natural incubation period of 1.5–3 years before the onset of clinical signs.

So far no evidence for the natural transmission of CWD to other species has been found. Cattle, sheep and goats have resided in research facilities together with CWD-affected animals for prolonged periods without developing the disease. However, experiments on the transmissibility of CWD to other species are ongoing and it is recommended that all meat and other offal from affected deer must not be used as food.

The clinical signs of CWD include emaciation, excessive salivation, behavioural changes such as loss of fear for humans, ataxia, head and ears drooping, weakness, increased thirst and urination, secondary pneumonia and trauma-induced lesions. Pathological lesions of the central nervous system are similar to other TSEs in that the disease causes degenerative changes to the brain, including vacuolation.

A confirmed diagnosis of CWD is made by necropsy examination of the brain tissue, immunohistochemistry to look for protease-resistant prion protein (PrPres) and/or Western immunoblotting.

Control of the disease in North American countries has been based on identification, isolation and slaughter of CWD-affected and contact animals.

Spongiform encephalopathies in domestic cats and exotic species

The diagnosis of feline spongiform encephalopathy in domestic cats is another example of the spread of BSE to another species. Transmission of these diseases between species, as we have seen above, is a reality even though the transmission tends to be 'inefficient', resulting in prolonged incubation periods relative to those following transmission within the 'original' species. The concern to a BSE-free country such as New Zealand is the negative publicity that accompanies a report of any TSE in animals and the risk of that disease being transferred to our cattle population via a TSE-infected animal. While cats imported directly from the UK pose the greatest risk, New Zealand also sources pet food from a number of overseas countries.

The Ministry for Primary Industries has alerted New Zealand veterinarians to this risk. Tables 21.8 and 21.9 detail cases of spongiform encephalopathies diagnosed in domestic cats and other exotic species in the UK.

The association of TSEs with human disease in recent years has stimulated an enormous amount of research into their biological nature and means of control. It is to be remembered that scrapie, the prototype TSE, has been endemic in some countries for centuries without known association with human disease. The relationship between BSE of cattle and vCJD in humans has raised the spectre of it 'back-crossing' into sheep (based on the scrapie theory of origin) and becoming a disaster to the sheep industry. Experimentally, sheep can be infected with BSE-infected meat and bone meal and develop clinical disease similar to scrapie. Of concern is the more extensive distribution of the BSE agent in artificially infected sheep compared with that in cattle. This means that it would be more difficult to ensure human safety by removing specified risk materials from the food chain were BSE to occur in sheep. However, there is confidence that international regulatory measures will prevent the spread of BSE beyond Europe and reduce the risk of contamination of the human food chain. Further, rapid advances in molecular biology have already given a better understanding of these diseases and will continue to do so.

Bluetongue

Bluetongue is a viral disease, primarily of sheep and cattle, which is transmitted by *Culicoides* midges. The disease is characterised by inflammation of the mucous membranes of the digestive and respiratory tracts, necrosis of skeletal muscles, placentitis, abortion and foetal malformation. Following the acute disease, surviving animals have a protracted convalescence. There are over 20 different serotypes of the virus, not all of which are pathogenic for sheep.

History

The virus of bluetongue, in common with the aetiological agent of African horse sickness, would appear to have originated in the African continent where it adapted itself to both vertebrate and invertebrate hosts.

With the introduction of highly susceptible Merino and

Diagnosis	No. of cases	Dates affected
Kudu	6	-
Gemsbok	1	1987
Nyala	1	1986
Oryx	2	1989–1992
Eland	6	1989–1995
Cheetah	5	1992–1998
Puma	3	1992–1999
Tiger	3	1995–1999
Ocelot	3	1994–1999
Bison (*Bison bison*)	1	1996
Ankole Cow	2	199?–1995
Lion	5	1995–2007

Table 21.8 Spongiform encephalopathies diagnosed in exotic species in the UK.

Cheetah total excludes one in Australia and one in the Republic of Ireland (both of these were litter mates born in Great Britain), and another two in France which were also born in Great Britain.

Year reported	No. of cases
1990	12
1991	12
1992	10
1993	11
1994	16
1995	8
1996	6
1997	6
1998	4
1999	2
2000	1
2001	1

Table 21.9 Spongiform encephalopathies diagnoses in domestic cats in the UK. (Source: Defra UK)

European breeds of sheep into the Cape Colony, at first by the Dutch East India Company between 1652 and 1783, and later in 1870, what may be presumed to have been accidental transmission by insects led to the recognition of the disease. A report dated 1876 referred to a febrile disease of sheep with morbidity of 30% and high mortality. The disease was recognised by soreness of the mouth and feet and was prevalent in low-lying areas.

Geographical distribution and spread

For many years it was accepted that the disease was confined to the African continent and existed in the following countries: Morocco, the Sudan, Chad, Nigeria, Central African Republic, Kenya, Tanzania, Zambia, Zimbabwe, Malawi, Namibia and South Africa.

The realisation that the serotypes of bluetongue virus vary considerably in virulence for sheep and other ruminants, and that mild and almost inapparent infection may occur, suggests that the disease may have prevailed at odd times outside of Africa. The first outbreak of this nature was in Cyprus in 1943 but it was considered that the disease had been present in a mild form since 1924.

A similar state of affairs seems to have existed in other countries such as Palestine and Syria, where bluetongue was diagnosed in 1943. Subsequently the disease has been recognised over a wide range of countries, including Turkey in 1944, and in the state of Texas in the USA in 1948. In the latter country the disease had spread to California by 1952 and by 1960 was present in 11 states. The disease is now widespread in the USA and bluetongue viral antibodies have been isolated from cattle, sheep, goats and wild ruminants in many states.

In 1956, the disease entered the continent of Europe where it was recognised in Portugal in both sheep and cattle. In the same year it was recorded in Spain. In 1959, bluetongue was diagnosed in Damani sheep in West Pakistan and later typical bluetongue occurred in the highly susceptible Merino sheep.

The first appearance of bluetongue in Japan was in cattle in 1959; there the disease was quite virulent and is said to have caused great havoc in the southern regions of the country. In India, an outbreak of bluetongue occurred in sheep in 1967 and goats and dairy cattle were also found to be seropositive.

Bluetongue virus was isolated from *Culicoides* midges in Australia in 1975, but clinical disease was not associated with the isolation. The virus was designated a new serotype and was shown experimentally to be moderately pathogenic for sheep. Serological surveys in Eastern Australia in 1978 and 1979 showed that bovine sera contained antibodies but clinical disease appeared to be rare, particularly in sheep. This may be because of the large cattle population, as *Culicoides* prefer to feed on cattle; the timing of shearing, as *Culicoides* prefer freshly shorn sheep; and the predominant breed of sheep (Merinos are less susceptible than British breeds).

Since 2006 bluetongue has been reported in Northern Europe. Typing of the virus suggests that its likely source of origin was sub-Saharan Africa, but it is unknown how it was introduced into Northern Europe. The first cases were reported in the Netherlands, resulting in up to 15% mortality in some flocks, and subsequently the disease was diagnosed in neighbouring regions of Belgium, France and Germany. In 2007, the disease spread rapidly through Northern Europe and it has been estimated that vector movement allowed it to spread an average of 16 km per week. In some affected flocks, up to 70% morbidity and 50% mortality rates were recorded. A worrying aspect of these outbreaks was that cattle, previously generally considered symptomless carriers of the virus, were also severely affected with up to 50% morbidity in some herds. Clinical signs of bluetongue were also seen in goats. In 2008, vaccination programmes became widespread and reduced the number of reported cases in most countries. In the UK, bluetongue was first reported in a cow in eastern England in September 2007 and was believed to have been introduced by airborne virus-infected midges from northern Europe. In eastern and southern England the spread of disease was rapid, although following the introduction of voluntary vaccination in 2008 the only cases reported in 2008 were in imported animals. Clinical cases in the UK were generally mild, but the restrictions on animal movement imposed by the disease resulted in economic losses.

Some species of *Culicoides* could possibly establish and survive in New Zealand. It is important to realise that the *Culicoides* species acting as vectors in northern Europe, including the UK, are different from the species in southern Europe and Africa (*C. pulicaris* and *C. obsoletus* vs *C. imicola*). Certification of freedom from bluetongue is required for the export of sheep meat and other sheep products.

Economic significance

It has been estimated by Blajan (1987) that bluetongue costs the world several billion US dollars annually. Dr Gareth Bath from South Africa has listed the economic effects of bluetongue as follows:

1. Deaths in unvaccinated flocks may be up to 20%. In European outbreaks, mortalities up to 50% have occurred.
2. Survivors have reduced weight gain, poor milk production and fleece-shedding.
3. Survivors are more susceptible to secondary disease.
4. Higher feed costs due to later marketing of sheep and sometimes downgrading of carcasses due to muscle damage.
5. Decreased reproductive performance due to temporary infertility of rams and, in ewes, poor conception, resorption, abortion or congenital malformation.
6. Suboptimal management procedures forced on the farmer to reduce the impact of bluetongue.
7. Costs incurred by control measures.
8. Zoosanitary procedures in force in many countries to prevent the entry of bluetongue or new strains of the disease.

As pointed out by Bath, the economic impact of bluetongue in a country depends on several factors. Those listed below would have particular significance for Australia and New Zealand.

1. The number of susceptible sheep, mainly breeds of European origin.
2. The number and prevalence of virulent bluetongue strains.
3. The suitability of the environment for the multiplication of bluetongue vectors.
4. The availability of primary virus multiplication hosts, i.e. cattle (most important), goats and wild game.

Epidemiology

The bluetongue viruses are arboviruses classified as *Orbivirus*. They are transmitted by biting midges, *Culicoides* spp. While living in the midge, the virus multiplies repeatedly. It is possible that other biting arthropods are capable of transmitting the virus mechanically, but the only one so far shown to be able to do so is the sheep ked *Melophagus ovinus*. The virus may also be transmitted by using the same needle on a number of sheep during a vaccination procedure. There is also evidence for transplacental transmission.

The virus infects sheep, cattle and wild ruminants. Goats may also become infected but appear far less susceptible than sheep. Sheep are not the preferred host for *Culicoides* and the virus multiplication will occur in a cycle between *Culicoides* and cattle (or game) long before the disease is seen in sheep. Its appearance in sheep is before the end of summer, when vector numbers are so high that secondary hosts like sheep are bitten.

European sheep breeds are most susceptible. Cattle are the main reservoir host and develop infections sometimes characterised by latency and periodic viraemia.

Pathogenesis

After inoculation of the bluetongue virus by the biting midge, the virus multiplies in lymph nodes draining the site of entry. This is followed by a viraemia and further dissemination of the virus throughout the body. At the peak of the viraemia, in sheep and cattle the fever is at its peak and the animals show a marked leucopenia. The incubation period following natural infection is believed to be in the region of 6–7 days.

The bluetongue virus has a high affinity for red blood cells and can persist in them for weeks. Following multiplication in lymphocytes, macrophages and the endothelial linings of blood vessels, characteristic lesions consisting of fluid exudation and many small haemorrhages develop. The virus can be transferred to the foetus via the placenta, causing death and malformation.

Clinical features

Bluetongue is essentially a seasonal disease, usually appearing from mid-summer and continuing through autumn until winter when insect activity becomes minimal. The manifestations of bluetongue can be very variable between areas, flocks, animals, seasons and different serotypes of the virus. It is therefore essential to look for disease signs and not the classical description of the disease alone. The disease becomes much more severe when sheep are exposed to direct sunlight and heat.

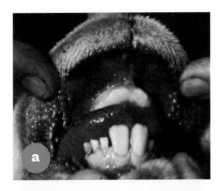
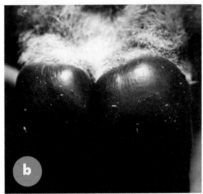

Figure 21.8 Bluetongue showing the swollen, reddened (a) lips and tongue and (b) coronets.

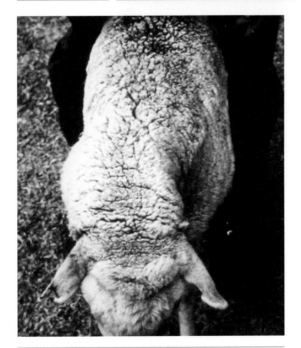

Figure 21.9 Torticollis as a result of bluetongue. (Photograph courtesy G Bath, South Africa)

In classical bluetongue, high fevers of 40.6–42°C occur. Hyperaemia and congestion of the visible mucosae around the nose, mouth and coronets closely resembles photosensitisation. Oedema of the face, ears, eyelids, lips and tongue may be inapparent to severe. Oedema of the lungs is very common and may result in dyspnoea and froth in the trachea. Ocular, nasal and oral discharges often form crusts which become infected. Haemorrhages appear in the mucous membranes of the mouth, and occasionally in severe cases the tongue becomes markedly swollen and oedematous and even protrudes from the mouth. It may be dark blue in colour (hence the name bluetongue) and the anterior part may be almost wholly stripped of its epithelium. There may also be lameness with reddening of the coronary band. Clinical signs indicative of muscular degeneration may occur and are recognised by extreme weakness, prostration and rapid emaciation. Haemorrhagic diarrhoea may develop, which is a poor prognostic sign.

In cases that survive for several days to weeks, the oedema, hyperaemia, pyrexia and ulcerations may disappear or become mild. Crusts about the nose and haemorrhages in the hooves may be the only remaining signs. Further signs that may develop in chronic cases are inhalation pneumonia, wool break and fleece shedding, hoof separation and wry neck (torticollis).

In some cases, especially young sheep and exotic breeds, the disease results in rapid death and no clinical signs may be seen. A number of sheep are infected without any visible signs, although these cases are usually febrile at some stage.

Prognosis

In mild cases the prognosis is generally favourable and recovery is usually rapid except for loss of condition. In severe cases the prognosis should be guarded. Animals that appear to be recovering may suddenly collapse and die. Depending on the degree of the buccal lesions and muscular involvement, animals may become very weak and debilitated and subjected to parasitism. Lambs especially take a long time to recover.

Under average field conditions the mortality rate usually varies between 2% and 30%. Most deaths occur from 1–8 days after the appearance of clinical signs. Lung oedema is a very common cause of death.

Pathology and diagnosis

In sheep the postmortem lesions vary greatly depending on the strain of the virus, the severity of the disease and the stage of the syndrome. The changes that occur are indicative of a severe inflammatory process. The oral and nasal mucosae are primarily affected and become oedematous, hyperaemic, haemorrhagic and ulcerated. The excoriations of the oral epithelium are covered with grey necrotic material. The tongue and mucous membranes of the mouth become swollen and may be dark blue.

Aspiration pneumonia is commonly seen, as is degeneration of the skeletal musculature. The lymph nodes draining the head are usually oedematous and haemorrhagic. The hyperaemia of the skin may be patchy, resulting in irregular crusty exanthematous areas and a localised dermatitis; generalised flushing of the skin may also occur and excoriations may develop on parts of the body that are subject to abrasion.

In pregnant animals there is a haemorrhagic necrotic placentitis. Depending on the stage of gestation, transplacental infection of the foetus may result in foetal death or an inflammatory reaction of the meninges and brain tissue, as well as developmental abnormalities.

Serum haematology and biochemistry reveal severe leucopenia involving lymphocytes and neutrophils, and elevated aspartate transaminase (AST) and creatinine phosphokinase (CPK) due to muscle damage. Antibodies can be demonstrated by a number of serological tests of which an enzyme-linked immunosorbent assay (ELISA) test is the most recognised. Polymerase chain reaction (PCR) has also been developed.

Control

The control of bluetongue requires consideration of the reservoirs of the virus, the vectors and the host animals. Because the virus has a wide host range and is transmitted by insects, control measures are based primarily on immunisation of susceptible animals and the prevention of contact with insect vectors. Attenuated vaccines are available and used extensively, but the existence of a variety of serotypes makes prophylactic immunisation difficult. Pregnant ewes, particularly those in the first trimester of pregnancy, should not be vaccinated.

In endemic situations, control is aimed at either lowering the chances of infection of the susceptible population or increasing its resistance to the disease. However, in the outbreaks of bluetongue in the UK surveillance areas were set up around infected properties; legislation allowed for movement restrictions within these areas and large numbers of animals were vaccinated with a multivalent vaccine.

Strategies to reduce the risk to susceptible sheep include early shearing so that there is reasonable wool coverage during the risk period, and avoiding grazing sheep in high-risk areas. The midges only feed at night and rarely come indoors, so stabling sheep at night is useful. Sheep can be grazed with cattle, and insecticidal ear tags or sprays may be used. Some sheep breeds are more resistant to the disease than others. In Africa the indigenous breeds such as the Ronderib Afrikander and the Namaqua sheep and similar breeds like the Black Head Persian, the Karakul and the Dorper are more resistant than other breeds.

Ovine enzootic abortion

New Zealand is fortunate to be free of enzootic abortion of ewes (EAE, chlamydial abortion), caused by a mammalian strain of *Chlamydophila (Chlamydia) abortus*. This organism can cause serious abortion problems in sheep. Australia is also free from the disease, but it is endemic in many sheep-raising countries of the world including the UK, Europe, the Middle East, South Africa and North America. Although the risk of introduction to New Zealand is not high, live sheep imported from anywhere other than Australia must be tested negative to *C. abortus* using the complement fixation test (CFT) before importation, and prior to use as embryo collection donors.

Chlamydophila abortus is zoonotic and can cause a serious flu-like disease and abortion in humans.

Transmission

The organism is present in infected placentae, foetuses and uterine fluids. Ewes that have previously aborted are immune to further enzootic abortions but may continue to shed *C. abortus* in vaginal discharges. The organism is transferred to uninfected animals by ingestion or inhalation of contaminated dust or fluid droplets. Susceptible pregnant ewes will abort if they are infected before the last month of pregnancy. Infection of ewes in late pregnancy means they will abort late in their next pregnancy. Ewe lambs may become infected *in utero* or during the neonatal period, and in some surviving ewe lambs the infection may lie dormant until they in turn abort during their first pregnancy. Rams are not thought to be involved in the transmission of the infection.

Clinical signs and diagnosis

The disease is characterised by abortion in the last 3 weeks of pregnancy, stillbirths or birth of weak lambs that may die soon after birth. Some infected ewes give birth to normal live lambs. Epidemiologically, the disease resembles campylobacteriosis in many ways. The ewe may develop a blood-stained vaginal discharge but remains otherwise healthy. Occasionally the placenta is retained and an associated metritis develops. Occasionally embryonic and foetal loss may be attributed to enzootic abortion.

Abortion rates in previously uninfected flocks may be 30% or higher. In partially immune flocks the abortion rate is around 5%. Affected sheep become immune after abortion. If this disease were to occur in New Zealand, it would have severe effects on individual farmers.

Pathology and diagnosis

Placentitis of variable severity is seen as discolouration and necrosis of cotyledons and oedema and thickening of the intercotyledonary tissue. The aborted foetus may have inflammatory foci in the liver, lungs and brain and the liver is often congested and ruptured during parturition. Diagnosis is by microscopy of suspect placentae or uterine discharges using a modified Ziehl-Neelson stain, PCR of tissue, CFT or ELISA testing of paired sera or isolation of the organism in embryonated eggs.

Control

During an abortion outbreak, routine hygiene procedures will help reduce the contamination. These include disposing of aborted materials and isolating affected ewes and their lambs. Long-acting oxytetracycline administered to ewes around 3 weeks pre-lambing will not eliminate the abortion problem, but may delay abortion and increase the proportion of viable lambs born.

The disease is usually introduced into a flock by the introduction of purchased sheep. Thus, it can be controlled by maintaining a closed flock or only purchasing replacements from accredited sources. A live vaccine is available and gives long-term protection following a single dose. A killed vaccine is also available. Vaccination will not prevent abortion in sheep already infected from the previous lambing time.

Were enzootic abortion to occur in New Zealand, confirmed cases would be dealt with primarily by quarantine and slaughter of infected animals. Overseas, vaccination is used.

Foot and mouth disease (FMD)

Foot and mouth disease is one of the most contagious diseases of domestic animals and affects all cloven-hooved animals. It is characterised by the formation of vesicles and erosions of the mouth, nose, feet and teats, although in sheep the clinical signs tend to be subtle. Foot and mouth disease is not usually fatal but it causes considerable production losses.

Of all the exotic diseases, FMD probably poses the greatest threat to New Zealand's agricultural industry. An outbreak would halt all exportation of animal products due to trade prohibitions or restrictions. Importation of the disease could conceivably occur (in order of likelihood) via refuse from ships or aircraft, illegal entry of infected animal products, or overseas travellers with contaminated clothing or footwear. It is probable that the disease would first occur in pigs following swill feeding of infected animal products.

To give an indication of the impact that an incursion of FMD might have on a country, during 2001 the United Kingdom experienced the worst outbreak of the disease in modern history. The index case occurred on a pig farm that practised swill feeding. It took nearly a year for official eradication, and during that time at least 4 million farm animals were slaughtered and disposed of. The outbreak was estimated to cost the government in excess of £8 billion. The size of the epidemic was due to a combination of events, including a delay in the diagnosis of the index case, the movement of infected sheep to market before the disease was first diagnosed, and the time of year. The virus was introduced at a time when there were many sheep movements around the country and weather conditions supported its survival.

Aetiology and distribution

The disease is caused by a *Picornavirus*, genus *Aphthovirus*.

There are seven distinct virus types, and each type is further subdivided into subtypes. It occurs in many parts of the world, including Africa, South America, the Middle East and Central Asia, with sporadic outbreaks occurring in many other countries, usually following accidental or illegal importation of infected animal products.

Epidemiology and transmission

The virus is relatively robust and may survive for long periods in infected animal products or in aerosols. It is sensitive to changes in pH and is inactivated by both acid and alkaline solutions. The virus is highly contagious and rapid transmission may occur, primarily by the respiratory route or following ingestion. Thus transmission could occur by contact with infected animals, by mechanical means such as vehicles, fomites and human activity, or by aerosol spread.

Infected animals shed virus in every body secretion and from clinical lesions. Viral excretion may occur for up to 4 days prior to the development of clinical disease, meaning that significant transmission can occur before the infection is detected. Pigs act as important amplifier hosts by excreting large amounts of virus, which may be spread by the airborne route. Sheep generally do not show dramatic clinical signs, and movement of clinically infected sheep with inapparent infections may help disseminate the disease. During the 2001 outbreak in the United Kingdom sheep were described as 'silent spreaders' of the disease.

Clinical signs

The incubation period of the disease is 2–8 days. The severity varies depending on the strain of the virus.

In sheep the clinical signs are mild and may be difficult to detect. Generally the first sign that is observed is lameness and the affected feet are hot and painful. There may be vesicles in the interdigital space, at the bulbs of the heel and along the coronary band. Affected animals are often febrile, although this is not always the case. Vesicles in the mouth are unusual and tend to heal rapidly. Those that do occur are usually on the caudal tongue and hard palate. Occasionally vesicles may form on the teats, vulva or prepuce. Sheep are sometimes described as 'silent shedders' due to the relative difficulty in detecting clinical signs in this species. The large FMD outbreak in the United Kingdom in 2001 emphasised the important role that

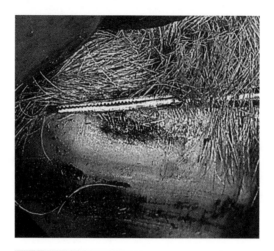

Figure 21.10 Foot and mouth disease in sheep, showing a small vesicle on the coronet.

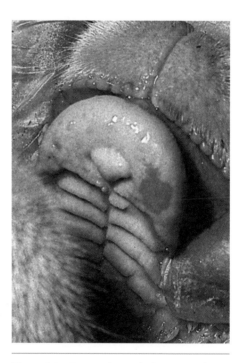

Figure 21.11 Foot and mouth disease in sheep, showing a ruptured vesicle on the dental pad.

Printed from the British MAFF book *Foot and Mouth Disease Ageing of Lesions* published by MAFF via Her Majesty's Stationery Office (HMSO). Crown copyright material is reproduced with the permission of the Controller of Her Majesty's Stationery Office.

sheep can play in the spread of this disease.

The disease in pigs and cattle tends to be more severe and is characterised by fever, anorexia, depression and the development of fluid-filled vesicles on the mouth and feet. The vesicles rapidly increase in size and rupture, leaving raw areas. Inappetence and lameness result in a considerable loss of condition. Vesicles may also form on the teats or vulva. Mortality is uncommon in adult animals.

Diagnosis

Foot and mouth disease should be suspected in any investigation where vesicles are a feature. Laboratory tests are required for confirmation and identification of the virus types involved. Confirmation is based on the recovery of the virus from vesicular fluids and epithelial tissue associated with the lesions, and detection of antigen or antibodies using serological tests such as ELISA. Due to the subtlety of clinical signs in sheep, ELISA testing is an important diagnostic aid.

Control

In countries where the disease is not endemic, outbreaks are dealt with in the first instance by eradication. This involves quarantine of infected properties and slaughter of affected animals and in-contact animals. On these properties, the premises are disinfected and not re-stocked for a defined period (usually 6 months). Control and movement-control areas are designated around the quarantine area to ban or restrict movement of susceptible livestock. Intense monitoring of at-risk herds and flocks is undertaken to detect any spread of disease. Gatherings of livestock, for example at sale yards, is banned. It is possible that tactical vaccination of susceptible animals in an area may also be used to help contain the disease.

Maedi-visna

Maedi-visna (maedi, progressive pneumonia) is a multi-organ disease of sheep caused by a lentivirus of the retrovirus family. Maedi is an Icelandic word meaning dyspnoea, and the name is now used internationally to describe a slowly progressive interstitial pneumonia of adult sheep. Visna means wasting, and is the name of a slowly progressive encephalomyelitis of adult sheep. The virus may also cause arthritis and mastitis. In general it is accepted that maedi-visna virus has a worldwide distribution, New Zealand and Australia being the only major sheep-raising countries where lentivirus infection has not been detected in sheep.

History

The history of the occurrence of maedi-visna in Iceland has some significant aspects with respect to the spread of slow virus diseases. It was in Iceland that the disease was first described as such, and it was the Icelanders Sigurdsson, Thormar and Palsson who first isolated the virus and later showed that maedi and visna were different manifestations of the same virus infections.

In 1933, Karakul sheep from Halle in East Germany were introduced to Iceland. The flock had originated in Buckara in Russia. As far as is known, no losses from diseases resembling maedi-visna or jaagziekte had ever been observed in the source flock in Germany. After a 2-month quarantine in Iceland the sheep, which were all healthy, were distributed to 14 farms in different parts of the country. With this importation maedi was without doubt introduced into Iceland. At least two of the rams in the imported flock carried the infection and gave rise to epizootics in two widely separated regions of the country, starting from farms where these rams were kept.

As well as maedi-visna, other contagious diseases previously not reported in Iceland have also been unintentionally introduced. These diseases are jaagziekte (sheep pulmonary adenomatosis, see later), Johne's disease and possibly scrapie.

Due to difficulties in diagnosis and masking by other diseases, maedi was not recognised until 6 years after the importation of the affected rams. By then the disease was widespread in many farms. Visna was first observed some years later than maedi and was found only in sheep flocks where maedi had already been causing losses for some years. Later it was shown that in sheep affected naturally with maedi, virus could also be demonstrated in the central nervous system of 25% of the autopsied animals.

Transmission

Sheep infected with maedi-visna virus are capable of transmitting the infection irrespective of the status of the disease. Transmission in a flock is predominantly between the ewes and their lambs by infected mononuclear cells in colostrum or milk. Horizontal transmission by aerosol does occur, especially in housed sheep, and transmission via respiratory secretions increases when sheep are co-infected with jaagziekte. Other pulmonary infections may also increase the horizontal transmission.

Intrauterine transmission can occur, but is rare. Transmission via ova or sperm cells has not been known. Cross-species transmission is very rare under natural conditions, but goat kids fed milk infected with maedi-visna virus become infected and lambs fed milk infected with caprine arthro-encephalitis virus become infected.

Maedi-visna is always introduced to a clean flock by an infected animal, e.g. the Karakul rams introduced into Icelandic sheep flocks and the horizontal transmission by ram-circles in Norway. Iatrogenic transmission can be prevented when one needle per animal is used for blood sampling procedures.

Clinical signs

Maedi

The clinical signs of maedi appear only in adult sheep, usually older than 3–4 years. The first sign is usually a slowly advancing listlessness and loss of condition. These signs are usually seen in pregnant or lactating ewes, and often become apparent when the sheep have been exposed to stress such as inclement weather.

An early sign is dyspnoea, particularly after exertion. The respiration becomes very rapid and shallow and the rate may be 80–120/min. As the disease progresses, the respiration even at rest becomes gradually more laboured. In contrast to jaagziekte, maedi never produces an appreciable amount of pulmonary fluid.

Ewes affected with maedi often give birth to small, weak lambs and their milk production is decreased.

Abortion may be seen in advanced cases. The progression of the disease may be delayed by good husbandry (i.e. feeding), but ultimately it becomes fatal. Sheep frequently succumb to secondary infections such as bacterial pneumonia. Affected sheep may survive 3–8 months after the first signs are noticed.

Visna

Visna, like maedi, is never found in sheep under 2 years of age. One of the first signs noticed is lagging behind the mob when the mob or flock is driven. Another early sign is a slight aberration of gait, especially in the hindquarters, in sheep made to trot. Gradually, stumbling and weakness of the hind-limbs becomes apparent.

At the same time there is a loss of weight and later the ability to extend the fetlocks is impaired, usually in one hind-limb before the other. Often sheep may be seen resting the distal end of the metatarsus of the affected limb on the ground. The paresis of the limbs progresses slowly and affected sheep tend to lie down even when grazing. Sometimes the disease progresses in waves with slight intervening remissions, but gradually the animal becomes paralytic in spite of remaining alert throughout. The course of the clinical disease is protracted; usually several months to a year may elapse before the stage of paraplegia is reached.

Pathology

Maedi

In maedi the lesions are confined to the thoracic cavity, except for those secondary to emaciation. The lungs are increased in size and, depending on the age of the lesions, may be 2–3 times the weight of normal lungs. The lung colour varies from dull greyish blue to greyish brown. Affected lungs are solid to the touch and the lesions are usually diffuse. The tracheobronchial and mediastial lymph nodes are always enlarged.

Histologically there is a chronic interstitial pneumonia characterised by lymphocytic infiltration of the alveolar septa, sometimes forming lymphoid follicles. Fibromuscular hyperplasia in alveolar walls is also a feature.

Visna

In sheep affected with visna, macroscopic lesions are seldom found unless there is concurrent maedi. There may be an atrophy of skeletal muscles and, exceptionally, a slight hyperaemia of the meninges may be seen. Microscopically, there is extensive microglial infiltration and malacia found mainly subependymally or near the meninges. In more chronic cases, marked demyelination may be seen.

Diagnosis

Neither the clinical signs nor the pathological findings are pathognomonic for maedi-visna, and from a practical point of view the only diagnostic methods are detection of antibodies against the virus. The majority of animals produce antibodies in response to infection, but the length of time from infection to seroconversion is unpredictable and may take months or even years. Furthermore, some infected animals remain antibody-negative. Consequently, negative test results cannot be used to ascertain freedom from infection in individual animals.

The serological tests used include an agar gel immunodiffusion test (AGID), an enzyme-linked immunosorbent assay (ELISA) or a complement fixation test (CFT). The AGID test has proven to be a simple and reliable flock test which is reproducible and suited for screening purposes. It is being gradually replaced by ELISA tests. Polymerase chain reaction (PCR) technology has also been developed.

Control

In Iceland the disease was controlled by dividing the country into different and fenced regions — sheep crossing the fences were slaughtered. During the years 1944–1953 all the infected regions, one by one, had to slaughter all sheep and the farms were re-stocked with lambs from disease-free areas. More than 100,000 sheep died from maedi-visna and 650,000 sheep were slaughtered in order to eradicate the disease. The total sheep population of Iceland is less than 1,000,000. The last occurrence of maedi-visna virus in Iceland was in 1965.

Since then, the knowledge of the disease and the causative agent has increased, and preventative control and eradication can be achieved using less drastic methods such as serological testing or sanitary procedures.

Voluntary control programmes based on serological testing are in operation in many European countries. The basis of the different programmes is the consecutive serological testing of flocks and stopping all contact between infected and accredited flocks.

In several countries, eradication programmes have been modified because of the high incidence of infection in many flocks. In these programmes, lambs are separated from their mothers (snatch lambing) immediately after birth, without allowing them to be suckled. The lambs are then fed cow colostrum and hand-reared on reconstituted milk powder until weaning. Serological testing is done at monthly intervals to the age of 6 months and at 3-monthly intervals thereafter. Lambs that react positively are eliminated.

Jaagziekte

Jaagziekte or sheep pulmonary adenomatosis (SPA) is a contagious neoplastic respiratory disease of adult sheep, probably caused by a slow-acting virus (retrovirus).

History

The disease has been recorded in Europe, South Africa, Asia, Britain, Iceland and Israel. Scotland appears to be a small focus of infection in Britain from which other outbreaks have arisen.

As with maedi-visna, the Icelandic experience is significant as the disease was almost certainly introduced into the country with the Karakul sheep that were also responsible for the introduction of the former disease in 1933. The first cases were noted about 1 year after the introduction of these sheep. During the next 2–3 years, about 60% of young breeding stock developed the disease and died. The heaviest death rate was in animals 1–3 years old. After 3–4 years the mortality rate in the flock dropped to under 10%, and when all sheep in the affected areas were slaughtered between 12 and 14 years after jaagziekte was introduced, only 2–3% of the animals showed typical lesions in the lungs. The disease declined with the occurrence of maedi-visna.

Aetiology

Two viruses have been associated with jaagziekte. The first, a herpesvirus, has been isolated from cases of the disease but not from normal animals. However, the disease cannot be reproduced with this virus. The other virus is a retrovirus, the particles of which have been observed in the cytoplasm of type II pneumocytes. Jaagziekte can be readily produced in lambs inoculated intratracheally with retrovirus containing lung-fluid concentrate. The disease is spread mainly as an aerosol and is favoured by close contact.

In South Africa the disease is reported where concentrated lambing is practised and where Karakul sheep in particular are yarded to select young milk lambs for slaughter.

Clinical signs

The incubation period is usually 6–8 months or longer, and clinical disease is usually seen in 3- to 4-year-old sheep. The first signs are associated with accumulation of excessive amounts of fluid in the lungs and include exercise intolerance, condition loss and dyspnoea. Breathing becomes accelerated particularly with exercise (e.g. if the flock is driven, affected sheep lag behind), but as the disease advances the respiration remains rapid. The breathing is accompanied by pumping flank movements and rhythmic jerking of the head. Animals will often collapse when driven. Characteristic rales are heard on auscultation and white froth is seen at the nostrils, particularly after sheep have been at rest. As the disease advances, white frothy fluid runs out of the nostrils if the hindquarters are raised while the head is lowered (wheelbarrow test).

Some sheep die only weeks after signs develop, but usually they live for 3–6 months. Many sheep become infected with a secondary bacterial pneumonia which may confuse the diagnosis.

Pathology and diagnosis

In jaagziekte the size of the lungs is the most remarkable feature: sometimes 3–4 times the normal size of a lung and the weight may be 2–3 kg. Milky froth usually fills the bronchi and the trachea.

The grey lung lesions that are typical of jaagziekte are found mainly in the apical and cardiac lobes and usually in the lower parts. They have a typical marbled appearance. The initial lesions of jaagziekte are often found in the diaphragmatic lobes. In advanced cases, lesions of different ages can often be found in the same lung. The younger lesions are greyish, translucent, rich in fluid and composed of several grey nodules 2–3 mm in diameter. Old lesions are homogeneous and white, like fibrous scar tissue.

Histopathological examination characteristically reveals neoplastic transformation of type II alveolar epithelial cells and epithelial cells of the small bronchi forming small papillary masses of cuboidal cells.

The disease is generally diagnosed by clinical signs which are described as pathognomonic, i.e. the severe nasal discharge. There are no serological tests available so confirmation of this disease must be made at necropsy.

Control

The only method of control is by slaughter of affected animals. This was practised successfully in Iceland along with the maedi-visna eradication programme. Iceland claimed freedom from jaagziekte in 1952. Prompt culling of unthrifty or dyspnoeic sheep and their offspring, and running young sheep separately from the main flock, may slow down the spread of the disease.

Schmallenberg virus

In late 2011 a new virus was identified in dairy cattle in Germany and was subsequently identified as causing congenital defects in perinatal lambs, kids and calves throughout Northern Europe. The spread throughout these regions in 2011 and 2012 appears to have been rapid, but by 2013 very few cases were seen, possibly because of the level of herd and flock immunity that had developed. The virus is an orthobunyavirus and is likely transmitted via *Culicoides* midges.

Clinical signs in newborn lambs include weakness, poor vision, various neurological signs and a range of congenital deformities including arthrogryposis, torticollis, scoliosis, kyphosis, brachygnathia inferior, and cerebellar, cerebral or spinal cord hypoplasia. Some affected lambs have a malformed head. These deformities vary likely depending on the stage of gestation when the infection occurred. Due to the deformities, dystocia of the dam is a common finding. Adult sheep and goats do not appear to show clinical signs associated with the disease, but in dairy cows fever, reduced milk yield, inappetence and diarrhoea have been reported.

Vaccines were rapidly developed for this disease, but uptake was limited and they are currently not commercially available. There has been no evidence for zoonotic transmission of this organism.

Other exotic diseases of sheep

The following diseases are described in brief because although they are very important in the countries where they occur, it is unlikely that they would ever occur in New Zealand. However, because of their occurrence in more tropical climates, some could be a risk to the Australian sheep industry. Further, the international quest for exotic material by some entrepreneurs within New Zealand and Australia supports the need for students and practising veterinarians alike to be aware of the range of exotic disease from which both Australia and New Zealand are fortunately free.

Ovine encephalomyelitis (louping ill)

Louping ill is an acute tick-borne encephalomyelitis that mainly affects sheep but may occasionally affect other animals and humans. It is unlikely to spread to Australia or New Zealand because of the absence of the host vector.

Aetiology and epidemiology

The causative agent is an arbovirus transmitted by the vector tick *Ixodes ricinus*. The tick is particularly prevalent during summer, and hence the disease mainly occurs at this time. Once it appears on a farm it will reappear every year. The number of 'abortive' infections is high and between 5% and 60% of sheep develop clinical signs after infection.

Pathogenesis

Following the infected tick bite, there is initial replication of the virus in the regional lymph node and then a viraemia and a febrile reaction for 3–5 days. After this period, the virus can no longer be detected in the blood but persists in the central nervous system and clinical signs may develop.

Clinical findings

The early signs of the initial pyrexia associated with slight depression often go unrecognised. A second pyrexia accompanies the onset of nervous signs about 5–7 days later. The nervous signs are variable and include head tremors, head pressing, an abnormal jerky gait progressing to paralysis, convulsions and death within 1–4 days.

Diagnosis in a severe outbreak may be made on clinical grounds alone, but confirmation depends on histology, serology and virus isolation. There is no effective treatment.

Control

The aim of control is to ensure that ewes are immune and that lambs are protected passively via colostrum. A vaccine is available and is given to ewes a month before lambing. A single injection will stimulate a high level of immunity for at least 2 years. It may also be necessary to protect ewe-lamb replacements by vaccination before summer when ticks become active. Other methods include tick control.

Two methods have been suggested for the eradication of louping ill, and both appear to be effective. These include de-stocking of sheep for a period of 2 years, during which time infected ticks die off naturally, or systematic mass vaccination over a period of 2 years.

Peste des petits ruminants

Peste des petits ruminants is a contagious viral disease of sheep and goats. It has clinical signs and lesions of the respiratory and alimentary systems, and in many ways resembles rinderpest. It has been reported in West and Central Africa and in the Middle East and India.

The peste des petits ruminants virus is of the genus *Morbillivirus* of the *Paramyxoviridae* and is related to canine distemper, human measles and rinderpest viruses.

Epidemiology

Peste des petits ruminants is a serious problem in West Africa, causing severe losses in sheep and goats. The disease occurs most commonly in lambs and hoggets, especially when they are moved from one region to another. In Nigeria, up to 20% of sheep and goats are seropositive to the virus and the proportion of positive reactors increases with the age of the population.

The disease is transmitted mainly by inhalation of aerosol virus particles from infected animals and the virus is excreted by infected animals by all routes. The clinical signs appear after a short incubation period of 5 days. The virus does not persist in the recovered animals, although the position of carrier animals is not known. Wild game may be carriers. The disease is highly contagious and quickly spreads through a flock.

Clinical signs

Peste des petits ruminants may occur in several forms. The morbidity is often nearly 100% and the mortality can be up to 90%. Severe peste des petits ruminants is characterised by fever, nasal catarrh, stomatitis, diarrhoea and death. The early lesions are similar to those of rinderpest, while chronic lesions are similar to scabby mouth. The course of the acute disease is about 5 days and usually results in death. The fever is followed by anorexia, and in surviving animals there is a severe ulcerative stomatitis with profuse mucopurulent discharges from the eyes and nose. A characteristic brown scab covers the lips, particularly at the commissures.

Pathology and diagnosis

The main lesions are found in the upper respiratory and alimentary tracts. They consist of epithelial erosions, ulcerations and encrustations of the external nares. Internal lesions are frequently complicated by bacterial infections resulting in rhinitis and bronchopneumonia. The entire mucosa of the mouth is usually affected and covered with necrotic desquamated epithelium. Diagnosis is dependent on clinical and postmortem features, although the disease can be confirmed by viral isolation.

Control

The main control of peste des petits ruminants is by vaccination. Because there is a close relationship between peste des petits ruminants and rinderpest viruses, the bovine tissue culture rinderpest vaccine is used in some countries to control peste des petits ruminants.

Rift Valley fever

Rift Valley fever is an acute, infectious, vector-transmitted viral disease of sheep, cattle, buffaloes and a wide range of other animals including humans. It is abortifacient and causes high losses in lambs and calves. It is believed to have spread from the Rift Valley in Kenya to other parts of Central Africa. The Rift Valley fever virus belongs to the family *Bunyaviridae*, genus *Phlebovirus*. It is a hepatotropic virus and grows readily in mice, sheep and all culture systems.

Transmission and infection

The virus is transmitted by biting arthropods; mosquitos are probably the most important vectors. Outbreaks of the disease occur at irregular intervals, with above-average rainfall being the most important factor because this favours multiplication of the vectors. Human infections are caused by exposure to contaminated meat or other animal materials. It can also be spread mechanically by such agents as contaminated syringes and needles. Once infected, animals develop a viraemia and the virus subsequently localises in the liver.

Clinical signs

The severity of the clinical signs depends on the species and the age of the host. The most severe signs are seen in lambs, calves and adult sheep and include massive body haemorrhages, jaundice, diarrhoea, skin erythema and severe abdominal pain. In lambs and calves the mortality rate may be up to 70%. In pregnant adult sheep and cattle the only evidence of disease may be widespread abortion, but in most instances some animals will die.

In humans, Rift Valley virus can be a somewhat vague disease characterised by fever, headaches and malaise, but severe hepatic, nervous and ocular symptoms may develop.

Pathology and diagnosis

At necropsy, there is massive haemorrhage throughout the carcass. The liver is covered in small grey-white areas of necrosis. The histological lesions of Rift Valley fever are pathognomonic and include focal or confluent hepatic necrosis. Ocular lesions, which often include retinal detachment, may be observed in human cases.

A clinical diagnosis can be confirmed by serological tests and virus isolation. Complement fixation testing, ELISA, immunodiffusion and immunofluoresence tests are all adequate for diagnosis. In addition, clinical illness with high mortality in young animals and a lower morbidity in adult animals is a significant feature of the disease and may be of diagnostic value.

Control

The control of Rift Valley fever is similar to the control of bluetongue. This includes the screening of holding areas to protect susceptible animals from the several species of mosquitoes that may transmit the virus. The application of residual insecticides to animals, yards and sheds is also helpful.

Two types of vaccine are available. A live vaccine is used for non-pregnant sheep and goats and gives long-lasting protection. An inactivated vaccine is used for pregnant sheep and for cattle but the period of protection is relatively short.

Heartwater

Aetiology

Heartwater is an important disease of sheep and goats in Africa. It is caused by the rickettsial organism *Cowdria ruminantium*, which is transmitted by the bont tick (*Amblyomma hebraeum*). *Cowdria ruminantium* infects reticuloendothelial cells, resulting in vasculitis with the development of bloody fluid and oedema in body cavities. Following exposure, animals develop immunity to the organism. Outbreaks may occur when susceptible animals are introduced to endemic areas, or when drought conditions reduce tick numbers resulting in a waning of the immunity of livestock. When climatic conditions change and tick numbers increase, the now-susceptible animals may show clinical signs.

Clinical features

The earliest clinical signs include fever, listlessness and inappetence, progressing to muscle tremors. Neurological signs such as increasing nervousness, circling and head-pressing develop, until eventually the affected animals develop seizures and die. Affected sheep also become photophobic.

Pathology and diagnosis

The characteristic feature of postmortem examination is the presence of straw- or blood-coloured fluid in the abdomen, thorax and pericardium. The internal organs may be heavy and filled with blood. The lungs are heavy and dark purple and there is usually haemorrhage on the inner and outer walls of the heart. The diagnosis can be confirmed by histopathological examination of the brain.

Treatment and prevention

Sheep found early in the course of the disease may be treated with tetracyclines. Animals born in endemic areas are generally immune by 1 month of age, and if this immunity is boosted from time to time by natural infection they should not develop clinical signs. Dipping may be undertaken to reduce tick numbers, although absolute control of ticks is not advisable. A vaccine is also available.

Capripox infections (sheep-pox, goat-pox, buffalo-pox and camel-pox)

The sheep and goat pox syndromes are the most severe pox diseases affecting domestic animals and are a cause of economic losses in many parts of the world. It was once believed that sheep-pox and goat-pox viruses were host-specific. However, it is now concluded that they are the same virus and the disease reflected is merely the individual host response to a particular strain. The previous host-related descriptions (i.e. sheep-pox and goat-pox) should be replaced by a single term, capripox, independent of the animal species involved. Capripox virus causes lamb and kid mortality, mastitis and abortion.

Aetiology

It is believed that the pox diseases originally came from one or more basic strains of virus, which, over the course of time, changed and became adapted to different hosts. The viruses of the *Poxviridae* family have a characteristic morphology by which they are readily identified. All the viruses are antigenically related. They survive for long periods of time in the environment, especially in scab material from skin lesions of recovered animals, which yield viable virus for up to 3 months.

Epidemiology and transmission

Capripox is endemic in the Near, Middle and Far East and North Africa. It is not present in the Republic of South Africa. Buffalo-pox has been reported in India, Indonesia, Italy, Pakistan, the former USSR and Egypt. The pox diseases are relatively rare among domestic animals in Europe and North America.

The transmission of pox virus occurs through close contact and inhalation. Contaminated premises may be infective for up to 6 months. Virulent capripox was eradicated in Europe over 100 years ago because of highly intensive agricultural practices. However, a combination of a dry environment, which favours environmental survival of the organism, and traditional nomadic pastoral systems of agriculture make the disease difficult to eradicate from areas such as the Near East.

Within endemic areas, capripox can usually be found throughout the year and a high level of flock immunity develops, restricting the severe disease to lambs and kids.

Clinical signs

In the field there is a wide range of clinical signs, most likely reflecting differences in host response and the virulence of the many virus strains. All ages of sheep and goats are affected although the disease is most severe in young animals. The incubation period is between 4 and 9 days.

Peracute disease in a naive population is characterised by high fever, a generalised haemorrhagic syndrome, widespread cutaneous ulceration and death within a few days. The morbidity may be over 75% and over 50% of affected animals will die. Young animals are particularly susceptible.

In acute infections the onset is usually sudden with high fever, naso-ocular discharges and salivation. Papules appear within 24 hours in mucous membranes of the nose, gums, lips, vulva and intradermally. Initially they are circumscribed, oedematous and hyperaemic but may become confluent. As the fever regresses the papules become encrusted with exudate, these eventually forming scabs. The scabs may become secondarily affected and are intensely irritant, causing animals to rub severely causing skin damage. The lesions are worst in the head, ears, axillae, groin, and perineum. Death may occur at any stage. Secondary bacterial pneumonia is common and the skin lesions in surviving animals leave permanent scars.

A more chronic or nodular form of capripox similar to bovine lumpy skin disease has been reported in sheep and goats. In the nodular form, vesicles rarely form and the lesions are thick and nodular (stone-pox and goat dermatitis). Subacute reactions are often missed.

Pathology and diagnosis

The main lesions in sheep and goats are on parts of the body not well covered with hair. The vesicular and nodular formations described above are characteristic of the disease. Lesions are also regularly found in the respiratory and alimentary tracts. Lesions in the lungs consist of depressed grey areas up to 3 cm in diameter, and secondary bacterial bronchopneumonia is often seen. Typical nodules are seen frequently in the lining of the abomasum.

The clinical diagnosis in endemic areas is not difficult during acute epizootics. However, in the more chronic situation the lesions may resemble scabby mouth (contagious ecthyma). The virus can be identified within 24 hours by direct fluorescent antibody technique. Other laboratory methods used in confirming a diagnosis include virus isolation, the detection of viral antigens in skin lesions and the demonstration of serum antibodies.

Control

In many endemic areas of the world, control is difficult due to the practice of nomadic pastoralism. However, capripox vaccines are available and are used to protect susceptible animals in endemic countries; in recent times the disease has been brought under control in Morocco and Tunisia, but is still important in other parts of Africa.

Nairobi sheep disease

Nairobi sheep disease is a tick-transmitted viral disease of sheep. It occurs in East Africa and is characterised by severe haemorrhagic gastroenteritis and lymph node hyperplasia. As with many viral diseases, adult sheep and goats gradually become immune to virus in enzootic areas. Animals reared in areas where the tick victor does not exist are particularly susceptible to the disease.

The Nairobi sheep disease virus has antigenic similarities to other arboviruses and belongs to the family *Bunyavirus,* genus *Nairovirus.* It is relatively resistant to environmental changes and can be stored for long periods.

Epidemiology and transmission

Nairobi sheep disease has been reported in Kenya, Uganda, Somalia, Tanzania and Zaire. Its occurrence is associated with the geographical distribution of *Rhipicephalus* tick vectors.

Sheep and goats are the species that are naturally susceptible to infection. Cattle can be infected experimentally but remain infected for only a few hours. The virus is pantropic in infected animals and is present in all body effusions.

Clinical signs

The disease may be mild with only a slight fever and no diarrhoea, or it may be very severe with fever and bloody dysentery. In some acute cases death occurs in 2–3 days. Animals are depressed, anorexic and usually have a mucopurulent nasal discharge which may contain blood. Respiration is rapid. The main feature of the acute disease is the bright to dark green watery diarrhoea accompanied by severe tenesmus and pain. Abortion may occur in pregnant ewes. The first fever peak is at 2–4 days; this may drop suddenly and be followed by a second fever peak up to 7 days later. Nasal discharge and conjunctivitis may also occur.

In all cases, if diarrhoea develops the prognosis is poor. The mortality may be as high as 70%.

Pathology and diagnosis

The main lesions are mucosal and serosal haemorrhages

and enteritis. Diagnosis can be confirmed by virus isolation or use of viral antigen AGID.

Control
Recovery from the disease usually results in a solid immunity. Information on control by vaccination is vague and attenuated vaccines are not yet commercially available. In most areas where the disease occurs, control is not undertaken. This is largely because of the expense of tick control in these regions. It is apparent that a great deal of work needs to be done both to understand and to combat this disease in enzootic situations.

Brucella melitensis (Malta or Mediterranean fever of humans)
Brucella melitensis causes brucellosis in goats, sheep and humans. The disease is quite different from *Brucella ovis* infection of rams and *Brucella abortus* infection of cattle.

Brucella melitensis infection occurs in Southern Europe, the Middle East, Malta, Spain, Portugal, Greece, Cyprus, Turkey, the former USSR, India, Pakistan, Southern USA, Mexico and South America. It probably occurs in Central Africa as well. *Brucella melitensis* is zoonotic. No human cases have been diagnosed in people permanently resident in New Zealand, but two cases have been diagnosed in returning New Zealanders who had been shearing small ruminants in Mediterranean countries. One case occurred in 1985 and the other in 1996.

Epidemiology
Although *B. melitensis* is primarily an infection of goats and sheep, it will infect cattle and pigs. Transmission between animals and different species is by direct ingestion. Infected, pregnant goats and sheep may abort or give birth to a normal kid or lamb, but in either event they discharge large numbers of brucellae into the environment. The disease is also transmitted to young animals via infected milk of the dam. In humans the disease is more often acquired by drinking milk from infected goats or sheep.

Pathogenesis
The pathogenesis is similar to *B. abortus* infection of cattle and depends on localisation of the organism in the lymph nodes, udder and uterus. Infection of the uterus during pregnancy results in placentitis with subsequent abortion.

Clinical signs
Abortion occurs during late pregnancy in infected animals. Initially there may be a few abortions followed by an abortion storm. *Brucella melitensis* may also cause mastitis in ewes and goats. Other signs seen in sheep and goats may include lameness due to osteoarthritis and synovitis. Orchitis may occur in rams and bucks.

Diagnosis
The diagnosis is similar to that of *B. abortus* and *B. ovis* infections. The organism can be cultured from infected milk and the excretions of animals that have aborted. There are also serological tests available to detect carrier animals.

Control
The control of the disease, were it to appear in either New Zealand or Australia, would be based on quarantine and slaughter of infected animals.

Screw-worm flies
The two species of blowfly *Chrysomyia bezziana* and *Cochliomyia hominivorax* are a potential risk to the Australian sheep and cattle industry because of their presence in southern New Guinea. The disease is considered very seriously by Australian veterinary authorities because of wide areas of country in both the Northern Territory and Queensland that would be suitable for screw-worm fly survival and multiplication. Alarmingly, screw-worm maggots have been found on ships visiting Australia on several occasions.

Screw-worm flies cause myasis in humans, cattle, sheep, goats and many other animals. They cause severe damage and a sudden and painful death to affected animals.

Life cycle
The female fly lays clusters of up to 500 eggs at the edge of the wound in the host (shearing cut, etc.). The screw-worm fly is very closely adapted to a specific parasitic life, namely breeding in the wounds of the host. It will not breed in dead carcasses. The larvae hatch in 10–12 hours and mature in 3–6 days, when they leave the host and pupate in the ground. The pupal stage lasts from 3–7 days to several weeks, according to the prevailing temperature. Hibernation commonly occurs in the pupal stage.

Clinical signs

Most cases occur during warm, rainy weather. The maggots penetrate into the tissues, which liquefy and extend the lesion. The wounds develop an offensive odour and a foul-smelling liquid oozes out. Most infestations are so severe that the animal is literally eaten alive, unless treated quickly.

Control

In areas where screw-worm fly exists it is necessary to treat all wounds with an insecticidal spray to prevent major losses. In the USA, a major programme was conducted in the 1950s to eradicate the screw-worm fly by the dissemination of irradiated, sterile male flies. The screw-worm fly mates only once and if mating takes place with a sterile male then no fertile eggs are produced. The massive campaign in the USA involved the release of 50 million irradiated flies a week, and required 40 tonnes of meat a week to feed the larvae.

Sheep scab

The cause of sheep scab is a microscopic mite, *Psoroptes ovis*. It is described as a cosmopolitan body-mite of domesticated sheep, cattle, horses and also donkeys and mules.

Sheep scab is a notifiable disease in New Zealand. It was recognised in imported sheep prior to 1850, and for the next half-century it was the main disease that hampered the development of sheep farming. The disease was not only devastating to production and cast a social stigma on the owners of scabby sheep, but its control was tedious in the extreme and the dipping procedure was a task that no modern farmer would tolerate. However, it is to their everlasting credit that despite not having an established veterinary authority at the time, successful eradication was achieved by farmer cooperation with local legislative councils (the New Zealand Department of Agriculture Veterinary Division was not established until 1893). New Zealand was declared free from sheep scab in 1894, although there was a single reoccurrence in Marlborough in 1896. Sheep scab has never occurred in New Zealand since. Australia is also free from the disease, having eradicated it in 1896. Great Britain was declared free of scab in 1952, but the mite reappeared in Britain in 1973 and despite the re-introduction of a compulsory dipping

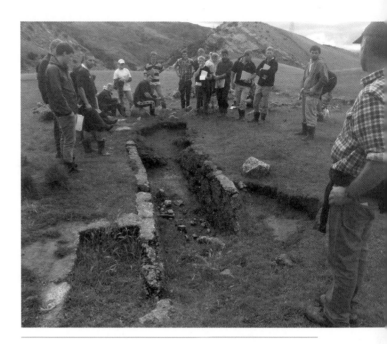

Figure 21.12 Remains of a typical scab eradication dip at Foxdown station, North Canterbury. Sheep were dipped in a solution of tobacco dust, sulphur and sometimes lime or arsenic. The tobacco was grown locally. The ingredients were boiled and the mixture poured into a dip kept at a temperature ranging from 100° to 120° Fahrenheit. To heat the dip, huge quantities of firewood had to be cut and burned. Immersion for 2 minutes was considered to kill *Psoroptes ovis*. A second dip 16 days later was necessary to kill mites hatched in the interval. Infected ground was left free of grazing for up to 6 months. (Photograph courtesy A. Fox, Foxdown, Scargill, North Canterbury)

programme, eradication has not been successful. In 1992 compulsory controls were abandoned and cases have continued to arise since in that country.

Life cycle and transmission

The eggs are laid on the skin and usually hatch in 1–3 days. Hatching may be deferred for up to 10 days. After hatching, the larvae feed for 2–3 days and then moult to the nymphal stage which lasts 3–4 days before moulting occurs. Small nymphs usually become males, and large nymphs females. The nymphs mate and the oviparous female begins laying a day later. The whole cycle can be as short as 9 days. The female may lay up to 90 eggs over 30–40 days. The nymphal stages may persist away from the animal for a few days, but the most important mode of transmission is by direct contact with infected animals.

Clinical features

Sheep scab lesions may occur on all parts of the body that are covered with wool or hair, but occur mainly on the shoulders, back and sides of woolled sheep. The mite and its lesions cause the sheep to bite its wool and rub incessantly. Exudation and encrustation of the skin and wool develop, with serious fleece damage. Sheep scab is most active in the autumn and winter, while latency tends to occur over summer. Diagnosis is relatively simple, but the latent lesions make it difficult to declare a large flock free from scab.

Control

Sheep scab can be controlled by dipping or by administration of macrocyclic lactone anthelmintics by injection. Were it to reappear in either New Zealand or Australia, strict quarantine procedures would need to be instigated until the disease was eradicated. However, once established in a country, excellent farmer cooperation as well as good surveillance is required for control and eradication.

Contagious agalactia

Contagious agalactia is a severe exotic disease of sheep and goats. It is caused by *Mycoplasma agalactiae* and other mycoplasmas, and occurs in parts of North Africa, Asia and Southern Europe.

It is a septicaemic disease and is transmitted from ewe to lamb(s) through the ewe's milk. The symptoms displayed are severe. Following incubation of up to 2 months, sheep show signs of fever and malaise and pregnant ewes may abort. Lactating ewes develop a severe bilateral mastitis and, if the ewes survive, the udder becomes fibrotic and atrophied. Affected sheep may become lame with arthritis affecting the carpal and tarsal joints, and they may also develop a unilateral or bilateral keratitis resulting in blindness.

Therapy is seldom effective, and although attenuated vaccines are available, their use interferes with disease-control programmes.

Q-fever

Q-fever is an important zoonotic disease which is sometimes fatal for humans. It is caused by *Coxiella burnetti* bacteria. In animals, signs of infection are mild and often inapparent. *Coxiella burnetti* is not present in New Zealand animals and is a notifiable organism under the Biosecurity Act 1993. Human cases reported in New Zealand have likely been due to overseas exposure.

A wide range of animal species are able to transmit the disease to humans, including cattle, sheep and goats, although alpacas, dogs and cats are other domestic species that may be infected. The organism has also been isolated from many other animals and birds. Its transmission is mainly by exposure to body fluids (placental fluid, blood, milk and urine), faeces and items such as straw wool and equipment contaminated by infected fluids. Tick transmission to humans is also possible but is believed to be rare.

Overseas, *C. burnetti* has been associated with abortion outbreaks in sheep and thus with live animal importations particular measures are taken to avoid this happening. These include quarantine and testing of live animals (except dogs and cats) and animal genetic material, and inspection and treatment of equipment that might potentially be contaminated. However, sheep may be seronegative yet still be shedding the bacteria, which poses a problem for live sheep imports.

REFERENCES

TRANSMISSIBLE SPONGIFORM ENCEPHALOPATHIES

Aguzzi A, Weissman C. A suspicious signature. *Nature* 383, 666-7, 1996

Anonymous. Scrapie: The lesson we must learn. *New Veterinary Journal* 26, 217, 1978

Anonymous. Bovine spongiform encephalopathy. *Veterinary Record* 122, 477-8, 1988

Anonymous. Feedstuffs confirmed as source of cow disease. *New Scientist* 129, 26, 1989

Anonymous. *Bovine Spongiform encephalopathy in Great Britain: A progress report June 2001.* Department for Environment, Food and Rural Affairs, 2001

Anonymous. Spongiform encephalopathy in cattle and deer. Reference No: 90/MQ/10. MAF, PO Box 2526, Wellington, New Zealand, 1990

Anonymous. Scrapie. OIE Terrestrial Manual 2016, Chapter 2.7.12, pp 1-11, 2016. Accessed at http://www.oie.int/fileadmin/Home/eng/Health_standards/tahm/2.07.12_SCRAPIE.pdf on 10 August 2017

Adlam GH. Scrapie: The risks in perspective. *New Veterinary Journal* 25, 359-60, 1977

Barlow RM. Slow virus diseases of sheep. *Proceedings of 15th Seminar of the Society of Sheep and Beef Cattle Veterinarians, New Zealand Veterinary Association*, 1-8, 1985

Black H. Obtaining brains for surveillance, the easy way. *Vetscript* 12, 6-7, 1999

Benestad SL, Mitchell G, Simmons M, Ytrehus B, Vikoren T. First case of chronic wasting disease in Europe in a Norwegian free-ranging reindeer. *Veterinary Research* 47, 2016

Brash AG. Scrapie in imported sheep in New Zealand. *New Veterinary Journal* 1, 27-30, 1952

Brotherston JG, Renwick CC, Stamp JT, Zlotnik I, Pattison IH. Spread of scrapie by contact to goats and sheep. *Journal of Comparative Pathology* 78, 9-17, 1968

Brown P, Rau HW, Johnson BK, Bacote AE, Gibbs Jr. CJ, Gajdusek DC. New studies on the heat resistance of hampster-adapted scrapie agent: Threshold survival after washing at 600°C suggests an inorganic template of replication. *PNAS* 97, 3418-21, 2000

Bruère AN. Scrapie a point of view. *New Zealand Veterinary Journal* 25, 259-60, 1977

Bruère AN. Scrapie in New Zealand — its history and what it could mean. *Proceedings of 15th Seminar of the Society of Sheep and Beef Cattle Veterinarians, New Zealand Veterinary Association*, 9-22, 1977

Bruère AN. Scrapie freedom — the New Zealand story. *Surveillance* 30(4) 3-7, 2003

Collinge J, Sidle KCL, Meads J, Ironside J, Hill AF. Molecular analysis of prion strain variation and the aetiology of 'new variant' CJD. *Nature* 383, 685-90, 1996

Cooke M. Observations on bovine spongiform encephalopathy and scrapie. *Surveillance* 16, 9-10, 1989

Cunningham AA, Wells GAH, Scott AC, Kirkwood JK, Barnett JEF. Transmissible spongiform encephalopathy in greater kudu (*Tragelaphus strepsiceros*). *Veterinary Record* 132, 68, 1993

Davies P. Transmissible spongiform encephalopathies (TSE) — an update. *Proceedings of the 31st Seminar of the Society of Sheep and Beef Cattle Veterinarians, New Zealand Veterinary Association*, 131-6, 2001

Dickinson AG. Scrapie in sheep & goats. *Slow virus diseases of animals & man*, edited by RH Kimberlin. North-Holland Publishing Co, Amsterdam/American Elsevier, New York, 1976

Dickinson AG, Stamp JT, Renwick CC. Maternal and lateral transmission of scrapie in sheep. *Journal of Comparative Pathology* 84, 19-25, 1974

Evans BC. *A history of agricultural production and marketing in New Zealand.* Keeling & Mundy Ltd, Palmerston North, New Zealand, 1969

Foster J, Toovey L, McKenzie C, Chong A, Parnham D, Drummond D, Hunter N. Atypical scrapie in a sheep in a closed UK flock with endemic classical natural scrapie. *Veterinary Record* 162, 723-5, 2008

Foster JD, Bruce M, McConnell I, Chree A, Fraser H. Detection of BSE infectivity in brain and spleen of experimentally infected sheep. *Veterinary Record* 138, 546-8, 1996

Foster JD, Hunter N, Williams A, Mylne MJA, McKelvey WAC, Hope J, Fraser H, Bostock C. Observations on the transmission of scrapie in experiments using embryo transfer. *Veterinary Record* 138, 559-62, 1996

Foster JD, Wilson M, Hunter N. Immunolocalisation of the prion protein (PrP) in the brains of sheep with scrapie. *Veterinary Record* 139, 512-15, 1996

Gibbs CJ, Amyx HL, Bacote A, Masters CL, Gajdusek DC. Oral transmission of Kuru, Creutzfeldt-Jakob disease and scrapie to nonhuman primates. *Journal of Infectious Diseases* 142, 205-8, 1980

Harrison PJ, Roberts GW. How now mad cow. *British Medical Journal* 304, 929-30, 1992

Hoinville IJ. A review of the epidemiology of scrapie in sheep. *Revue scientifique et technique / Office international des épizooties* 15, 827-52, 1996

Hourrigan J, Klingsporn A, Clark WW, de Camp M. Epidemiology of scrapie in the United States. *Slow transmissible diseases of the nervous system*, edited by SB Prusiner and WJ Hadlow, pp 331-56. Academic Press, New York, 1979

Hunter N, Moore L, Hosie BD, Dingwall WS, Greig A. Association between natural scrapie and PrP genotype in a flock of Suffolk sheep in Scotland. *Veterinary Record* 140, 59-63, 1997

Johnstone A. The roles of Laboratory Network and the practitioner in transmissible spongiform encephalopathy surveillance. *Vetscript* 10, 18-19, 1997

Kimberlin RH. Scrapie. *British Veterinary Journal* 137, 105-12, 1981

Kimberlin RH. BSE stocktaking. *Surveillance* 18, 15-16, 1991

Kirkwood JK, Wells GAH, Cunningham AA, Jackson ST, Scott AC, Dawson M, Wilesmith JW. Scrapie-like encephalopathy in a greater kudu which had not been fed ruminant-derived protein. *Veterinary Record* 130, 365-7, 1992

Kittelberger R, Chaplin MJ, Simmons MM, Ramirez-Villaescusa A, McIntyre L, MacDiarmid SC, Hannah MJ, Jenner J, Bueno R, Bayliss D, Black H, Pigott CJ, O'Keefe JS. Atypical scrapie/Nor98 in a sheep from New Zealand. *Journal of Veterinary Diagnostic Investigation* 22, 863-75, 2010

Luhken G, Buschmann A, Brandt H, Eiden M, Groschup MH, Erhardt G. Epidemiological and genetical differences between classical and atypical scrapie cases. *Veterinary Research* 38, 65-80, 2007

MacDiarmid S. Aspects of scrapie and bovine spongiform encephalopathy. *Surveillance* 16, 11-12, 1989

McIntryre L, Brangenberg, N. Exotic disease focus: Chronic wasting disease. *Surveillance* 36(1), 5-6, 2009

M'Fadyean J. Scrapie. *Journal of Comparative Pathology* 31, 102-31, 1918

Mohri S, Farquhar CF, Somerville RA, Jeffrey M, Foster J, Hope J. Immunodetection of a disease specific PrP fraction in scrapie-affected sheep and BSE-affected cattle. *Veterinary Record* 131, 537-9, 1992

Munday BL. Spongiform encephalopathies — or are there such things as infectious proteins? *Surveillance* 19, 19-21, 1992

Parry HB. *Scrapie disease of sheep*, edited byOppenheimer DR. Academic Press, London, 1983

Parsonson IM. Scrapie: Recent trends. *Australian Veterinary Journal* 74, 383-7, 1996

Stockman S. Scrapie: An obscure disease of sheep. *Journal of Comparative Pathology* 26, 317-27, 1913

Surveillance (1991) 18 (3):22-3: Scrapie

Taylor DM. Scrapie agent decontamination: Implications for bovine spongiform encephalopathy. *Veterinary Record* 124, 291-2, 1989

Taylor DM, Fraser H, McConnell I, Brown DA, Lamza KA, Smith GRA. Decontamination studies with the agent of bovine spongiform encephalopathy and scrapie. *Archives of Virology* 139, 313-26, 1994

Taylor DM, Fernie K, McConnell I, Ferguson CE, Steele PJ. Solvent extraction as an adjunct to rendering: The effect on BSE and scrapie agents of hot solvents followed by dry heat and steam. *Veterinary Record* 143, 6-9, 1998

Taylor DM. Inactivation of transmissible degenerative encephalopathy agents: A review. *Veterinary Journal* 159, 10-17, 2000

Wells GAH, Scott AC, Johnson CT, Gunning RF, Hancock RD, Jeffrey M, Dawson M, Bradley R. A novel progressive spongiform encephalopathy in cattle. *Veterinary Record* 121, 419-20, 1987

Williams ES, Young S. Chronic wasting disease of captive mule deer; a spongiform encephalopathy. *Journal of Wildlife Diseases* 16, 89-98, 1980

Williams ES, Young S. Spongiform encephalopathy of Rocky Mountain elk. *Journal of Wildlife Diseases* 18, 465-71, 1982

Williams ES, Miller MW. Chronic wasting disease in deer and elk in North America. *Revue scientifique et technique / Office international des épizooties* 21, 305-16, 2002

Wisniewski HM, Sigurdarson S, Rubenstein R, Kascsak RJ, Carp RI. Mites as vectors in scrapie. *Lancet* 347, 1114, 1996

Wood DJM, Mason JB, Chapman HM. Scrapie scruples. *New Zealand Veterinary Journal* 26, 190-1, 1978

Wood JL, McGill IS, Done SH, Bradley R. Neuropathology of scrapie: A study of the distribution patterns of brain lesions in 222 cases of natural scrapie in sheep, 1982-1991. *Veterinary Record* 140, 167-74, 1997

Woodbury M. *Chronic wasting disease update.* University of Sakatchewan, Research & development programme. Extension service. February, 2001

Wrathall AE, Brown KFD, Sayers AR, Wells GAH, Simmons MM, Farrelly SSJ, Bellerby P, Squirrell J, Spencer YI, Wells M, Stack MJ, Bastiman B, Pullar D, Scatcherd J, Heasman L, Parker J, Hannam DAR, Helliwell DW, Chree A, Fraser H. Studies of embryo transfer from cattle clinically affected by bovine spongiform encephalopathy (BSE). *Veterinary Record*, 365-78, 2002

BLUETONGUE

Bath GF. Bluetongue. *Proceedings of the Society of Sheep and Beef Cattle Veterinarians, New Zealand Veterinary Association* 19, 349-57, 1989

Bath GF, de Wet J. *Sheep and goat diseases*. Tafelburg Publishers Ltd, Cape Town, South Africa, 2000

Blajan L. World production and utilisation of products of animal origin. *Revue scientifique et technique / Office international des épizooties* 6, 849-83, 1987

Beveridge WIB. Bluetongue in Animal Health in Australia. *Volume 1 Viral diseases of livestock*, pp 10-15. Australian Bureau of Animal Health. Australian Government Publishing Service Canberra, 1981

Erasmus BJ. Bluetongue in sheep and goats. *Australian Veterinary Journal* 51, 165-70, 1975

Hateley G. Bluetongue in northern Europe: The story so far. *In Practice* 31, 202-9, 2009

Losos GJ. Bluetongue. *Infectious tropical diseases of domestic animals*, pp 409-51, edited by Logos GJ. Longman Scientific and Technical, Canada, 1986

Maclachlan NJ. Bluetongue: History, global epidemiology and pathogenesis. *Preventive Veterinary Medicine* 102, 107-111, 2011

Menzies FD, McCullough SJ et al. Evidence for transpalcental and contact transmission of bluetongue virus in cattle. *Veterinary Record* 163, 203-9, 2008

Neville EM. The use of cattle to protect sheep from bluetongue infection. *Journal of the South African Veterinary Association* 49, 129-30, 1978

Osburn BI. Bluetongue. *Diseases of sheep* (3rd ed.), pp 393-397. Blackwell Science, 2000

OVINE ENZOOTIC ABORTION
Bath G, de Wet J. *Sheep and goat diseases.* Tafelberg Publishers Ltd, Capetown, South Africa, 2000

Surveillance

(1996) 23: 6	Special issue — exotic diseases
(1997) 24(2): 18-19	Chlamydial abortion in sheep

FOOT AND MOUTH DISEASE
Anonymous. The 2001 FMD epidemic: How the disease took hold. *Veterinary Record* 149, 721-2, 2001

Barnett PV, Cox SJ. The role of small ruminants in the epidemiology and transmission of foot-and-mouth disease. *Veterinary Journal* 158, 6-13, 1999

Donaldson AI, Sellers RF. Foot and mouth disease. *Diseases of sheep* (4th ed), edited by Aitken I, pp 282-7 Blackwell Science, Oxford, 2007

Hyslop NS. The epizootiology and epidemiology of foot and mouth disease. *Advances in Veterinary Science* 14, 261-307, 1970

Pharo HJ. Foot-and-mouth disease: An assessment of the risks facing New Zealand. *New Zealand Veterinary Journal* 50, 46-55, 2002

Sanson RL. The epidemiology of foot-and-mouth disease: Implications for New Zealand. *New Zealand Veterinary Journal* 22, 41-53, 1994

Surveillance

(1988) 15(4): 5-7	Exotic diseases issue
(1991) 18(3): 13-15	Exotic diseases issue
(1996) 23: 8-9	Exotic diseases issue

MAEDI-VISNA
Hoff-Jorgensen R. Maedi-visna. *Proceedings of the 2nd International Congress for Sheep Veterinarians, Sheep and Beef Cattle Society of the New Zealand Veterinary Association,* Massey University, Palmerston North, 1989

Houwers DJ. Experimental maedi-visna control in the Netherlands. *Slow viruses in sheep, goats and cattle,* pp 115-121. Commission of European Communities Report EUR 8076 EN, 1985

Palsson PA. *Slow virus diseases of animals and man,* pp 17-43, edited by Kimberlin RH. North-Holland Publishing C. Amsterdam/American Elsevier, New York, 1976

Palsson PA. Maedi/Visna of sheep in Iceland. *Slow viruses of sheep, goats and cattle: Agriculture Commission of European Communities,* pp 3-19, edited by Sharp JM, Hoff-Jorgensen R. Office for Official Publications of the European Communities, Luxembourg, 1985

Pritchard GC, McConnell I. Maedi-visna. *Diseases of sheep* (4th ed), edited by Aitken I, pp 217-23, Blackwell Science, Oxford, 2007

Williams-Fulton NR, Simard CL. Evaluation of two management procedures for the control of maedi-visna. *Canadian Journal of Veterinary Research* 53, 419-23, 1989

Zwahlen R. The presence of lentivirus infections in Swiss goat herds. *Slow viruses in sheep, goats and cattle: Agriculture Commission of European Communities,* pp 153-38. Commission of European Communities Report EUR 8076 EN, 1985

JAAGZIEKTE
Palsson PA. Maedi/Visna of sheep in Iceland. *Slow viruses of sheep, goats and cattle: Agriculture Commission of European Communities,* edited by Sharp JM, Hoff-Jorgensen R., pp 3-10. Office for Official publications of The European Communities, Luxembourg, 1985

Wandera JG. Sheep pulmonary adenomatosis (jaagziekte). *Advances in Veterinary Science* 15, 251, 1971

SCHMALLENBERG VIRUS
Beer M, Contraths FJ, Van Der Poel WHM. 'Schmallenberg virus' — a novel orthobunyavirus emerging in Europe. *Epidemiology and Infection* 141, 1-8, 2013

Lievaart-Peterson K, Luttikhold SJM, Van den Brom R, Vellema P. Schmallenberg virus infection in small ruminants — first review of the situation and prospects in Northern Europe. *Small Ruminant Research* 106, 71-6, 2012

PESTE DES PETITS RUMINANTS
Scott GR. Rinderpest and peste des petits ruminants. *Virus diseases of food animals. A world geography of epidemiology and control. Disease Monographs, Volume 2,* edited by Gibbs EPJ, pp401-32. Academic Press, New York, 1981

Taylor WD, Barrett T. Peste des petits ruminants and rinderpest. *Diseases of sheep* (4th ed), edited by Aitken I, pp 460-8. Blackwell Science, Oxford, 2007

RIFT VALLEY FEVER
Bath GF. Rift valley fever. *Diseases of sheep* (4th ed), edited by Aitken I, pp 460-72. Blackwell Science, Oxford, 2007

Easterday BC. Rift Valley fever. *Advances in veterinary science,* Volume 10, edited by Brandly CA, Cornelius, C., pp 65-77. Academic Press, New York, 1965

Sellers RF. Rift Valley fever. *Virus diseases of food animals. A world geography of epidemiology and control. Disease Monographs, Volume 2,* edited by Gibbs EPJ, pp 674-80. Academic Press, New York, 1981

HEARTWATER
Bath G, de Wet J. *Sheep and goat diseases.* Tafelberg Publishers Ltd, Cape Town, South Africa, 2000

CAPRIPOX INFECTIONS
Davies FG. Sheep and goat pox. *Virus diseases of food animals. A world geography of epidemiology and control. Disease Monographs, Volume 2,* edited by Gibbs EPJ, pp 733-49. Academic Press, New York, 1981

Kitching RP. Sheep pox. *Diseases of sheep* (4th ed), edited by Aitken I, pp 302-6. Blackwell Science, Oxford, 2007

NAIROBI SHEEP DISEASE
Losos GJ. Nairobi sheep disease. *Infectious tropical diseases of domestic animals,* 540-8. Longman Scientific and Technical, 1986

Q-FEVER
Frazer J, Rooney J. Exotic disease focus: Q-fever. *Surveillance* 36(1) 3-4, 2009

Reichel MP, Ross GP. Targeted survey for exotic ovine abortifacients in New Zealand. *Surveillance* 25 (3) 9, 1998

Index

Numbers in **bold** denote illustrations. Those marked 'f' denote figures.

A

abamectin 172–3
abomasal bloat 90
abortion 10, 54–7, 63–75, 73–4, 299, 377–8
abscesses 22, 23, **23**, 298–9, **298–9** see also specific abscesses
acidosis 191
Acremonium 51
Actinobacillus seminis 26, 34–6, **35**
acute fibrinous pneumonia see pneumonia
acute necrotising pneumonia see pneumonia
adenoviruses 99, **100f**
agalactia 267
agar gel immunodiffusion test 225, 382
Aggregatibacter actinomycetemcomitans 34
Akabane virus & disease 72, 73, 303
albendazole **181f**
albumin & albumin copper 134, 146
algal poisoning 309, 315
alkali disease 114, 115
All-trace Trace Element Bolus 143
alpacas 294
amaurosis 302
amino-acetonitrile derivatives 10, 172–3
amino acids 114
ammonia 20–2, 195–6
amoxicillin 85
anaemia 107, 125, 138, 139, 162
androstenediones 51, 52
Androvax 51–2, **52f**
anthelmintic drenching 53, 121, 164, **164f**, 169–79, **170f, 171f** see also drenching
anthelmintics 10, 130, 305
anthrax 289
anti-inflammatory drugs see specific diseases; specific medicines
antibiotics see specific diseases; specific medicines
apricot stain 326
Arcanobacterium pyogenes 249
Argentine stem weevil 295
arthritis 87, 248–9, 287
arthrogryposis 72
ataxia 85, 137, 138, 198, 287, 293, 303–4 see also gait; swayback
Australian and New Zealand College of Veterinary Scientists 11
avermectins 172

B

Bacillus anthracis 289
Bacillus licheniformis 72
Bacillus species 63, 324
bacterial meningitis 298–9
balano-posthitis 20–2, **21**
basic slag 198
Batten's disease 303
bearings **343,** 343–5
Beef and Lamb New Zealand 44
bent leg 104–5
benzimidazoles 10, 172, 177, 181, 182
benzoyl phenyl ureas 336
Bibersteinia 99, **100f**
bilateral epididymal spermiostasis 26
bilateral spermiostases 26
birds, transmission of disease 63
birthweight see lambs, growth rates
black disease 181, 277–8
black fungus tip 324
black mastitis 266
blackleg 87, 275–6, **276**
blind staggers 114

blood tests see specific diseases
blowflies 331–3, **332f,** 388–9
blue banding 326
bluetongue 373–7, **376**
body condition scoring 96, **96f, 97f,** 207–29 see also ewes; hoggets; lambs; two-tooth
bone diseases 138–9, **139**
Booroola breed 48, 49
border disease see hairy shaker disease
Border Leicester breed 303
Borderdale breed 303
Bordetalla parapertussis 100, **100f**
botulism 271, 278–9
Bovicola ovis 327, 333–5, **334f**
bovine adenovirus type 7 **100f**
bovine spongiform encephalopathy 357, 368–73, **369f, 371f**
bowie **99f,** 104–5
brachygnathia 213, 222, **222**
bradshot 271, 277
bradyzoites 68
brain abscesses 298–9, **299,** 302
Branhamella ovis 253
brassica crops 83–4, 145, 146, 148, 317, 318
Brassica napus 72, 309, 315
braxy 271, 277
breeding sheep see ewes; lambs; rams; specific breeds; specific diseases & conditions
broken mouth 213, 219–21, **220, 221**
Broomfield Corriedale breed 241
brown and green banded stains 326
browntop 104–5, 115, 146, **147f**
Brucella melitensis 73, 388
Brucella ovis 26–34, **34f**
brucellosis 30
Bunostomum 157, **165f**
Bunyaviridae, genus *Phlebovirus* 385

Bunyavirus, genus *Nairovirus* 387-8
bur medick 315
bush sickness 113, 122, 129

C

cadmium 134
caeruloplasmin. 134-5, **135f**
caesarean section 193
calcined magnesite 197
calcium 194-5, **196f,** 216
    calcium borogluconate 193, 195, 197, 199, 202
    calcium carbonate calculi 351
calculus 214
Caldow technique 221
Calliphora spp 331-3, **332f**
Campylobacter coli 63
Campylobacter fetus fetus 63-5, **65**
Campylobacter jejuni 63, 64
campylobacteriosis 10, 63-5, **65,** 84
canary yellow 326
cancers 228, **228,** 322-3, **323**
capripox infections 386-7
caseous lymphadenitis 259-62, **260,** 340
cataracts 256
cats 65-7, 118, 372-3
cattle
    anthrax 289
    bluetongue 373-7
    bovine spongiform encephalopathy 357-8, 368-73
    Brucella melitensis 388
    cattle tick 335
    dermatophilosis 316
    facial eczema 314
    feed, problems from 113-50, **136f, 137f, 138,** 200, 288, 294, 296, 297
    flies & mites 388, 389
    foot & mouth disease 378, 380
    footrot 237, 239
    Histophilus somni septicaemia 286
    intestinal infections 275, 279
    Johne's disease 223-8
    leptospirosis 347, 348
    listeriosis 299
    Nairobi sheep disease 387
    poisoning 298, 315
    Q-fever 390
    Rift Valley fever 385
    Schmallenberg virus 383
    tuberculosis 350
    yellow fat 352
Causmag (magnesium oxide) 197
cell-mediated immune tests 226
cereal feeding *see* grain & cereal feeding
cerebellar abiotrophy 304
cerebellar cortical atrophy 303
cestodes 181-2
Chabertia 157, **165f, 177f**
cheesy gland 259-62, **260,** 340
chemoprophylaxis 67
Cheviot breed 132, 352, 359-60
chicory 131
Chlamydophila 253-5, **253f**
Chlamydophila abortus 63
Chlamydophila (Chlamydia) abortus 73, 377-8
chondrodysplasia gene 346, **346**
chorea 70
Chorioptes bovis 22, 335
chorioptic mange 22-3
chromogen 352
chronic non-progressive pneumonia *see* pneumonia
chronic ovine laryngitis 348-9
chronic wasting disease 372
Chrysomya rufifacies 331-3, **332f**
Chrysomyia bezziana 388-9
ciliostasis 100
circling 293
Circus approximans 63
Claviceps purpurea 309
clear drenches 172
cloprosterol 58
closantel 173, **181f**
clostridial diseases & infections 10, 261, 271-81, **271f,** 279-81, 340
Clostridium botulinum 278-9
Clostridium chauvoei 275-6
Clostridium novyi 277-8
Clostridium novyi type *B* 181, 276
Clostridium perfringens 265, 279
Clostridium perfringens type B 278
Clostridium perfringens type C 278
Clostridium perfringens type D 272-4, 301
Clostridium septicum 275-6
Clostridium sordellii 279
Clostridium tetani 274-5
clovers 50, 94-5, **95f,** 146-7, **147f,** 266, 309, 315
coagulase-negative staphylococci 265
coast disease 113, 122, 129
cobalamines 123 *see also* cobalt deficiency
cobalt deficiency 99, 113, 122-30, **124f,** 125-9, **125f, 126f, 127, 127f, 128f,** 302
coccidiosis 87, 182
Cochliomyia hominivorax 388-9
cockle 327, 333
coenurosis 305
Coenurus cerebralis 305
collagen dysplasia disease 323
Combi Clamp **18**
complement fixation test 30-2, 34, 382
congenital abnormalities 303-5
congenital defects 85, **85f**
congenital toxoplasmosis 304
conjunctivitis 87, 253-5, **253f, 254**
contagious agalactia 390
contagious ecthyma 319-21, **319f, 320, 321**
contagious ophthalmia 87, 253-5, **253f, 254**
contagious pustular dermatitis 248, 319-21, **319f, 320, 321**
Cooperia 157, 165, **165f, 177f**
Coopworth breed 9, 43, 46, 303-4, 365
copper 217
    copper calcium edetate 143
    copper glycinate 143

copper oxide capsules 143
deficiency 87, 113, 116, 130–45, **140f, 142f,** 304, 324
toxicity 143–4
Coriaria 297–8
Corriedale breed 9, 106, 303, 309, 315, 348
corticosteroids 193
Corynebacterium pseudotuberculosis 259–61, 265, 340
Corynebacterium renale 20–2
coumesterol 50
Cowdria ruminantium 385–6
Coxiella burnetti 390
Creutzfeldt–Jakob disease, variant 357, 371–2
Crohn's disease 224
cryptorchidism 26, **27**
cryptosporidiosis 183
cud staining 105
Culicoides midges 373–5, 383
cutaneous aesthesia 323
cycstine calculi 351
cypermethrin 336
cyromazine 336
Cysticercus ovis 182
Cysticercus tenuicollis 182
cytochrome oxidase 135, **135f**

D

daft lamb disease 303
Damalinia ovis 333–5, **334f**
danthonia 104–5
dead matter 94–5, **95f**
decoquinate 67
deer
   Brucella ovis 27–32
   cattle tick 335
   chronic wasting disease 372
   dermatophilosis 316
   feed, problems from 116–7, 122, 124–5, 137, 138, **139,** 141–3, 145, 149–50, 294
   footrot 237, 239
   Johne's disease 224, 226

leptospirosis 347
parasites 169, 180
poisoning 198
scabby mouth 319
spongiform encephalopathy 357
tuberculosis 350
Yersiniosis 108
deltamethrin 336
dentition 209–23, **210f, 211–3, 214f, 215, 219–23**
   clinical terminology 214
   defective development 216–7
   dental abnormality syndrome 223
   dental caries 222
   dentigerous cyst (odontogenic cyst) 222, **222**
   enamel defects 214, 216, 218–9, **219**
   jaw conformation **222,** 222–3, **223**
   milk teeth 210–1
   periodontal (parodontal) disease 219–21, **220, 221**
   permanent teeth 211–3, **211–3,** 217–8
   tooth wear 214–7, **215**
depression 117, 198, 200, 287, 289, 300
dermatitis 321–2
dermatophilosis 309, 316–9, **316f, 317, 318,** 325–6, 340
Dermatophilus 332
Dermatophilus congolensis 248, 316–9, **316f, 317, 318**
dextrose/glucose therapy 193
diammonium phosphate (DAP) 198–9
diarrhoea *see* specific diseases
diazinon 336
Dichelobacter nodosus 235, 238–41
dicyclanil 336
diet 82, 83–4, 88–9, **94f,** 199–201, 218, 350–1 *see also* ewes; hoggets; lambs; pasture & shelter; rams; two-tooth; specific deficiencies; specific diseases; specific feeds
diflubenzuron 336
dipping 103, 248–9, 259, 276, 298, 318, 333–41

diseases
   clinical procedures 12–5
   definition 11–2
docking 83, 87, 248–9, 274–6, 280, 298, 323, 345
doggy wool 327
dogs 87, 118
dopamine-B-hydroxylase **135f**
Dorper breed 324
Dorset breed 45, 315
Dorset Horn breed 43
drenching 142, 148–9, 157, 162, 166–7, 314 *see also* anthelmintic drenching
Drysdale breed 303
dysentery *see* specific diseases
dyspnoea 191
dystocia 82, **82, 83f,** 88

E

East Friesian breed 44–5, **45f,** 94, 348, 366
Echinococcus granulosus 182
economic effects *see* specific diseases
ectoparasites 331–41
ectoparasiticides 333
Eimeria crandallis 182
Eimeria ovinoidalis 182
embryogenesis 54–7 *see also* abortion
enamel defects *see* dentition
encephalopathy 304
endectocides 172
enteric listeriosis 288–9
enteric salmonellosis 69
enteritides 87
enteritis **68,** 299
enterotoxaemia 87, 271–4, **272, 273,** 288, 301, 302
entropion 254, 255
enzootic abortion 377–8 *see also* abortion
enzootic ataxia *see* swayback
enzootic pneumonia *see* pneumonia
enzyme-linked immunosorbent assay 30–2, 34, 382

Eperythrozoon ovis &
    eperythrosoonosis **99f,** 107–8
epidermolysis bullosa 323
epididymitis 17, 22, 26–36, **29,** 287
ergot 72
ergotism 309
Erodium moschatum 309
Erodium spp 315
Erysipelothrix arthritis 248–9
Erysipelothrix rhusiopathiae 87,
    248–9, 339–40
erythema 311
erythrocyte copper complex 134
erythrocytic superoxide dismutase
    134
erythromycin 240
Escherichia coli 249, 253, 265, 299
Escherichia coli endotoxaemia 84–5
euthanasia 208
ewes *see also* specific diseases &
    conditions
    abortion & embryogenesis 54–7, **56**
    bodyweight & nutrition 48–9, **49f,**
        52, **136f,** 190–1, **190f,** 194–7,
        199–202, 207–29, 216
    breeding, ovulation & reproductive
        performance **41f,** 42–53, **42f,**
        43f, 44f, 47f, 48f, 57, 117–8,
        139–40, 194, **343,** 343–5
    genetic makeup 49
    immunisation 52–3, **52f,** 56, 64–5,
        67, 69
    mating 53–5, **54f, 55f,** 88
    pregnancy termination 57–8
exports, live sheep 102, 103, 238
exposure 85–7, **86f** *see also* pasture &
    shelter; stress
exposure-starvation syndrome 201–3
exudative diathesis 118
eye diseases 253–6 *see also* specific
    diseases

F

facial eczema 50, **99f,** 103, 229, 309,
    310–5, **312, 313**

faecal egg count reduction test 176–7,
    228–9
falling disease 138
familial episodic ataxia 304
fasciola hepatica & fascioliasis 179–81,
    181f, 229, **229**
feet & hooves
    foot abscess 235, 244–7, **244f, 246f**
    foot and mouth disease 248, **378,**
        378–80
    foot bathing 237, 238, 240–3, 247
    foot diseases **99f,** 235–50, 323 *see*
        also lameness; specific foot
        diseases
    foot paring 240, 242, 243
    footrot 87, 235–6, 237–44, 332
    toe abscess 235, 244, 245, 247–8
    toe granuloma 235, 248
ferrets 118
fertility *see also* ewes; lambs; rams;
    semen
fetlock knuckling 293
Finn breed 44–5, **45f,** 48, 49, 94, 312,
    366
fleece 9, 70, 98, 135, 138–9, 192, 324
    disorders 309–26, **310f,** 325, **325f**
    fleece rot 326, 332, 340
    parasites 163–4
flourine 198–9, 216–7, 218–9
fluid therapy 193
flunixin meglumine 193
flystrike 317, 331–3, **332f,** 335–41
focal symmetrical encephalomalacia
    273, 301, 302
foliar spraying 130
folic acid 123
Footvax 241
formalin 240–3, 245, 247
formiminoglutamic acid 129
fostering lambs 90
fungi toxins 50–1
Fusarium 50
Fusobacterium necrophorum 87, 235,
    244, 247, 248, 250, 298, 349

G

gait 116, 135, 200, 279, 293–5, 304, 305,
    362, 381 *see also* ataxia
Galba (Lymnaea) truncatula 180
gamma glutamyl transferase (GGT) 50
gangrenous mastitis 266
gastrointestinal nematode parasitism
    157–79, **158–68, 170f, 171f, 177f,**
    228–9
gel diffusion test (GDT) 30, 32, 34
gid 305
gingivitis 219
glucocorticoid dexamethasone 58
glucose 202
    glucose/dextrose therapy 193
    glucose solutions 195
glutathione peroxidase 118
glycerine 321
goats
    agalactia 267
    anthrax 289
    bluetongue 374–5
    braxy 277
    Brucella melitensis 388
    Brucella ovis 27
    caseous lymphadenitis 259, 261
    Chorioptic mange 22
    chronic wasting disease 372
    contagious agalactia 390
    dermatophilosis 316
    feed, problems from 82–3, 123–4,
        145, 146
    footrot 237, 239, 242, 243
    heartwater 385
    jaagziekte 383
    Johne's disease 224
    listeriosis 299, 301, 388
    maedi-visna 381
    parasites 168, 175, 179
    peste des petits 384
    pinkeye 253
    poisoning 198
    pox 386–7
    Rift Valley fever 385
    scabby mouth 319

screw-worm flies 388
spongiform encephalopathies 357, 359, 361, 364, 367–8
toxoplasmosis 65–7
white muscle disease 116–7
goitre & goitrogens 83–4, 87, 145–50, **149**
gonadotrophin 47
grain & cereal feeding 199–201, 218, 350–1
Gram-negative coccobacillus. 28
Gram-negative pleomorphic bacteria 26, 34–6
grass 94–5, **95f**, 131
grass tetany 195–8
green and brown banded stains 326
green-feed oats 106
gulls 63, 68, 300
gum recession 214
gummy 214
Gymnorhina tibicen 63

H

Haemaphysalis longicornis 335
haemoconcentration 192
haemoglobinuria 107
Haemonchus 87, 157, 159, 161, 162, 164, **165f, 166,** 169, 173, 174, **177f**
Haemophilus agni 34, 286
Haemophilus somnus 34, 286
haemorrhage 87
hairy maggot fly 331–3, **332f**
hairy shaker disease 56, **70,** 70–1, 84, 303, 304–5
Hampshire breed 346, **346,** 348
hard udder 267
hawks 63
hay mites 360
hay & silage 48, 72, 98, 132, **132f,** 300
head tremors 293, 295
heart failure 138
Heartwater 385–6
heat stress *see* stress
heel abscess *see* feet & hooves
Helicobacter spp 71

hepatic encephalopathy 298
hepatosis diatetica 118
hereditary chondrodysplasia 346, **346**
herpesvirus 382–3
hide defects 327
histopathology 31
Histophilus ovis 34, 286
Histophilus somni 26, 34–6, 265, 286–8
hoggets *see also* lambs; two-tooth; specific diseases & conditions
  clinical examination 98–9
  diseases & health 96–108, 96–110
  growth 93–6, **93f, 94f, 95f,** 105
  oestrous activity 44–5, **45f**
homozygous recessive genotype 346, **346**
hooves *see* feet & hooves
hormonal induction, oestrus 46–7
horses 118, 294
hydatids 182
hyperaemia 317
Hypericum perforatum 309, 315
hyperketonaemia 191–2
hyperphosphataemia 199
hypertonic solutions 303
hypocalcaemia 194–5, 199, 305
hypocuprosis **134f,** 140
hypoglycaemia 89, 190–2
hypomagnesaemia 195–8, **196f, 198,** 302, 305, 370
hypomyelinogenesis 139
hypospadias 20
hypothermia 89 *see also* stress

I

ill thrift *see* diet
immune response 118
indirect fluorescent antibody test 67
infectious necrotic hepatitis 181, 277–8
infective bulbar necrosis *see* foot abscess
inflammation 118
inherited defects *see* congenital defects
injections *see* specific diseases
insect growth regulators 336, 339
insecticides 22–3 *see also* specific insecticides
interdigital fibromas 248
internal parasites *see* gastrointestinal nematode parasitism; parasites; specific parasites
International Embryo Transfer Society 360
International Sheep Veterinary Congresses 11
intra-ruminal boluses 121
intra-ruminal capsules 130
Inverdale breed 49
inverted eyelids 254, 255
iodine & iodine deficiency 83–4, 87, 113, 145–50, **147f, 149,** 321
iron
  dietary 133, **134f**
  iron dextran 90
itchmite 335
ivermectin 22–3, 177, 179, 337
Ixodes ricinus 384

J

jaagziekte 380, 382–3
jaw conformation *see* dentition
jetting wand treatments **338,** 338–9, **339f**
Johne's disease 223–8, **226, 227,** 380

K

kale 147
kangaroo gait 293, 305
keratitis *see* entropion; pink eye
ketoacidosis 192
ketonuria 192
ketosis *see* pregnancy toxaemia
kidneys 85, 119, 134, 198–9
Klebsiella pneumoniae 265
Krebs cycle 123
kudu 369, 373

L

lacrimation 254, 255
lactation 87, 89–90
lactic acidosis 199–201
lambing sickness *see* pregnancy toxaemia
lambs *see also* hoggets; specific diseases & conditions
    growth rates 10, 88, **95f**, 105, **164f**
    lambing 41–61, **47f**, 88–90
    lambing percentages 10, 41–2, 48–53, **48f**, 94
    survival & mortality 77–91, **78f, 81f**, 147–8
lamellar suppuration *see* feet & hooves
lameness 229 *see also* feet & hooves; specific foot diseases
laminitis 249–50
Larus dominicanus 63, 68
laryngeal chondritis 348–9
lead poisoning 298
legumes 115, 124, 131
Leicester breed 365
lentivirus 380–2
Leptospira 63
Leptospira borgpetersenii serovar Hardjobovis 347–8, **348**
Leptospira interrogans serovar Pomona 57, 72, 347–8, **348**
leptospirosis 347–8, **348**
levamisole 172, 177
lice 333–5, **334f**, 335–41
lime 133, 138
Lincoln breed 365
lincomycin-spectinomycin 240
Linognathus ovillus 107, 333–5, **334f**
Linognathus pedalis 333–5, **334f**
liquid nitrogen 245
Listeria 63, 72
Listeria monocytogenes 299–300
Listeria spp 288–9
listeriosis 293, 299–300, **300,** 302
Listronotus bonariensis 295
litter size **48f**, 49, 80–1, 88
live sheep exports 102, 103, 238
liver 125, 127, **127f, 128f**, 131, 140–1, **141f**, 277–8, 311–2, **313**
    biopsy 149–50
    copper **145f**
    liver flukes 179–81, 229, **229**, 277
liveweights *see* hoggets, growth
lolitrem B 295
Lolium perenne 295
Lotus corniculatus 315
louping ill 384
lucerne 50, 288, 315
Lucilia 336
Lucilia cuprina 331–3, **332f**
Lucilia sericata 331–3, **332f**
lumpy wool 316–9, **316f, 317, 318**
lung abscesses 229
lungworm 103
lupin 309
lupinosis 315
Lupinus angustifolius 309
lymph glands 259–62, **260,** 340
lymphadenitis 68
lympho 259–62, **260,** 340
lysyl oxidase 135, **135f**

M

macrocarpa 72
macrocyclic lactones 10, 172, 179
maedi 380–2
magnesium 195–6, **196f**
    magnesium sulphate 195, 197, 202
magpie 63
Mairoa dopiness 113, 122, 129
maleruption 214
malignant oedema 87, 276–7
malonate 123
malposition 214
Malta fever 388
mammary glands 265–7
Mana Island 9
mange *see* specific manges
Manneheimia haemolytica 99, 100, **100f**
Mannheimia (Pasteurella) haemolytica 265
mastitis 265–7, 319
mating *see* ewes; rams
Medicago polymorpha 315
Medicago sativa 315
Medicago species 50
Mediterranean fever 388
melatonin 46
Melophagus ovinus 107, 335, 365
meningitis, bacterial 298–9
meningoencephalitis 287, 299–300
mercury 134
Merino breed 9, 365
    diseases & health *see* specific diseases
    ewes 43, 46, 49, 117
    rams 22, 23, 26, 140
    wool & skin 22, 139, 327, 332
metabolic diseases 305
metabolisable energy (ME) 94–5, **95f**
methyl malonate 123
methyridine 10
metritis 63, **68,** 68–9
Michel chip 255
Micrococcus spp 265
microphthalmia 256
milbemycins 172
milk fever 194–5
milk of magnesia 200
milk testing, iodine 148
mites 335, 360
molybdenised superphosphate 144
molybdenum 132–3, 138, **139,** 144, 217
monensin 67
monepantel 172–3
Moniezia expansa 181–2
Moniezia spp 272
monorchidism 26
morantel 172
Morbillivirus 384
Morton Mains 124
Morton Mains disease 113, 122, 129
moxidectin 22–3, 173, 178, 241
mulberry heart disease 118
mulga 351
myasis 388

Mycobacterium avium subsp.
paratuberculosis 224–5
Mycobacterium bovis 350
Mycoplasma agalactiae 267, 390
Mycoplasma arganini **100f**
Mycoplasma conjunctivae 253–5
Mycoplasma ovipneumoniae 100, **100f**
*Mycoplasma ovis see Eperythrozoon
ovis* & eperythrosoonosis
Mycoplasma spp 265
mycotic dermatitis 316–9, **316f, 317, 318**
mycotoxins 50
myopathy *see* white muscle disease
Myoporum laetum 309, 315

N

Nairobi sheep disease 387–8
navel infection **83f**, 84, 87
necropsy *see* specific diseases
necrosis **68,** 68–9 *see also* specific diseases
nematode parasitism 87, 125, 157–9, **158–68, 170f, 171f, 177f,** 181–3, 208, 228–9
Nematodirus 87, 157–9, 161, 164, **165f,** 173, 177
Nematodirus filicollis 161
Nematodirus spathiger 161
neonatal ataxia 87, 132, 138, 139, 293, 304
Neospora caninum 57, 63, 71–2, **73**
Neotyphodium (Acremon-ium) lolii 295
neuraxonal dystrophy 303–4
neurological disorders 293–305, **294f**
new grass 72
New Zealand Romney breed 9, 43
ngaio poisoning 309, 315
nitrate poisoning 72
Norway 98/atypical scrapie 367–8
nutrition *see* diet
nystagmus 293

O

oats, green 72

odontogenic cyst 222, **222**
oedema 311
Oesophagostomum **165f, 177f**
oestradiol benzoate 58
oestrous activity *see* ewes; hoggets
Office International des Epizooties 363
opisthotonus 301
oral dosing 130
Orbivirus 375
orf 319–21, **319f, 320, 321**
organophosphates 333, 336
organophosphorus compounds 22–3
organophosphorus poisoning 298
orthobunyavirus 383
osteochondrosis 138, **139**
Ostertagia 87 *see* Teladorsagia
Ovastim 51–2
overshot jaw 222–3, **223**
ovine adenovirus type 6 **100f**
ovine brucellosis 17
ovine ceroid-lipofuscinosis 303
ovine encephalomyelitis 384
ovine infectious keratoconjunctivitis 87, 253–5, **253f, 254**
ovine interdigital dermatitis 235–7, **236, 237,** 242, 244–7
ovine segmental axonopathy 304
ovine spongiform leucoencephalopathy 304
Ovis Management 182
oxalate calculi 351
oxfendazole **181f**
oxyclozanide **181f**
oxytetracycline *see* specific diseases

P

parainfluenza virus type 3 99, **100f**
parakeelya 351
Paramyxoviridae 384
parapituitary abscesses 299
parasites 10, **99f,** 106, 132, 157–83, 216, 295, 324 *see also* nematode parasitism; specific parasites;

specific remedies
ectoparasites 309
external 331–41
parasitic diseases 305
parasiticides 22–3 *see also* specific parasiticides
parasitoid wasps 340
parenteral administration, of copper 143, 144
Pasteurella multocida 265
Pasteurella species 299
Pasteurellaceae & *Pasteurella* 99, **100f**
pasteurellosis *see* pneumonia
pasture & shelter 88–9, **88f,** 94–5, **95f, 98f,** 202–3, 227, 266–7, 313 *see also* diet; specific breeds; specific diseases
fertilisers 197–8
parasites 167–72, **168f,** 178
trace elements **115f,** 124–4, **126f,** 129–30, 131, **132f, 147f**
pathology *see* specific diseases
Patterson Merino breed 241
Pawera red clover 50
pelt defects 327
penicillin *see* specific diseases
penis & prepuce 20–2
pentobarbitone 208
peptidyglycine α-animating monooxygenase **135f**
peracute disease 386–7
peramine 295
Perendale breed 9, 43, 101, 303–4, 352, 365
periodontal (parodontal) 214
periodontal (parodontal) disease 219–21, **220, 221**
Persian breed 43
peste des petits ruminants 384–5
pestiviruses 70
Peyer's patches 225
Peyronella glomerata 324
Phalaris
Phalaris staggers 123, 125, 293, 296
poisoning 296–7

Phalaris arundinacea 296–7
Phalaris tuberosa 296–7
phenothiazine, fine-particle 10
pheromones 45
Phomopsis leptostromiformis 315
phosphate calculi 350
phospholipid glutathione peroxidase 118
phosphorus 106, 132, 138, 163, 194–5, 198, 213, 216
photomotor reflex 293
photoperiod control 46
photophobia 254
photosensitisation 309, 311, 312, 315, 317
phylloerythrin excretion 309
phyto-oestrogen-induced calculi 351
phyto-oestrogens 50
Picornavirus, genus *Aphthovirus* 378–9
pigs 87, 118, 275, 347
pink eye 87, 253–5, **253f, 254**
pink rot 324
pink tip 326
Pithomyces chartarum 50, 311–5
pizzle rot 20–2, **21**
placentitis 69
plantain 131
plasma amino acids 134
plasma caeruloplasmin 134
pleurisy 99, 100
plunge-dips 339–40, **340**
pneumonia 99–104, **99f, 100f, 101f, 103f**, 229, 287, 340, 376–7, 380–2
Poa spp 146, **147f**
pocket 214
poisoning 294, **294f,** 309
    algal 309, 315
    lead 298
    ngaio 309, 315
    nitrate 72
    organophosphorus 298
    Phalaris 296–7
    St John's wort 309, 315
    storksbill 309, 315

tutin 297–8
tutu 297–8
polioencephalomalacia 123, 125, 293, 301–3
Poll Dorset breed 304
poll strike 332
polymerase chain reaction 225–6, 382
Pomona *see Leptospira interrogans* serovar Pomona
poor thrift *see* diet
Portulaca spp 351
post-dipping lameness 339–40
post-parturient haemoglobinuria 138
posterior paralysis 293
postmortems *see* specific diseases
potassium 196, 198
    potassium aluminium sulphate 318–9
poultry 118
pour on treatments **338,** 338–9, **339f**
pox infections 386–7
Poxviridae 319–21, **319f, 320, 321,** 386–7
praziquantel 173, 182
predation 87
pregnancy disease *see* pregnancy toxaemia
pregnancy toxaemia 189–94, **191f, 192,** 245, 293, 305
prepuce & penis 20–2, **21**
prions 358
proclination 214
progestagen 47
prognathia 213, 214, 222–3, **223**
propetamphos 336
propionic acid 123
prostaglandin 58
PrP gene 359
pruritis 311, 362
Pseudomonas aeruginosa 265, 322, **322,** 325–6, **325f,** 340
Pseudosuccinea (Lymnaea) columella 180
Psorobia (Psorergates) ovis 335
Psoroptes ovis 335, 389–90

pulpy kidney *see* enterotoxaemia
purple stain 326
pyelonephritis **83f**
pyrimidine derivatives 336

Q
Q-fever 73, 390

R
rabbits 224
radiology 246
ragwort toxicity 123
Ramguard 51
rams *see also* specific diseases & conditions
    breeding 17–20, **18,** 53–5, **54f, 55f,** 140
    genitalia 17–38
    harnesses 54
    teaser rams 45–6
rape 72
    rape scald 309, 315, 317
rectal prolapse 345, **345**
red foot 323
redgut 288
reed canary grass 296–7
Regulin 46
respiratory syncytial virus **100f**
retroclination 214
retrovirus 382–3
rickets **99f,** 105–7, **106**
Rickettsia conjunctivae 253
ricobendazole **181f**
Rift Valley fever 73, 385
ringworm 324
Romney breed 9, 365
    caseous lymphadenitis 261
    diseases & health 105, 224, 228, 287, 303–4, 348, 349, 352
    ewes & breeding 42, **42f,** 43–4, 46, 49, 71, 78, 89
    eye diseases 255, 256
    poor thrift 217, 218
    rams 22, 23, 26, 45
    wool & skin 22, 85, 314, 322, 323, 325

Romney Marsh breed 9, **9**
Rothera's test 192
rumen acidosis 199–201
rumen impaction 199–201
ruminant metabolism **123f, 124f**
ryegrass 72, 106, 146–7, **147f**
    ryegrass staggers **99f**, 293, 294–6

S

Salmonella abortus ovis 63, 73
Salmonella bovis-morbificans 69, 283
Salmonella Brandenburg 63, **68,** 68–9, 283
Salmonella Hindmarsh 69, 283
Salmonella typhimurium 69, 283
salmonella, vaccines 10
salmonellosis 283–6, **284, 285**
salt licks 142
Salvexin +B 69
sarcocystosis 183
scabby mouth 87, 248, 266, 309, 319–21, **319f, 320, 321**
scald 235
Schmallenberg virus 383
SciQuest 11
Scottish Blackface breed 132
scourable diffuse yellow 326
scouring *see* specific diseases
scrapie 357–73, **357f, 359f– 362f, 363, 364f, 366f, 367, 368f, 369f, 371f–3f,** 380
screw-worm flies 388–9
scrotal mange 22–3
scrotal mange mite 335
scrotum 22–3
segmental aplasia 26, **26**
selenium deficiency 56, 82–3, 87, 99, 113, 114–22, **115f, 117, 119f, 120f,** 148
semen 18–9, 23, 24–5, 28–31, 53, 66 *see also* rams
septicaemia 286–8, 299
serological tests *see* specific diseases
serum methylmalonic acid (MMA) 129
sex 88

shearing 94, 266, 317–20, 324, 341, 388
    benefits 25, 52, 82, 193, 333–7, 339, 344
    ill effects 102–3, 194–5, 259–62, 322, 374, 377
    stress 46–8, 189–90, 201–3
    wounds to sheep 20, 22, 28, 275, 327, 340
sheep *see also* ewes; hogget; lambs; rams; two-tooth
    sheep *Brucella ovis* flock accreditation scheme 32–3, **33f**
    sheep ked 335
    sheep meat markets 9–10
    sheep pulmonary adenomatosis 382–3
    sheep scab 335, **389,** 389–90
shelly hoof 250
shelter *see* pasture & shelter
shower treatments 339–40
silage & hay 48, 72, 98, 132, **132f,** 300
silica calculi 350
silver 134
Sip gene 359
skin disorders 309–26, **310f**
sleepy sickness *see* pregnancy toxaemia
slow-release rumen bullets 143
small-intestinal carcinoma 228, **228**
sodium 196, 198
    sodium lactate solution 217
    sodium lauryl sulphate 237, 240
soils *see* pasture & shelter
solubilisation hypothesis 217
sorghums 146
South Dorset Down breed 323
South Hampshire breed 303
Southdown breed 309, 315, 348, 349
Southland pneumonia *see* pneumonia
sperm *see* semen
spider lamb syndrome 346, **346**
spinal abscesses 298, **298**
spinal reflex arcs 294
spinosad 336
spirochaetes 236

spiroindoles 172–3
Spongiform encephalopathies 357–73, **357f, 359f– 362f, 363, 364f, 366f, 367, 368f, 369f, 371f–3f**
sporidesmin 311–5
spraying
    crops 130 *see also* topdressing
    treatments **338,** 338–9, **339f**
Squamous cell carcinoma 322–3, **323**
St John's wort poisoning 309, 315
Staphylococcal mastitis 266
Staphylococcus 249
Staphylococcus aureus 253, 265–6, 298, 299, 321–2
steatitis 118
steely wool 324
stoats 224
stocking rate conversion factors table **13f**
Stomoxys calcitrans 107
storksbill poisoning 309, 315
Strawberry cotyledons **68**
Streptococcus dysgalactiae 249
Streptococcus spp 265, 299
streptomycin *see* specific diseases
stress 46, 56, 89, 102, 190, 266
stringy yolk 326–7
struck 271, 278
sturdy 305
succinate 123
Suffolk breed 303–4, 323, 346, **346,** 348, 359–60, 363, 365–6
sulphonamides 67
sulphur 115, 131, 132–3, 301
superoxide dismutase **135f**
superphosphates 104, 105, 115, 122, 126, 132, 134, 144, 198
supparative pneumonia *see* pneumonia
suppurative arthritis 249
Surveillance 84, 124, 271
swayback 87, 132, 138, 139, 293, 304
swedes 146–7
synthetic pyrethroids 336

T

tachyzoites 68
Taenia hydatigena 182
Taenia multiceps 305
Taenia ovis 182
tapeworms 181-2, 272
Tauranga disease *see* bush sickness
teeth *see* dentition
Teladorsagia (Ostertagia) 157, 159, 161, 163, 164, **164f, 165f,** 173, 176, **177f,** 179
temperature *see* exposure; pasture & shelter; stress
testes **23,** 23-36, **25, 26, 27, 29, 35**
    testicular atrophy 24-6
    testicular degeneration 24-6, **25**
    testicular hypoplasia 26
testosterone treatment 22
tetanus 87, **274,** 274-5
tetany 107
tetracyclines 85
tetrathiomolybdate 133
Texel breed 88, 256, 348, 349
Theileria orientalis 335
thiabendazole 177
thiamine 301-2, 302-3
thiocyanate 83-4, 146
thiouracil 83-4
thistles 319
thyroglobulin 146
thyroid gland 145-6
thyroxine (T4) 145-6, 148
tick-borne fever 73
ticks 87, 384, 385-6, 387-8
tilmicosin 240, 255
toe abscess 235, 244, 245, 247-8
toe granuloma 235, 248
topdressing 143
    cobaltised superphosphate 129-30
    potassic (phosphatic fertiliser toxicity) 197, **198,** 198-9
    selenium 122
toxic nephrosis 199
Toxoplasma gondii 63, 65-8. **65f, 66f, 67**

toxoplasmosis 10, 56, 84
    congenital 304
Toxovax 67
trace-elements 10, 82-3, 87, **99f,** 113-50 *see also* specific remedies
Trachymene glaucifolia 105
trauma 72
trefoil dermatitis 309, 315
trematodes 179-81
Treponema species 236
tri-iodothyronine (T3) 145-6, 148
triazine derivatives 336
Tribrissen injection 48% 67
tricarboxylic acids 191
Trichophyton verrucosum 324
Trichostrongylus 157, **158,** 159, 161, 162-3, **164f, 165f,** 173, 176, **177f**
triclabendazole 181, **181f**
triflumuron 336
Trifolium pratense 50
Trifolium subterraneum 50
trotting gait 293, 295
Trueparella pyogenes 236
Trueparella (Arcanobacter) pyogenes 298, 299
Trueparella (Arcanobacterium) pyogenes 244, 248
Trueperella pyogenes 87, 265, 266
tuberculosis 349-50
turnips 72
tutin poisoning 297-8
tutu poisoning 297-8
twin lamb disease *see* pregnancy toxaemia
two-tooth 85 *see also* hogget; specific diseases & conditions
    ewes 43-6, 49, **49f,** 52-6, **54f,** 66, 77, 88-9
    growth 93
    rams 19-20, 23
tyrosinase 135, **135f**
tyrosine 146

U

udders *see* mammary glands

ultrasound scanning 41, 48, 52, 56-7, **57f, 58f, 59f,** 77
under-nutrition syndrome 189-90
undershot jaw 222, **222**
uraemia 192
urethral process obstruction 20
urinary methylmalonic acid 129
urine tests, iodine 148
urolithiasis 350-2

V

vaccines *see* ewes, immunisation; specific diseases
vaginal prolapse **343,** 343-5
varicocele 23, 26
veterinarians 10-1 *see also* specific diseases & conditions; specific sheep
    clinical procedures 12-5
VetLearn 11
VetScholar 11
vibriosis & vibrio *see Campylobacter fetus fetus*
visna 380-2
vitamin B12 122-4, 125, 127-30, **127f, 128f**
vitamin E 87, 114, 118

W

wasting disease 113, 122, 129
water
    treatments in 130, 131, 142, 314, 321, 339
    water maceration 235
watery mouth 84-5
weather *see* exposure; pasture & shelter; stress
Welsh Mountain breed 43, 132
Wesselbron disease 73
white drenches 172
white liver disease 123, 125, 309, 316
white muscle disease 82-3, 87, 113, 114, 116-7, **117,** 118
white parsnip 105
Wiltshire breed 304

wool *see also* fleece
    markets 9
    wool break **324f,** 325
wormwise.co.nz 166

X
xanthine calculi 351
xanthophylls 352

Y
yellow banding 326
yellow fat 352, **352**
Yersinia pseudotuberculosis 108
Yersinia & yersiniosis 63, **99f,** 108
yoghurt 90

Z
zearalenone 50–1, **51f**
Ziehl-Neelsen method 31
zinc 134, 313–4
zinc oxide 314
zinc sulphate 237, 240–3, 247, 314, 318, 322, 340

About the authors

DAVE WEST BVSc (Massey), PhD (Massey), FACVSc Emeritus Professor, was formerly at the Institute of Veterinary Animal and Biomedical Sciences, Massey University, Palmerston North, New Zealand.

NEIL BRUÈRE ONZM, BVSc (Sydney), PhD (Glasgow), DVSc (Sydney), FACVSc Emeritus Professor, was previously Professor of Veterinary Medicine and Clinical Pharmacology and formerly Head of Department, Veterinary Sciences, at Massey University, Palmerston North, New Zealand.

ANNE RIDLER BVSc (Massey), PhD (Massey), is Associate Professor in Sheep and Beef Cattle Health and Production at the School of Veterinary Science, Massey University, Palmerston North, New Zealand.

For more information about our books please visit

www.masseypress.ac.nz